Cardiovascular
Pharmacotherapeutics

MANUAL

SECOND EDITION

Cardiovascular Pharmacotherapeutics

MANUAL

Edited by:

William H. Frishman, M.D.

The Barbara & William Rosenthal Professor and Chair, Department of Medicine
Professor of Pharmacology
New York Medical College
Director of Medicine
Westchester Medical Center
Valhalla, New York

Edmund H. Sonnenblick, M.D.

Edmond J. Safra Distinguished Professor of Medicine
Chief Emeritus, Division of Cardiology
Albert Einstein College of Medicine
Montefiore Medical Center
Bronx, New York

Domenic A. Sica, M.D.

Professor of Medicine & Pharmacology
Chairman, Section of Clinical Pharmacology
Division of Nephrology
Medical College of Virginia
Virginia Commonwealth University
Richmond, Virginia

McGraw-Hill
Medical Publishing Division

New York Chicago San Francisco Lisbon London Madrid Mexico City
Milan New Delhi San Juan Seoul Singapore Sydney Toronto

Cardiovascular Pharmacotherapeutics Manual, Second Edition

Copyright © 2004, 1998 by *The McGraw-Hill Companies, Inc.* All rights reserved. Printed in the United States of America. Except as permitted under the United States Copyright Act of 1976, no part of this publication may be reproduced or distributed in any form or by any means, or stored in a data base or retrieval system, without the prior written permission of the publisher.

1 2 3 4 5 6 7 8 9 0 DOC/DOC 0 9 8 7 6 5 4 3

ISBN 0-07-137363-2

This book was set in Times Roman by PV&M Publishing Solutions.
The editors were Darlene Cooke and Nicky Fernando.
The production supervisor was Catherine H. Saggese.
The cover designer was Janice Bielawa.
The index was prepared by Jerry Ralya.
RR Donnelley was the printer and binder.

This book is printed on acid-free paper.

Library of Congress Cataloging-in-Publication Data

Cardiovascular pharmacotherapeutics, manual. — 2nd ed. / edited by
  William H. Frishman, Edmund H. Sonnenblick, Domenic A. Sica.
    p. ; cm.
  Companion v. to: Cardiovascular pharmacotherapeutics. 2003.
  Includes bibliographical references and index.
  ISBN 0-07-137363-2
    1. Cardiovascular agents—Handbooks, manuals, etc. I. Frishman, William H.,
  1946– . II. Sonnenblick, Edmund H, 1932– . III. Sica, Dominic A.
  IV. Cardiovascular pharmacotherapeutics.
    [DNLM: 1. Cardiovascular Agents—pharmacology—Handbooks.
  2. Cardiovascular Diseases—drug therapy—Handbooks. 3. Cardiovascular
  System—drug effects—Handbooks. QV 39 C26772 2004]
  RM345.C3768 2004
  616.1′061—dc21
                                                                    2003051207

INTERNATIONAL EDITION ISBN 0-07-121223-X

Copyright © 2004. Exclusive rights by the McGraw-Hill Companies, Inc., for manufacture and export. This book cannot be reexported from the country to which it is consigned by McGraw-Hill. The International Edition is not available in North America.

Contents

SPECIAL TOPICS SECTION

APPENDICES

Angela Cheng-Lai, William H. Frishman, Adam Spiegel, and Pamela Charney

Contributors

Jonathan Abrams, M.D.
Department of Medicine/Division of Cardiology
University of New Mexico School of Medicine
Albuquerque, New Mexico
(Chapter 9)

Yogesh K. Agarwal, M.D.
Department of Medicine/Division of Cardiology
New York Medical College/Westchester Medical Center
Valhalla, New York
(Chapter 18)

Masoud Azizad, M.D.
Department of Medicine
USC School of Medicine
Santa Barbara Cottage Hospital
Santa Barbara, California
(Chapter 18)

Erdal Cavusoglu, M.D.
Department of Medicine/Division of Cardiology
Mt. Sinai School of Medicine and Bronx VA Medical Center
New York, New York
(Chapter 7)

Pamela Charney, M.D.
Department of Medicine
Norwalk Hospital
Norwalk, Connecticut
and
Obstetrics & Gynecology and Women's Health
Albert Einstein College of Medicine
Bronx, New York
(Appendices)

Judy W. M. Cheng, Pharm.D.
Department of Pharmacy
Mt. Sinai Medical Center
New York, New York
and
Arnold & Marie Schwartz College of Pharmacy
   & Health Sciences of Long Island University
Brooklyn, New York
(Chapters 19 & 20)

Angela Cheng-Lai, Pharm.D.
Departments of Pharmacy & Medicine
Montefiore Medical Center
Bronx, New York
(Appendices)

Jay D. Coffman, M.D.
Department of Medicine
Boston University School of Medicine
Boston Medical Center
Boston, Massachusetts
(Chapter 22)

Robert T. Eberhardt, M.D.
Department of Medicine/Division of Cardiology
Boston University School of Medicine
Boston Medical Center
Boston, Massachusetts
(Chapter 22)

Robert Forman, M.D.
Department of Medicine/Division of Cardiology
Albert Einstein College of Medicine/Montefiore Medical Center
Bronx, New York
(Chapter 14)

William H. Frishman, M.D.
Departments of Medicine & Pharmacology
New York Medical College/Westchester Medical Center
Valhalla, New York
(Chapters 1-11, 13-21, 23-25, & Appendices)

Todd W. B. Gehr, M.D.
Department of Medicine/Division of Nephrology
Medical College of Virginia of
    Virginia Commonwealth University
Richmond, Virginia
(Chapters 5 & 6)

Michael H. Gewitz, M.D.
Department of Pediatrics/Division of Pediatric Cardiology
New York Medical College
Children's Hospital at Westchester Medical Center
Valhalla, New York
(Chapters 24 & 25)

Hilary Hotchkiss, M.D.
Department of Pediatrics/Division of Pediatric Nephrology
Mt. Sinai School of Medicine & Hospital Center
New York, New York
(Chapter 17)

Daniel W. Kang, M.D.
Department of Medicine
University of Hawaii
Tripler Army Medical Center
Honolulu, Hawaii
(Chapter 18)

Peter R. Kowey, M.D.
Department of Medicine/Division of Cardiology
Jefferson Medical College
Philadelphia, Pennsylvania
and
Lankenau Hospital & Main Line Health System
Wynnewood, Pennsylvania
(Chapter 12)

Lawrence R. Krakoff, M.D.
Department of Medicine
Mt. Sinai School of Medicine
New York, New York
and
Englewood Hospital Center
Englewood, New Jersey
(Chapters 10 & 11)

Thierry H. LeJemtel, M.D.
Department of Medicine/Division of Cardiology
Albert Einstein College of Medicine/Montefiore Medical Center
Bronx, New York
(Chapter 8)

Robert G. Lerner, M.D.
Department of Medicine/Division of Hematology
New York Medical College/Westchester Medical Center
Valhalla, New York
(Chapter 13)

Walter G. Levine, Ph.D.
Department of Molecular Pharmacology
Albert Einstein College of Medicine
Bronx, New York
(Chapter 1)

B. Robert Meyer, M.D.
Department of Medicine
Weill Medical College of Cornell University
New York, New York
and
New York Presbyterian Medical Center
New York, New York
(Chapter 3)

Eric L. Michelson, M.D.
Astra Zeneca LP
Wayne, Pennsylvania
and
Jefferson Medical College
Philadelphia, Pennsylvania
(Chapter 12)

Nauman Naseer, M.D.
Department of Medicine/Division of Cardiology
New York Medical College/Westchester Medical Center
Valhalla, New York
(Chapter 25)

Joel M. Neutel, M.D.
University of California-Irvine School of Medicine
Integrated Research
Orange, California
(Chapter 16)

Lionel H. Opie, M.D.
Cape Heart Centre Medical School
Cape Town, South Africa
(Chapter 21)

Stephen J. Peterson, M.D.
Departments of Medicine & Pharmacology/
    Division of General Internal Medicine
New York Medical College/Westchester Medical Center
Valhalla, New York
(Chapter 23)

Neil S. Shachter, M.D.
Department of Medicine
Columbia University College of Physicians & Surgeons
New York Presbyterian Medical Center
New York, New York
(Chapter 15)

Ronald L. Shazer M.D.
Cedars-Sinai Medical Center
Department of Medicine
Los Angeles, California
(Chapter 25)

Domenic A. Sica, M.D.
Department of Medicine/Division of Nephrology & Clinical Pharmacology
Medical College of Virginia
    of Virginia Commonwealth University
Richmond, Virginia
(Chapters 4-7, 19, & 21)

Stephen T. Sinatra, M.D.
Department of Medicine/Division of Cardiology
University of Connecticut School of Medicine &
    Eastern Connecticut Health Network
Farmington, Connecticut
(Chapter 23)

Tatjana N. Sljapic, M.D.
Department of Medicine/Division of Cardiology
Lankenau Hospital
Wynnewood, Pennsylvania
(Chapter 12)

Edmund H. Sonnenblick, M.D.
Department of Medicine/Division of Cardiology
Albert Einstein College of Medicine/Montefiore Medical Center
Bronx, New York
(Chapter 8)

Adam Spiegel, D.O.
Department of Medicine
Stony Brook Health Sciences Center/Stony Brook University Hospital
Stony Brook, New York
(Appendices)

Michael A. Weber, M.D.
Office of the Dean & Department of Medicine
SUNY Health Science Center-Brooklyn
Brooklyn, New York
(Chapter 16)

Paul Woolf, M.D.
Department of Pediatrics/Division of Pediatric Cardiology
New York Medical College
Children's Hospital at Westchester Medical Center
Valhalla, New York
(Chapter 24)

Joyce Wu, M.D.
Department of Pediatrics
University of Washington School of Medicine
Children's Hospital Regional Medical Center
Seattle, Washington
(Chapter 24)

Preface

This is the companion handbook to the second edition of *Cardiovascular Pharmacotherapeutics*. The chapters and appendices in the handbook were prepared by the authors of the corresponding chapters and appendices found in the larger book. In addition, the handbook contains a chapter on the treatment of endocarditis, not found in the larger text. The handbook was designed to provide a concise, portable reference source on cardiovascular drug treatment for healthcare providers and students who cannot always access the larger textbooks. However, it is not intended to replace the more detailed reference sources in cardiology, adult medicine, and pharmacology.

ACKNOWLEDGMENTS

The editors would like to express their gratitude to the authors who contributed to the handbook. We would also like to thank our editorial assistant and secretary, Joanne Cioffi-Pryor, for her expertise in helping to put this handbook together as well as both editions of the larger textbook. We are appreciative of all the hard work provided by McGraw-Hill and its editorial and production staff in seeing this project through to its successful completion. Finally, we would like to acknowledge the constant support of our families and the encouragement of our students and trainees who continue to inspire us.

William H. Frishman, M.D.
Edmund H. Sonnenblick, M.D. •
Domenic A. Sica, M.D.
November 2003

1 | Basic Principles of Clinical Pharmacology Relevant to Cardiology

Walter G. Levine   William H. Frishman

This chapter focuses on some of the basic pharmacologic principles that influence the manner by which cardiovascular drugs manifest their pharmacodynamic and pharmacokinetic actions. A discussion of drug receptor pharmacology is followed by a review of drug disposition, drug metabolism, excretion, and effects of disease states on pharmacokinetics.

RECEPTORS

For nearly 100 years, it has been recognized that, to elicit a response, a drug must interact with a receptor, the interface between drug and body, and the principal determinant of drug selectivity. The receptor (a) recognizes and binds the drug, (b) undergoes changes in conformation and charge distribution, and (c) transduces information inherent in the drug structure (extracellular signal) into intracellular messages, resulting in a change in cellular function. A receptor may be any functional macromolecule and is often a receptor for endogenous regulatory substances, such as hormones or neurotransmitters.

Nature of Receptors

Receptors typically are proteins, lipoproteins, or glycoproteins including (a) regulatory proteins that mediate the action of endogenous substances such as neurotransmitters, hormones, etc.; (b) enzymes, which typically are inhibited by drugs; (c) transport proteins such as Na^+, K^+-ATPase; and (d) structural proteins such as tubulin.

1. Gated channels involve synaptic transmitters (e.g., acetylcholine, norepinephrine) and drugs mimicking their action. These receptors regulate ion flow through membranes, altering transmembrane potentials. The well-characterized nicotinic acetylcholine receptor is a protein consisting of five subunits, two of which selectively bind acetylcholine, thus opening the Na^+ channel through conformational alterations. In the absence of agonist, the channel remains closed. Other drugs, e.g., certain anxiolytics, act similarly at Cl^- channels regulated by γ-aminobutyric acid. The time sequence is extremely fast (milliseconds).
2. G proteins (which interact with guanine nucleotides) diffuse within the cell membrane and interact with more than one receptor. They regulate enzymes, such as adenyl cyclase, or ion channels. Their large number and great diversity may account for drug selectivity in some cases. A prominent example is the role of a specific G protein in the regulation of muscarinic receptors in cardiac muscle. Activation enhances potassium permeability, causing hyperpolarization and depressed electrical activity.
3. Transmembrane enzymes, e.g., protein tyrosine kinases, recognize ligands such as insulin and several growth factors. These bind to an extracellular

1

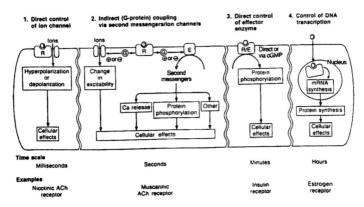

FIG. 1-1 Scheme for the four major tyes of drug receptors and linkage to their cellular effects. E, enzyme; G, G protein; R, receptor molecule.

domain of the receptor and allosterically activate the enzyme site at the cytoplasmic domain, thus enabling phosphorylation of receptor tyrosines. The signaling process proceeds to phosphorylation of other intracellular proteins, which also involves serine and threonine. Downregulation of these receptors is frequently seen, thereby limiting the intensity and duration of action of the ligand (drug).

4. With intracellular receptors, the lipophilic drug (agonist) penetrates the plasma membrane and binds selectively to an intracellular macromolecule. The drug–receptor complex subsequently binds to DNA-modifying gene expression. Response time is slow (up to several hours), and the duration of hours or days after disappearance of the drug is due to turnover time of the proteins expressed by the affected gene.

The four major classes of receptors are depicted in Fig. 1-1. Transmembrane signal transduction also involves several second-messenger systems that respond to receptor activation. These systems include (a) cyclic adenosine monophosphate, which is formed by the action of ligand-activated adenyl cyclase on adenosine triphosphate and, through activation of selective protein kinases, mediates numerous hormonal and drug responses. (b) Phosphatidyl inositol, which, through hydrolysis by phospholipase C within the cell membrane, yields water-soluble inositol triphosphate, which enters the cell and releases bound Ca^{2+}, and (c) lipid-soluble diacylglycerol, which remains in the membrane, where it activates protein kinase C.

Kinetics of Drug–Receptor Interactions

Drug or agonist interacts with its receptor as follows:

$$A + R \underset{k_2}{\overset{k_1}{\rightleftharpoons}} AR$$

where R is the unoccupied receptor and AR is the drug–receptor complex.

According to the law of mass action, the forward reaction rate is given by $k_1[A][R]$, and the reverse reaction rate is given by $k_2[AR]$.

The dissociation constant $\{Kd\} = ([A][R])/[AR]$ relates to k_2/k_1. The binding (affinity) constant $\{Ka\} = 1/Kd$ relates to k_1/k_2.

Each constant is characteristic of a drug and its receptor.

Drug–receptor interactions may involve any type of bond: van der Waals, ionic, hydrogen, or covalent. The interaction is usually of the weaker, reversible type, because covalent binding would effectively destroy receptor function (which may be desirable in the case of an irreversible inhibitor such as the cholinesterase inhibitors, echothiophate, and parathion). Affinity for receptors varies considerably in a teleologically satisfactory manner. Postsynaptic receptors have low affinity for endogenous neurotransmitters released in high concentrations into the synaptic cleft. In contrast, intracellular steroid receptors have high affinity for hormones, which are found in the circulation in very low concentration.

Quantitative Considerations

If one measures an effect at different drug doses (concentrations) and plots the drug response versus the dose, a rectangular hyperbola is obtained (Fig. 1-2A). Because quantitative comparisons among drugs and types of receptors are best described in terms of the dose eliciting 50% maximal response (ED_{50}), it is necessary to plot the response versus the log dose. In this way, the ED_{50} can be determined more accurately (Fig. 1-2B), because it is found in a relatively linear part of the curve. This relation is valid when a graded response is discernible.

The log dose–response curve also can be used to distinguish competitive from noncompetitive inhibition, which is characteristic of many commonly used drugs. Competitive inhibition implies that the agonist and antagonist compete for binding at the active site of the receptor (e.g., β-adrenergic receptor blocking drugs are competitive inhibitors at β-adrenergic receptor sites). Binding of the antagonist to the active site induces no biological response but causes a shift to the right of the log dose–response curve, indicating that more agonist is required to attain a maximal response (Fig. 1-3A). Conversely, a noncompetitive inhibitor binds at a site other than the active one, thus preventing the agonist from inducing a maximal response at any

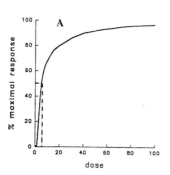
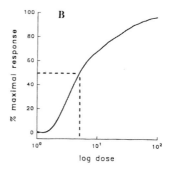

FIG. 1-2 Theoretical dose (concentration)–response curves. *A*. Arithmetic dose scale. *B*. Log dose scale. Dashed lines, determination of 50% effect.

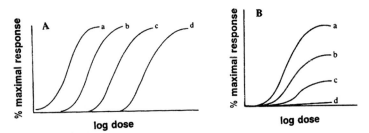

FIG. 1-3 Log dose–response curves illustrating competitive (*A*) and non-competitive (*B*) forms of antagonisms. In *A*, a is the curve for agonist alone; b, c, and d are curves obtained in the presence of increasing concentration of a competitive inhibitor. In *B*, a is the curve for agonist alone; b, c, and d are the curves obtained in the presence of increasing concentrations of a noncompetitive inhibitor.

dose (Fig. 1-3B). There also may be blockade of an action distal to the active site of the receptor. For example, verapamil and nifedipine are calcium channel blockers and prevent influx of calcium ions, thus nonspecifically blocking smooth muscle contraction.

A partial agonist induces a response qualitatively similar to that of the true agonist but far less than the maximal response. Of critical importance is the lack of full response to the agonist in the presence of the partial agonist, the latter thereby acting as an inhibitor. The nonselective beta blocker pindolol exhibits prominent partial agonist activity. The original hope that such a drug would be valuable in cardiac patients with asthma or other lung diseases has not been fulfilled.

Two fundamental properties of drugs, efficacy (intrinsic activity) and potency, must be distinguished (Fig. 1-4A). A partial agonist, unable to elicit a full response, has lower efficacy than does the true agonist. *Efficacy* is actually a property of the drug–receptor complex, because the efficacy of a drug may change from one receptor system to another. *Potency* refers to the concentration or dose of drug required to elicit a standard response. Figure 1-4B

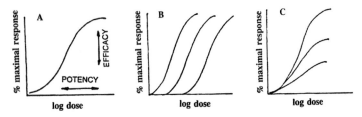

FIG. 1-4 *A*. Log dose–response curves distinguishing potency from efficacy (intrinsic activity). *B*. Response to three drugs with similar efficacies but different potencies. *C*. Response to three drugs with similar potencies but different efficacies. In each case, the receptor system is the same.

shows that a series of drugs acting on the same receptor and differing in potency may possess similar efficacy; with increasing dose, each can induce the same maximal response. Figure 1-4C shows the log dose–response curves for several agonists with similar potencies but with different efficacies. Potency is often considered to be a function of the drug–receptor binding constant. Clinically, a drug that undergoes extensive first-pass metabolism is rapidly inactivated or has other impediments to accessing its receptor and may actually require a high dose despite demonstration of high receptor affinity in vitro. High potency in itself is not a therapeutic advantage for a drug. The therapeutic index must always be considered. A twofold increase in potency may be accompanied by a similar increase in toxicity, thus yielding no advantage.

A fundamental tenet in receptor theory is that a receptor must be "occupied" by an agonist to elicit a biological response and that the biological response is proportional to the number of receptors occupied. However, the ultimate response—changes in blood pressure, renal function, secretion, etc.—may not exhibit a simple proportional relationship owing to the complexity of postreceptor events. The spare-receptor theory states that a maximal response may be attained before occupancy of all receptors at a particular site. This is strictly a quantitative concept because the spare (unoccupied) receptors do not differ qualitatively from other receptors at the same site. Spare receptors may represent 10% to 99% of the total and may allow agonists of low affinity to exert a maximal effect.

Modulation of receptor function is frequently seen. Downregulation is the decrease in the number of receptors upon chronic exposure to an agonist, resulting in lower sensitivity to the agonist. The receptor number may later normalize. For example, administration of a dobutamine infusion to patients with cardiac failure often leads to loss of efficacy of the drug due to downregulation of myocardial β-adrenoceptors. Upregulation was first illustrated by denervation supersensitivity. Sympathetic denervation reduces the amount of neurotransmitter (norepinephrine) to which the postsynaptic adrenoceptor is exposed. Over some period, the receptor population increases, resulting in a heightened sensitivity to small doses of agonist. Drug-induced depletion of sympathetic neurotransmitter (reserpine, guanethidine) elicits a similar response. The increase in cardiac β-receptors during hyperthyroidism increases the sensitivity of the heart to catecholamines. Thus, thyrotoxicosis is accompanied by tachycardia, which responds to propranolol.

DRUG DISPOSITION AND PHARMACOKINETICS

Although binding of a drug to its receptor is required for most drug effects, the amount bound is a small fraction of the total within the body. The mechanisms controlling the movement, metabolism, and excretion of total drug within the body are critical. The dose, route of administration, onset and duration, intensity of effect, frequency of administration, and, often, toxic side effects depend on these mechanisms.

Passage of Drugs Across Cell Membranes

Movement of nearly all drugs within the kidney requires transport across cell membranes by filtration (kidney glomeruli), active transport (renal tubules), passive transport, and facilitated diffusion. Most drugs cross most membranes under most conditions by simple diffusion. Passive flux of molecules down a concentration gradient is given by Fick's law:

$$\text{flux (molecules per unit time)} = C_1 - C_2 \frac{(\text{area} \times \text{permeability coefficient})}{\text{thickness}}$$

where C_1 and C_2 are the higher and lower concentrations, respectively; area is the area of diffusion; permeability coefficient is the mobility of molecules within the diffusion pathway; and thickness describes the diffusion path.

Therefore, rate and direction of passage depend on (a) concentration gradient across the membrane of unbound drug and (b) lipid solubility of drug. Most drugs, being weak organic bases or acids, will be ionized or un-ionized depending on their pK and the pH of their environment. The *un-ionized* form, being more lipid soluble, readily diffuses across the membrane, whereas the *ionized* form is mainly excluded from the membrane. This principle is adhered to most rigidly in the brain, where the tight gap junctions in cerebral capillaries prevent intercellular diffusion of hydrophilic drugs, thus creating the so-called blood–brain barrier. Drugs having a charge at physiologic pH, e.g., terfenadine (Seldane) and neostigmine, are generally excluded from the brain. In contrast, in the liver, blood passes through sinusoids that are highly fenestrated, thereby allowing plasma constituents, including charged and noncharged drugs, to pass readily into the interstitial space and have direct contact with the liver cells, where selectivity for drug transport is far weaker.

Absorption

Absorption of drugs from sites of administration follows the general principles described above. Other factors include solubility, rate of dissolution, concentration at site of absorption, circulation to site of absorption, and area of the absorbing surface.

Routes of Drug Administration

Sublingual Route

Sublingual administration avoids destruction due to the acidic environment of the stomach and bypasses the intestine and liver, thereby avoiding loss through absorption and enzymatic destruction (first-pass effect). It is used for nitroglycerin (angina pectoris), ergotamine (migraine), and certain testosterone preparations (avoids prominent first-pass effects).

Oral Route

In addition to the convenience of this route, the structure, surface area, and movement of the intestines are conducive to absorption, which takes place throughout the gastrointestinal (GI) tract. Rules for passive transport are applicable; pH gradient along the tract influences absorption of drugs with different pKs. Aqueous and lipid solubilities of a drug may be competing factors, i.e., a drug may be lipid soluble, favoring absorption, but so insoluble in water that absorption is very poor or erratic. Rate of absorption is regulated in part by intestinal blood flow, which serves to remove drug from the absorption site, thus maintaining a high GI tract–blood concentration gradient and gastric emptying time (most drugs are absorbed mainly in the intestine). Absorption varies with pH, presence and nature of food, mental state, GI and other diseases, endocrine status, and drugs that influence GI function.

Drugs may be extensively (high extraction) or minimally (low extraction) cleared from the portal and systemic circulations by the liver. The extent of removal is referred to as the *extraction ratio*. It follows that the rate of plasma clearance of high-extraction drugs is very sensitive to hepatic blood flow. An increase or decrease in hepatic blood flow will enhance or depress, respectively, drug clearance from the plasma. Conversely, variations in hepatic blood flow have minimal influence on removal of low-extraction drugs, because so little is removed per unit time. Diminished hepatic extraction capacity, as seen in severe liver disease and aging, can significantly decrease the first-pass effect and plasma disappearances of high-extraction drugs.

Rectal Route

This route is reserved mainly for infants, cases of persistent vomiting, and the unconscious patient. Absorption follows rules for passive transport but is often less efficient than in other parts of the GI tract. Because blood flow in the lower part of the rectum connects directly with the systemic circulation, portions of rectally administered drugs bypass the first-pass effect.

Pulmonary Route

The pulmonary route is used primarily for gaseous and volatile drugs and for nicotine and other drugs of abuse, such as crack cocaine. These are rapidly absorbed due to their high-lipid solubility, small molecular size, and vast alveolar surface area (approximately 200 m^2).

Transdermal Route

This route has come into vogue for the administration of certain cardiac, central nervous system (CNS), and endocrine drugs for a slow, sustained effect. The large surface area (2 m^2) and blood supply of the skin (30%) are conducive to absorption. Advantages include more stable blood levels, avoidance of first-pass effect, better compliance because frequency of administration is greatly diminished, no injection risks, and elimination of variability in oral absorption. The drug must be relatively potent, i.e., effective in low dose, sufficiently lipid, and water soluble to penetrate the several layers of the skin; it also must be nonirritant and stable for several days. Inflammation, by increasing cutaneous blood flow, enhances drug absorption. Drugs administered by the transdermal route include scopolamine, nitrate, clonidine, and estradiol.

Injection

This route avoids the first-pass effect. The *intravenous* route allows rapidity of access to the systemic circulation and a degree of accuracy for dosage not possible with other routes. *Intramuscular* and *subcutaneous* routes require absorption into the systemic circulation at rates dependent on the lipid solubility of the drug and circulation to the injected area. Epinephrine may be added to subcutaneous injection to constrict blood vessels and thus retard absorption. Drugs also can be administered into regional circulations through *indwelling catheters* (e.g., vascular growth factors) and injected directly into the vascular endothelium and myocardium (e.g., gene therapy, cell therapy).

Bioavailability

There are two aspects of this concept: (a) absolute bioavailability, or the proportion of administered drug gaining access to the systemic circulation after oral as opposed to intravenous administration, thus reflecting the first-pass effect; and (b) relative bioavailability of different preparations of the same drug.

By plotting plasma concentration versus time, one can calculate the area under the curve, a measure of bioavailability (Fig. 1-5).The curve also indicates peak plasma levels and time to attain peak levels. Bioequivalent preparation should be identical in each of these parameters. However, considerable variation may be seen among different preparations, thus reflecting extent and rate of drug release from its dosage form (pill, capsule, etc.) within the GI tract. Factors that may affect bioavailability include conditions within the GI tract, pH, food, disease, other drugs, metabolism, and/or binding within the intestinal wall and liver. Ideally, preparations should be tested for bioavailability under identical conditions in the same subject. The narrower the therapeutic index of a drug, the greater the concern for variation in bioavailability.

Distribution to Tissues

Vascularity and plasma concentration of drug are the main determinants of tissue distribution. Organs receiving a high blood supply, e.g., kidney, brain, and thyroid, are rapidly exposed to drugs, whereas bone and adipose tissue receive only a minor fraction of the dose. High plasma concentrations of drugs result in high tissue levels due to mass action and passive diffusion across cell membranes. Lipid-soluble drugs readily pass the placenta, thus enabling distribution to and possible action on the developing fetus. Therefore, the use of any drug is not recommended during pregnancy; thiazide diuretics and warfarin, among others, are particularly discouraged. Redistribution of drugs can influ-

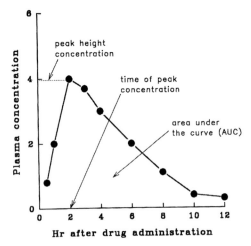

FIG. 1-5   Theoretical plasma levels of drug as a function of time. The curve is used to determine bioavailability, because it illustrates peak concentration, time of peak concentration, and area under the curve (AUC).

ence pharmacologic response. For example, it is well established that the actions of benzodiazepines and thiopental are terminated not by metabolism or excretion but by redistribution of the drugs away from the brain.

Site-specific drug delivery would enhance therapeutic effectiveness and limit side and toxic effects. This has been achieved for very few drugs, because normal body mechanisms are generally conducive to wide distribution to sites unrelated to the desired drug receptors. A type of organ targeting is seen with prodrugs such as L-dopa, which is converted to the active form, dopamine, in the CNS, and sulfasalazine, which is converted to the active salicylate by gut bacteria within the lower bowel.

Binding to Plasma Proteins

Most drugs are bound to plasma proteins to some extent. Albumin binds a wide spectrum of drugs, particularly those with acidic and neutral characteristics. Binding is usually nonspecific, although some selective sites are known. Basic drugs also may bind to albumin, but mainly to α_1-acid glycoprotein, an acute-phase reactant protein. Lipoproteins also bind some lipophilic and basic compounds. Many highly specific proteins exist that bind thyroxine, retinol, transcortin, etc., but these are of little consequence for drugs and other xenobiotics.

Binding to plasma proteins is always reversible, and the half-time of binding and release is exceedingly short (measured in milliseconds). Thus, even in the case of extensive (tight) binding, it is rapidly reversible under physiologic conditions. Because concentration gradients, which determine the rate of passive transport across membranes, are based solely on free drug, it follows that binding to plasma proteins slows the rate of removal of drug from plasma by diminishing the concentration gradient across capillary cell membranes. Thus, access to all extravascular sites, receptors, metabolism, storage, and excretion are to a great extent regulated by plasma protein binding. It follows that the half-lives of many drugs correlate with the extent of binding. In contrast, active transport, as in the proximal tubule, is unaffected by plasma protein binding. For example, nifedipine, which is 96% bound to plasma proteins, has a half-life of only 1.8 h. In this case, the protein-bound portion of the drug serves as a readily accessible reservoir due to rapid reversibility of binding.

Hepatic extraction is sensitive to plasma protein binding. For low-extraction drugs, binding is of considerable importance, whereas hepatic uptake of high extraction drugs is little influenced by binding.

Displacement of drugs from binding sites increases the proportion of free drug in the plasma and, hence, the effective concentration of the drug in extravascular compartments. Similarly, increasing the dose of a drug beyond binding capacity disproportionately increases the unbound fraction within the plasma and may lead to undesired pharmacologic effects. Plasma-binding proteins may be decreased in concentration or effectiveness under the following conditions:

- Albumin: Burns, nephrosis, cystic fibrosis, cirrhosis, inflammation, sepsis, malnutrition, neoplasia, aging, pregnancy, stress, heart failure. Uremia causes decreased binding of acidic but not basic drugs.
- α_1-Acid glycoprotein: Aging, oral contraceptives, pregnancy.

The possibility of altered drug disposition should be considered in each case.

Volume of Distribution

Under ideal conditions, drugs are considered to be distributed in one or more of the body fluid compartments. The apparent volume of distribution (Vd) is the body fluid volume that appears to contain the drug.

$$Vd = \frac{dose}{plasma\ concentration\ (after\ equilibration)}$$

For example, Vd = plasma volume (e.g., heparin) implies extensive binding of the drug to plasma proteins, with the bulk of the drug remaining in the plasma. Vd = total body water (e.g., phenytoin, diazepam) implies that the drug is evenly distributed throughout the body. However, one should avoid associating Vd values with a specific anatomic compartment, because binding at extravascular sites (e.g., procainamide, verapamil, metoprolol) may significantly affect Vd determinations. Their importance lies in the fact that Vd can change with age, sex, disease, etc. Thus, changes in plasma protein synthesis, skeletal muscle mass, adipose tissue mass, adipose:muscle ratio, and body hydration will be reflected in Vd and may markedly alter the therapeutic and toxic responses to a drug. Values of Vd, if used intelligently, can provide information on body distribution of a drug, changes in body water compartments, implications for intensity of effect, and rate of elimination.

Half-Life and Clearance

The half-life ($t_{1/2}$) of a drug is the time for the plasma concentration to be decreased by one-half. It is usually independent of route of administration

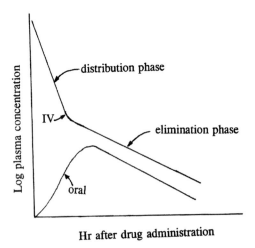

FIG. 1-6 Theoretical plasma disappearance curve for a drug after intravenous or oral administration. During the elimination phase, the straight line obtained from a semilog plot reflects first-order kinetics.

and dose. Assuming equilibration among all body fluid compartments, it theoretically is a true reflection of the $t_{1/2}$ within the total body and correlates closely with duration of action. The $t_{1/2}$ is derived from a first-order reaction calculated from a semilog plot of the plasma concentration versus time during the elimination phase, which reflects metabolism and excretion of the drug (Fig. 1-6). Linearity of this phase reflects exponential kinetics (first order), in which plasma concentrations of drug do not saturate the rate-limiting step in elimination. The process may be expressed as a rate constant, k, the fractional change per unit time. The factors $t_{1/2}$ and k are related by the following equation:

$$t_{1/2} \times k = 0.693(\ln 0.5)$$

or

$$t_{1/2} = 0.693/k$$

After oral administration, the initial period is called the *absorption phase*. Here too, $t_{1/2}$ is calculated from the elimination phase. In a few cases (alcohol, phenytoin, high-dose aspirin), the rate-limiting step is saturated, and plasma disappearance rate is zero order. For phenytoin, this phase may lead to difficulty in controlling blood levels to maintain efficacy and avoid toxicity.

Total body clearance (Cl_{τ}) is an expression of the fluid Vd cleared per unit time. It is calculated as the product of the elimination rate constant and the Vd.

$$Cl_{\tau} = kVd$$

It follows that

$$t_{1/2} = \frac{0.693 \text{ Vd}}{Cl}$$

This concept assumes clearance from a single body fluid compartment and is the sum of renal and hepatic clearances. Disease states, aging, and other conditions in which Vd may be altered would change clearance. Clearance can be used to determine correct dosage when the desired plasma concentration has been predetermined but changes in physiologic parameters governing drug disposition have occurred, thus altering clearance.

$$\text{Dosage} = Cl \times C_{ss}$$

where Cl is clearance and C_{ss} is the steady-state plasma drug concentration. Dosage therefore is a replacement of cleared drug.

Caution Because clearance is calculated from Vd, a theoretical rather than a physiologic term, the number derived may not be truly physiologic. In therapeutics, it is the change of clearance that is a marker for altered drug disposition.

Steady-State Kinetics

During chronic oral administration of a drug, its steady-state plasma level is not a set concentration but a fluctuating concentration, reflecting periodic absorption and continual removal. When drug administration is begun, in accord with first-order kinetics, the elimination rate gradually increases with increasing plasma levels, and, eventually, a steady state is attained

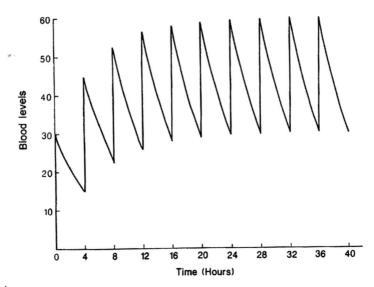

FIG. 1-7 Blood level–time profile for a drug, with a half-life of 4 h, administered every 4 h. The plateau effect determines that 95% of the final mean blood level is attained in four to five half-lives.

where input equals output. This is the plateau effect (Fig. 1-7). It can be shown that

- 50% of steady state is attained after one half-life
- 75% of steady state is attained after two half-lives
- 87.5% of steady state is attained after three half-lives
- 93.75% of steady state is attained after four half-lives

The rule of thumb is that steady state is attained in four to five half-lives. After drug withdrawal, the converse of the plateau effect is seen; i.e., plasma levels are reduced by

- 50% in one half-life
- 75% in two half-lives
- 87.5% in three half-lives
- 93.75% in four half-lives

When a long half-life, e.g., 14 h, and therapeutic demands preclude waiting four to five half-lives to attain desired plasma concentration of drug, a loading dose (LD) is used, calculated as follows:

$$LD = (Vd \times C)/F$$

where Vd is the apparent volume of distribution, C is the desired plasma concentration, and F is the fraction of oral dose that reaches the systemic circulation (first-pass effect).

This formula is based on the need to fill the entire Vd to the desired concentration as rapidly as possible. The dose is limited by toxicity, distribution rate, and other variables.

For a drug given by intravenous infusion, LD = infusion rate $\times$ $t_{1/2}$.

DRUG METABOLISM (BIOTRANSFORMATION)

Mechanisms and Pathways

Most drugs and other xenobiotics are metabolized before excretion. Although •
most drugs are ultimately converted to inactive products, many are transformed to pharmacologically active metabolites. In some instances, a drug is
metabolized via several pathways, some of which represent inactivation,
whereas others involve activation to toxic product(s).

For many drugs, the first step (phase I) is catalyzed by the cytochrome P450
(mixed-function oxidase) system of the endoplasmic reticulum (microsomal
fraction). Cytochrome P450 is actually a large family of isozymes, members
of which vary with species, sex, and age. Each has its own spectrum of substrates and can be independently influenced by induction and inhibition.

The mixed-function oxidase system exists mainly in the liver but has been
detected in nonhepatic tissue, particularly at other sites of xenobiotic entry,
e.g., lung, skin, etc. Total metabolism in these tissues is a fraction of that of
the liver. Nevertheless, because environmental chemicals often enter the body
through the lungs and skin, these tissues are of considerable importance in
their metabolism.

Major phase I pathways, microsomal and nonmicrosomal, include (a)
aliphatic and aromatic hydroxylation, (b) N-dealkylation, (c) O-dealkylation,
(d) sulfoxidation, (e) N-hydroxylation (commonly associated with toxic activation of aromatic amines, including a number of chemical carcinogens), (f) azo
and nitro reductions, (g) O-methylation, and (h) hydrolysis by plasma esterase.

Conjugation (synthetic) pathways (phase II) often but not always follow
phase I. They include (a) acylation, a common pathway for aliphatic and aromatic primary amines; (b) glucuronide formation; (c) sulfate formation; and
(d) glutathione conjugate formation. Phase II reactions increase drug polarity
and charge and thus promote renal excretion (see below).

Glutathione conjugation is a major inactivation mechanism for toxic metabolic intermediates of numerous drugs. For example, in normal dosage, a
toxic metabolite of acetaminophen is effectively removed as a glutathione
conjugate. In extreme overdose (10 to 15 g), the demand for glutathione exceeds its rate of hepatic biosynthesis, and the accumulation of toxic intermediate leads to liver toxicity and, in rare cases, necrosis and death. Toxicity
is treated with acetylcysteine, which serves to restore liver glutathione.

Factors Affecting Drug Metabolism

Species

Species is a major problem in drug development and research.

Age

Few drugs are studied in young children before their approval by the U.S.
Food and Drug Administration, thus presenting a considerable challenge in
the treatment of this population. In the neonate, factors affecting drug disposition include prolonged gastric emptying time, fluctuating gastric pH,
smaller muscle mass, greater cutaneous absorption of toxic substances (e.g.,
hexachlorophene), changing body water:fat ratio, less effective plasma protein binding, poor hepatic drug metabolism, and low renal blood flow. Drugs
that pass the placenta present problems of disposition to the fetus. The newborn often exhibits a deficiency in glucuronyl transferase, which catalyzes the

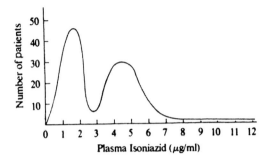

FIG. 1-8 Bimodal distribution of patients into rapid and slow acetylators of isoniazid. Slow acetylators are homozygous for an autosomal recessive gene.

essential step in bilirubin excretion. If this deficiency goes unappreciated, kernicterus may ensue. The postneonatal period is also a time of rapid structural and physiologic changes, including the capacity to metabolize drugs. Therefore, calculation of dosage based solely on body weight or surface area may not always be appropriate. In the elderly, one sees diminished renal plasma flow and glomerular filtration rate, decreased hepatic phase I but not phase II drug metabolism, diminished Vd due to loss of body water compartment, decreased muscle mass, decreased or increased adipose tissue, and decreased first-pass effect.

Genetic Factors

Marked differences in rates of drug metabolism are often attributable to genetic factors. Approximately 50% of the male population in the United States acetylates aromatic amines, such as isoniazid, rapidly and the other half acetylates slowly (Fig. 1-8). The slow acetylator phenotype is inherited as an autosomal recessive trait. Neither slow nor fast acetylation is an advantage, because the toxicities of isoniazid (peripheral neuropathies, preventable by pyridoxine administration) and its acetylated metabolite (hepatic damage) are known. Other affected drugs include procainamide, hydralazine, and sulfasalazine.

A small percentage (<1%) of the population has an abnormal form of plasma pseudo-esterase and is unable to hydrolyze succinylcholine at the normal rapid rate, leading to an exaggerated duration of action. Three forms of cytochrome P450 (CYP2D6, CYP2C19, and CYP2C9) exhibit polymorphism. The phenotypes are slow and rapid metabolizers of many drugs: CYP2D6—debrisoquin, tricyclic antidepressants, phenformin, dextromethorphan, and several beta blockers; CYP2C19—mephenytoin; and CYP2C9—warfarin. Some 3% to 10% of the population has the slow trait, inherited in an autosomal recessive fashion.

Nutritional Deficiency

Multiple manifestations of malnutrition may significantly affect drug disposition. These include changes in GI and renal functions, body composition (fluids, electrolytes, fat, protein, etc.), hepatic drug metabolism, endocrine function, and immune response. This is most likely among economically depressed populations and in diseases such as cancer, which are often accompanied by malnutrition. Obviously, hepatic or renal disease can have major consequences for drug disposition. Half-lives for many drugs increase in cirrhosis, hepatitis, obstructive jaundice, nephritis, and other types of kidney failure. Liver disease may result in altered hepatic blood flow, decreased extraction, or depressed metabolizing enzymes. Kidney disease may be manifest as altered renal blood flow and depressed glomerular filtration, active transport, or passive reabsorption. In cardiac failure, the decreased blood supply to most organs means delayed and incomplete absorption of drugs. In contrast, decreased Vd may mean higher plasma drug levels and, as a consequence, exaggerated responses to drug.

Induction

Chronic exposure to any of a large number of drugs and other environmental chemicals induces the synthesis of specific forms of cytochrome P450; conjugation with glucuronic acid and glutathione also may be affected. The duration of action of some drugs is thereby shortened, their blood levels are lowered, and their potency is diminished. The half-lives of drugs with low hepatic extraction are mainly affected, whereas drugs not metabolized by these enzymes are not affected. Examples of well-known inducing agents are lipid-soluble drugs such as phenobarbital, phenytoin, rifampin, and ethanol; glucocorticoids; and environmental pollutants such as benzo(a)pyrene and other polycyclic hydrocarbons formed in cigarette smoke, polychlorinated biphenyls, and dioxin. The effect of smoking on plasma drug levels is shown in Fig. 1-9.

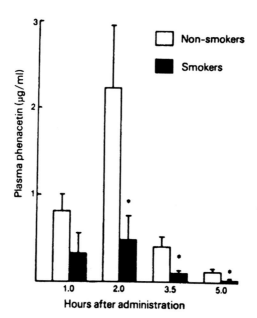

FIG. 1-9   Blood levels of phenacetin in smoking and nonsmoking populations, reflecting the inducing effect of components of cigarette smoke on drug-metabolizing enzymes.

Inhibition

Inhibition of drug metabolism will have the opposite effect, leading to a prolonged half-life and an exaggerated pharmacologic response. Drugs well known for their inhibitory effects include chloramphenicol, cimetidine, allopurinol, and monoamine oxidase inhibitors. Alcohol acutely depresses certain drug metabolism pathways (although, chronically, it induces them) and may lead to enhanced and prolonged effects of other drugs. Erythromycin and ketoconazole block the conversion of terfenadine (Seldane), a prodrug, to its active metabolite. Because the parent compound is arrhythmogenic, serious cardiac toxicity may be seen with such drug combinations. For this reason, terfenadine has been banned, although its active metabolite is marketed as fexofenadine (Allegra), which lacks cardiotoxicity and CNS effects. It is suspected that there are many more such inhibitory drugs, but it is difficult to predict a priori when inhibition will occur.

Metabolism by Intestinal Microorganisms

The abundant flora of the lower gut includes many organisms capable of metabolizing drugs and their metabolic derivatives. Because the microflora consist mainly of obligate anaerobes and the gut environment is anaerobic, only pathways not requiring oxygen are seen. These bacteria make a significant contribution to drug metabolism, and suppression of the gut flora by oral antibiotics or other drugs will appreciably alter the fate and thus the effects of many other drugs. The various pathways include hydrolysis of glucuronides, sulfates, and amides; dehydroxylation; deamination; and azo and nitro reductions.

Enterohepatic Circulation

Many conjugated drugs are transported into the bile and pass into the intestine. Intestinal microorganisms hydrolyze the conjugate (glucuronides in particular), yielding the original, less polar compound, which can then be reabsorbed. This cycle tends to repeat itself and makes a major contribution to maintenance of drugs and certain endogenous compounds within the body. For example, bile salts are 90% re-circulated through this mechanism. Suppression of gut bacteria by oral antibiotics will appreciably affect the half-lives and thus the plasma levels of compounds that undergo extensive enterohepatic circulation.

EXCRETION

All drugs are ultimately eliminated from the body via one route or another. Elimination rate, as reflected in plasma disappearance rate for most drugs, is generally proportional to the total amount in the body, according to first-order kinetics.

1. The *kidney* is the major organ of excretion for most drugs and associated metabolites. Its large blood supply (25% of cardiac output) is conducive to efficient excretion. Drugs not bound to plasma proteins are filtered in the glomeruli with nearly 100% efficiency. Reabsorption within the tubule is mainly by passive diffusion. Thus, highly charged drugs (or metabolites)

will be poorly reabsorbed and readily excreted. Changes in tubular pH alter excretion rates by influencing the net charge on the compound. Appropriate manipulation of urinary pH is helpful in facilitating excretion in cases of drug overdose. For example, raising the pH increases excretion of phenobarbital, an organic acid, whereas lowering the pH increases excretion of amphetamine, an organic base. Active transport of organic anions and cations takes place in the tubules. Penicillin, a weak organic acid, is actively pumped into the tubule's lumen by the tubular anion transport system, an action readily suppressed by probenecid, an inhibitor of the anion pump. Renal failure presents a major therapeutic problem due to accumulation of drug and toxic metabolites. Hemodialysis filters out unbound drugs from the plasma, thus assisting clearance. Drugs bound in extravascular areas are less affected by dialysis.

2. *Biliary* excretion is usually reserved for highly polar compounds with molecular weights greater than 500 kDa. Bile empties into the duodenum, and drugs passing via this route are frequently reabsorbed in the intestinal tract (see Enterohepatic Circulation). Unlike the mechanisms involving urine, those of bile formation and biliary excretion are poorly understood. Biliary secretion is greatly but not entirely dependent on bile salt transport. Bile salts may facilitate or inhibit biliary excretion of drugs, depending on the drug and the concentration of bile salts.

3. *Lungs* are the excretion route for many general anesthetics and other volatile substances. A clever use of the lungs as a route of excretion is the "aminopyrine breath test." Aminopyrine that has been labeled with radioactive carbon in its methyl moiety is administered. It is demethylated by the liver's P450 system, ultimately forming radioactive carbon dioxide, which is then collected from the expired air and counted. The amount of radioactivity is a reflection of hepatic drug metabolism and has been used as a noninvasive assessment of liver function in, e.g., liver cirrhosis. In recent years, erythromycin has been used as the test substance.

4. Considerable concern has been raised regarding drugs in breast milk in view of the increase in the past two decades in the number of nursing mothers. Drug entry into plasma is affected by pK of drug, pH of milk and plasma, binding to plasma and milk proteins, and fat composition of milk. Drugs enter the milk by passive diffusion. The pH of milk (6.5 to 7.0) and milk's changing volume and high content of fat globules and unique proteins influence drug secretion, especially for lipid-soluble compounds. Drugs known to be secreted into milk include cardiovascular drugs (hydralazine, digoxin), CNS drugs (caffeine, amitriptyline, primidone, ethosuximide), drugs of abuse (nicotine, narcotics, cocaine), and others (metronidazole, medroxyprogesterone, nor-testosterone). This does not necessarily imply an incompatibility between nursing and taking any of these drugs. However, drugs contraindicated or to be used with caution during lactation include alcohol, amiodarone, atropine, chlorpromazine, cimetidine, cocaine, cyclosporine, doxorubicin, lithium, morphine, nitrofurantoin, phenytoin, phenindione, salicylates, tetracyclines, and tinidazole. At present, drugs must be evaluated individually when deciding on the safety of nursing infants. Similar considerations are valid for cow's milk, because these animals may be given drugs to increase milk production.

Another route of excretion being developed for noninvasive assessment of blood levels of drugs is saliva. For some drugs, a known equilibrium exists between the plasma and saliva. Although the work is only in its infancy, one can foresee the day when, if plasma levels are required, a patient will simply spit for the doctor rather than being stuck with a needle five or six times.

ADDITIONAL READINGS

Berndt WO, Stitzel RE: Excretion of drugs, in Craig CR, Stitzel RE (eds): *Modern Pharmacology*, 4th ed. Boston, Little Brown, 1994, p 47.

Bourne HR, Roberts JM: Drug receptors and pharmacodynamics, in Katzung BG (ed): *Basic and Clinical Pharmacology*, 8th ed. Norwalk, Appleton & Lange, 2001, p 9.

Cheng JWM: Cytochrome P450-mediated cardiovascular drug interactions. *Heart Dis* 2:254, 2000.

Correia MA: Drug biotransformation, in Katzung BG (ed): *Basic and Clinical Pharmacology*, 8th ed. Norwalk, Appleton & Lange, 2001, p 51.

Fleming WW: Mechanisms of drug action, in Craig CR, Stitzel RE (eds): *Modern Pharmacology*, 4th ed. Boston, Little Brown, 1994, p 9.

Godin DV: Pharmacokinetics: disposition and metabolism of drugs, in Munson PL, Mueller RA, Breese GR (eds): *Principles of Pharmacology: Basic Concepts and Clinical Applications*. New York, Chapman & Hall, 1995, p 39.

Gram TE: Drug absorption and distribution, in Craig CR, Stitzel RE (eds): *Modern Pharmacology*, 4th ed. Boston, Little Brown, 1994, p 19.

Gram TE: Metabolism of drugs, in Craig CR, Stitzel RE (eds): *Modern Pharmacology*, 4th ed. Boston, Little, Brown, 1994, p 33.

Gwilt PR: Pharmacokinetics, in Craig CR, Stitzel RE (eds): *Modern Pharmacology*, 4th ed. Boston, Little Brown, 1994, p 55.

Holford NHG, Benet LZ: Pharmacokinetics and pharmacodynamics: rational dose selection and the time course of drug action, in Katzung BG (ed): *Basic and Clinical Pharmacology*, 8th ed. Norwalk, Appleton & Lange, 2001, p 35.

Hollenberg MD, Severson DL: Pharmacodynamics: drug receptors and receptors/mechanisms, in Munson PL, Mueller RA, Breese GR (eds): *Principles of Pharmacology: Basic Concepts and Clinical Applications*. New York, Chapman & Hall, 1995, p 7.

Levine WG: Basic principles of clinical pharmacology relevant to cardiology, in: Frishman WH, Sonnenblick EH, Sica DA (eds): *Cardiovascular Pharmacotherapeutics*, 2nd ed. New York, McGraw-Hill, 2003, p 3.

Nierenberg DW, Melmon KL: Introduction to clinical pharmacology and rational therapeutics, in Carruthers SG, Hoffman BB, Melmon KL, Nierenberg DW (eds): *Melmon & Morrelli's Clinical Pharmacology*, 4th ed. New York, McGraw-Hill, 2000, p 3.

Opie LH, Frishman WH: Adverse cardiovascular drug interactions and complications, in Fuster V, Alexander RW, O'Rourke RA, et al (eds): *Hurst's the Heart*, 11th ed. New York, McGraw-Hill, In press.

Rang HP, Dale MM, Ritter HM, Gardner P: *Pharmacology*. New York, Churchill Livingstone, 1995.

Sokol SI, Cheng-Lai A, Frishman WH, Kaza CS: Cardiovascular drug therapy in patients with hepatic diseases and patients with congestive heart failure. *J Clin Pharmacol* 40:11, 2000.

2 | α- and β-Adrenergic Blocking Drugs

William H. Frishman

Catecholamines are neurohumoral substances that mediate a variety of physiologic and metabolic activities in humans. The effects of the catecholamines ultimately depend on their chemical interactions with receptors, which are discrete macromolecular structures on the plasma membrane. Differences in the ability of the various catecholamines to stimulate a number of physiologic processes were the criteria used by Ahlquist in 1948 to separate these receptors into distinct types: α- and β-adrenergic. Subsequent studies have found that β-adrenergic receptors exist as three discrete subtypes: β_1, β_2, and β_3 (Table 2-1). It is now appreciated that there are two subtypes of α receptors, designated α_1 and α_2 (see Table 2-1). At least three subtypes of α_1- and α_2-adrenergic receptors are known, but distinctions in their mechanisms of action and tissue location have not been well defined.

This chapter examines the adrenergic receptors and the drugs that can inhibit their function. The rationale for use and clinical experience with α- and β-adrenergic drugs in the treatment of various cardiovascular disorders is also discussed.

ADRENERGIC RECEPTORS: HORMONAL AND DRUG RECEPTORS

The effects of an endogenous hormone or exogenous drug depend ultimately on physiochemical interactions with macromolecular structures of cells called *receptors*. Agonists interact with a receptor and elicit a response; antagonists interact with receptors and prevent the action of agonists.

In the case of catecholamine action, the circulating hormone or drug ("first messenger") interacts with its specific receptor on the external surface of the target cells. The drug hormone–receptor complex, mediated by a G protein called Gs, activates the enzyme adenyl cyclase on the internal surface of the plasma membrane of the target cell, which accelerates the intracellular formation of cyclic adenosine monophosphate (cAMP). Cyclic AMP–dependent protein kinase ("second messenger") then stimulates or inhibits various metabolic or physiologic processes. Catecholamine-induced increases in intracellular cAMP are usually associated with stimulation of β-adrenergic receptors, whereas the stimulation of α-adrenergic receptors is mediated by a G protein known as Gi and is associated with lower concentrations of cAMP and possibly increased amounts of guanosine 3′5′-monophosphate in the cell. These changes may result in the production of opposite physiologic effects from those of catecholamines, depending on what adrenergic receptor system is activated.

Until recently, most research on receptor action bypassed the initial binding step and the intermediate steps and examined the accumulation of cAMP or the end step, the physiologic effect. Currently, radioactive agonists or antagonists (radioligands) that attach to and label the receptors have been used to study binding and hormone action. The cloning of adrenergic receptors has also revealed important clues about receptor function.

TABLE 2-1 Characteristics of Subtypes of Adrenergic Receptors*

Receptor	Tissue	Response
α_1[†]	Vascular smooth muscle, genitourinary smooth muscle	Contraction
	Liver[‡]	Glycogenolysis; gluconeogenesis
	Heart	Increased contractile force; arrhythmias
α_2[†]	Pancreatic islets (β cells)	Decreased insulin secretion
	Platelets	Aggregation
	Nerve terminals	Decreased release of norepinephrine
	Vascular smooth muscle	Contraction
β_1	Heart	Increased force and rate of contraction and atrioventricular nodal conduction velocity
	Juxtaglomerular cells	Increased renin secretion
β_2	Smooth muscle (vascular, bronchial, gastrointestinal, and genitourinary)	Relaxation
	Skeletal muscle	Glycogenolysis; uptake of K^+
	Liver[‡]	Glycogenolysis; gluconeogensis
β_3[#]	Adipose tissue	Lipolysis, thermogenesis

* This table provides examples of drugs that act on adrenergic receptors and of the location of subtypes of adrenergic receptors.
† At least three subtypes of each α_1- and α_2-adrenergic receptor are known, but their mechanisms of action and tissue locations have not been clearly defined.
‡ In some species (e.g., rat), metabolic responses in the liver are mediated by α_1-adrenergic receptors, whereas in others (e.g., dog), β_2-adrenergic receptors are predominantly involved. Both types of receptors appear to contribute to responses in human beings.
# Metabolic responses in adipocytes and certain other tissues with atypical pharmacologic characteristics may be mediated by this subtype of receptor. Most β-adrenergic receptor antagonists (including propranolol) do not block these responses.
Source: Adapted with permission from Hoffman BB, Taylor P: Neurotransmission: The autonomic and somatic motor nervous sytems, in Hardman JG, Limbird LE (eds): *Goodman & Gilman's The Pharmacological Basis of Therapeutics,* 10th ed. New York; McGraw-Hill, 2001, p 115.

α-ADRENERGIC BLOCKERS

Clinical Pharmacology

When an adrenergic nerve is stimulated, catecholamines are released from their storage granules in the adrenergic neuron, enter the synaptic cleft, and bind to α receptors on the effector cell. A feedback loop exists by which the amount of neurotransmitter released can be regulated: accumulation of catecholamines in the synaptic cleft leads to stimulation of α receptors in the neuronal surface and inhibition of further catecholamine release. Catecholamines from the systemic circulation can also enter the synaptic cleft and bind to presynaptic or postsynaptic receptors.

Initially it was believed that α_1 receptors were limited to postsynaptic sites, where they mediated vasoconstriction, whereas the α_2 receptors existed only at the prejunctional nerve terminals and mediated the negative feedback control of norepinephrine release. The availability of compounds with high specificity for α_1 or α_2 receptors demonstrated that, whereas presynaptic α receptors are almost exclusively of the α_2 subtype, the postsynaptic receptors are made up of comparable numbers of α_1 and α_2 receptors. Stimulation of the postsynaptic α_2 receptors causes vasoconstriction. However, a functional difference does exist between the two types of postsynaptic receptors. The α_1 receptors appear to exist primarily within the region of the synapse and respond preferentially to neuronally released catecholamine, whereas α_2 receptors are located extrasynaptically and respond preferentially to circulating catecholamines in the plasma.

Drugs having α-adrenergic blocking properties are of several types.

1. Nonselective alpha blockers having prominent effects on the α_1 and α_2 receptors (e.g., the older drugs such as phenoxybenzamine and phentolamine). Whereas virtually all of the clinical effects of phenoxybenzamine are explicable in terms of α blockade, this is not the case with phentolamine, which also possesses several other properties, including a direct vasodilator action and sympathomimetic and parasympathomimetic effects.
2. Selective α_1 blockers having little affinity for α_2 receptors (e.g., prazosin, terazosin, doxazosin, and other quinazoline derivatives). It is now clear that these drugs, originally introduced as direct-acting vasodilators, exert their major effect by reversible blockade of postsynaptic α_1 receptors. Other selective α_1 blockers include indoramin, trimazosin, and urapidil (Table 2-2). Urapidil is of interest because of its other actions, which include stimulation of presynaptic α_2-adrenergic receptors and a central effect.
3. Selective α_2 blockers (e.g., yohimbine) have been used primarily as tools in experimental pharmacology. Yohimbine is now marketed in the United States as an oral sympatholytic and mydriatic agent. Male patients with impotence of vascular, diabetic, or psychogenic origin have been treated successfully with yohimbine.
4. Blockers that inhibit α- and β-adrenergic receptors (e.g., carvedilol, labetalol). Carvedilol and labetalol are selective α_1 blockers. Because these agents are much more potent as β blockers than as α blockers, they are discussed in greater detail in the section on β blockers.

TABLE 2-2 Pharmacokinetics of Selective α_1-Adrenergic Blocking Drugs

Selective α_1 blocker	Daily dose mg	Frequency/ day	Bioavailability (% of oral dose)	Plasma half-life (h)	Urinary excretion (% of oral dose)
Doxazosin	1–16	1	65	10–12	NA
Indoramin*	50–125	2–3	NA	5	11
Prazosin	2–20	2–3	44–69	2.5–4	10
Terazosin	1–20	1	90	12	39
Trimazosin*	100–500	2–3	61	2.7	NA

* Investigational drug.
Key: NA, not available.
Source: Adapted with permission from Luther RR: New perspectives on selective α_1-blockade. *Am J Hypertens* 2:729, 1989.

5. Agents having α-adrenergic blocking properties but whose major clinical use appears unrelated to these properties (e.g., chlorpromazine, haloperidol, quinidine, bromocriptine, amiodarone, and ketanserin, a selective blocking agent of serotonin-2 receptors). It has been demonstrated that verapamil, a calcium-channel blocker, also has α-adrenergic blocking properties. Whether this is a particular property of verapamil and its analogues or is common to all calcium-channel blockers is not clear. Also to be clarified is whether verapamil-induced α blockade occurs at physiologic plasma levels and helps to mediate the vasodilator properties of the drug.

All the α blockers in clinical use inhibit the postsynaptic α_1 receptor and result in relaxation of vascular smooth muscle and vasodilation. However, the nonselective α blockers also antagonize the presynaptic α_2 receptors, allowing for increased release of neuronal norepinephrine. This results in attenuation of the desired postsynaptic blockade and spillover stimulation of the β receptors and, consequently, in troublesome side effects such as tachycardia and tremulousness and increased renin release. The α_1-selective agents that preserve the α_2-mediated presynaptic feedback loop prevent excessive norepinephrine release and thus avoid these adverse cardiac and systemic effects.

Because of these potent peripheral vasodilatory properties, one would anticipate that even the selective α_1 blockers would induce reflex stimulation of the sympathetic and renin-angiotensin system in a manner similar to that seen with other vasodilators such as hydralazine and minoxidil. The explanation for the relative lack of tachycardia and renin release observed after prazosin, terazosin, and doxazosin may be due in part to the drugs' combined action of reducing vascular tone in resistance (arteries) and capacitance (veins) beds. Such a dual action may prevent the marked increases in venous return and cardiac output observed with agents that act more selectively to reduce vascular tone only in the resistance vessels. The lack of tachycardia with prazosin, terazosin, and doxazosin use also has been attributed by some investigators to a significant negative chronotropic action of the drugs independent of their peripheral vascular effects.

Use in Cardiovascular Disorders

Hypertension

Increased peripheral vascular resistance is present in most patients with long-standing hypertension. Because dilation of constricted arterioles should result in lowering of elevated blood pressure, interest has focused on the use of α-adrenergic blockers in the medical treatment of systemic hypertension. Except for pheochromocytoma, the experience with nonselective α blockers in the treatment of hypertension was disappointing because of accompanying reflex stimulation of the sympathetic and renin-angiotensin system, resulting in frequent side effects and limited long-term antihypertensive efficacy. However, the selective α_1 blockers prazosin, doxazosin, and terazosin have been shown to be effective antihypertensive agents.

Prazosin, doxazosin, and terazosin decrease blood pressure in the standing and supine positions, although blood pressure decrements tend to be somewhat greater in the upright position. Because their antihypertensive effect is accompanied by little or no increase in heart rate, plasma renin activity, or circulating catecholamines, prazosin, doxazosin, and terazosin have been found useful as first-step agents in hypertension. Monotherapy with these agents, however, promotes sodium and water retention in some patients, although it is less pronounced than with other vasodilators. The concomitant use of a diuretic prevents fluid retention and in many cases markedly enhances the antihypertensive effect of the drugs. In clinical practice, prazosin, doxazosin, and terazosin have their widest application as adjuncts to one or more established antihypertensive drugs in treating moderate to severe hypertension. Their effects are additive to those of diuretics, beta blockers, α-methyldopa, and the direct-acting vasodilators. The drugs cause little change in glomerular filtration rate or renal plasma flow and can be used safely in patients with severe renal hypertension. There is no evidence for attenuation of the antihypertensive effect of prazosin, doxazosin, or terazosin during chronic therapy, unless sodium and water retention occurs.

In large comparative clinical trials, the efficacy and safety of α_1 blockers have been well documented. In the Treatment of Mild Hypertension Study, doxazosin, 2 mg/day given over 4 years, reduced blood pressure as much as agents from other drugs classes. In a large Veterans Administration Study in which patients with severe hypertension were studied, prazosin, 20 mg daily given over 1 year, had a treatment effect that was significantly greater than that with placebo. Doxazosin, 2 to 8 mg daily, was one of the drugs used in the Antihypertensive and Lipid Lowering Treatment to Prevent Heart Attack Trial, which was designed to compare various antihypertensive agents and their effects on coronary morbidity and mortality in high-risk antihypertensives 55 years and older. Doxazosin was withdrawn from this trial after an interim analysis showed a 25% greater rate of a secondary end point, combined cardiovascular disease, in patients on doxazosin than in those on chlorthalidone, largely driven by congestive heart failure. Based on this study, α_1 blockers should not be considered as first-line monotherapy treatment for hypertension but may be considered as part of a combination regimen to provide maximal blood pressure control.

Selective α blockers appear to have neutral or even favorable effects on plasma lipids and lipoproteins when administered to hypertensive patients. Investigators have reported mild reductions in levels of total cholesterol, low-density lipoprotein and very–low-density lipoprotein cholesterol, and triglycerides and elevations in levels of high-density lipoprotein cholesterol and insulin sensitivity with prazosin, doxazosin, and terazosin. With long-term use, selective α_1 blockers also appear to decrease left ventricular mass in patients with hypertension and left ventricular hypertrophy.

Several prazosin, doxazosin, and terazosin analogues have been developed (e.g., trimazosin) that in preliminary clinical trials have also shown promise as antihypertensive agents. Doxazosin and terazosin have a longer duration of action than does prazosin and have been shown to produce sustained blood pressure reductions with single daily administration. Prazosin, doxazosin, and terazosin are available for clinical use in the United States.

Congestive Heart Failure

α-Adrenergic blocking drugs appear particularly attractive for use in the treatment of heart failure because they hold the possibility of reproducing balanced reductions in resistance and capacitance beds. In fact, phentolamine was one of the first vasodilators shown to be effective in the treatment of heart failure. The drug was infused into normotensive patients with persistent left ventricular dysfunction after a myocardial infarction and found to induce a significant fall in systemic vascular resistance accompanied by considerable elevation in cardiac output and a reduction in pulmonary artery pressure. Because of its high cost and the frequent side effects that it produces, especially tachycardia, phentolamine is no longer used in the treatment of heart failure. Oral phenoxybenzamine also has been used as vasodilator therapy in heart failure; like phentolamine, it has been replaced by newer vasodilator agents.

Studies evaluating the acute hemodynamic effects of prazosin in patients with congestive heart failure consistently have found significant reductions in systemic and pulmonary vascular resistances and left ventricular filling pressures associated with increases in stroke volume. In most studies, there was no change or a decrease in heart rate. The response pattern seen with prazosin is similar to that observed with nitroprusside with the exception that the heart rate tends to be higher with the use of nitroprusside; therefore, the observed increases in cardiac output are also higher with nitroprusside.

Controversy still exists as to whether the initial clinical and hemodynamic improvements seen with prazosin are sustained during long-term therapy. Whereas some studies have demonstrated continued efficacy of prazosin therapy after chronic use, others have found little hemodynamic difference between prazosin- and placebo-treated patients. Some investigators believe that whatever tolerance to the drug does develop is most likely secondary to activation of countervailing neurohumoral forces; if the dose is raised and the tendency toward sodium and water retention is countered by appropriate increases in diuretic dose, prazosin is likely to remain effective. Others argue that sustained increases in plasma renin activity or plasma catecholamines are not seen during long-term therapy and that tolerance is not prevented or reversed by a diuretic. Some clinical studies have suggested that patients with initially high plasma renin activity experience attenuation of beneficial hemodynamic effects more frequently. What appears clear is the need to evaluate patients individually as to the continued efficacy of their prazosin therapy. Whether there are subgroups of patients with heart failure (e.g., those with highly activated sympathetic nervous systems) who are more likely to respond to prazosin or other α blockers remains to be determined.

A multicenter study from the Veterans Administration hospitals has shown that prazosin, when compared with placebo therapy, did not reduce mortality with long-term use in patients with advanced forms of congestive heart failure. In the same study, a favorable effect on mortality was seen with an isosorbide dinitrate–hydralazine combination.

Doxazosin and metoprolol were combined and compared with metoprolol alone in the treatment of patients with chronic heart failure. After 3 months of continuous therapy, both treatment groups showed similar and significant reductions in systemic vascular resistance and heart rate, with significant increases in cardiac index, ejection fraction, and exercise capacity. It was concluded that the combination of doxazosin and metoprolol was no better than metoprolol alone.

There is increasing evidence that α_1-adrenergic receptors, different from those of other tissues, also exist in the myocardium and that an increase in the force of contraction may be produced by stimulation of these sites. The mechanism of α-adrenergic positive inotropic response is unknown. What the biologic significance of α-adrenergic receptors in cardiac muscle is and whether these receptors play a role in the response to α-blocker therapy in congestive heart failure also remain to be determined.

Angina Pectoris

α-Adrenergic receptors help mediate coronary vasoconstriction. It has been suggested that a pathologic alteration of the α-adrenergic system may be the mechanism of coronary spasm in some patients with variant angina. In uncontrolled studies, the administration of α-adrenergic blockers, acutely and chronically, has been shown as effective in reversing and preventing coronary spasm. However, in a long-term, randomized, double-blind trial, prazosin exerted no obvious beneficial effect in patients with variant angina. The demonstration of an important role for the postsynaptic α₂ receptors in determining coronary vascular tone may help explain prazosin's lack of efficacy. Further study in this area is anticipated.

Arrhythmias

It has been postulated that enhanced α-adrenergic responsiveness occurs during myocardial ischemia and that it is a primary mediator of the electrophysiologic derangements and resulting malignant arrhythmias induced by catecholamines during myocardial ischemia and reperfusion. In humans, there have been favorable reports of the use of an α blocker in the treatment of supraventricular and ventricular ectopy. Whether there is a significant role for α-adrenergic blockers in the treatment of cardiac arrhythmias will be determined through further clinical study.

Use in Other Disorders

Pheochromocytoma

Alpha blockers have been used in the treatment of pheochromocytoma to control the peripheral effects of the excess catecholamines. In fact, intravenous phentolamine was used as a test for this disorder, but the test is now rarely done because of reported cases of cardiovascular collapse and death in patients who exhibited exaggerated sensitivity to the drug. It is still rarely used in cases of pheochromocytoma-related hypertensive crisis. However, for long-term therapy, oral phenoxybenzamine is the preferred agent. β-Blocking agents also may be needed in pheochromocytoma for control of tachycardia and arrhythmias. A β blocker of any kind, but primarily the nonselective agents, should not be initiated before adequate α blockade because severe hypertension may occur as a result of the unopposed α-stimulating activity of the circulating catecholamines.

Shock

In shock, hyperactivity of the sympathetic nervous system occurs as a compensatory reflex response to reduced blood pressure. Use of α blockers in shock has been advocated as a means of lowering peripheral vascular resistance and increasing vascular capacitance and not antagonizing the cardiotonic effects of the sympathomimetic amines. Although investigated for many years for the treatment of shock, α-adrenergic blockers are not approved for this purpose. A prime concern of the use of α blockers in shock is that the rapid drug-induced increase in vascular capacitance may lead to inadequate cardiac filling and profound hypotension, especially in the hypovolemic patient. Adequate amounts of fluid replacement before the use of an alpha blocker can minimize this possibility.

Pulmonary Hypertension

The part played by endogenous circulating catecholamines in the maintenance of pulmonary vascular tone appears to be minimal. Studies evaluating the effects of norepinephrine administration on pulmonary vascular resistance have found that the drug has little or no effect. The beneficial effects on the pulmonary circulation that phentolamine and other α blockers have demonstrated in some studies most likely is due primarily to their direct vasodilatory actions rather than to α blockade. Like other vasodilators, in patients with pulmonary hypertension due to fixed anatomic changes, α blockers can produce hemodynamic deterioration secondary to their systemic vasodilatory properties.

Bronchospasm

Bronchoconstriction is mediated in part through catecholamine stimulation of α receptors in the lung. It has been suggested that in patients with allergic asthma, a deficient β-adrenergic system or enhanced α-adrenergic responsiveness could result in α-adrenergic activity being the main mechanism of bronchoconstriction. Several studies have shown bronchodilation or inhibition of histamine and allergen- or exercise-induced bronchospasm with a variety of α blockers. Additional studies are needed to define more fully the role of α blockers for use as bronchodilators.

Arterioconstriction

Oral α-adrenergic blockers can produce subjective and clinical improvement in patients experiencing episodic arterioconstriction (Raynaud's phenomenon). α Blockers also may be of value in the treatment of severe peripheral ischemia caused by an α agonist (e.g., norepinephrine) or ergotamine overdose. In cases of inadvertent infiltration of a norepinephrine infusion, phentolamine can be given intradermally to avoid tissue sloughing.

Benign Prostatic Obstruction

α-Adrenergic receptors have been identified in the bladder neck and prostatic capsule of male patients. In clinical studies, use of α blockers in patients with benign prostatic obstruction has resulted in increased urinary flow rates and reductions in residual volume and obstructive symptoms. The drugs prazosin, terazosin, and doxazosin are approved as medical therapies for benign prostatic hypertrophy. Also available is tamsulosin, a long-acting partially selective blocker of the α_1 subtype that mediates prostatic smooth muscle tone and appears to be as effective as other α_1 blockers in the treatment of prostatism, but with little effect on blood pressure.

Clinical Use and Adverse Effects

Oral phenoxybenzamine has a rapid onset of action, with the maximal effect from a single dose seen in 1 to 2 h. The gastrointestinal absorption is incomplete, and only 20% to 30% of an oral dose reaches the systemic circulation in active form. The half-life of the drug is 24 h, with the usual dose varying between 20 and 200 mg daily in one or two doses. Intravenous phentolamine is initially started at 0.1 mg/min and is then increased at increments of 0.1 mg/min every 5 to 10 min until the desired hemodynamic effect is reached. The drug has a short duration of action of 3 to 10 min. Little is known about the pharmacokinetics of oral phentolamine used long-term. The main side effects of the drug include postural hypotension, tachycardia, gastrointestinal disturbances, and sexual dysfunction. Intravenous infusion of norepinephrine can be used to combat severe hypotensive reactions. Oral phenoxybenzamine is approved for use in pheochromocytoma.

Prazosin is almost completely absorbed after oral administration, with peak plasma levels achieved at 2 to 3 h. The drug is 90% protein bound. Prazosin is extensively metabolized by the liver. The usual half-life of the drug is 2 h to 4 h; in patients with heart failure, the half-life increases to the range of 5 to 7 h.

The major side effect of prazosin is the first-dose phenomenon—severe postural hypotension occasionally associated with syncope seen after the initial dose or after a rapid dose increment. The reason for this phenomenon has not been clearly established but may involve the rapid induction of venous and arteriolar dilatation by a drug that elicits little reflex sympathetic stimulation. It is reported more often when the drug is administered as a tablet rather than as a capsule, possibly related to the variable bioavailability or rates of absorption of the two formulations. (In the United States, the drug is available in capsule form.) The postural hypotension can be minimized if the initial dose of prazosin is not higher than 1 mg and if it is given at bedtime. In treating hypertension, a dose of 2 to 3 mg/day should be maintained for 1 to 2 weeks, followed by a gradual increase in dosage titrated to achieve the desired reductions in pressures, usually up to 20 to 30 mg/day, given in two or three doses. In treating heart failure, larger doses (2 to 7 mg) may be used to initiate therapy in recumbent patients, but the maintenance dose is also usually not higher than 30 mg. Higher doses do not seem to produce additional clinical benefit.

Other side effects of prazosin include dizziness, headache, and drowsiness. The drug produces no deleterious effects on the clinical course of diabetes mellitus, chronic obstructive pulmonary disease, renal failure, or gout. It does not adversely affect the lipid profile.

Terazosin, which has been approved for once-daily use in hypertension, may be associated with a lesser incidence of first-dose postural hypotension than prazosin. The usual recommended dose range is 1 to 5 mg administered once a day; some patients may benefit from doses as high as 20 mg daily or from split dosing.

Doxazosin is also approved as a once-daily therapy for systemic hypertension. The initial dosage of doxazosin is 2 mg once daily. Depending on the patient's standing blood pressure response, the dosage may then be increased to 4 mg and, if necessary, to 8 or 16 mg to achieve the desired reduction in blood pressure. Doses beyond 4 mg increase the likelihood of excessive postural effects, including syncope, postural dizziness or vertigo, and postural hypotension.

The α_2 blocker yohimbine, 5.4 mg orally, is used four times daily to treat male impotence. Urologists have used yohimbine for the diagnostic classification of certain cases of male erectile dysfunction. Increases in heart rate and blood pressure, piloerection, and rhinorrhea are the most common adverse reactions. Yohimbine should not be used with antidepressant drugs.

β-ADRENERGIC BLOCKING DRUGS

β-Adrenergic blocking drugs, which constitute a major pharmacotherapeutic advance, were conceived initially for the treatment of patients with angina pectoris and arrhythmias; however, they also have therapeutic effects in many other clinical disorders including systemic hypertension, hypertrophic cardiomyopathy, mitral valve prolapse, silent myocardial ischemia, migraine, glaucoma, essential tremor, and thyrotoxicosis. β Blockers have been effective in treating unstable angina and for reducing the risk of cardiovascular mortality and nonfatal reinfarction in patients who have survived an acute myocardial infarction. β Blockade is a potential treatment modality, with or without thrombolytic therapy, for reducing the extent of myocardial injury and mortality during the hyperacute phase of myocardial infarction.

Recently, various β blockers have been approved for use in patients with New York Heart Association class II to IV heart failure who are receiving angiotensin-converting enzyme (ACE) inhibitors, diuretics, and digoxin to reduce the progression of disease and mortality.

β-Adrenergic Receptor

Radioligand labeling techniques have greatly aided the investigation of adrenoreceptors, and molecular pharmacologic techniques have positively delineated the β-adrenoceptor structure as a polypeptide with a molecular weight of 67,000 kDa.

In contrast to the older concept of adrenoreceptors as static entities in cells that simply serve to initiate the chain of events, newer theories hold that the adrenoceptors are subject to a wide variety of controlling influences resulting in dynamic regulation of adrenoceptor sites and/or their sensitivity to catecholamines. Changes in tissue concentration of receptor sites likely are involved in mediating important fluctuations in tissue sensitivity to drug action. These principles may have significant clinical and therapeutic implications. For example, an apparent increase in the number of β adrenoceptors, and thus a supersensitivity to agonists, may be induced by chronic exposure to antagonists. With prolonged adrenoceptor-blocker therapy, receptor occupancy by catecholamines can be diminished and the number of available receptors can be increased. When the β-adrenoceptor blocker is withdrawn suddenly, an increased pool of sensitive receptors will be open to endogenous catecholamine stimulation. The resultant adrenergic stimulation could precipitate unstable angina pectoris and/or a myocardial infarction. The concentration of β adrenoceptors in the membrane of mononuclear cells decreases significantly with age.

Using radioligand techniques, a decrease in β-adrenoceptor sites in the myocardium has been demonstrated in patients with chronic congestive heart failure. An apparent reduction in β adrenoceptors and/or β-adrenoceptor function also has been associated with the development of refractoriness or desensitization to endogenous and exogenous catecholamines, a phenomenon likely caused by the prolonged exposure of these adrenoceptors to high levels of catecholamines. This desensitization phenomenon is caused not by a change in receptor formation or degradation but rather by catecholamine-induced changes in the conformation of the receptor sites, thus rendering them ineffective. More recently, it has been determined that one of the most important mechanisms for explaining the rapid regulation of β-adrenergic receptor function is agonist stimulation of receptor phosphorylation, which leads to decreased sensitivity to further catecholamine stimulation. When the receptors are phosphorylated by protein kinases, the end result is a decreased coupling to Gs and decreased stimulation of adenyl cyclase. A receptor-directed protein kinase, β-adrenergic receptor kinase, phosphorylates the receptors only when they are occupied by an agonist. It was subsequently discovered that β-adrenergic receptor kinase is a member of at least six protein-regulated receptor kinases that can phosphorylate and regulate a wide variety of G-protein–coupled receptors. Phosphorylation of the receptor is not sufficient to fully desensitize receptor function. A second reaction must occur, which involves an "arresting protein" known as arrestin. Agonists also produce reversible sequestration (internalization) of receptors. β-Adrenoceptor blocking drugs do not induce desensitization or changes in the conformation of receptors but do block the ability of catecholamines to desensitize receptors.

Basic Pharmacologic Differences among β-Adrenoceptor Blocking Drugs

More than 100 β-adrenoceptor blockers have been synthesized during the past 35 years, and more than 30 are available worldwide for clinical use. Selectivity for two subgroups of the β-adrenoceptor population also has been exploited: β_1 receptors in the heart and β_2 receptors in the peripheral circulation and bronchi. More controversial has been the introduction of β-blocking drugs with α-adrenergic blocking actions, different amounts of selective and nonselective intrinsic sympathomimetic activity (partial agonist activity), calcium-channel blocker activity, antioxidant actions, effects on nitric oxide production, and nonspecific membrane stabilizing effects. There are also pharmacokinetic differences between β-blocking drugs that may be of clinical importance.

Sixteen β-adrenoceptor blockers are now marketed in the United States for cardiovascular disorders: propranolol for angina pectoris, arrhythmias, systemic hypertension, migraine prophylaxis, essential tremor, and hypertrophic cardiomyopathy and for reducing the risk of cardiovascular mortality in survivors of an acute myocardial infarction; nadolol for hypertension and angina pectoris; timolol for hypertension and for reducing the risk of cardiovascular mortality and nonfatal reinfarction in survivors of myocardial infarction and in topical form for glaucoma; atenolol for hypertension and angina and in intravenous and oral formulations for reducing the risk of cardiovascular mortality in survivors of myocardial infarction; metoprolol for hypertension, angina pectoris, moderate congestive heart failure, and in intravenous and oral formulations for reducing the risk of cardiovascular mortality in survivors of acute myocardial infarction; penbutolol, bisoprolol, and pindolol for treating hypertension; betaxolol and carteolol for hypertension and in a topical form for glaucoma; acebutolol for hypertension and ventricular arrhythmias; intravenous esmolol for supraventricular arrhythmias; sotalol for ventricular and atrial arrhythmias; labetalol for hypertension and in intravenous form for hypertensive emergencies; and carvedilol for hypertension and moderate to severe congestive heart failure. In addition, oxprenolol has been approved for use in hypertension but has never been marketed in the United States. Currently under investigation are two ultra–short-acting β blockers for use in patients with arrhythmia, landiolol and ONO-1011, and nebivolol for hypertension.

Despite the extensive experience with β blockers in clinical practice, there have been no studies suggesting that any of these agents has major advantages or disadvantages in relation to the others for treatment of many cardiovascular diseases. When any available blocker is titrated properly, it can be effective in patients with arrhythmia, hypertension, or angina pectoris. However, one agent may be more effective than other agents in reducing adverse reactions in some patients and for managing specific situations.

Potency

β-Adrenergic receptor blocking drugs are competitive inhibitors of catecholamine binding at β-adrenergic-receptor sites. The dose–response curve of the catecholamine is shifted to the right; that is, a given tissue response requires a higher concentration of agonist in the presence of β-blocking drugs. β_1-Blocking potency can be assessed by the inhibition of tachycardia produced by isoproterenol or exercise (the more reliable method in the intact organism); the potency varies from compound to compound (Table 2-3). These differences in potency are of no therapeutic relevance, but they do explain the different drug doses needed to achieve effective β-adrenergic blockade in initiating therapy in patients or in switching from one agent to another.

Structure–Activity Relations

The chemical structures of most β-adrenergic blockers have several features in common with the agonist isoproterenol, an aromatic ring with a substituted ethanolamine side chain linked to it by an $-OCH_2$ group. The β blocker timolol has a catecholamine-mimicking side chain but a more complex ring structure.

TABLE 2-3 Pharmacodynamic Properties of β-Adrenergic Blocking Drugs

	β_1 blockade potency ratio (propranolol =1.0)	Relative β_1 selectivity	Intrinsic sympathomimetic activity	Membrane-stabilizing activity
Acebutolol	0.3	+	+	+
Atenolol	1.0	++	0	0
Betaxolol	1.0	++	0	+
Bisoprolol*	10.0	++	0	0
Carteolol	10.0	0	+	0
Carvedilol†	10.0	0	0	++
Esmolol	0.02	++	0	0
Labetalol‡	0.3	0	+	0
Metoprolol	1.0	++	0	0
Nadolol	1.0	0	0	0
Nebivolol#	10.0	++	0	0
Oxprenolol	0.5–1.0	0	+	+
Penbutolol	1.0	0	+	0
Pindolol	6.0	0	++	+
Propranolol	1.0	0	0	++
Sotalol§	0.3	0	0	0
Timolol	6.0	0	0	0
Isomer-D-propranolol	—	—	—	++

* Bisoprolol is also approved as a first-line antihypertensive therapy in combination with a very low-dose diuretic.
† Carvedilol has peripheral vasodilating activity and additional α_1-adrenergic blocking activity.
‡ Labetalol has additional α_1-adrenergic blocking activity and direct vasodilatory activity.
# Nebivolol can augment vascular nitric oxide release.
§ Sotalol has an additional type of antiarrhythmic activity.
Key: ++, strong effect; +, modest effect; 0, absent effect.
Source: Adapted with permission from Frishman WH: *Clinical Pharmacology of the β-Adrenoceptor Blocking Drugs,* 2nd ed. Norwalk, Appleton-Century-Crofts, 1984.

Most β-blocking drugs exist as pairs of optical isomers and are marketed as racemic mixtures. Almost all the β-blocking activity is found in the negative (−) levorotatory stereoisomer. The two stereoisomers of β-adrenergic blockers are useful for differentiating between the pharmacologic effects of β blockade and membrane-stabilizing activity (possessed by both optical forms). The positive (+) dextrorotatory stereoisomers of β-blocking agents have no apparent clinical value except for D-nebivolol, which has β-blocking activity, and D-sotalol, which appears to have type III antiarrhythmic properties. Penbutolol and timolol are marketed only in the L form. As a result of asymmetric carbon atoms, labetalol and nebivolol have four stereoisomers and carvedilol has two. With carvedilol, β-blocking effects are seen in the (−) levorotatory stereoisomer and α-blocking effects in both the (−) levorotatory and (+) dextrorotatory stereoisomers.

Membrane-Stabilizing Activity

At concentrations well above therapeutic levels, certain β blockers have a quinidine-like or local anesthetic membrane-stabilizing effect on the cardiac action potential. This property is exhibited equally by the two stereoisomers of the drug and is unrelated to β-adrenergic blockade and major therapeutic antiarrhythmic actions. There is no evidence that membrane-stabilizing activity is responsible for any direct negative inotropic effect of the β blockers because drugs with and without this property equally depress left ventricular function. However, membrane-stabilizing activity can manifest itself clinically with massive β-blocker intoxications.

β_1 Selectivity

β-Adrenoceptor blockers may be classified as selective or nonselective according to their relative abilities to antagonize the actions of sympathomimetic amines in some tissues at lower doses than those required in other tissues. When used in low doses, β_1-selective blocking agents such as acebutolol, betaxolol, bisoprolol, esmolol, atenolol, and metoprolol inhibit cardiac β_2 receptors but have less influence on bronchial and vascular β adrenoceptors (β_2). In higher doses, however, β_1-selective blocking agents also block β_2 receptors. Accordingly, β_1-selective agents may be safer than nonselective ones in patients with obstructive pulmonary disease, because β_2 receptors remain available to mediate adrenergic bronchodilatation. Even selective β blockers may aggravate bronchospasm in certain patients, so these drugs generally should not be used in patients with bronchospastic disease.

A second theoretical advantage is that, unlike nonselective β blockers, β_1-selective blockers in low doses may not block the β_2 receptors that mediate dilatation of arterioles. During infusion of epinephrine, nonselective β blockers can cause a pressor response by blocking β_2-receptor–mediated vasodilatation because α-adrenergic vasoconstrictor receptors are still operative. Selective β_1 antagonists may not induce this pressor effect in the presence of epinephrine and may lessen the impairment of peripheral blood flow. Leaving the β_2 receptors unblocked and responsive to epinephrine may be functionally important in some patients with asthma, hypoglycemia, hypertension, or peripheral vascular disease treated with β-adrenergic blocking drugs.

Intrinsic Sympathomimetic Activity (Partial Agonist Activity)

Certain β-adrenoceptor blockers possess intrinsic sympathomimetic activity (partial agonist activity) at β_1-adrenoceptor receptors sites, β_2-adrenoceptor receptors sites, or both. In a β blocker, this property is identified as a slight cardiac stimulation that can be blocked by propranolol. The β blockers with this property slightly activate the β receptor in addition to preventing the access of natural or synthetic catecholamines to the receptor. Dichloroisoprenaline, the first β-adrenoceptor blocking drug synthesized, exerted such marked partial agonist activity that it was unsuitable for clinical use. However, compounds with less partial agonist activity are effective β-blocking drugs. The partial agonist effects of β-adrenoceptor blocking drugs such as pindolol differ from those of the agonist epinephrine and isoproterenol in that the maximum pharmacologic response that can be obtained is low, although the affinity for the receptor is high. In the treatment of patients with arrhythmias, angina pectoris of effort, and hypertension, drugs with mild to moderate partial agonist activity appear to be as efficacious as β blockers lacking this property. It is still debated whether the presence of partial agonist activity in a β blocker constitutes an overall advantage or disadvantage in cardiac therapy. Drugs with partial agonist activity cause less slowing of the heart rate at rest than do propranolol and metoprolol, although the increments in heart rate with exercise are similarly blunted. These β-blocking agents reduce peripheral vascular resistance and also may cause less depression of atrioventricular conduction than drugs lacking these properties. Some investigators claim that partial agonist activity in a β blocker protects against myocardial depression, adverse lipid changes, bronchial asthma, and peripheral vascular complications, as caused by propranolol. The evidence to support these claims is not conclusive, and more definitive clinical trials are necessary to resolve these issues.

α-Adrenergic Activity

Labetalol is a β blocker with antagonistic properties at α and β adrenoceptors, and it has direct vasodilator activity. Labetalol has been shown to be 6 to 10 times less potent than phentolamine at α-adrenergic receptors and 1.5 to 4 times less potent than propranolol at β-adrenergic receptors; it is itself 4 to 16 times less potent at α than at β adrenoceptors. Like other β blockers, it is useful in the treatment of hypertension and angina pectoris. Unlike most β blockers, the additional α-adrenergic blocking actions of labetalol lead to a reduction in peripheral vascular resistance that may maintain cardiac output. Whether concomitant α-adrenergic blocking activity is actually advantageous in a β blocker remains to be determined.

Carvedilol is another β blocker having additional α-blocking activity. Compared with labetalol, carvedilol has a ratio of α_1 to β blockade of 1:10. On a milligram-to-milligram basis, carvedilol is about two to four times more potent than propranolol as a β blocker. In addition, carvedilol has antioxidant and antiproliferative activities. Carvedilol has been used for the treatment of hypertension and angina pectoris and has been shown to be effective as a treatment for patients having symptomatic heart failure.

Direct Vasodilator Activity

Bucindolol is a nonselective β blocker that also has direct peripheral vasodilatory activity. It has undergone clinical evaluation as a treatment for symptomatic congestive heart failure and provides less benefit than other β blockers approved for this indication.

Nebivolol is a β_1-selective adrenergic receptor antagonist with a unique ability to increase vascular nitric oxide production, and the drug is currently being evaluated as a treatment for hypertension.

Pharmacokinetics

Although the β-adrenergic blocking drugs as a group have similar therapeutic effects, their pharmacokinetic properties are markedly different. Their varied aromatic ring structures lead to differences in completeness of gastrointestinal absorption, amount of first-pass hepatic metabolism, lipid solubility, protein binding, extent of distribution in the body, penetration into the brain, concentration in the heart, rate of hepatic biotransformation, pharmacologic activity of metabolites, and renal clearance of a drug and its metabolites, which may influence the clinical usefulness of these drugs in some patients. The desirable pharmacokinetic characteristics in this group of compounds are a lack of major interindividual differences in bioavailability and in metabolic clearance of the drug and a rate of removal from active tissue sites that is slow enough to allow longer dosing intervals.

The β blockers can be divided by their pharmacokinetic properties into two broad categories: those eliminated by hepatic metabolism, which tend to have relatively short plasma half-lives, and those eliminated unchanged by the kidney, which tend to have longer half-lives. Propranolol and metoprolol are lipid soluble, are almost completely absorbed by the small intestine, and are largely metabolized by the liver. They tend to have highly variable bioavailability and relatively short plasma half-lives. A lack of correlation between the duration of clinical pharmacologic effect and plasma half-life may allow these drugs to be administered once or twice daily.

In contrast, agents such as atenolol and nadolol are more water soluble, are incompletely absorbed through the gut, and are eliminated unchanged by the kidney. In addition to longer half-lives, they tend to have less variable bioavailability in patients with normal renal function, thereby allowing one dose a day. The longer half-lives may be useful in patients who find compliance with frequent β-blocker dosing a problem.

Long-acting sustained-release preparations of propranolol and metoprolol are available. A delayed-release long-acting chronotherapeutic propranolol formulation has been approved for clinical use. Studies have shown that long-acting propranolol and metoprolol can provide a much smoother curve of daily plasma levels than can comparable divided doses of conventional immediate-release formulations.

Ultra–short-acting β blockers are now available and may be useful when a short duration of action is desired (e.g., in patients with questionable congestive heart failure). One of these compounds, esmolol, a β_1-selective drug (see Table 2-3), has been shown to be useful in the treatment of perioperative hypertension and supraventricular tachycardias. The short half-life (approximately 15 min) relates to the rapid metabolism of the drug by blood and hepatic esterases. Metabolism does not seem to be altered by disease states. A propranolol nasal spray that can provide immediate β blockade has been tested in clinical trials, as has a new sublingual immediate-release formulation (esprolol).

The specific pharmacokinetic properties of individual β-adrenergic blockers (first-pass metabolism, active metabolites, lipid solubility, and protein binding) may be clinically important. When drugs with extensive first-pass metabolism are taken by mouth, they undergo so much hepatic biotransformation that relatively little drug reaches the systemic circulation. Depending on the extent of first-pass effect, an oral dose of β blocker must be larger than an intravenous dose to produce the same clinical effects. Some β-adrenergic blockers are transformed into pharmacologically active compounds (acebutolol, nebivolol) rather than into inactive metabolites. The total pharmacologic effect therefore depends on the amount of the drug administered and its active metabolites. Characteristics of lipid solubility in a β blocker have been associated with the ability of the drug to concentrate in the brain, and many side effects of these drugs, which have not been clearly related to β blockade, may result from their actions on the central nervous system (CNS; lethargy, mental depression, and hallucinations). It is still not certain whether drugs that are less lipid soluble cause fewer of these adverse reactions.

There are genetic polymorphisms that can influence the metabolism of various β-blocking drugs, which include propranolol, metoprolol, timolol, and carvedilol. A single codon difference of CYP2D6 may explain a significant proportion of interindividual variation of propranolol's pharmacokinetics in Chinese subjects. There is no effect of exercise on propranolol's pharmacokinetics.

Relations between Dose, Plasma Level, and Efficacy

Attempts have been made to establish a relation between the oral dose, the plasma level measured by gas chromatography, and the pharmacologic effect of each β-blocking drug. After administration of a certain oral dose, β-blocking drugs that are largely metabolized in the liver show large interindividual variation in circulating plasma levels. Many explanations have been proposed to explain wide individual differences in the relation between plasma concentrations of β blockers and any associated therapeutic effect. First, patients may have different levels of "sympathetic tone" (circulating catecholamines and active β-adrenoceptor binding sites) and thus may require different drug concentrations to achieve adequate β blockade. Second, many β blockers have flat plasma–drug level response curves. Third, active drug isomers and active metabolites are not specifically measured in many plasma assays. Fourth, the clinical effect of a drug may last longer than the period suggested by the drug's half-life in plasma because recycling of the β blocker between the receptor site and neuronal nerve endings may occur. Despite the lack of correlation between plasma levels and therapeutic effect, there is some evidence that a relation does exist between the logarithm of the plasma level and the β-blocking effect (blockade of exercise- or isoproterenol-induced tachycardia). Plasma levels have little to offer as therapeutic guides except for ensuring compliance and diagnosis of overdose. Pharmacodynamic characteristics and clinical response should be used as guides in determining efficacy.

Clinical Effects and Therapeutic Applications

The therapeutic efficacy and safety of β-adrenoceptor blocking drugs has been well established in patients with angina pectoris, cardiac arrhythmias, congestive cardiomyopathy, and hypertension and for reducing the risk of mortality and possibly nonfatal reinfarction in survivors of acute myocardial infarction. These drugs may be useful as a primary protection against cardio-

TABLE 2-4 Reported Cardiovascular Indications for β-Adrenoceptor Blocking Drugs

Hypertension* (systolic and diastolic)
Isolated systolic hypertension in the elderly
Angina pectoris*
"Silent" myocardial ischemia
Supraventricular arrhythmias*
Ventricular arrhythmias*
Reducing the risk of mortality and reinfarction in survivors of acute myocardial infarction*
Reducing the risk of mortality after percutaneous coronary* revascularization
Hyperacute phase of myocardial infarction*
Dissection of aorta
Hypertrophic cardiomyopathy*
Reversing left ventricular hypertrophy
Digitalis intoxication (tachyarrhythmias)*
Mitral valve prolapse
QT interval–prolongation syndrome
Tetralogy of Fallot
Mitral stenosis
Congestive cardiomyopathy*
Fetal tachycardia
Neurocirculatory asthenia

* Indications formally approved by the US Food and Drug Adminiatration.

vascular morbidity and mortality in hypertensive patients. The drugs are also used for a multitude of other cardiac (Table 2-4) and noncardiac uses.

Cardiovascular Effects

Effects on elevated systemic blood pressure β-Adrenergic blockers are effective in reducing the blood pressure of many patients with systemic hypertension (Tables 2-5 and 2-6), including elderly patients with isolated systolic hypertension, and have been cited as a first-line treatment by the Seventh Report of the Joint National Committee on Prevention, Detection, Evaluation and Treatment of High Blood Pressure. However, a recent meta-analysis showed that the beneficial effects on clinical outcomes with diuretic treatment used as monotherapy in the elderly were more favorable than those observed with β blockers.

TABLE 2-5 Proposed Mechanisms to Explain the Antihypertensive Actions of β-Blockers

Reduction in cardiac output
Inhibition of renin
Central nervous system effects
Effects on prejunctional β receptors: reductions in norepinephrine release
Reduction in peripheral vascular resistance
Improvement in vascular compliance
Reduction in vasomotor tone
Reduction in plasma volume
Resetting of baroreceptor levels
Attenuation of pressor response to catecholamines with exercise and stress

Source: Reproduced with permission from Frishman WH: β-Adrenergic blockers. *Med Clin North Am* 72:37, 1988.

TABLE 2-6 Pharmacodynamic Properties and Cardiac Effects of β-Adrenoceptor Blockers

	Relative β₁ selectivity	ISA	MSA	HR rest/exer	MC rest	BP rest/exer	AV conduction rest	Antiarrhythmic effect
Acebutolol	+	+	+	↔↓/↓	→	↓/↓	→	+
Atenolol	++	0	0	↓/↓	→	↓/↓	→	+
Betaxolol	++	0	+	↓/↓	→	↓/↓	→	+
Bisoprolol	++	0	0	↓/↓	→	↓/↓	→	+
Carteolol	0	+	0	↔↓/↓	↓↔	→	↓↔	+
Carvedilol†	0	0	++	↓/↓	↔→/	↓/↓	→	+
Esmolol	++	0	0	↔↓/↓	→	↓/↓	↓↔	+
Labetalol‡	+	0	0	↓/↓	↓↔	↓/↓↓	→	+
Metoprolol	++	0	0	↔↓/↓	→	↓/↓	→	+
Nadolol	0	0	0	↓/↓	→	↓/↓	↓↔	+
Nebivolol#	++	0	0	↔↓/↓	↓↔	↓/↓	↓↔	+
Oxprenolol	0	+	+	↔↓/↓	↓↔	↓/↓	↓↔	+
Penbutolol	0	+	0	↔↓/↓	↔↔	↓/↓	↓↔	+
Pindolol	0	++	+	↓/↓	→	↓/↓	→	+
Propranolol	0	0	++	↓/↓	→	↓/↓	→	+
Sotalol	0	0	0	↓/↓	→	↓/↓	→	+
Timolol	0	0	0	↓/↓	→	↓/↓	→	+
Isomer-D-propranolol	0	0	++	↔/↔	↔↓§	↔/↔	↔↓§	+§

*β₁ selectivity is seen only with low therapeutic drug concentrations. With higher concentrations, β₁ selectivity is not seen.
† Carvedilol has peripheral vasodilating activity and additional α₁-adrenergic blocking activity.
‡ Labetalol has additional α₁-adrenergic blocking activity and direct β₂ vasodilatory activity.
# Nebivolol can augment vascular nitric oxide release.
§ Effects of D-propranolol with doses in human beings are well above the therapeutic level. The isomer also lacks β-blocking activity.
Key: AV, atrioventricular; BP, blood pressure; HR, heart rate; ISA, intrinsic sympathomimetic activity; MC, myocardial contractility; MSA, membrane stabilizing activity; rest/exer, resting and exercise; +, modest effect; ++, strong effect; 0, absent effect; ↑, elevation; ↓, reduction; ↔, no change.

Most recently, it was shown that losartan has a more favorable effect than atenolol on cardiovascular morbidity and mortality and a similar reduction in blood pressure in hypertensive patients with left ventricular hypertrophy. A prospective cohort study associated antihypertensive therapy with β blockers with a greater incidence of type II diabetes than treatment with ACE inhibitors, diuretics, and calcium blockers. However, this increased risk of diabetes must be weighed against the proven benefit of β blockers in reducing the risk of cardiovascular events.

There is no consensus as to the mechanism(s) by which these drugs lower blood pressure. It is probable that some or all of the following proposed mechanisms play a part. β Blockers without vasodilatory activity appear to be more efficacious in white patients and younger patients than in elderly and/or black patients.

Negative chronotropic and inotropic effects Slowing of the heart rate and some decrease in myocardial contractility with β blockers lead to a decrease in cardiac output, which in the short and long terms, may lead to a reduction in blood pressure. These factors might be of particular importance in the treatment of hypertension related to high cardiac output and increased sympathetic tone.

Differences in effects on plasma renin The relation between the hypotensive action of β-blocking drugs and their ability to reduce plasma renin activity remains controversial. Some β-blocking drugs can antagonize sympathetically mediated renin release, although adrenergic activity is not the only mechanism by which renin release is mediated. Other major determinants are sodium balance, posture, and renal perfusion pressure.

The important question remains: Is there a clinical correlation between the β blocker's effect on the plasma renin activity and the lowering of blood pressure? Investigators have found that "high renin" patients do not respond or may even show a rise in blood pressure, and that "normal renin" patients have less predictable responses. In high-renin hypertensive patients, it has been suggested that renin may not be the only factor maintaining the high blood pressure state. At present, the exact role of renin reduction in blood pressure control is not well defined.

Central nervous system effect There is now good clinical and experimental evidence to suggest that β blockers cross the blood–brain barrier and enter the CNS. Although there is little doubt that β blockers with high lipophilicity (e.g., metoprolol, propranolol) enter the CNS in high concentrations, a direct antihypertensive effect mediated by their presence has not been well defined. Also, β blockers that are less lipid soluble and less likely to concentrate in the brain appear to be as effective in lowering blood pressure as propranolol.

Peripheral resistance Nonselective β blockers have no primary action in lowering peripheral resistance and indeed may cause it to rise by leaving the α-stimulatory mechanisms unopposed. The vasodilating effect of catecholamines on skeletal muscle blood vessels is β_2 mediated, suggesting possible therapeutic advantages in using β_1-selective blockers, agents with partial agonist activity, and drugs with α-blocking activity. Because β_1 selectivity diminishes as the drug dosage is raised and because hypertensive patients generally have to be given far larger doses than are required simply to block the β_1 receptors alone, β_1 selectivity offers the clinician little, if any, real specific advantage in the treatment of hypertension.

Effects on prejunctional receptors Apart from their effects on postjunctional tissue β receptors, it is believed that blockade of prejunctional β receptors may be involved in the hemodynamic actions of β-blocking drugs. The stimulation of prejunctional α_2 receptors leads to a reduction in the quantity of norepinephrine released by the postganglionic sympathetic fibers. Conversely, stimulation of prejunctional β receptors is followed by an increase in the quantity of norepinephrine released by the postganglionic sympathetic fibers. Blockade of prejunctional β receptors therefore should diminish the amount of norepinephrine released, leading to a weaker stimulation of postjunctional α receptors—an effect that would produce less vasoconstriction. Opinions differ on the contributions of presynaptic β blockade to a reduction in the peripheral vascular resistance and the antihypertensive effects on β-blocking drugs.

Other proposed mechanisms Less well-documented effects of β blockers that may contribute to their antihypertensive actions include favorable effects on arterial compliance, venous tone and plasma volume, membrane-stabilizing activity, and resetting of the baroreceptors.

Genetic polymorphisms of the β_1 and β_2 receptors and other genetic markers have been implicated as a cause for systemic hypertension and the responsiveness of patients to treatment with β blockers.

Effects in Angina Pectoris

Ahlquist demonstrated that sympathetic innervation of the heart causes the release of norepinephrine by activating β adrenoreceptors in myocardial cells (see Table 2-6). This adrenergic stimulation causes an increment in heart rate, isometric contractile force, and maximal velocity of muscle fiber shortening, all of which lead to an increase in cardiac work and myocardial oxygen consumption. In contrast, the decrease in intraventricular pressure and volume caused by the sympathetic-mediated enhancement of cardiac contractility tends to reduce myocardial oxygen consumption by reducing myocardial wall tension (Laplace's law). Although there is a net increase in myocardial oxygen demand, this is normally balanced by an increase in coronary blood flow. Angina pectoris is believed to occur when oxygen demand exceeds supply, i.e., when coronary blood flow is restricted by coronary atherosclerosis. Because the conditions that precipitate anginal attacks (exercise, emotional stress, food, etc.) cause an increase in cardiac sympathetic activity, it might be expected that blockade of cardiac β adrenoreceptors would relieve the anginal symptoms. It is on this basis that the early clinical studies with β-blocking drugs in patients with angina pectoris were initiated.

Three main factors—heart rate, ventricular systolic pressure, and the size of the left ventricle—contribute to the myocardial oxygen requirements of the left ventricle. Of these, heart rate and systolic pressure appear to be important (the product of heart rate multiplied by the systolic blood pressure is a reliable index to predict the precipitation of angina in a given patient). However, myocardial contractility may be even more important.

The reduction in heart rate effected by β blockade has two favorable consequences: (1) a decrease in blood pressure, thus reducing myocardial oxygen needs, and (2) a longer diastolic filling time associated with a slower heart rate, allowing for increased coronary perfusion. β Blockade also reduces exercise-induced blood pressure increments, the velocity of cardiac contraction, and oxygen consumption at any patient workload. Pretreatment heart rate variability or low exercise tolerance may predict which patients will respond best to treatment with β blockade. Despite the favorable effects on heart rate, the blunting of myocardial contractility with β blockers may also be the primary mechanism of their antianginal benefit.

Studies in dogs have shown that propranolol causes a decrease in coronary blood flow. However, subsequent experimental animal studies have demonstrated that β-blocking–induced shunting occurs in the coronary circulation, thus maintaining blood flow to ischemic areas, especially in the subendocardial region. In human beings, concomitantly with the decrease in myocardial oxygen consumption, β blockers can cause a reduction in coronary blood flow and a rise in coronary vascular resistance. On the basis of coronary autoregulation, the overall reduction in myocardial oxygen needs with β blockers may be sufficient cause for this decrease in coronary blood flow.

Virtually all β blockers—whether or not they have partial agonist activity, α-blocking effects, membrane-stabilizing activity, and general or selective beta-blocking properties—produce some degree of increased work capacity without pain in patients with angina pectoris. Therefore, it must be concluded that this results from their common property: blockade of cardiac β receptors. D- and L-propranolol have membrane-stabilizing activity, but only L-propranolol has significant β-blocking activity. The racemic mixture (D- and L-propranolol) causes a decrease in heart rate and force of contraction in dogs, whereas the D-isomer has hardly any effect. In human beings, D-propranolol, which has "membrane" activity but no β-blocking properties, has been found to be ineffective in relieving angina pectoris even at very high doses.

β Blockers are recommended as the initial therapy for long-term management of angina pectoris.

Although exercise tolerance improves with β blockade, the increments in heart rate and blood pressure with exercise are blunted, and the rate–pressure product (systolic blood pressure × heart rate) achieved when pain occurs is lower than that reached during a control run. The depressed pressure–rate product at the onset of pain (about 20% reduction from control) is reported to occur with various β-blocking drugs, likely related to decreased cardiac output. Thus, although there is increased exercise tolerance with beta blockade, patients exercise less than might be expected. This increased tolerance also may relate to the action of β blockers in increasing left ventricular size, thus causing increased left ventricular wall tension and increased oxygen consumption at a given blood pressure.

Combined Use of Beta Blockers with Other Antianginal Therapies in Angina Pectoris

Nitrates Combined therapy with nitrates and β blockers may be more efficacious for the treatment of angina pectoris than the use of either drug alone. The primary effects of β blockers are to cause a reduction in resting heart rate and the response of heart rate to exercise. Because nitrates produce a reflex increase in heart rate and contractility owing to a reduction in arterial pressure, concomitant β-blocker therapy is extremely effective because it blocks this reflex increment in the heart rate. Similarly, the preservation of diastolic coronary flow with a reduced heart rate will be beneficial. In patients with a propensity for myocardial failure who may have a slight increase in heart size with the β blockers, the nitrates will counteract this tendency by reducing heart size as a result of its peripheral venodilator effects. During the administration of nitrates, the reflex increase in contractility that is mediated through the sympathetic nervous system will be checked by the presence of β blockers. Similarly, the increase in coronary resistance associated with β-blocker administration can be ameliorated by the administration of nitrates.

Calcium-entry blockers Calcium-entry blockers are a group of drugs that block transmembrane calcium currents in vascular smooth muscle to cause arterial vasodilatation (see Chap. 4). Some calcium-entry blockers (diltiazem, mibefradil, and verapamil) also slow the heart rate and reduce atrioventricular (AV) conduction. Combined therapy with β-adrenergic and calcium-entry blockers can provide clinical benefits for patients with angina pectoris who remain symptomatic with either agent used alone. Because adverse cardiovascular effects can occur, patients being considered for such treatment must be carefully selected and observed.

Angina at Rest and Vasospastic Angina

Angina pectoris can be caused by multiple mechanisms, including coronary vasospasm, myocardial bridging, and thrombosis, which appear to be responsible for ischemia in a significant proportion of patients with unstable angina and angina at rest. Therefore, β blockers that primarily reduce myocardial oxygen consumption but fail to exert vasodilating effects on coronary vasculature may not be totally effective in patients in whom angina is caused or increased by dynamic alterations in coronary luminal diameter. Despite potential dangers in rest and vasospastic angina, β blockers have been used successfully as monotherapy and in combination with vasodilating agents in many patients. The drugs also have been shown to favorably affect C-reactive protein concentrations in the blood, an important disease marker for active coronary artery disease.

Electrophysiologic and Antiarrhythmic Effects

Adrenoceptor-blocking drugs have two main effects on the electrophysiologic properties of specialized cardiac tissue (Table 2-7). The first effect results from specific blockade of adrenergic stimulation of cardiac pacemaker potentials. In concentrations causing significant inhibition of adrenergic receptors, β blockers produce little change in the transmembrane potentials of cardiac muscle. By competitively inhibiting adrenergic stimulation, however, β blockers decrease the slope of phase 4 depolarization and the spontaneous firing rate of sinus or ectopic pacemakers and thus decrease automaticity. Arrhythmias occurring in the setting of enhanced automaticity—as seen in myocardial infarction, digitalis toxicity, hyperthyroidism, and pheochromocytoma—therefore would be expected to respond well to β blockade.

The second electrophysiologic effect of β blockers involves membrane-stabilizing action, also known as *quinidine-like* or *local anesthetic* action, which is observed only at very high dose levels. This property is unrelated to inhibition of catecholamine action and is possessed equally by the D- and L-isomers of the drugs (D-isomers have almost no β-blocking activity). Characteristic of this effect is a reduction in the rate of rise of the intracardiac

TABLE 2-7 Antiarrhythmic Properties of β Blockers

β Blockade
    Electrophysiology: depress excitability and conduction
    Prevention of ischemia: decrease automaticity, inhibit reentrant
      mechanisms
Membrane-stabilizing effects
    Local anesthetic "quinidine-like" properties: depress excitability, prolong
      refractory period, delay conduction
    Clinically: probably not significant
Special pharmacologic properties
    β_1 selectivity, intrinsic sympathomimetic activity (do not appear to
      contribute to antiarrhythmic effectiveness)

Source: Reproduced with permission from Frishman WH: *Clinical Pharmacology of the β-Adrenoceptor Blocking Drugs*, 2nd ed. Norwalk, Appleton-Century-Crofts, 1984.

action potential without an effect on the spike duration of the resting potential. Associated features include an elevated electrical threshold of excitability, a delay in conduction velocity, and a significant increase in the effective refractory period. This effect and its attendant changes have been explained by inhibition of the depolarizing inward sodium current. There is a greater antifibrillatory effect when β blockers are combined with some other antiarrhythmics.

Sotalol is unique among the β blockers in that it possesses class III antiarrhythmic properties, causing prolongation of the action potential period and thus delaying repolarization. Clinical studies have verified the efficacy of sotalol in the control and prevention of atrial and ventricular arrhythmias, but additional investigation will be required to determine whether its class III antiarrhythmic properties contribute significantly to its efficacy as an antiarrhythmic agent. A clinical study demonstrated an increased mortality risk with D-sotalol, the stereoisomer with type III antiarrhythmic activity and no β-blocking effect.

There is a quantitative difference between men and women in response to D, L-sotalol, which may explain the greater propensity of women to drug-induced torsades de pointes. To ensure patient safety with sotalol use, it has been suggested that patients be admitted to the hospital for initiation of treatment.

The most important mechanism underlying the antiarrhythmic effect of β blockers, with the possible exclusion of sotalol, is believed to be β blockade with resultant inhibition of pacemaker potentials. The contribution of membrane-stabilizing action does not appear to be clinically significant. In vitro experiments with human ventricular muscle have shown that the concentration of propranolol required for membrane stabilizing is 50 to 100 times the concentration that is usually associated with inhibition of exercise-induced tachycardia and at which only β-blocking effects occur. Moreover, D-propranolol, which possesses membrane-stabilizing properties but no β-blocking action, is a weak antiarrhythmic even at high doses, whereas β blockers devoid of membrane-stabilizing action (atenolol, esmolol, metoprolol, nadolol, pindolol, etc.) have been shown to be effective antiarrhythmic drugs. Differences in the overall clinical usefulness of β blockers for arrhythmia are related to their other associated pharmacologic properties.

TABLE 2-8 Effects of β Blockers in Various Arrhythmias

Supraventricular

Sinus tachycardia: treat underlying disorder; excellent response to β blocker if needed to control rate (e.g., ischemia).

Atrial fibrillation: reduce rate, rarely restore sinus rhythm, may be useful in combination with digoxin

Atrial flutter: reduce rate, sometimes restore sinus rhythm

Atrial tachycardia: effective in slowing ventricular rate, may restore sinus rhythm; useful in prophylaxis.

Maintain patients in normal sinus rhythm after electrocardioversion of atrial and ventricular arrhythmias.

Ventricular

Premature ventricular contractions: good response to β blockers, especially digitalis induced, exercise (ischemia) induced, mitral valve prolapse, or hypertrophic cardiomyopathy

Ventricular tachycardia: effective as quinidine, most effective in digitalis toxicity or exercise (ischemia) induced

Ventricular fibrillation: electrical defibrillation is treatment of choice; can be used to prevent recurrence in cases of excess digitalis or sympathomimetic amines; appear to be effective in reducing the incidence of ventricular fibrillation and sudden death postmyocardial infarction.

Source: Reproduced with permission from Frishman WH: *Clinical Pharmacology of the β-Adrenoceptor Blocking Drugs*, 2nd ed. Norwalk, Appleton-Century-Crofts, 1984.

Therapeutic Uses in Cardiac Arrhythmias

β-Adrenergic blocking drugs have become an important treatment modality for various cardiac arrhythmias (Table 2-8) when used alone and in combination with other antiarrhythmic drugs. Although it has long been believed that β blockers are more effective in treating supraventricular arrhythmias than ventricular arrhythmias, this may not be the case. These agents can be quite useful in the treatment of ventricular tachyarrhythmias in the setting of myocardial ischemia, mitral valve prolapse, and for other cardiovascular conditions (see Chap. 12). A high prevalence of antibodies against β_1 and β_2 adrenoceptors has been observed in patients with atrial arrhythmias, ventricular arrhythmias, and conduction disturbances.

Effects in Survivors of Acute Myocardial Infarction

β-Adrenergic blockers have beneficial effects on many determinants of myocardial ischemia (Table 2-9). The results of placebo-controlled, long-term treatment trials with some β-adrenergic blocking drugs in survivors of acute myocardial infarction have demonstrated a favorable effect on total mortality; cardiovascular mortality, including sudden and non-sudden cardiac deaths; and the incidence of nonfatal reinfarction. These beneficial results with β-blocker therapy can be explained by the antiarrhythmic (see Table 2-9) and the anti-ischemic effects of these drugs. β-Adrenergic blockers also have been postulated to reduce the risk of atherosclerotic plaque fissure and subsequent thrombosis. Two nonselective β blockers, propranolol and timolol, have been approved for reducing the risk of mortality in infarct survivors when started 5 to 28 days after an infarction. Metoprolol and atenolol, two β_1-selective blockers, are approved for the same indication and can be used intravenously in the hyperacute phase of a myocardial infarction. The α- β-blocker carvedilol has been approved for use in survivors of acute myocardial infarction with evidence of left ventricular dysfunction. β Blockers also have been suggested as a treatment for reducing the extent of myocardial injury and mortality during the hyperacute phase of myocardial infarction, but their exact role in this situation remains unclear. Intravenous and oral atenolol has been shown to be effective in causing a modest reduction in early mortality when given during the hyperacute phase of acute myocardial infarction. Atenolol and metoprolol reduce early infarct mortality by 15%, an effect that may be improved when β-adrenergic blockade is combined with acute thrombolytic therapy. Metoprolol and atenolol combined with acute thrombolysis has been evaluated in the TIMI-II and GUSTO studies. Immediate β-blocker therapy given to patients with acute myocardial infarction who have received tissue-type plasminogen activator has been associated with a significant reduction in the frequency of intracranial hemorrhage. Despite all the evidence showing that β blockers are beneficial in patients surviving myocardial infarction, they are considerably underused in clinical practice.

Recent studies have shown the cost effectiveness of using beta blockers in a larger percentage of the postinfarction population, including the elderly, diabetics, and patients with mild to moderate chronic obstructive pulmonary disease. β Blockers also have been shown to be effective in patients after coronary revascularization and in those with diminished ejection fraction postmyocardial infarction. Attempts should be made to increase β-blocker use in clinical practice. Treatment with lower doses of β blockers than those used in large clinical trials is associated with at least as great a reduction in mortality as treatment with higher doses. In patients surviving a myocardial infarction in whom larger doses of β blockers might be contraindicated, the use of smaller doses should be encouraged. Studies have examined the use of β-blockade by paramedics, before hospital admission, with some benefit observed.

"Silent" Myocardial Ischemia

In recent years, investigators have observed that not all myocardial ischemic episodes detected by electrocardiography (ECG) are associated with detectable symptoms. Positron emission tomography imaging techniques have validated

TABLE 2-9 Possible Mechanisms by Which β Blockers Protect the Ischemic Myocardium

Reduction in myocardial consumption, heart rate, blood pressure, and myocardial contractility
Augmentation of coronary blood flow; increase in diastolic perfusion time by reducing heart rate, augmentation of collateral blood flow, and coronary flow reserve, and redistribution of blood flow to ischemic areas
Prevention of attenuation of atherosclerotic plaque, rupture, and subsequent coronary thrombosis
Alterations in myocardial substrate utilization
Decrease in microvascular damage
Stabilization of cell and lysosomal membranes
Shift of oxyhemoglobin dissociation curve to the right
Inhibition of platelet aggregation
Inhibition of myocardial apoptosis, allowing natural cell regeneration to occur

the theory that these silent ischemic episodes are indicative of true myocardial ischemia. Compared with symptomatic ischemia, the prognostic importance of silent myocardial ischemia occurring at rest and/or during exercise has not been determined. β Blockers are as successful in reducing the frequency of silent ischemic episodes detected by ambulatory ECG monitoring as they are in reducing the frequency of painful ischemic events.

Congestive Cardiomyopathy

The ability of intravenous sympathomimetic amines to affect an acute increase in myocardial contractility through stimulation of the β-adrenergic receptor had prompted the hope that the use of oral catecholamine analogues could provide long-term benefit for patients with severe heart failure. However, recent observations concerning the regulation of the myocardial adrenergic receptor and abnormalities of β-receptor–mediated stimulation of the failing myocardium have caused a critical reappraisal of the scientific validity of sustained β-adrenergic receptor stimulation. Evidence suggests that β-receptor blockade may, when tolerated, have a favorable effect on the underlying cardiomyopathic process, perhaps by upregulation and preservation of β-receptor signaling.

Recently it has been shown that excess catecholamine stimulation of β receptors can result in receptor desensitization by the phosphorylation of inhibitory β-adrenergic receptor kinases with β-receptor uncoupling from Gs due to β-arrestin activity. In addition, agonist anti–$β_1$-adrenergic receptor autoantibodies have been described in patients with heart failure, which can also cause receptor desensitization.

Enhanced sympathetic activation is seen consistently in patients with congestive heart failure and is associated with decreased exercise tolerance, hemodynamic abnormalities, and increased mortality. Increases in sympathetic tone can potentiate the patient's renin-angiotensin system, leading to increased salt and water retention, arterial and venous constriction, and increments in ventricular preload and afterload. Catecholamines in excess can increase heart rate and cause coronary vasoconstriction. They can adversely influence myocardial contractility on the cellular level and cause myocyte hypertrophy and vascular remodeling. Catecholamines can stimulate growth and provoke oxidative stress in terminally differentiated cardiac cells; these two factors can trigger the process of programmed cell death known as *apoptosis*. They can increase the risk of sudden death in patients with congestive heart failure by adversely influencing the electrophysiologic properties of the failing heart.

Controlled trials over the past 25 years with several different β blockers in patients with ischemic and nonischemic cardiomyopathies have shown that these drugs can improve symptoms, ventricular function, and functional capacity and reduce the need for hospitalization. A series of placebo-controlled clinical trials with the α- and β-blocker carvedilol showed a morbidity and mortality benefit in patients with New York Heart Association class II to IV heart failure when the drug was used in addition to diuretics, ACE inhibitors, and digoxin. Carvedilol also has been studied in symptomatic patients with low ejection fraction after an acute myocardial infarction, with a benefit shown on all-cause and cardiovascular mortality and recurrent nonfatal myocardial infarction. It has been shown that patients treated with inotropic therapy (milrinone) can be titrated on carvedilol after reaching a stable state, with subsequent weaning of the inotrope.

Placebo-controlled studies also have been done showing the benefit of using the β_1-selective blockers, metoprolol (sustained-release) and bisoprolol, in patients with class II to III heart failure. Sustained-release metoprolol was recently approved as a once-daily treatment for patients with congestive cardiomyopathy. A trial with the β-blocker and vasodilator bucindolol showed less benefit than with other β blockers used to treatment congestive heart failure, demonstrating that all β blockers may not be interchangeable for this indication. The recently completed Carvedilol or Metoprolol European Trial (COMET) comparing the α- and β-blocker carvedilol to metoprolol in heart failure patients found a 17% reduction in mortality with carvedilol versus metoprolol, but no significant difference in the coprimary end points of death or hospitalization. The dose and formulation type for metoprolol have been speculated on as possible explanations for these findings.

The mechanisms of benefit with β-blocker use are not known as yet. Possible mechanisms for β-blocker benefit in chronic heart failure are listed in Table 2-10 and include the upregulation of impaired β-receptor expression in the heart, alteration of myocardial gene expression, augmentation of the cardiac natriuretic peptides, and improvement in impaired baroreceptor functioning, which can inhibit excess sympathetic outflow. It has been suggested that long-term therapy with β blockers improves the left atrial contribution to left ventricular filling and normalizes the abundance of myocyte Ca^{2+} regulatory proteins with improved Ca^{2+} handling.

TABLE 2-10 Possible Mechanisms by Which β-Adrenergic Blockers Improve Ventricular Function in Chronic Congestive Heart Failure

Upregulation of β receptors
Direct myocardial protective action against catecholamine toxicity
Improved ability of noradrenergic sympathetic nerves to synthesize norepinephrine
Decreased release of norepinephrine from sympathetic nerve endings
Decreased stimulation of other vasoconstrictive systems including renin–angiotensin–aldosterone, vasopressin, and endothelin
Potentiation of kallikrein–kinin system and natural vasodilatation (increase in bradykinin)
Antiarrhythmic effects raising ventricular fibrillation threshold
Protection against catecholamine-induced hypokalemia
Increase in coronary blood flow by reducing heart rate and improving diastolic perfusion time; possible coronary dilation with vasodilator β blocker
Restoration of abnormal baroreflex function
Prevention of ventricular muscle hypertrophy and vascular remodeling
Antioxidant effects (carvedilol?)
Shift from free fatty acid to carbohydrate metabolism (improved metabolic efficiency)
Vasodilation (e.g., carvedilol)
Antiapoptosis effect allowing myocardial cell regeneration to occur
Improved left atrial contribution to left ventricular filling
Modulation of postreceptor inhibitory G proteins
Normalization of myocyte Ca^{2+} regulatory proteins and improved Ca^{2+} handling
Increasing natriuretic peptide production
Attenuation of inflammatory cytokines
Restoring cardiac calcium release channel (ryanodine receptor)

Other Cardiovascular Applications

Although β blockers have been studied extensively in patients with angina pectoris, arrhythmias, and hypertension, they have been shown to be safe and effective in diabetic patients and for other cardiovascular conditions (see Table 2-4), some of which are described below.

Hypertrophic cardiomyopathy β-Adrenergic receptor blocking drugs have been proven effective in therapy for patients with hypertrophic cardiomyopathy and idiopathic hypertrophic subaortic stenosis. These drugs are useful in controlling the symptoms of dyspnea, angina, and syncope. β Blockers also have been shown to lower the intraventricular pressure gradient at rest and with exercise.

The outflow pressure gradient is not the only abnormality in hypertrophic cardiomyopathy; more important is the loss of ventricular compliance, which impedes normal left ventricular function. It has been shown by invasive and noninvasive methods that propranolol can improve left ventricular function in this condition. The drug also produces favorable changes in ventricular compliance while it relieves symptoms. Propranolol has been approved for this condition and may be combined with the calcium-entry blocker verapamil in patients who do not respond to the β blocker alone.

The salutary hemodynamic and symptomatic effects produced by propranolol derive from its inhibition of sympathetic stimulation of the heart. There is no evidence that the drug alters the primary cardiomyopathic process; many patients remain in or return to their severely symptomatic state, and some die despite its administration.

Mitral valve prolapse This auscultatory complex, characterized by a non-ejection systolic click, a late systolic murmur, or a midsystolic click followed by a late systolic murmur, has been studied extensively over the past 15 years. Atypical chest pain, malignant arrhythmias, and nonspecific ST- and T-wave abnormalities have been observed with this condition. By decreasing sympathetic tone, β-adrenergic blockers have been shown to be useful for relieving the chest pains and palpitations that many of these patients experience and for reducing the incidence of life-threatening arrhythmias and other ECG abnormalities.

Dissecting aneurysms β-adrenergic blockade plays a major role in the treatment of patients with acute aortic dissection. During the hyperacute phase, β-blocking agents reduce the force and velocity of myocardial contraction (dP/dt) and, hence, the progression of the dissecting hematoma. Moreover, such administration must be initiated simultaneously with the institution of other antihypertensive therapy, which may cause reflex tachycardia and increases in cardiac output, factors that can aggravate the dissection process. Initially propranolol is administered intravenously to reduce the heart rate to slower than 60 beats/min. Once a patient is stabilized and long-term medical management is contemplated, the patient should be maintained on oral β-blocker therapy to prevent recurrence.

It has been demonstrated that long-term β-blocker therapy also may reduce the risk of dissection in patients prone to this complication (e.g., Marfan's syndrome). Systolic time intervals are used to assess the adequacy of β blockade in children with Marfan's syndrome.

Tetralogy of Fallot By reducing the effects of increased adrenergic tone on the right ventricular infundibulum in tetralogy of Fallot, β blockers have been shown to be useful for the treatment of severe hypoxic spells and hyper-cyanotic attacks. With chronic use, these drugs also have been shown to prevent prolonged hypoxic spells. These drugs should be looked on as palliative only because definitive surgical repair of this condition is usually required.

QT interval–prolongation syndrome The syndrome of ECG QT-interval prolongation is usually a congenital condition associated with deafness, syncope, and sudden death. Abnormalities in sympathetic nervous system functioning in the heart have been proposed as explanations for the electro-physiologic aberrations seen in these patients. Propranolol and other β blockers appear to be the most effective drugs for the treatment of this syndrome. They reduce the frequency of syncopal episodes in most patients and may prevent sudden death. These drugs reduce the ECG QT interval. Patients not responding to β blockers should be candidates for implantable defibrillators.

Regression of left ventricular hypertrophy Left ventricular hypertrophy induced by systemic hypertension is an independent risk factor for cardiovascular mortality and morbidity. Regression of left ventricular hypertrophy with drug therapy is feasible and may improve patient outcome. β-Adrenergic blockers can cause regression of left ventricular hypertrophy, as determined by echocardiography, with or without an associated reduction in blood pressure.

Atherogenesis β Blockers may have a direct anti-atherosclerotic effect at a dose well below commonly prescribed regimens. The mechanisms underlying this beta-blocker benefit is not known. An effect on reactive oxygen species has been proposed. Recently it was shown that chronic propranolol treatment does not favorably influence the course of patients having abdominal aortic aneurysms.

Syncope Vasovagal syncope is the most common form of syncope observed. Upright tilt-table testing with isoproterenol can help differentiate vasovagal syncope from other forms. β Blockers, including those with partial agonist properties, have been shown to be useful for relieving symptoms and normalizing abnormal tilt-table tests in patients with syncope, with some studies showing no benefit. The mechanism for benefit with β blockers may be an interruption of the Bezold-Jarisch reflex or an enhancement of peripheral vasoconstriction by blockade of β_2-adrenergic receptors.

Myocardial protection during surgery β Blockers can protect patients at high risk for myocardial ischemia during and after major surgery. Prior β-blocker therapy also has been shown to have a cardioprotective effect in limiting creatine kinase-MB release after percutaneous coronary interventions, associated with a lower mortality at intermediate-term follow up. However, a recent observational study did not support the contention that β blockade can favorably influence creatine kinase-MB rise during angioplasty.

Noncardiovascular Applications

β-Adrenergic receptors are ubiquitous in the human body, and their blockade affects a variety of organ and metabolic systems. Some noncardiovascular uses of β blockers (glaucoma, migraine headache prophylaxis, and essential tremor) have been approved by the US Food and Drug Administration. The combination of nitrates and β blockers has been shown to be effective in preventing bleeding from esophageal varices.

Adverse Effects of β Blockers

Evaluation of adverse effects is complex because of the use of different definitions of side effects, the kinds of patients studied, study design features, and different methods of ascertaining and reporting adverse side effects from study to study. Overall, the types and frequencies of adverse effects attributed to various β-blocker compounds appear similar. The side effect profiles resemble those seen with concurrent placebo treatments, thus attesting to the remarkable safety margin of the β blockers.

Adverse effects fall in two categories: (1) those from known pharmacologic consequences of β-adrenoceptor blockade and (2) other reactions apart from β-adrenoceptor blockade.

The first type includes asthma, heart failure, hypoglycemia, bradycardia and heart block, intermittent claudication, and Raynaud's phenomenon. The incidence of these adverse effects varies with the β blocker used.

Side effects of the second category are rare. They include an unusual oculomucocutaneous reaction and the possibility of carcinogenesis.

Adverse Cardiac Effects Related to β-Adrenoceptor Blockade

Congestive heart failure Despite benefit in many patients with congestive cardiomyopathy, blockade of β receptors may cause congestive heart failure in an enlarged heart with impaired myocardial function, when excessive sympathetic drive is essential to maintain the myocardium on a compensated Starling curve and when left ventricular stroke volume is restricted and tachycardia is needed to maintain cardiac output.

Thus, any β-blocking drug may be associated with the development of heart failure. Further, heart failure may be augmented by increases in peripheral vascular resistance produced by nonselective agents (e.g., propranolol, timolol, and sotalol). It has been claimed that β blockers with intrinsic sympathomimetic activity and α-blocking activity are better in preserving left ventricular function and less likely to precipitate heart failure.

In patients with impaired myocardial function who require β-blocking agents, digitalis, ACE inhibitors, and diuretics can be used.

Sinus node dysfunction and atrioventricular conduction delay Slowing of the resting heart rate is a normal response to treatment with β-blocking drugs with and without intrinsic sympathomimetic activity. Healthy persons can sustain a heart rate of 40 to 50 beats/min without disability unless there is clinical evidence of heart failure. Drugs with intrinsic sympathomimetic activity do not lower the resting heart rate to the same degree as propranolol, but all β-blocking drugs are contraindicated (unless an artificial pacemaker is present) in patients with sick sinus syndrome.

If there is a partial or complete AV conduction defect, the use of a β-blocking drug may lead to a serious bradyarrhythmia. The risk of AV impairment may be less with β blockers that have intrinsic sympathomimetic activity.

Overdosage Suicide attempts and accidental overdosing with β blockers are being described with increasing frequency. Because β-adrenergic blockers are competitive pharmacologic antagonists, their life-threatening effects (bradycardia, myocardial and ventilatory failure) can be overcome with an immediate infusion of β-agonist agents such as isoproterenol and dobutamine. In situations where catecholamines are not effective, intravenous glucagon, amrinone, or milrinone have been used.

Close monitoring of cardiorespiratory function is necessary for at least 24 h after the patient responds to therapy. Patients who recover usually have no long-term sequelae, but they should be observed for the cardiac signs of sudden β-blocker withdrawal.

β-*Adrenoceptor blocker withdrawal* After abrupt cessation of chronic β-blocker therapy, exacerbation of angina pectoris and, in some cases, acute myocardial infarction and death have been reported. Observations made in multiple double-blind randomized trials have confirmed the reality of a propranolol withdrawal reaction. The mechanism for this reaction is unclear. There is some evidence that the withdrawal phenomenon may be due to the generation of additional β-adrenoceptors during the period of β-adrenoceptor blockade. When the β-adrenoceptor blocker is then withdrawn, the increased β-receptor population readily results in excessive β-receptor stimulation, which is clinically important when the delivery and use of oxygen are finely balanced, as occurs in ischemic heart disease. Other suggested mechanisms for the withdrawal reaction include heightened platelet aggregation, an elevation in thyroid hormone activity, and an increase in circulating catecholamines. A β-blocker withdrawal phenomenon with an increased risk for death also has been described in patients with heart failure who are withdrawn from β blockers.

Adverse Noncardiac Side Effects Related to β-Adrenoceptor Blockade

Effect on ventilatory function The bronchodilatory effects of catecholamines on the bronchial β_2-adrenoceptors are inhibited by nonselective β blockers (e.g., propranolol, nadolol). β-Blocking compounds with partial agonist activity, β_1 selectivity, and α-adrenergic blocking actions are less likely to increase airways resistance in asthmatics. However, β_1 selectivity is not absolute and may be lost with high therapeutic doses, as shown with atenolol and metoprolol. It is possible in treating asthma to use a β_2-selective agonist (such as albuterol) in certain patients with concomitant low-dose β_1-selective blocker treatment. In general, all β blockers should be avoided in patients with bronchospastic disease.

Peripheral vascular effects (Raynaud's phenomenon) Cold extremities and absent pulses have been reported more frequently in patients receiving β blockers for hypertension than in those receiving methyldopa. Among the β blockers, the incidence was highest with propranolol and lower with drugs having β_1 selectivity or intrinsic sympathomimetic activity. In some instances, vascular compromise has been severe enough to cause cyanosis and impending gangrene. This result is likely due to the reduction in cardiac output and blockade of β_2-adrenoceptor–mediated skeletal muscle vasodilatation, resulting in unopposed β-adrenoceptor vasoconstriction. β-Blocking drugs with β_1 selectivity or partial agonist activity will not affect peripheral vessels to the same degree as propranolol.

Raynaud's phenomenon is one of the more common side effects of propranolol treatment. It is more troublesome with propranolol than with metoprolol, atenolol, or pindolol, probably because of the β_2-blocking properties of propranolol.

Patients with peripheral vascular disease who suffer from intermittent claudication occasionally report worsening of the claudication when treated with β-blocking drugs. Whether drugs with β_1 selectivity or partial agonist activity can protect against this adverse reaction has not been determined.

Hypoglycemia and hyperglycemia   Several investigators have described severe hypoglycemic reactions during therapy with β-adrenergic blocking drugs. Some of the patients affected were insulin-dependent diabetics, whereas others were nondiabetic. Studies of resting normal volunteers have demonstrated that propranolol produces no alteration in blood glucose values, although the hyperglycemic response to exercise is blunted. β Blockers can increase the incidence of type II diabetes. Weight gain (average, 1.2 kg) and insulin resistance have been reported with chronic β-blocker use.

The enhancement of insulin-induced hypoglycemia and its hemodynamic consequences may be less with β_1-selective agents (where there is no blocking effect on β_2 receptors) and agents with intrinsic sympathomimetic activity (which may stimulate β_2 receptors).

There is also marked diminution in the clinical manifestations of the catecholamine discharge induced by hypoglycemia (tachycardia). These findings suggest that β blockers interfere with compensatory responses to hypoglycemia and can mask certain "warning signs" of this condition. Other hypoglycemic reactions, such as diaphoresis, are not affected by β-adrenergic blockade.

Hyperlipidemia   Nonselective β-blocking agents can raise triglycerides and reduce high-density lipoprotein cholesterol. This effect may not be seen with agents having partial agonist or α-blocking activity.

Central nervous system effects   Dreams, hallucinations, insomnia, and depression can occur during therapy with β blockers. These symptoms provide evidence of drug entry into the CNS and may be more common with the highly lipid-soluble β blockers (propranolol, metoprolol), which presumably penetrate the CNS better. It has been claimed that β blockers with less lipid solubility (atenolol, nadolol) cause fewer CNS side effects. This claim is intriguing, but its validity has not been corroborated by other extensive clinical experiences.

Miscellaneous Side Effects

Diarrhea, nausea, gastric pain, constipation, and flatulence have been noted occasionally with all β blockers (2% to 11% of patients). Hematologic reactions are rare. Rare cases of purpura and agranulocytosis have been described with propranolol. β-Blocker use early in pregnancy has been associated with fetal growth retardation (see Appendix 3).

A devastating blood pressure rebound effect has been described in patients who discontinued clonidine while being treated with nonselective β-blocking agents. The mechanism for this may be related to an increase in circulating catecholamines and an increase in peripheral vascular resistance. Whether β_1-selective or partial agonist β blockers have similar effects after clonidine withdrawal has not been determined. This has not been a problem with labetalol.

TABLE 2-11 Drug Interactions That May Occur with β-Adrenoceptor Blocking Drugs

Drug	Pharmacokinetic	Pharmacodynamic	Precautions
Alcohol	Enhanced first-pass hepatic degradation	None	May need increased doses of lipid-soluble agents
α-Adrenergic blockers		Increased risk for first-dose hypotension	Use with caution
Aluminum hydroxide gel	Decreased β-blocker absorption	None	Clinical efficacy rarely altered
Amiodarone	None	Enhanced negative chronotropic activity	Monitor response
Aminophylline	Mutual inhibition		Observe patient's response
Ampicillin	Impaired GI absorption leading to decreased β-blocker bioavailability		May need to increase β-blocker dose
Angiotensin II receptor blockers (losartan)	None	Enhanced blood pressure effects and bronchospasm	Monitor response
Antidiabetics	Enhanced and blunted responses seen	None	Monitor for altered diabetic response
ACE inhibitors	None	Enhanced blood pressure effects and bronchospasm	Monitor response
Calcium	Decreases β-blocker absorption		May need to increase β-blocker dose
Calcium channel blockers	Decreased hepatic clearance of lipid-soluble and water-soluble β blockers; decreased clearance of calcium blockers	Potentiation of AV nodal negative inotropic and hypotensive responses	Avoid use if possible, although few patients show ill effects
Cimetidine	Decreased hepatic clearance of lipid-soluble β blockers	None	Combination should be used with caution
Clonidine	None	Nonselective agents exacerbate clonidine withdrawal phenomenon	Use only β₁-selective agents or labetalol
Diazepam	Diazepam metabolism reduced		Observe patient's response

(continued)

51

TABLE 2-11 (continued) Drug Interactions That May Occur with β-Adrenoceptor Blocking Drugs

Drug	Pharmacokinetic	Pharmacodynamic	Precautions
Digitalis glycosides	None	Potentiation of bradycardic and AV blocks	Observe patient's response; interactions may benefit angina patients with abnormal ventricular function
Epinephrine	None	Severe hypertension and bradycardia	Administer epinephrine cautiously; cardioselective β blocker may be safer
Ergot alkaloids	None	Severe hypertension and peripheral artery hyperperfusion have been seen, although β blockers are commonly coadministered	Observe patient's response; few patients show ill effects
Fluvoxamine	Decreased hepatic clearance of propranolol		Use with caution
Glucagon	Enhanced clearance of lipid-soluble β blockers	None	Monitor for reduced response
Halofenate			Observe for impaired response to β blockade
Hydralazine	Decreased hepatic clearance of lipid-soluble β blockers	Enhanced hypotensive response	Cautious coadministration
Indomethacin and ibuprofen	None	Reduced efficacy in treatment of hypertension	Observe patient's response
Isoproterenol	None	Cancels pharmacologic effect	Avoid concurrent use or choose β_1-selective blocker
Levodopa		Antagonism of hypotensive and positive inotropic effects of levodopa	Monitor for altered response; interaction may have favorable results
Lidocaine	Decreased hepatic clearance of lidocaine by lipid-soluble β blockers.	Enhanced lidocaine toxicity	Combination should be used with caution; use lower doses of lidocaine
Methyldopa		Hypertension during stress	Monitor for hypertensive episodes

Monoamine oxidase inhibitors	Uncertain	Enhanced hypotension	Manufacturer of propranolol considers concurrent use contraindicated
Nitrates	None	Enhanced hypotension	Monitor response
Omeprazole	None	None	None
Phenobarbital	Increased hepatic metabolism of β blockers		May need to increase lipid soluble β-blocker dose
Phenothiazines	Increased phenothiazine and β-blocker blood levels	Additive hypotensive response	Monitor for altered response; especially with high doses of phenothiazine
Phenylpropanolamine		Severe hypertensive reaction	Avoid use, especially in hypertension controlled by both methyldopa and β blockers
Phenytoin		Additive ventricular depressive effects	Use with caution
Reserpine	Not marked	Depression, possible enhanced sensitivity to β-adrenergic blockade	Monitor closely
Ranitidine		None	Observe response
Smoking	Enhanced first-pass metabolism	None	May need to increase dose of lipid-soluble β blockers
Sulindac and naproxen	None	None	
Tricyclic antidepressants		Inhibits negative inotropic and chronotropic effects; enhanced hypotension	Use with caution with sotalol because of additive effects on ECG QT interval
Tubucuraine		Enhanced neuromuscular blockade	Observe response in surgical patients, especially after high doses of propranolol
Type I antiarrhythmics	Propafenone and quinidine decrease clearance of lipid-soluble β blockers	Disopyramide is a potent negative inotropic and chronotropic agent	Cautious coprescription: use with sotalol can be dangerous because of additive effects on ECG QT interval
Warfarin	Decreased clearance of warfarin	None	Monitor response

Key: ACE, angiotensin-converting enzyme; AV, atrioventricular; ECG, electrocardiogram; GI, gastrointestinal.

TABLE 2-12 Clinical Situations That Would Influence the Choice of a β-Blocking Drug

Condition	Choice of β blocker
Asthma, chronic bronchitis with bronchospasm	Avoid all β blockers, if possible, but small doses of β_1-selective blockers can be used; β_1 selectivity is lost with higher with doses; drugs with partial agonist activity and labetalol with α-adrenergic blocking properties can also be used
Congestive heart failure	Drugs with partial agonist activity, β_1 selectivity (metoprolol) and vasodilatory activity (carvedilol, labetalol) may have an advantage, although all β blockers should be used with caution.
Angina	In patients with angina at low heart rates, drugs with partial agonist activity are probably contraindicated; patients who have angina at high heart rates but who have resting bradycardia may benefit from a drug with partial agonist activity; in vasospastic angina, labetalol may be useful; other β blockers should be used with caution
Atrioventricular conduction defects	β Blockers are generally contraindicated, but drugs with partial agonist activity and labetalol can be tried with caution
Bradycardia	β Blockers with partial agonist activity and labetalol have less of a pulse-slowing effect and are preferable.
Raynaud's phenomenon, intermittent claudication, cold extremities	β_1-Selective blocking agents (labetalol, carvedilol) and agents with partial agonist activity may have an advantage
Depression	Avoid propranolol; substitute a β blocker with partial agonist activity
Diabetes mellitus	β1-Selective blocking agents and partial agonist drugs are preferable
Thyrotoxicosis	All agents will control symptoms, but agents without partial agonist activity are preferred
Pheochromocytoma	Avoid all β blockers unless an α blocker is given first; labetalol may be used as a treatment of choice
Renal failure	Use reduced doses of compounds largely eliminated by renal mechanisms (nadolol, sotalol, atenolol) and drugs whose bioavailability is increased in uremia (propranolol); also consider possible accumulation of active metabolites (propranolol, nebivolol)
Insulin and sulfonylurea use	There is a danger of hypoglycemia that may decrease when using drugs with β_1 selectivity
Clonidine	Avoid nonselective β blockers; there is a severe rebound effect with clonidine withdrawal
Oculomucocutaneous syndrome	Stop drug; substitute with any β blocker
Hyperlipidemia	Avoid nonselective β blockers; use agents with partial agonism, β_1 selectivity or α-blocking activity

Source: Reproduced with permission from Frishman WH: *Clinical Pharmacology of the β-Adrenoceptor Blocking Drugs,* 2nd ed. Norwalk, Appleton-Century-Crofts, 1984.

Adverse Effects Unrelated to β-Adrenoceptor Blockade

Oculomucocutaneous syndrome A characteristic immune reaction, the oculomucocutaneous syndrome—affecting one or both eyes, mucous and serous membranes, and the skin, often in association with a positive antinuclear factor—has been reported in patients treated with practolol and has curtailed its clinical use. Close attention has been focused on this syndrome because of fears that other β-adrenoceptor blocking drugs may be associated with this syndrome.

Drug–Drug Interactions

β Blockers are commonly employed, and the list of commonly used drugs with which they can interact is extensive (Table 2-11). Most of the reported interactions have been associated with propranolol, the best studied β blocker, and may not necessarily apply to other drugs in this class.

How to Choose a β Blocker

The various β-blocking compounds given in adequate dosage appear to have comparable antihypertensive, antiarrhythmic, and antianginal effects. Therefore, the β-blocking drug of choice in an individual patient is determined by the pharmacodynamic and pharmacokinetic differences between the drugs in conjunction with the patient's other medical conditions (Table 2-12).

ADDITIONAL READINGS

Abrams J, Frishman WH, Bates SM, et al: Pharmacologic options for treatment of ischemic disease, in Antman EM (ed): *Cardiovascular Therapeutics. A Companion to Braunwald's Heart Disease,* 2nd ed. Philadelphia, WB Saunders, 2002, pp 97–153.

The ALLHAT Officers and Coordinators for the ALLHAT Collaborative Research Group: Major cardiovascular events in hypertensive patients randomized to doxazosin vs chlorthalidone. The Antihypertensive and Lipid-Lowering Treatment to Prevent Heart Attack Trial (ALLHAT). *JAMA* 283:1967, 2000.

Averbach AD, Goldman L: β-Blockers and reduction of cardiac events in noncardiac surgery. Clinical applications. *JAMA* 287:1445, 2002.

Broeders MAW, Doevendans PA, Bekkers BCAM, et al: Nebivolol: A third-generation β blocker that augments vascular nitric oxide release. Endothelial beta$_2$-adrenergic receptor-mediated nitric oxide production. *Circulation* 102:677, 2000.

The CAPRICORN Investigators: Effect of carvedilol on outcome after myocardial infarction in patients with left ventricular dysfunction: The CAPRICORN randomised trial. *Lancet* 357:1385, 2001.

Chan AW, Quinn MJ, Bhatt DL, et al: Mortality benefit of beta-blockade after successful elective percutaneous coronary intervention. *J Am Coll Cardiol* 40:669, 2002.

CIBIS-II Investigators and Committee: The Cardiac Insufficiency Bisoprolol Study II (CIBIS-II): A randomised trial. *Lancet* 353:9, 1999.

Exner DV, Reiffel JA, Epstein AE, et al, and the AVID Investigators: Beta blocker use and survival in patients with ventricular fibrillation or symptomatic ventricular tachycardia: The Antiarrhythmics versus Implantable Defibrillators (AVID) trial. *J Am Coll Cardiol* 34:325, 1999.

Fihn SD, Williams SV, Daley J, Gibbons RJ: Guidelines for the management of patients with chronic stable angina: Treatment. *Ann Intern Med* 135:616, 2001.

Foody JM, Farrell MH, Krumholz HM: β-Blocker therapy in heart failure. Scientific review. *JAMA* 287:883, 2002.

Frishman WH: *Clinical Pharmacology of the β-Adrenoceptor Blocking Drugs,* 2nd ed. Norwalk, Appleton-Century-Crofts, 1984.

Frishman WH: Secondary prevention of myocardial infarction: the roles of β-adrenergic blockers, calcium-channel blockers, angiotensin converting enzyme inhibitors, and aspirin, in Willich SN, Muller JE (eds): *Triggering of Acute Coronary Syndromes.* The Netherlands, Kluwer, 1996, p 367.

Frishman WH: Carvedilol. *N Engl J Med* 339:1759, 1998.

Frishman WH: Alpha- and beta-adrenergic blocking drugs, in Frishman WH, Sonnenblick EH, Sica DA (eds): *Cardiovascular Pharmacotherapeutics,* 2nd ed. New York, McGraw-Hill, 2003, p 67–97.

Frishman WH: Role of β-adrenergic blockade, in Fuster V, Topol EJ, Nabel EG (eds): *Atherosclerosis and Coronary Artery Disease,* 2nd ed. New York, Lippincott Williams & Wilkins, in press.

Frishman WH, Alwarshetty M: Beta-adrenergic blockers in systemic hypertension: Pharmacokinetic considerations related to the JNC-VI and WHO-ISH guidelines. *Clin Pharmacokinet* 41:505, 2002.

Frishman WH, Cavusoglu E: β-Adrenergic blockers and their role in the therapy of arrhythmias, in Podrid PJ, Kowey PR (eds): *Cardiac Arrhythmias: Mechanisms, Diagnosis and Management.* Baltimore, Williams & Wilkins, 1995, p 421–433.

Frishman WH, Cheng-Lai A, Chen J (eds): *Current Cardiovascular Drugs,* 3rd ed. Philadelphia, Current Medicine, 2000, p 120.

Frishman WH, Furberg CD, Friedewald WT: β-Adrenergic blockade for survivors of acute myocardial infarction. *N Engl J Med* 310:30, 1984.

Frishman WH, Opie LH, Sica DA: Adverse cardiovascular drug interactions and complications, in Fuster V, Alexander RW, O'Rourke RA (eds): *Hurst's the Heart,* 11th ed. New York, McGraw-Hill, 2003, in press.

Frishman WH, Sica DA: β-Adrenergic blockers, in Izzo JL Jr., Black HR (eds): *Hypertension Primer,* 3rd ed. Dallas, American Heart Association, 2003, 417.

Gheorghiade M, Goldstein S: β-Blockers in the post-myocardial infarction patient. *Circulation* 106:394, 2002.

Gibbons RJ, Chatterjee K, Daley J, et al: ACC/AHA/ACP-ASIM guidelines for the management of patients with chronic stable angina: Executive summary and recommendations. A report of the American College of Cardiology/American Heart Association Task Force on Practice Guidelines (Committee on Management of Patients with Chronic Stable Angina). *Circulation* 99:2829, 1999.

Goldstein S: Benefits of β-blocker therapy for heart failure. Weighing the evidence. *Arch Intern Med* 162:641, 2002.

Heidenreich PA, McDonald KM, Hastie T, et al: Meta-analysis of trials comparing β blockers, calcium antagonists, and nitrates for stable angina. *JAMA* 281:1927, 1999.

Hjalmarson A, Goldstein S, Fagerberg B, et al, for the MERIT-HF Study Group: Effects of controlled-release metoprolol on total mortality, hospitalizations, and well-being in patients with heart failure. The Metoprolol CR/XL Randomized Intervention Trial in Congestive Heart Failure (MERIT-HF). *JAMA* 283:1295, 2000.

Hoffman BB, Taylor P: Neurotransmission: The autonomic and somatic motor nervous systems, in Hardman JG, Limbird LE (eds): *Goodman & Gilman's the Pharmacological Basis of Therapeutics,* 10th ed. New York, McGraw-Hill, 2001, p 115.

LeJemtel TH, Sonnenblick EH, Frishman WH: Diagnosis and medical management of heart failure, in Fuster V, Alexander RW, O'Rourke RA (eds): *Hurst's the Heart,* 11th ed. New York, McGraw-Hill, 2003, in press.

Lindholm LH, Ibsen H, Devereux RB, et al: Cardiovascular morbidity and mortality in patients with diabetes in the Losartan Intervention for Endpoint Reduction in Hypertension Study (LIFE), a randomized trial against atenolol. *Lancet* 359:1004, 2002.

Lowes BD, Gilbert EM, Abraham MT, et al: Myocardial gene expression in dilated cardiomyopathy treated with beta blocking agents. *N Engl J Med* 346:1357, 2002.

MERIT-HF Study Group: Effect of metoprolol CR/XL in chronic heart failure: Metoprolol CR/XL Randomised Intervention Trial in Congestive Heart Failure (MERIT-HF). *Lancet* 353:2001, 1999.

Messerli FH, Grossman E, Goldbourt U: Are β blockers efficacious as first-line therapy for hypertension in the elderly? *JAMA* 279:1903, 1998.

Moss AJ, Zareba W, Hall WJ, et al: Effectiveness and limitations of β blocker therapy in congenital long QT syndrome. *Circulation* 101:616, 2000.

Opie LH, Yusuf S: Beta-blocking agents, in Opie LH, Gersh BJ (eds): *Drugs for the Heart*, 5th ed. Philadelphia, WB Saunders, 2001, p 1.

Packer M, Coats AJS, Fowler MB, et al, for the Carvedilol Prospective Randomized Cumulative Survival Study Group: Effect of carvedilol on survival in severe chronic heart failure. *N Engl J Med* 344:1651, 2001.

Perez-Stable EJ, Halliday R, Gardiner PS, et al: The effects of propranolol on cognitive function and quality of life: A randomized trial among patients with diastolic hypertension. *Am J Med* 108:359, 2000.

Pfisterer M, Cox JL, Granger CB, et al, for the GUSTO-I Investigators: Atenolol use and clinical outcomes after thrombolysis for acute myocardial infarction: The GUSTO-I experience. *J Am Coll Cardiol* 32:634, 1998.

Phillips KA, Shlipak MG, Coxson P, et al: Health and economic benefits of increased β blocker use following myocardial infarction. *JAMA* 284:2748, 2000.

Pool JL: α-Adrenoceptor blockers, in Izzo JL Jr, Black HR (eds): *Hypertension Primer*, 3rd ed. Dallas, American Heart Association, 2003, p 421.

Poole-Wilson PA, Swedberg K, Cleland JG et al for the Carvedilol or Metoprolol European Trial Investigators: Comparison of carvedilol and metoprolol on clinical outcomes in patients with chronic heart failure in the Carvedilol or Metoprolol European Trial (COMET): Randomised controlled trial. *Lancet* 362:7, 2003.

Sica DA, Frishman WH, Manowitz N: Pharmacokinetics of propranolol after single and multiple dosing with sustained-release propranolol or propranolol CR (Innopran XL), a new chronotherapeutic formulation. *Heart Dis* 5:176, 2003.

3 | Cholinergic and Anticholinergic Drugs

B. Robert Meyer   William H. Frishman

The term *parasympathetic nervous system* refers to those portions of the peripheral autonomic nervous system that begin as preganglionic fibers in one of three distinct regions of the central nervous system (CNS), exit the CNS in the cranial or the sacral regions, and have their postganglionic fibers distributed in a variety of organs throughout the body. One of the three sites of origin for parasympathetic fibers is the midbrain. Fibers originating here join the third cranial nerve and course to the ciliary ganglion. At this ganglion they synapse, and postganglionic fibers innervate the iris and ciliary body. The second site of origin for the parasympathetic system is in the medulla. Fibers originating here join the seventh, ninth, and tenth cranial nerves to exit the CNS. These preganglionic fibers distribute in the pattern of each of these nerves. Fibers in the tenth nerve (the vagus) are distributed to ganglia associated with various visceral organs, including the heart and gastrointestinal tract. The third and final source of parasympathetic outflow is in the sacral portion of the spinal cord. Preganglionic fibers from this site lead to connections with the bladder, bowel, and pelvic organs.

The anatomic organization of the parasympathetic system differs from that of the sympathetic system. The preganglionic fibers of the parasympathetic system extend from their sites of origin in the CNS to the end organ they are innervating. Ganglia of the parasympathetic system are relatively smaller than those of the sympathetic system, and the postganglionic fibers that emerge from these ganglia are short and localized to a specific organ. The sympathetic system has preganglionic fibers that synapse in large paravertebral ganglia and has an extensive and diffuse postganglionic network that distributes to multiple organs of the body.

Inherent in the structural organization of the parasympathetic system is the ability to act at specific organs to cause very specific responses via localized discharges. In general, where the sympathetic system tends to diffusely stimulate activity through its widespread postganglionic network, the effects of the parasympathetic system are to act at specific organs to accommodate periods of rest and recovery. The system lowers heart rate, increases gastrointestinal motility, stimulates bladder emptying, increases biliary contraction, and lowers blood pressure. The parasympathetic nervous system is exclusively cholinergic in character (using acetylcholine as a transmitter), whereas in the sympathetic system the postganglionic fibers are almost exclusively adrenergic. Acetylcholine receptors were first recognized as being of two basic types in 1914, when Dale noted that, although acetylcholine could stimulate all types of cholinergic receptors, certain effects could be blocked by the administration of atropine. Effects that are blocked by atropine are termed *muscarinic effects*, named after a substance isolated from the poisonous mushroom *Amanita muscaria,* which produces these pharmacologic properties. These effects correspond almost directly to the actions of the parasympathetic system. After atropine blockade, higher doses of acetylcholine can elicit another constellation of effects that appear to be very similar to the properties of nicotine. Dale called these *nicotinic effects*.

Modern investigation into the muscarinic receptors that constitute the parasympathetic system has demonstrated that there are at least five major subtypes of muscarinic receptors (Table 3-1). All muscarinic receptors act via G proteins. Types 1, 3, and 5 activate a G protein that in turn stimulates phospholipase C. Phospholipase C then hydrolyzes phosphatidyl inositol. Ultimately, activation of these receptors leads to increased intracellular calcium concentration. Type 2 and 4 receptors activate a different G protein that inhibits adenylate cyclase, activates K^+ channels, and may also suppress voltage controlled Ca^{2+} channels.

The most important subgroup of muscarinic receptors for the cardiovascular system are the M2, or cardiac receptors. Activation of these receptors and alteration of potassium transport produce the negative chronotropic and inotropic effects noted in Table 3-1. Most muscarinic receptors are located in the specialized conduction tissue of the heart, and direct innervation of the myocardium itself is sparse. Effects of muscarinic stimulation lead to a decreased rate of spontaneous depolarization of the sinoatrial node, a consequent delay in the achievement of threshold potential, and a slowing of spontaneous firing. The rate of conduction in the atrioventricular (AV) node is also decreased, and the refractory period to repetitive stimulation is prolonged. The effects of muscarinic receptors on the contractility of the ventricle are substantially less intense than those on the conduction system. Blockade of cholinergic receptors produces positive inotropic effects; negative inotropic effects with cholinergic stimulation can be demonstrated in experimental situations. The clinical relevance of the aforementioned effects remains unknown. All effects of muscarinic stimulation are enhanced in the context of activation of the sympathetic nervous system. M3 receptors have vasodilatory properties. Because direct muscarinic innervation of the vasculature has not been demonstrated and acetylcholine is a local neurotransmitter, the exact role of these receptors as part of the parasympathetic nervous system is debatable. It appears that the pharmacologic effect of M3 receptors is mediated by receptor-mediated local release of nitric oxide.

Drugs that act at muscarinic receptors can do so by a number of mechanisms to produce their effects. The most common mechanisms of action and the relevant drugs are shown in Table 3-2.

DRUGS THAT ENHANCE MUSCARINIC ACTIVITY

Choline Esters

Acetylcholine itself is not a useful drug. It has been used in heart failure patients in experimental studies to assess peripheral vascular function (endothelial release of nitric oxide). It also has been used in patients with coronary artery disease during angiography to assess endothelial function. Its pharmacologic properties are nonselective and include the stimulation of all muscarinic and nicotinic sites. Therefore, an attempt has been made to develop synthetic analogues of acetylcholine that would have greater selectivity for specific subpopulations of muscarinic receptors. The only clinically useful agents that have emerged thus far from this effort are bethanechol and

TABLE 3-1 Types of Muscarinic Receptors

Receptor	Location	Effect	Mechanism	Agonists	Antagonist
M1 (neural)	Cortex, hippocampus	Memory?	Stimulates phospholipase C	Acetylcholine Oxytremorine McNa343	Atropine Pirenzepine
	Gastric parietal cells	Gastric acid secretion	Increased intracellular Ca^{2+}		
M2 (cardiac)	Enteric ganglia SA node	GI motility Slowed spontaneous depolarization	Inhibition of adenylate cyclase Activation of K^+ channels	Acetylcholine	Atropine, gallamine, AF-DX116
	Atrium	Shortened action, potential duration, decreased contractile force			
	AV node	Decreased speed of conduction			
	Ventricle	Decreased contractile force			
M3	Smooth muscle	Contraction	Increased phospholipase C	Acetylcholine	Atropine
	Vascular endothelium	Vasodilatation		Vasodilation via nitric oxide	Hexahydro-siladifenidol
	Secretory glands	Increased secretion			
M4	CNS	?	Like M2 via adenylate cyclase	Acetylcholine	?Himbacine
M5	CNS	?	?Increased phospholipase C	Acetylcholine	?

Key: AV, atrioventricular; CNS, central nervous system; GI, gastrointestinal; SA, sinoatrial.

TABLE 3-2 Mechanisms of Action of Drugs Active at Muscarinic Receptors

Mechanism of action	Effect	Drug	Comments
Choline esters	Mimic effect of acetylcholine at receptors	Bethanechol Methacholine Edrophonium	Moderate selectivity (see text)
Anticholin-esterases	Enhance effect of acetylcholine at receptors	Physostigmine Pyridostigmine Neostigmine Rivastigmine Donepezil Tacrine	Nicotinic and muscarinic effects are present
Muscarinic receptor antagonists	Compete for binding at postsynaptic receptor	Atropine Scopolamine	Minimal structural selectivity for different muscarinic receptor Selectivity reflects distribution/density of receptors Selectivity may be enhanced by route of administration

methacholine. Bethanechol is relatively selective for the urinary bladder and gastrointestinal tract. It has very little activity at M2 receptors in the heart. Methacholine is potentially useful in the diagnosis of reactive airway disease and has some activity at cardiac receptors. Pilocarpine is a naturally occurring muscarinic agent that has agonist properties principally at muscarinic receptors in the eye and in the gastrointestinal tract. Selective M1 receptor agonists have been developed for use in patients with Alzheimer's disease, with little evidence to date for their effectiveness.

Anticholinesterase Agents

The effects of acetylcholine at postsynaptic sites are a function of the concentration of the transmitter at the postsynaptic receptor site. The compound is inactivated by the enzyme acetylcholinesterase, which is readily demonstrable at high concentrations at the postsynaptic sites. Some of the enzyme is bound to the membrane at the synaptic cleft itself, and some floats free in the medium. Acetylcholine effects can be enhanced and prolonged by the inhibition of the action of acetylcholinesterase. Clinically available anticholinesterases are listed in Table 3-2. These agents reversibly inhibit cholinesterase activity at all receptor sites; therefore, their pharmacologic effects reflect not only muscarinic but also nicotinic actions. All of these drugs also inhibit the activity of butyryl-cholinesterase. This pseudocholinesterase is present in many sites of the body, including the liver and plasma. Anticholinesterase drug effects constitute an enhancement of the vagal stimulus on the heart. This leads to a shortening of the effective refractory period, a decrease in sinoatrial- and AV-nodal conduction times, and a diminution of cardiac output. This is modified somewhat by effects at nicotinic receptors. In addition, with persistent stimulation, a paradoxical decrease in effect will occur. Therefore, with high doses and longer duration of action, a paradoxical decrease in acetylcholine effect can be seen. All of these agents have significant potential for noncardiac effects, including gastrointestinal (increased contraction, acidity, propulsion), skeletal muscle (enhanced activity), and pulmonary effects (enhanced bronchoconstriction).

The anticholinesterase with the shortest duration of action is edrophonium. When given intravenously, it has an onset of effect within 30 to 60 s and a duration of effect that is generally shorter than 10 min, although longer durations of action may be seen in some susceptible individuals. Given this pharmacodynamic profile, edrophonium has been used for the acute diagnosis of myasthenia gravis and for the diagnosis and acute termination of paroxysmal supraventricular tachycardia. Cardiac disease is listed by the manufacturer of edrophonium as a reason for caution in its use, and the US Food and Drug Administration has not approved the drug for use in the management of cardiac disease. However, many clinicians have used the drug's capacity to produce acute and intense muscarinic effects as a way of diagnosing atrial arrhythmias after other routine measures have failed. Occasionally, edrophonium is used for the acute control of heart rate, e.g., slowing heart rate in the context of an evaluation of demand pacemaker functioning. As a single dose, edrophonium should not exceed 10 mg. In older or sicker patients, the maximal dose may need to be reduced to 5 to 7 mg. When the goal of therapy is to gradually decrease heart rate, the drug may be administered in 2-mg boluses up to a total dosage of 10 mg. Significantly higher doses of the drug have been used safely in other clinical contexts.

Recent articles have suggested that the diagnostic use of edrophonium in cardiovascular disease may be extended to include its administration during tilt-table testing as part of the evaluation for possible vasovagal syncope. It is also used in the diagnostic evaluation of patients with atypical chest pain syndromes in which response to acid infusion and edrophonium administration may identify those with esophageal sources of pain.

Edrophonium is a quaternary drug whose affinity is limited to peripheral nervous system synapses. In contrast, the new cholinesterase inhibitors that have been introduced for the treatment of Alzheimer's disease (tacrine, donepezil, rivastigmine, and galantamine) cross the blood–brain barrier to inhibit cholinesterase metabolism in the CNS.

Other anticholinesterases include physostigmine, pyridostigmine, neostigmine, and ambenonium. These drugs generally have not been found to have any significant role in the management of cardiovascular disease. However, they are used in other areas of medicine; therefore, it is important to be familiar with the indications for their use and their potential cardiac side effects. Perhaps the most important use for some of these drugs is in the immediate reversal of neuromuscular blockade during general anesthesia. They will reverse the effects of nondepolarizing muscular blocking agents such as tubocurarine, metocurine, gallamine, vecuronium, atracurium, and pancuronium. When titrated appropriately with close monitoring of their effects on neuromuscular blockade, the cardiac effects of these drugs are generally not a problem. On occasion, however, they may produce the syndrome of excessive parasympathetic effect. Because they have no effect on the muscle blockade produced by depolarizing agents such as succinylcholine or decamethonium, these drugs should not be used in that context.

Ambenonium, pyridostigmine, and neostigmine are commonly used for the management of myasthenia gravis. They also may be used to improve bladder function postoperatively.

Physostigmine is used in topical ophthalmic medications for the treatment of glaucoma. Because this drug is a tertiary amine and penetrates into the CNS more than other agents in this class, there has been sporadic interest in its potential use in enhancing cholinergic transmission in the CNS for patients with Alzheimer's disease.

DRUGS THAT DIMINISH MUSCARINIC ACTIVITY

Muscarinic Receptor Antagonists

Atropine is the best known of the muscarinic receptor antagonists. Atropine has a dose-related effect on muscarinic receptors. At its lowest doses, a relatively selective effect on salivary secretion and sweating is demonstrated; at higher doses, it exhibits cardiac effects and more diffuse anticholinergic effects that include nicotinic and muscarinic blockade. Atropine's dose–response curve is described in Table 3-3. It has been reported that Chinese individuals show an increased sensitivity to atropine that is independent of resting vagal and sympathetic tone. At low doses (<0.5 mg), it may produce a paradoxical and usually mild slowing of heart rate. The mechanism for this mild bradycardia has been debated. It has been attributed by some investigators to a central stimulation of vagal afferents. At higher doses, atropine causes a progressive vagolytic effect on the heart, with increased heart rate, decreased refractory period of the AV node, and increased AV conduction velocity. Atropine is indicated for use in the acute treatment of severe symptomatic bradycardia, particularly in the context of acute myocardial infarction. On rare occasions, when it may be hypothesized that endogenous sympathetic activity is suppressed by parasympathetic effects of vagal stimulation, atropine has been thought to precipitate ventricular arrhythmias. For this reason, it is clear that the drug should not be used casually; its use should be restricted to cases of severe symptomatic bradycardia.

Because atropine counteracts bradycardia or heart block produced by acetylcholine or its analogues, it can be used to counteract the cardiac effects of any syndromes in which vagal nerve stimulation plays an important role. The drug therefore can block the bradycardia and hypotension seen in vasovagal syndromes. Because atropine is available only as a parenteral injection and because its effects are relatively brief, it is useful only for acute reversal of bradyarrhythmias and has no role in chronic management of these conditions.

A selective muscarinic antagonist for the M2 receptor is available (tryptamine), which has the potential for use in treating cholinergic bradycardia.

Atropine has also been investigated recently for its potential utility as an adjunct to dobutamine-stress echocardiography. Atropine has been given as a secondary medication for the enhancement of cardiac response, for which dobutamine infusion has limited success in producing the desired tachycardia, in particular for patients receiving beta blockers. In this regard, acetylcholine

TABLE 3-3 Dose–Effect Relation for Atropine

Dose (mg)	Pharmacologic effect
0.0–0.5	Mild bradycardia, dry mouth, decreased sweating
0.5–1.0	Cardioacceleration, very dry mouth, some pupillary dilation
1.0–2.0	Tachycardia (potentially symptomatic), very dry mouth, pupillary dilation, blurred vision
>3.0	All of the preceding, except more marked, and including erythematous, hot skin, increased intestinal tone, urinary retention; at highest doses, excitement and agitation lead to delirium or ultimately to coma, accompanied by fevers and scarlet skin

has been seen to induce ventricular tachycardia when employed as part of a spasm provocation test.

There are other drugs with muscarinic blocking effects like those of atropine, but they have not had a significant role in cardiovascular therapy. Instead, their use has been largely confined to delivery systems designed to provide therapeutic benefit without cardiac effects. Ipratropium bromide (Atrovent) and tiotropium (Spiriva) are quaternary ammonium compounds with atropine-like effects that are commonly used as inhalational agents for the reversal of cholinergically mediated bronchoconstriction. Ipratropium bromide has had its greatest clinical utility in the management of patients with chronic obstructive pulmonary disease. As a quaternary ammonium compound, ipratropium is very inefficiently absorbed from the pulmonary vascular bed. Approximately 1% of a dose is absorbed systemically. Most of this absorption is probably secondary to oral absorption of swallowed drug. It is possible that, on rare occasions, systemic effects from this drug might be seen.

Scopolamine continues to be available as a parenteral drug, but it is very rarely used. Its most common use at this time is in a transdermal patch preparation that delivers a low, continuous dose of drug over a 2- to 3-day period for the treatment of motion sickness. On occasion—due to changes in the permeability of skin, excessive dosing (several patches at once), or careless handling of the patches—a significant systemic effect from this drug can be seen. Transdermal scopolamine has been investigated as an antiarrhythmic drug in patients with acute myocardial infarction and congestive heart failure, but it is not indicated for these conditions.

ADDITIONAL READINGS

Bonner TI, Buckley NJ, Young AC, Brann MR: Identification of a family of muscarinic receptor genes. *Science* 237:527, 1987.

Brown JH, Taylor P: Muscarinic receptor agonists and antagonists, in Hardman JG, Limbird LE (eds): *Goodman & Gilman's the Pharmacological Basis of Therapeutics,* 10th ed. New York, McGraw-Hill, 2001, p 155.

Caulfield MP: Muscarinic receptors: Characterization, coupling and function. *Pharmacol Ther* 58:319, 1993.

Hoffman BB, Taylor P: Neurotransmission: The autonomic and somatic motor nervous systems, in Hardman JG, Limbird LE (eds): *Goodman & Gilman's the Pharmacological Basis of Therapeutics,* 10th ed. New York, McGraw-Hill, 2001, p 115.

Levine RR, Birdsall NJM (eds): Subtypes of muscarinic receptors: V. *Life Sci* 52 (suppl):405, 1993.

Marine JE, Watanabe MA, Smith TW, Monahan KM: Effects of atropine on heart rate turbulence. *Am J Cardiol* 89:767, 2002.

Meisner JS, Shirani J, Alaeddini J, et al: Use of pharmaceuticals in noninvasive cardiovascular diagnosis. *Heart Dis* 4:315, 2002.

Meyer BR, Frishman WH: Cholinergic and anticholinergic drugs, in Frishman WH, Sonnenblick EH, Sica DA (eds): *Cardiovascular Pharmacotherapeutics,* 2nd ed. New York, McGraw-Hill, 2003, pp 99–103.

Sueda S, Saeki H, Otani T, et al: Major complications during spasm provocation tests with an intracoronary injection of acetylcholine. *Am J Cardiol* 85:391, 2000.

Taylor P: Anticholinesterase agents, in Hardman JG, Limbird LE (eds): *Goodman & Gilman's the Pharmacological Basis of Therapeutics,* 10th ed. New York, McGraw-Hill, 2001, p 175.

Tio RA, Monnink SHJ, Amoroso G, et al: Safety evaluation of routine intracoronary acetylcholine infusion in patients undergoing a first diagnostic coronary angiogram. *J Investig Med* 50:133, 2002.

4 | Calcium Channel Blockers

William H. Frishman   Domenic A. Sica

The calcium channel blockers are a heterogeneous group of drugs with widely variable effects on heart muscle, sinus node function, atrioventricular (AV) conduction, peripheral blood vessels, and coronary circulation. Ten of these drugs—nifedipine, nicardipine, nimodipine, nisoldipine, felodipine, isradipine, amlodipine, verapamil, diltiazem, and bepridil—are approved in the United States for clinical use. Other agents under investigation that are available for clinical use outside the United States include barnidipine, benidipine, cilnidipine, clevidipine, lacidipine, lercanidipine, and manidipine.

PHYSIOLOGIC BACKGROUND

Calcium ions play a fundamental role in the activation of cells. An influx of calcium ions into the cell through specific ion channels is required for myocardial contraction, for determining peripheral vascular resistance through calcium dependent-regulated tone of vascular smooth muscle, and for helping to initiate the pacemaker tissues of the heart, which are activated largely by the slow calcium current.

The concept of calcium channel inhibition originated in 1960, when it was noted that prenylamine, a newly developed coronary vasodilator, depressed cardiac performance in canine heart and lung preparations. Initial studies with verapamil showed that it exerted negative inotropic effects on the isolated myocardium in addition to having vasodilator properties. These potent negative inotropic effects seemed to differentiate these drugs from the classic coronary vasodilators, such as nitroglycerin and papaverine, which have little, if any, myocardial depressant activity. Unlike β-adrenergic antagonists, many of the calcium antagonists depress cardiac contractility without altering the height or contour of the monophasic action potential and thus can interfere with excitation and contraction coupling. Reversible closure of specific calcium ion channels in the membrane of the mammalian myocardial cell was suggested as the explanation of these observed effects.

Subsequently, the effects of verapamil on atrial and ventricular intracellular potentials were studied. Antiarrhythmic compounds were classified into local anesthetics, which decreased the maximum rate of depolarization; beta blockers; and a third class, which prolonged the duration of the cardiac action potential. However, none of these electrophysiologic actions could explain the antiarrhythmic effect of verapamil. Thus, a fourth class of antiarrhythmic drug, typified by verapamil, was proposed, with effects separate from those of sodium channel inhibitors and beta blockers. The antiarrhythmic actions and negative inotropic effects of verapamil have been shown to be mediated predominantly through interference with calcium conductance.

CHEMICAL STRUCTURE AND PHARMACODYNAMICS

Structure of the Calcium Channel Blockers

Diltiazem is a benzothiazepine derivative that is structurally unrelated to other vasodilators. Nifedipine is a dihydropyridine derivative unrelated to the nitrates, which is lipophilic and is inactivated by light. Nicardipine, amlodipine, felodipine, isradipine, nisoldipine, and nimodipine are also dihydropyridine derivatives similar in structure to nifedipine. Verapamil [(+)verapamil] has some structural similarity to papaverine. Bepridil, which is currently available for treatment of angina pectoris, is not related chemically to other cardioactive drugs.

Differential Effects on Slow Channels

The most important characteristic of all calcium channel blockers is their ability to selectively inhibit the inward flow of charge-bearing calcium ions when the calcium ion channels become permeable. Previously, the term *slow channel* was used, but it has recently been recognized that the calcium ion current develops faster than previously thought and that there are at least two types of calcium channels, L and T. The conventional calcium channel, which has been known for a long time to exist, is called the L channel. It is blocked by all the calcium channel antagonists and has its permeability increased by catecholamines. The T-type channel appears at more negative potentials than the L-type channel and likely plays an important role in the initial depolarization of sinus and AV nodal tissues. The function of the L-type channel is to admit the substantial amount of calcium ions required for initiation of contraction via calcium release from the sarcoplasmic reticulum. Mibefradil is the first calcium channel blocker that has selective blocking properties on the T-type channel in addition to its blocking effects on the L-type channel. Specific blockers for the T-type channel are not yet available, but they are expected to inhibit the sinus and AV nodes profoundly.

Bepridil possesses all the characteristics of the traditional calcium antagonists. In addition, the drug appears to affect the sodium channel (fast channel) and possibly the potassium channel, producing a quinidine-like effect. Bepridil specifically inhibits maximal upstroke velocity, i.e., the influx of sodium in appropriate load dosages. The effect of bepridil on the maximum rate of depolarization has been examined; the action potential height does not change, but the action potential duration extends in a quinidine-like manner.

CARDIOVASCULAR EFFECTS

Effects on Muscular Contraction

Calcium is the primary ionic link between neurologic excitation and mechanical contraction of cardiac, smooth, and skeletal muscles. Actin and myosin are the protein filaments that slide past one another in the adenosine triphosphate-dependent contractile process of all muscle cells. In myocardial cells, the regulatory proteins tropomyosin and troponin inhibit this process. When the myocardial cell membrane repolarizes, calcium enters the cell (L channel) and triggers the release of additional calcium from internal stores within the sarcoplasmic reticulum. Calcium released from this large intracellular reservoir then initiates contraction by combining with the inhibitors troponin and tropomyosin. Previously hidden active sites on actin molecules are then available for binding by myosin.

Effects on Coronary and Peripheral Arterial Blood Vessels

The contraction of vascular smooth muscle such as that found in the coronary arteries is slightly different from the contraction of cardiac and skeletal muscles (Table 4-1). Myosin must be phosphorylated, and calmodulin is the regulatory protein to which calcium binds. In addition, vascular smooth muscle cells have significantly less intracellular calcium stores than do myocardial cells and so rely more heavily on the influx of extracellular calcium.

The observation that calcium channel blockers are significantly more effective in inhibiting contraction in coronary and peripheral arterial smooth muscles than in cardiac and skeletal muscles is of great clinical importance. This differential effect is explained by the observation that arterial smooth muscle is more dependent on external calcium entry for contraction, whereas cardiac and skeletal muscles rely on a recirculating internal pool of calcium. Because calcium entry blockers are membrane-active drugs, they reduce the entry of calcium into cells and therefore exert a much greater effect on vascular wall contraction. This preferential effect allows calcium entry blockers to dilate coronary and peripheral arteries in doses that do not severely affect myocardial contractility or have little, if any, effect on skeletal muscle.

It has been shown recently that dihydropyridines can induce the release of nitric oxide (NO) from the vascular endothelium of various blood vessels. In addition, in several preparations, including micro- and macrovasculature, the sensitivity of the vasorelaxing effects of the dihydropyridines to inhibitors of NO synthase, such as L-N^G-nitro-arginine or L-nitro-arginine-methyl-ester, has been demonstrated. These findings for a dual mode of action of dihydropyridines—i.e., the direct relaxing effect by inhibition of the smooth muscle L-type calcium ion channel and the indirect relaxing effect by the release of NO from vascular endothelium—may explain the highly potent vasodilatory actions of these drugs. In addition, an anti-endothelin action of calcium channel blockers has been described, as has an inhibitory effect on matrix metalloproteinase 1.

Effects on Veins

The calcium channel blockers seem to be less active in veins than in arteries and are ineffective at therapeutic doses (in contrast to nitrates) for increasing venous capacitance.

Effects on Myocardial Contractility

Force generation during cardiac muscle contraction depends in part on calcium influx during membrane depolarization (see Table 4-1). In isolated myocardial preparations, all calcium channel antagonists have been demonstrated to exert potent negative inotropic effects. In guinea pig atria exposed to drug concentration of 1026 mol/L, the order of potency for depressing the maximal rate of force development during constant pacing was found to be nifedipine and then verapamil and diltiazem. In dog papillary muscle, developed tension also was decreased most markedly by nifedipine; the relative potencies (on a weight basis) of verapamil and diltiazem were $1/15$ and $1/40$, respectively. The negative inotropic effect of the calcium channel antagonists are dose dependent. The excitation–contraction coupling of vascular smooth muscle is three to ten times more sensitive to the action of calcium channel antagonists than is that of myocardial fibers. Hence, the relatively low doses of these drugs used in vivo to produce vasodilatation or beneficial antiarrhythmic effects may not produce significant negative inotropic effects. Further, in intact animals and human beings, the intrinsic negative inotropic properties of these compounds are greatly modified by a baroreceptor-mediated reflex augmentation of β-adrenergic tone consequent to vasodilatation

TABLE 4-1 Pharmacologic Effects of Calcium Channel Blockers

	Heart rate		Conduction		Myocardial coronary	Peripheral contractility	CO	Coronary BF	MVO$_2$ demand
	Acute	Chronic	SA node	AV node					
Diltiazem	↓	↓	↓	↓	↑	↓	V	↑	↓
Bepridil	↓	↓	↓	↓	V↑	—	V	↑	↓
Verapamil	↓	↓	↓	↓	↑	↓↓	V	↑	↓
Amlodipine	↑	↓—	—	—	—	↓↓	↑—	↑	↓
Felodipine	↑	↑—	—	—	—	↓↓	↑—	↑	↓
Isradipine	↑	↑—	—	—	—	↓↓	↑—	↑	↓
Nicardipine	↑	↑—	—	—	↑	↓↓	↑—	↑	↓
Nifedipine	↑	↑—	—	—	—	V↓	↑—	↑	↓
Nimodipine	↑	↑—	—	—	—	↓↓	↑—	↑	↓
Nisoldipine	↑	↑—	—	—	—	↓↓	↑—	↑	↓

Key: —, no change; ↑, increase; ↓, decrease; AV, atrioventricular; BF, blood flow; CO, cardiac output; MVO$_2$, myocardial oxygen; SA, sinoatrial; V, variable.

Source: Reproduced with permission from Frishman WH, Stroh JA, Greenberg SM, et al: Calcium channel blockers in systemic hypertension. *Med Clin North Am* 71:449, 1988.

and a decrease in blood pressure. Nifedipine and other dihydropyridines, which exert the greatest vasodilator effects among these agents, accordingly produce the strongest reflex β-adrenergic response and the one most likely to offset the negative inotropic activity of the drugs and lead to enhancement of ventricular performance. Although this mechanism plays an important role in patients with normal or nearly normal left ventricular function, it is unlikely to play a similar role in patients with severe congestive heart failure, in whom the baroreceptor sensitivity is markedly attenuated. Regarding the newer calcium channel blockers, the hemodynamic profile of amlodipine was compared with those of verapamil and diltiazem in conscious normotensive rats. Verapamil and diltiazem were negatively inotropic. Amlodipine decreased left ventricular contractility only at the highest dose used.

Electrophysiologic Effects

Although verapamil, nifedipine, diltiazem, and bepridil depress cardiac contractility with only quantitative differences (see Table 4-1), their effects on the electrophysiology of the heart are different qualitatively. Local anesthetic actions of bepridil, diltiazem, and particularly verapamil may account for some of these differences. Nifedipine and other dihydropyridines have a more selective action at the slow channels, whereas verapamil and diltiazem, at least at higher doses, also inhibit currents in the fast channels in the manner of the local anesthetics. Bepridil has definite class I antiarrhythmic properties.

Verapamil and diltiazem prolong the conduction and refractoriness in the AV node; the A-H interval is lengthened more than is the H-V interval. In therapeutic concentrations, there are no demonstrable actions on the rate of depolarization or the repolarization phases of the action potentials in atrial, ventricular, and Purkinje fibers. The rate of discharge of the sinus node, which depends on the calcium ion current, is depressed by all calcium channel blockers. In vivo, this effect can be compensated or overcompensated for by activation of baroreceptor reflexes, which increase sympathetic nervous activity.

The antiarrhythmic actions of verapamil and diltiazem relate to their effects on nodal cardiac tissues. In sinoatrial (SA) and AV nodal cells, the drugs modify slow-channel electropotentials in three ways: (a) there is a decrease in the rate of rise and slope of diastolic slow depolarization and an increase in the membrane threshold potential, which reduces the rate of firing in the cell; (b) the action potential upstroke is decreased in amplitude, which slows conduction; and (c) the duration of the action potential is increased. These electrophysiologic effects are dose related, and above the clinical range electrical standstill may occur in SA and AV nodal cells. These and other observations support the concept that slow-channel activity is important in the generation of pacemaker potential in the SA node.

Verapamil and diltiazem also exert a depressant effect on the AV node and in low concentrations prolong the effective refractory period. Unlike β-adrenergic blocking drugs and vagomimetic interventions, which depress AV node transmission by altering autonomic impulse traffic, verapamil and diltiazem prolong AV nodal refractoriness directly. However, verapamil may have additional vagomimetic effects.

PHARMACOKINETICS

Although calcium entry blockers are classified together, there are differences in their pharmacokinetic properties (Table 4-2). Differences in completeness

TABLE 4-2 Additional Pharmacokinetic Characteristics of Calcium Channel Blockers

Agent	Dosage Oral	Dosage IV	Onset of action (min) Oral	Onset of action (min) IV	Therapeutic PC (ng/mL)	Site of metabolism	Active metabolites	Excretion (%)
Diltiazem	30–90 mg q6–8 h	75–150 mg 10–20 mg	<30	<10	50–200	Deacetylation N-deacetylation O-demethylation Major hepatic first-pass effect	Yes	60 (fecal) 2–4 (unchanged in urine)
Diltiazem SR	60–120 mg q12 h		30–60		50–200			Yes
Diltiazem IV		0.25 mg/kg (20 mg)						
Diltiazem CD	180–360 mg q24 h		30–60		50–200		Yes	
Diltiazem XR	180–540 mg q24 h		30–60		40–200		Yes	
Diltiazem ER	120–540 mg q24 h				40–200		Yes	
Diltiazem LA	180–420 mg q24 h				40–200		Yes	
Verapamil	80–120 mg q6–12 h	150 µg/kg 10–20 mg	<30	<5	>100	N-dealkylation O-demethylation Major hepatic first-pass effect	Yes	15 (fecal) 70 (renal) 3–4 (unchanged in urine)
Verapamil SR	240–480 mg q12 or 24 h	<30	>50				Yes	15 (fecal) 70 (renal) 3–4 (unchanged in urine)

Drug	Dose							Elimination
Verelan (Verapamil SR)	120–480 mg q24 h				>50		Yes	16 (fecal) 70 (renal) 3–4 (unchanged in urine)
Verelan PM	200–400 mg q24 h							
Coer Verapamil	180–540 mg q24 h		4–5 h				Yes	16 (fecal) 70 (renal) 3–4 (unchanged in urine)
Verapamil IV		5–10 mg (0.075–0.15 mg/kg) 5–15 µg/kg						
Nifedipine	10–40 mg q6–8 h		<20	3 SL	25–100	A hydroxycarbolic acid and a lactone with no known activity Major hepatic first-pass effect	No	20–40 (fecal) 50–80 (renal) <0.1 (unchanged in urine)
Nifedipine CC Nifedipine GITS	30–90 mg/d 30–180 mg q24 h		<60 2 h		25–100		No No	
Nicardipine	10–20 mg tid	1.15 mg/h	<20	<5	28–50	Major hepatic first-pass effect	No	30 (fecal) 60 (renal) <1 (unchanged in urine)
Nicardipine SR	30–60 mg bid		20		28–50			35 (fecal) 60 (renal) <1 (unchanged in urine)
Nicardipine IV Nimodipine	60 mg q4 h	5–15 mg/h	4–5 h <30	<2–3	60–800 7	Hepatic Major hepatic first-pass effect	No No	

(continued)

TABLE 4-2 (continued) Additional Pharmacokinetic Characteristics of Calcium Channel Blockers

Agent	Dosage Oral	Dosage IV	Onset of action (min) Oral	Onset of action (min) IV	Therapeutic PC (ng/mL)	Site of metabolism	Active metabolites	Excretion (%)
Nisoldipine ER	20–40 mg q24 h					Hepatic hydroxylation	Yes	80 (renal) <1 (unchanged in urine)
Amlodipine	5–10 mg q24 h		90–120 in vitro		6–10	Oxidation extensive but slow hepatic metabolism	No	20–25 (fecal) 60 (renal) 10 (unchanged in urine)
Isradipine	2.5–10 mg q12 h		120			Hepatic de-esterification and aromatization	No	30 (fecal) 70 (renal) 0 (unchanged in urine)
Isradipine CR	5–20 mg q24 h		2–3 h					25–30 (fecal) ‖ 60–65 (renal)
Felodipine ER	5–20 mg q24 h		2–5 h		2–20 nmol/L	Hepatic microsomal P450 system oxidation Major hepatic first-pass effect	No	10 (fecal) 60–70 (renal) <0.5 (unchanged in urine and feces)
Bepridil	200–400 mg		30–60		1200–3500		Yes	70 (renal) 20 (fecal)

Key: ↓↓, decrease; bid, twice daily; CC, core coat; CD, controlled delivery; CR, continuous release; ER, extended release; GITS, gastrointestinal therapeutic system; IV, intravenous; LA, long acting; PC, plasma concentrations; PM, evening hours; q, every; SL, sublingual; SR, sustained release; tid, thrice daily; XR, extended release.
Source: Adapted with permission from Frishman WH, Sonnenblick EH: Calcium channel blockers, in Schlant RC, Alexander RW (eds): Hurst's the Heart, 8th ed. New York, McGraw-Hill, 1994, p 1291.

of gastrointestinal absorption, amount of first-pass hepatic metabolism, protein binding, extent of distribution in the body, and the pharmacologic actions of different metabolites may influence the clinical usefulness of these drugs in different patients.

Because many of the calcium channel blockers are relatively short acting, they are now available in various sustained-release delivery systems: diffusion type (diltiazem, verapamil), bio-erosion (diltiazem, nifedipine, nicardipine), osmosis (verapamil, isradipine, nifedipine), and diffusion erosion (felodipine). Nisoldipine was approved as a once-daily therapy in the coat-core formulation, and verapamil became available in two different delayed-onset sustained-release drug delivery systems. Diltiazem is currently available in a delayed-onset graded-release formulation. Nitrendipine is being evaluated as a transdermal formulation.

After administration of a certain oral dose, the calcium entry blocking drugs, which are metabolized largely in the liver, show greater interindividual variations in circulating plasma levels. In angina pectoris and hypertension, wide individual differences also exist in the relation between plasma concentrations of calcium entry blockers and the associated therapeutic effect.

Various dihydropyridine calcium channel blockers (felodipine, nifedipine, nisoldipine) should not be administered with grapefruit juice or Seville orange juice, because these juices have been shown to interfere with the drug's metabolism, resulting in about a threefold mean increase in C_{max} and an almost twofold mean increase in area under the plasma concentration versus time curve.

The pharmacokinetics of calcium channel blockers are minimally affected by renal failure. Further, the drugs are not dialyzable. The predictability of the kinetic profile of the calcium channel blockers in renal failure simplifies their use in end-stage renal disease.

CLINICAL APPLICATIONS

The calcium channel blockers are available in the United States for the treatment of patients with angina pectoris (diltiazem, nifedipine, amlodipine, nicardipine, verapamil, bepridil), for chronic treatment of systemic hypertension (verapamil, isradipine, diltiazem, amlodipine, nicardipine, nisoldipine, felodipine), for the management of hypertensive emergencies and perioperative hypertension (intravenous nicardipine), for treatment and prophylaxis of supraventricular arrhythmias (verapamil, diltiazem), and for reducing morbidity and mortality in patients with subarachnoid hemorrhage (nimodipine). These drugs are also being evaluated and used for a multitude of other cardiovascular and noncardiovascular conditions.

Angina Pectoris

The antianginal mechanisms of calcium entry blockers are complex (Table 4-3). The drugs exert vasodilator effects on the coronary and peripheral vessels and depressant effects on cardiac contractility, heart rate, and conduction; all these actions may be important in mediating the antianginal effects of the drugs. These drugs not only are mild dilators of epicardial vessels not in spasm but also markedly attenuate sympathetically mediated and ergonovine-induced coronary vasoconstriction; these actions provide a rational basis for effective-

TABLE 4-3 Hemodynamic Effects of Calcium Entry Blockers on
Myocardial Oxygen Supply and Demand*

	Verapamil	Nifedipine	Diltiazem	Bepridil
Demand				
Wall tension	↑↔	↔ reflex	↔	↔
Systolic blood pressure	↓	↓	↓	↔
Ventricular volume	↑	↔	↔	↔
Heart rate	↓↔	↑ reflex	↓↔	↓↔
Contractility	↓↓	↓	↓	↓
Supply				
Coronary blood flow	↑	↑↑	↑	↑
Coronary vascular resistance	↓	↓↓	↓	↓
Spasm	↓	↓	↓	↓
Diastolic perfusion time	↑↔	↓	↑↔	↑↔
Collateral blood flow	↔	↑	↑	↔

*Heart rate may increase sharply but decreases with long-term use.
Key: ↑, increase; ↓, decrease; ↔, no apparent effect.
Source: Adapted from Frishman WH, Sonnenblick EH: Calcium channel blockers, in Schlant RC, Alexander RW (eds): Hurst's the Heart, 8th ed. New York, McGraw-Hill, 1994, p 1291.

ness of the drugs in vasospastic ischemic syndromes. In patients with exertional angina pectoris, the peripheral vasodilator actions of diltiazem and verapamil and the inhibitory effects on the sinus node serve to attenuate the increases in double product that normally accompany and serve to limit exercise.

Stable Angina Pectoris

Multiple double-blind, placebo-controlled studies have clearly confirmed the efficacy of diltiazem, nifedipine, amlodipine, nicardipine, verapamil, and bepridil in stable angina pectoris, with patients showing a reduction in chest pain attacks and nitroglycerin consumption and improved exercise tolerance. Calcium entry blockers, for the most part, appear to be as safe and effective as beta blockers and nitrates when used as monotherapies. They also can be used as single-dose therapies in hypertensive patients with angina.

In choosing between a calcium channel antagonist and a β-adrenergic blocking drug in the management of patients with effort-related symptoms, it is apparent that some patients do better with one drug than with the other, although beta blockers are considered the preferred first-line therapy. Unfortunately, little is known about how to predict with confidence the superior agent in a specific patient without a therapeutic trial. However, verapamil and diltiazem can be used as effective alternatives in patients who remain symptomatic despite therapy with beta blockers and as first-time antianginal drugs in patients with contraindications to beta blockade; the use of nifedipine as a first-line drug in its original formulation was limited by the reflex tachycardia and potential aggravation of angina that accompanied its use. However, this is not a problem with the nifedipine gastrointestinal therapeutic system formulation or with amlodipine.

Diltiazem is also approved as a once-daily treatment for angina pectoris in a sustained-delivery formulation. A delayed-release, sustained-release formulation of verapamil has been compared with atenolol, amlodipine, and the combination of amlodipine plus atenolol in patients with angina pectoris and has been shown to be as effective in improving exercise tolerance and markers of silent ischemia.

Bepridil is available in doses of 200 to 400 mg once daily for use in patients with angina pectoris who are refractory to other antianginal drug therapy. Close monitoring of patients with this drug is necessary at the onset of therapy, because a small percentage of patients can have a prolongation of the QT interval on the electrocardiogram (ECG). Bepridil can be combined with a beta blocker, if necessary.

The comparative effects of abrupt withdrawal of verapamil and propranolol in patients with angina pectoris have been studied. Ten percent of patients with stable effort-related symptoms experienced a severe clinical exacerbation of the anginal syndrome upon withdrawal of propranolol; no patient experienced rebound symptoms when verapamil was abruptly discontinued. There also appear to be no major withdrawal reactions with nifedipine and diltiazem.

Angina at Rest

Patients with angina at rest have a wide spectrum of disorders, ranging from those with variant angina (ST-segment elevation) associated with angiographically normal coronary arteries to those with unstable angina with ST-segment depression or elevation associated with multivessel coronary artery disease. Studies have suggested that coronary vasospasm and or thrombosis plays a major role in the pathogenesis of ischemia in most patients with angina at rest, regardless of the coronary anatomy. In clinical trials, calcium channel antagonists were effective in this syndrome because of their ability to block spontaneous and drug-induced spasm.

The comparative efficacy of verapamil and propranolol was assessed in a randomized, double-blind, crossover trial in rest angina. Only verapamil reduced symptomatic and asymptomatic episodes of ischemia. These findings are consistent with the concept that coronary vasospasm plays a crucial role in patients with angina at rest; in contrast, rather than providing any benefit, propranolol may exacerbate vasospastic phenomena.

Another study assessed the comparative efficacy of verapamil and nifedipine. Verapamil and nifedipine proved equally effective, and neither drug depressed ventricular function at rest or during exercise. Accordingly, in the management of patients with variant angina, the choice of a calcium antagonist is likely to be determined not so much by which drug is more effective but by which agent is better tolerated by an individual patient.

The usefulness of calcium channel antagonists as an adjunctive therapy in the long-term management of unstable angina was demonstrated in a double-blind, placebo-controlled, randomized clinical trial showing that the addition of nifedipine to patients receiving nitrates and propranolol can reduce the number of patients with unstable anginal syndromes requiring surgery for relief of pain; the incidence of sudden death and myocardial infarction was similar in the two groups. However, clinical benefits were largely confined to patients whose pain was accompanied by ST-segment elevation. Current guidelines suggest that calcium channel blockers be used as adjunctive therapy in patients with unstable angina.

Combination Therapy in Angina Pectoris

Combination therapy with nitrates and or beta blockers may be more efficacious for the treatment of angina pectoris than one drug used alone. The hemodynamic effects of a calcium blocker/beta blocker combination are

TABLE 4-4 Hemodynamic Effects of Calcium Entry Blockers, Beta Blockers, and Combination Treatment

	Calcium blockers	Beta blockers	Combination
Heart rate	↓↔↑ reflex	↓	↓↔
Contractility	↓↔ reflex	↓	↓↔
Wall tension	↓	↔	↓
Systolic blood pressure	↓	↓	↓
Left ventricular volume	↓↔	↑	↑↔
Coronary resistance	↓	↑↔	↓↔

Key: ↑, increase; ↓, decrease; ↔, no change.
Source: Reproduced with permission from Frishman WH: Beta-adrenergic blockade in the treatment of coronary artery disease, in Hurst JW (ed): *Clinical Essays on the Heart.* New York, McGraw-Hill, 1984. p 48.

shown in Table 4-4. Because adverse effects can occur from this combination (heart block, severe bradycardia, congestive heart failure), patients must be carefully selected and observed. The hemodynamic effects of combined nitrate/calcium channel blocker therapy are shown in Table 4-5. Hypotension should be avoided. Different calcium channel blockers also may be combined (nifedipine with verapamil or diltiazem) with added benefit; however, compared with monotherapy, side effects may be prohibitive.

Arrhythmias

Sinus Tachycardia

In an intensive care setting, intravenous diltiazem has been used successfully to treat sinus tachycardia in critically ill patients in whom beta blockers were contraindicated.

TABLE 4-5 Hemodynamic Rationale for Combining Nitrates and Calcium Channel Blockers in Angina Pectoris

	Nitrates	Calcium channel blockers	Combination
Heart rate	↑ reflex	↓↔↑	↔↑ reflex
Blood pressure	↓	↓	↓↓
Heart size	↓	↓↔↑	0
Contractility	↑ reflex	↓	0
Venomotor tone	↓	0	↓
Peripheral resistance	↓	↓	↓↓
Coronary resistance	↓	↓	↓↓
Coronary blood flow	↑	↑	↑↑
Collateral blood flow	↑	↑	↑↑

Key: ↑, increase; ↓, decrease; ↓↓?, questionable additive effects; ↔, no change.
Source: Reproduced with permission from Frishman WH: Beta-adrenergic blockade in the treatment of coronary artery disease, in Hurst JW (ed): *Clinical Essays on the Heart.* New York, McGraw-Hill, 1984, p 48.

TABLE 4-6 Effects of Diltiazem and Verapamil in Treatment
of Common Arrhythmias

Effective	Ineffective
Sinus tachycardia	Nonparoxysmal automatic atrial
Supraventricular tachycardia	tachycardia
AV nodal reentrant PSVT	Atrial fibrillation and flutter in WPW
Accessory pathway reentrant	syndrome (ventricular rate may not
PSVT SA nodal reentrant PSVT	decrease)
Atrial reentrant PSVT	Ventricular tachyarrhythmias*
Atrial flutter (ventricular rate	
decreases but arrhythmia will	
only occasionally convert)	
Atrial fibrillation (ventricular rate	
decreases but arrhythmia will only	
occasionally convert)	

* There is only limited experience in this area.
Key: AV, atrioventricular; PSVT, paroxysmal supraventricular tachycardia;
SA, sinoatrial; WPW, Wolff-Parkinson-White syndrome.
Source: Reproduced with permission from Frishman WH, LeJemtel TH:
Electropharmacology of calcium channel antagonists in cardiac arrhythmias.
Pace 5:402, 1982.

Atrial Fibrillation

Except in rare situations, verapamil and diltiazem are ineffective in converting
acute and chronic atrial fibrillations to normal sinus rhythm, and verapamil
does not prevent long-term tachycardia-induced atrial electrical remodeling
(Table 4-6). However, diltiazem and verapamil (oral and intravenous) are
effective for decreasing and controlling ventricular rate during atrial fibrillation by prolonging AV nodal conduction and refractoriness, thereby increasing
AV block at rest and during exercise. Clinical trials with verapamil in patients
with atrial fibrillation have indicated that its ability to decrease ventricular rate
appears to be unrelated to the chronicity of the arrhythmia, its etiology, or the
patient's age. Verapamil appears to be more effective than digoxin in slowing
the rapid ventricular rate in response to physical activity. Diltiazem or verapamil can be used orally in combination with digoxin in treating rapid heart
rates in patients with acute and chronic atrial fibrillation and flutter.

It has been demonstrated that verapamil treatment can maintain normal
sinus rhythm in patients undergoing electrocardioversion for atrial fibrillation.
Pretreatment with diltiazem has been shown to prevent atrial arrhythmias
after thoracic surgery.

Paroxysmal Supraventricular Tachycardia

Virtually all cases of supraventricular tachycardia (SVT) due to intranodal
reentry and those related to circus movement type of tachycardia in preexcitation respond promptly and predictably to intravenous verapamil or diltiazem,
whereas only about two-thirds of ectopic atrial tachycardias convert to sinus
rhythm after adequate doses of the drug (see Table 4-6). Intravenous verapamil and diltiazem are highly efficacious in treating reentry paroxysmal
SVT regardless of etiology or age. The recommended dosage range of vera-

pamil for terminating paroxysmal SVT in adults is 0.075 to 1.5 mg/kg infused over 1 to 3 min and repeated at 30 min. In patients with myocardial dysfunction, the dose should be reduced. Children have been treated safely with a regimen of 0.075 to 0.15 mg. The recommended dose of diltiazem is 0.25 mg/kg infused over 2 min and repeated at 0.35 mg/kg after 15 min.

There have been few clinical studies comparing intravenous verapamil and diltiazem with other standard regimens in the treatment of paroxysmal SVT. However, in a number of clinical situations, verapamil and diltiazem may offer an advantage over digitalis preparations or β-adrenergic blockers. For instance, verapamil is preferable in cases in which there is an urgent need to terminate paroxysmal SVT, because it can produce therapeutic responses within 3 min of infusion, whereas the effects of digoxin are not evident for approximately 30 min. Also, if drug therapy fails to achieve normal sinus rhythm, the short duration of action of verapamil and diltiazem permits earlier cardioversion without some of the dangers that accompany electrical cardioversion during digoxin therapy. Verapamil and diltiazem also offer distinct advantages over β-adrenergic blocking drugs in patients whose arrhythmias are associated with chronic obstructive lung disease or peripheral vascular disease.

Oral verapamil has been approved for prophylaxis against paroxysmal SVT in doses of 160 to 480 mg/day, and the treatment experiences have yielded favorable results. Diltiazem is not yet approved in oral form as an antiarrhythmic agent.

Atrial Flutter

The immediate effect of intravenous verapamil and diltiazem in atrial flutter in most patients is an increase in AV block that slows the ventricular response, rarely followed by a return to sinus rhythm (see Table 4-6). In some, the response occurs through the development of atrial fibrillation with a controlled ventricular response. A single intravenous dose of verapamil or diltiazem has been found to be of diagnostic value in differentiating rapid atrial flutter from paroxysmal SVT when these two arrhythmias are indistinguishable on the ECG. If the rhythm is atrial flutter, the AV block increases immediately, revealing the true nature of the arrhythmia. Oral verapamil also has been used to convert paroxysmal atrial flutter and reduce the rapid ventricular rates associated with this arrhythmia.

Preexcitation

Verapamil and diltiazem have been found to induce reversion of most cases of accessory pathway SVT. From intracardiac recordings of electrical activity during programmed electrical stimulation of the heart, data have become available regarding the actions of verapamil on the electrophysiologic properties of the accessory pathway in overt cases of the Wolff-Parkinson-White syndrome. The drug has a minimal effect on the antegrade and retrograde conduction times and on the refractory period. Verapamil and diltiazem, therefore, terminate accessory pathway paroxysmal SVT in the same manner as they do AV nodal reentrant paroxysmal SVT: by slowing AV nodal conduction and increasing refractoriness. The minimal effect of verapamil and diltiazem on the electrophysiologic properties of the bypass tract is consistent with the observation that the drug is ineffective in atrial fibrillation, thereby complicating Wolff-Parkinson-White syndrome, in which fibrillatory impulses, as with digoxin, conduct predominantly through the anomalous pathway. Under these circumstances, radiofrequency catheter ablation of the accessory pathways appears to be the therapy of choice.

Ventricular Arrhythmias

Intravenous verapamil and diltiazem provide no apparent benefit in ventricular arrhythmias except in acute myocardial infarction. Oral verapamil has no demonstrated role in the management of ventricular tachyarrhythmias. However, bepridil, with its class I antiarrhythmic activity, has been shown to be effective in the short- and long-term control of ventricular arrhythmias. Dihydropyridines do not appear to have a proarrhythmic effect in patients with myocardial ischemia.

Precautions in Treating Arrhythmias

A diseased SA node is much more sensitive to slow channel blockers and may be depressed to the point of atrial standstill. Sinus arrest also can occur without overt evidence of sick sinus syndrome. Calcium channel blockade also may suppress potential AV nodal escape rhythms that need to arise if atrial standstill occurs. In patients with the bradytachy form of sick sinus syndrome, digoxin or β-adrenoceptor blocking drugs probably should not be combined with verapamil or diltiazem in the prophylaxis of tachyarrhythmias unless a demand ventricular pacemaker is first inserted.

Systemic Hypertension

Calcium channel blockers are effective in the treatment of systemic hypertension and hypertensive emergencies. Calcium channel blocking drugs can be considered potential first-line therapy for initiating treatment in many patients with chronic hypertension. A vast experience in the United States has been collected from use of verapamil, diltiazem, nifedipine, amlodipine, nicardipine, felodipine, nisoldipine, and isradipine in patients with hypertension. Verapamil, nicardipine, nifedipine, nisoldipine, felodipine, and diltiazem are available in the United States in conventional and sustained-release oral formulations, allowing once- and twice-daily dosing. Verapamil and diltiazem are available in unique delayed-onset sustained-release delivery systems to provide a peak blood level at the time of blood pressure elevation during awakening.

Multiple studies have evaluated the effects of calcium channel blockers in elderly patients with isolated systolic hypertension (ISH). The Systolic Hypertension in Europe Study (SYST-EUR) was limited to patients 60 years and older with a resting systolic pressure of 160 to 219 mm Hg and a diastolic pressure below 95 mm Hg. Patients were randomized to receive nitrendipine or placebo. If additional blood pressure control was necessary, patients received an angiotensin-converting enzyme (ACE) inhibitor and then a diuretic. Compared with placebo, nitrendipine therapy was associated with significant reductions in the rate of stroke, major cardiovascular events, and cognitive disorders. Based on this study, the guidelines presented in the sixth report of the Joint National Committee on Detection, Evaluation and Treatment of High Blood Pressure included the use of dihydropyridine calcium antagonists in addition to thiazide diuretics as first-line treatment for ISH in the elderly.

The Systolic Hypertension in China (SYST-CHINA) study also looked at nitrendipine as a first-line treatment modality compared with placebo in elderly patients with ISH. Compared with placebo, nitrendipine was associated with a reduction in stroke events, major cardiovascular events, and mortality.

The Stage I Systolic Hypertension in the Elderly was a pilot trial that enrolled elderly patients (>55 years) with mild (stage I) systolic hypertension (140 to 155 mm Hg), a population not studied in Systolic Hypertension in the Elderly Program, SYST-EUR, or SYST-CHINA. Felodipine was compared with placebo in an attempt to reduce systolic blood pressure by 10%. Felodipine was shown to be more effective than placebo in reducing blood pressure. In addition, the drug was shown to reduce ventricular wall thickness and improve ventricular function. Amlodipine also has been shown to be as useful as chlorthalidone in reducing blood pressure in patients with stage I hypertension.

Many studies have compared various calcium channel blockers with other antihypertensive drugs in older subjects with combined systolic and diastolic hypertension. The Second Swedish Trial in Old Patients with Hypertension (STOP-2) enrolled 6614 patients ranging in age from 70 to 84 years with a supine blood pressure of 180/105 mm Hg or higher. The original STOP trial compared the effects of diuretics and beta blockers in elderly hypertensives in terms of cardiovascular morbidity and mortality. STOP-2 compared these two treatments with a calcium channel blocker (felodipine or isradipine) or an ACE inhibitor (enalapril or lisinopril). There was no difference between the three treatment groups with respect to the combined end points of fatal stroke, fatal myocardial infarction, and other cardiovascular diseases. There was a lower incidence of nonfatal myocardial infarction and congestive heart failure in the ACE inhibitor group than in the other treatment modalities. In the International Nifedipine Study Intervention as a Goal in Hypertension Treatment (INSIGHT), 6321 elderly patients 55 to 80 years of age were randomized to double-blind treatment with the long-acting nifedipine gastrointestinal therapeutic system or the combination drug co-amilozide (hydrochlorothiazide and amiloride). The study end points were overall cardiovascular morbidity and mortality, and both treatments appeared equally effective in preventing vascular events. In the Nordic Diltiazem Study, 10,881 patients 50 to 74 years of age with systemic hypertension were randomized to receive first-line therapy with diltiazem, diuretics, or a beta blocker. Diltiazem was as effective as the other treatments in reducing the incidence of combined study end points of stroke, myocardial infarction, and other cardiovascular death. Another smaller study was conducted among Japanese patients 60 years or older (National Interventional Cooperative Study in Elderly Hypertensives). Inclusion criteria were systolic blood pressure of 160 to 220 mm Hg and diastolic blood pressure below 115 mm Hg after a 4-week placebo period and no history of cardiovascular complications. The number of cardiovascular events was low due to the small sample size and to the inclusion criteria. There was no difference in combined cardiovascular end points. In the Prospective Randomized Evaluation of Diltiazem CD Trial, 8000 patients 55 years or older were randomized to receive diltiazem or chlorthalidone. The results have not yet been published.

Studies have demonstrated the efficacy of calcium channel blockers used alone or in combination in elderly patients when compared with alternative medications.

The Hypertension Optimal Treatment (HOT) trial studied 18,790 patients 50 to 80 years of age. The study examined whether maximal reduction of diastolic blood pressure with antihypertensive drugs and aspirin could cause a further reduction in cardiovascular events (myocardial infarction or stroke) or be associated with harm (J-curve hypothesis). Felodipine, a long-acting dihydropyridine, was used as the first-line treatment for all patients, and aspirin (75 mg) or placebo was also given. An ACE inhibitor, a beta blocker, and a thiazide diuretic could be given to achieve the desired diastolic blood pressure goal. The study results reported maximal protection with antihypertensive therapy when a diastolic blood pressure of 82.6 mm Hg was achieved; in diabetic patients, an additional reduction in diastolic blood pressure (<80 mm Hg) was needed to achieve maximal benefit. A J-curve response was not observed despite major reductions in blood pressure. The HOT study had greater success in achieving blood pressure targets among the oldest subjects, with a low incidence of medication side effects.

The Antihypertensive and Lipid-Lowering Treatment to Prevent Heart Attack Trial (ALLHAT), sponsored by the National Heart, Lung, and Blood Institute, was one of the largest prospective, randomized studies ever undertaken. The study enrolled 42,418 patients older than 55 years. The goal of the study was to compare four antihypertensive interventions—long-acting calcium antagonist (amlodipine), ACE inhibitor (lisinopril), diuretic (chlorthalidone), and alpha blocker (doxazosin)—in terms of their ability to impact coronary artery disease related events (among other secondary cardio- and cerebrovascular outcomes). Fifty percent of the patients also received pravastatin to test the benefits of lowered cholesterol in older patients. The study showed that amlodipine performs admirably in comparison with chlorthalidone relative to all end points other than new-onset congestive heart failure. Based on the ALLHAT findings, calcium channel blockers can be considered an acceptable treatment alternative in diuretic-intolerant patients. However, ALLHAT did not explore the issue of adding calcium channel blockers to ongoing diuretic therapy. There is experimental support for such a combination in reducing blood pressure, more so than with either component alone.

The Controlled-Onset Verapamil Investigation of Cardiovascular Events trial (CONVINCE) compared a delayed/slow-release verapamil delivery system with atenolol or hydrochlorothiazide in 15,000 hypertensive patients 55 years or older. The study was stopped by the sponsor for cost reasons, and the accumulated data from the trial showed no advantage of using this verapamil delivery system on morbid and mortal cardiovascular events.

The calcium channel blockers reduce systolic and diastolic pressures, with minimal side effects, including orthostasis. They can cause left ventricular hypertrophy to regress in patients with hypertension. These drugs also may exhibit antiadrenergic and natriuretic activities and can normalize the abnormal coronary vasomotion often observed in hypertensive patients. They can be combined with other antihypertensive drugs, if necessary (beta blockers, ACE inhibitors, and diuretics).

There is also a growing experience with combination calcium channel blocker therapy in hypertension. Innovative combination antihypertensive formulations have been evaluated in clinical trials and are now available: enalapril and extended-release diltiazem, benazepril and amlodipine, trandolapril and extended-release verapamil, and extended-release felodipine and enalapril.

Calcium channel blockers are equally effective in black and white patients and in the young and the old. Women may have greater blood pressure–lowering effects than men with comparable doses of drug. They do not lower the pressures of normotensive patients. These drugs may be most useful in patients with low-renin, salt-dependent forms of hypertension. In addition, they have been shown to be useful in treating patients with hypertension after heart and kidney transplant.

Hypertension with Concomitant Diabetes

Compared with placebo, nitrendipine has been shown to reduce the risk for subsequent cardiovascular events and mortality. In the SYST-EUR study, 10.5% of patients had diabetes mellitus. Among those, systolic blood pressure was slightly higher than among patients without diabetes. Compared with placebo, the relative risk reductions were 73% for fatal and nonfatal strokes and 76% for cardiovascular mortality, which clearly exceeded the benefit seen in nondiabetic patients. Although not statistically significant, there was a 57% reduction in relative risk for myocardial infarction. In line with these findings are the results of the SYST-CHINA trial, with a large risk reduction among the subgroup of patients with diabetes.

Although calcium channel blockers in diabetic subjects are associated with a clear risk reduction compared with placebo, the results of studies in which calcium channel blockers were compared with other blood pressure–lowering drugs, in particular ACE inhibitors, appear to be less favorable. In the Appropriate Blood Pressure Control in Diabetes trial, nisoldipine was compared with enalapril among patients with non–insulin-dependent diabetes with or without hypertension. Among the primary aims of the study was to test the effect of the calcium channel blocker nisoldipine on risk of cardiovascular events. The trial was terminated early because, in the subgroup of patients with hypertension receiving nisoldipine, there was a significant excess in myocardial infarction. Compared with enalapril, the secondary end point of fatal versus nonfatal myocardial infarction was strongly increased (25 vs. 5). However, these data have been questioned as to the accuracy of the assignment to drug-specific end points group.

Similarly, in the Fosinopril Versus Amlodipine Cardiovascular Events Randomized Trial (FACET), compared with fosinopril, patients randomized to calcium channel blockers had a twofold excess in combined cardiovascular end points (27 vs. 14). However, in a subanalysis of the STOP-2 trial that included a large number of patients with diabetes mellitus, the potential disadvantage of calcium channel blockers compared with other treatments was less evident.

Compared with placebo, calcium antagonists apparently reduce the risk for clinical end points among patients with diabetes and hypertension; but in head-to-head comparison, there is evidence that ACE inhibitors are superior to calcium blockers in reducing cardiovascular end points and for reducing the rate of progression of proteinuric renal disease. However, the superiority of other treatments over calcium blockers may be small or even absent.

Hypertension with Heart Disease

Despite the widespread use of calcium channel blockers for the treatment of systemic hypertension, there are questions regarding their relative cardioprotective efficacy as compared with other antihypertensive agents.

In 1995, there were two published reports suggesting an increased risk of myocardial infarction and mortality in hypertensive patients receiving the short-acting calcium channel blockers (verapamil, diltiazem, nifedipine) as treatment compared with patients receiving other antihypertensive therapies that included diuretics and beta blockers. These reports were case control studies that had significant methodologic flaws built into their experimental design. A great debate appeared in the medical literature regarding the safety of calcium channel blockers as a class for treating hypertension. Based on the available evidence, the U.S. Food and Drug Administration has advised physicians not to use the short-acting calcium channel blockers for treating hypertension, but it placed no restrictions on the first-line supplementary use of sustained-release calcium channel blocker formulations or longer-acting formulations available for this indication when there appears to be no apparent harm with their use.

In the treatment of hypertension, dihydropyridine calcium blockers appear to be as efficacious as diuretics in reducing cardiovascular and cerebrovascular morbidity and mortality. In hypertensive patients with angina, beta blockers should be the initial treatment of choice, with calcium blockers used as an add-on treatment or as an alternative monotherapy in individuals intolerant of beta blockers. In patients with hypertension and heart failure, ACE inhibitors, beta blockers, and diuretics are the treatment of choice, with calcium blockers as a possible add-on treatment. In patients with diabetes, there is strong evidence for the use of ACE inhibitors or angiotensin II blockers over calcium blockers. The ACE inhibitors also seem to provide a greater venoprotective effect, which makes them useful agents in the correction of calcium blocker-related peripheral edema.

In patients without evidence of coronary artery disease, heart failure, renal disease, or diabetes, calcium channel blockers can be considered a first-line therapy with efficacy similar to that of other antihypertensive agents.

Hypertensive Emergencies and Perioperative Hypertension

Some of the calcium channel blockers also have been shown to be beneficial and safe in patients with severe hypertension and hypertensive crises. Single oral, sublingual, and intravenous doses of these drugs have rapidly and smoothly reduced blood pressure in adults and children without causing significant untoward effects. The absolute reduction in blood pressure with treatment appears to be inversely correlated with the height of the pretreatment blood pressure level, and few episodes of hypotension have been reported. Continuous hemodynamic monitoring of patients does not seem necessary in most instances. Intravenous nicardipine is approved for clinical use in the treatment of hypertensive emergencies and perioperative hypertension. Its clinical utility compared with that of other parenteral treatments including other intravenous calcium blockers (clevidipine) remains to be determined.

Silent Myocardial Ischemia

In addition to their favorable effects in relieving painful episodes of myocardial ischemia, the calcium blockers are effective in relieving transient myocardial ischemic episodes (detected by ECG) that are unrelated to symptoms (silent myocardial ischemia). Diltiazem, nifedipine (low dose), amlodipine, and verapamil alone and in combination with beta blockers and nitrates have been shown to be effective in reducing the number of ischemic episodes and their duration. The prognostic importance of relieving silent myocardial ischemia with calcium blockers and other treatments was evaluated in a study sponsored by the National Heart Lung and Blood Institute, the Asymptomatic Coronary Ischemia Pilot.

Myocardial Infarction

Several experimental studies have indicated that nifedipine, verapamil, and diltiazem can reduce the size of myocardial necrosis induced in experimental ischemia. Ischemia can lead to diminished adenosine triphosphate production, which eventually can affect the sodium and calcium ion pumps, with the ultimate consequence of calcium ion accumulation in the cytoplasm and calcium overload in the mitochondria. Calcium channel blockers can diminish myocardial oxygen consumption and inhibit the influx of calcium ions to the myofibrils and thus favorably influence the outcome of experimental coronary occlusion. These experimental observations have been the basis for the suggested use of calcium channel blockers to reduce or contain the extent of myocardial infarction during acute coronary artery occlusions in human beings and as an adjunct to cardioplegia during open heart surgery. However, there have been no adequate studies in human beings to support these approaches.

Compared with the established protective actions of some beta-blocking drugs used intravenously or orally, the results with calcium channel blockers (diltiazem, lidoflazine, nifedipine, verapamil) have not been as favorable. The results of a meta-analysis examining the effects of immediate-release nifedipine in patients surviving myocardial infarction even suggested the potential for harm, which also prompted a debate in the literature regarding the safety of calcium channel blockers as a treatment class for patients surviving myocardial infarction.

The plausibility of these mortality results with calcium blockers are supported by a failure to show a beneficial effect on infarct size, development of myocardial infarctions, or reinfarctions in most trials of patients with myocardial infarctions or unstable angina. A trial using diltiazem in patients with non–Q-wave infarction reported a reduction in recurrent myocardial infarction in the diltiazem-treated patients but no reduction in mortality. In a larger trial with diltiazem in infarction survivors, no favorable effects on mortality were seen. A subgroup of patients with left ventricular dysfunction did worse with diltiazem therapy than with placebo; however, diltiazem therapy appeared effective in patients with relatively normal left ventricular function. Similarly, a more recent study did show benefit of verapamil compared with placebo in infarction survivors, with less benefit observed in patients with left ventricular dysfunction.

A double-blind study compared oral diltiazem and aspirin with aspirin alone (Incomplete Infarction Trial of European Research Collaborators Evaluating Prognosis Post-Thrombolysis) in patients with myocardial infarction who had received thrombolytic therapy. The study enrolled 874 subjects, and treatment with diltiazem did not reduce the cumulative occurrence of cardiac death, nonfatal reinfarction, or refractory ischemia during a 6-month follow-up, but it did reduce composite end points of nonfatal cardiac events, particularly the need for myocardial revascularization. In another study, intravenous diltiazem was given as an adjunct to thrombolysis in acute myocardial infarction and shown to have protective effects, with no effect on coronary artery patency and left ventricular function and perfusion.

Prophylactic use of calcium channel blockers to improve patient survival after myocardial infarction cannot be recommended as a first-line therapy unless there are specific indications for using these drugs. However, in patients with contraindications to β-adrenergic blockade, one can consider using verapamil or diltiazem in survivors of myocardial infarction who have good ventricular function. Bepridil use may put postinfarction patients at an increased risk.

Hypertrophic Cardiomyopathy

Propranolol remains the therapeutic agent of choice for symptomatic patients with hypertrophic cardiomyopathy. The beneficial effects produced by propranolol derive from its blocking of sympathetic stimulation of the heart.

Clinical studies have shown that the administration of verapamil can also improve exercise capacity and symptoms in many patients with hypertrophic cardiomyopathy. The exact mechanism by which verapamil produces these beneficial effects is not known. Acute and chronic verapamil administration reduces left ventricular outflow obstruction, but examination of indices of left ventricular systolic function during chronic therapy showed that this effect does not result from a reduction in left ventricular hypercontractility. Because patients with hypertrophic cardiomyopathy also exhibit abnormal diastolic function, it is likely that improvement in diastolic filling may be responsible in part for the benefit conferred by verapamil. Enhanced early diastolic filling and improvement in the relation between diastolic pressure and volume might be expected to result in an increase in left ventricular end-diastolic volume, which would decrease the Venturi forces that act to move the anterior mitral valve leaflet across the outflow tract toward the septum. This decrease would cause a diminution of obstruction, reducing left ventricular pressure and myocardial wall stress and thus raising the threshold at which symptoms occur.

In a large study of patients with hypertrophic cardiomyopathy refractory to beta blockers, verapamil proved to be effective on a long-term basis, with almost 50% of patients showing a significant improvement in exercise tolerance, an improvement in symptoms, or a reduction in myocardial ischemia. Approximately 50% of patients, who were considered to be candidates for surgery because of moderately severe symptoms unresponsive to propranolol, showed significant improvement on verapamil, and surgery was no longer considered necessary.

Other studies have reported that chronic administration of verapamil can not only improve symptoms in patients with hypertrophic cardiomyopathy but also reduce the left ventricular muscle mass and the ventricular septal thickness measured by echocardiographic and ECG analyses. Verapamil and nifedipine were shown to improve the impaired left ventricular filling characteristics. This beneficial effect on left ventricular diastolic relaxation has not occurred after propranolol.

There may be serious and fatal complications of verapamil treatment in patients with hypertrophic cardiomyopathy. These complications result from the accentuated hemodynamic or electrophysiologic effects of the drug. It is not clear whether the fatal complications occur as a result of verapamil-induced reduction in blood pressure with a resultant increase in left ventricular obstruction or the negative inotropic effects of the drug. Verapamil probably should not be used in patients with clinical congestive heart failure. The loss of sequential atrial ventricular depolarization caused by the electrophysiologic effects of the drug could also compromise cardiac function. The adverse electrophysiologic effects are often transient; however, they could prevent the use of larger drug doses that might provide better relief.

If the calcium entry blocking effects of verapamil are responsible for its therapeutic actions in hypertrophic cardiomyopathy, other drugs in this class also may be useful. However, the results of a double-blind trial comparing verapamil with nifedipine indicated that verapamil is more effective than nifedipine in improving exercise tolerance and clinical symptoms. Diltiazem recently was shown to improve active diastolic function in patients with hypertrophic cardiomyopathy; however, certain patients had a marked increase in outflow obstruction.

Congestive Cardiomyopathy

The potent systemic vasodilatory actions of nifedipine and other dihydro-pyridine calcium entry blockers make them potentially useful as afterload-reducing agents in patients with left ventricular failure. Unlike other vasodilatory drugs, however, nifedipine also exerts a direct negative inotropic effect on the myocardium that is consistent with its ability to block transmembrane calcium transport in cardiac muscle cells. The suc-cessful use of nifedipine as a vasodilator in patients with left ventricular failure would depend on its effect to reduce ventricular afterload exceeding its direct negative inotropic actions, thereby leading to an improvement in hemodynamics and forward flow.

Studies evaluating the effect on hemodynamics of nifedipine used in combi-nation with other vasodilators in patients with heart failure have uniformly demonstrated significant reductions in systemic vascular resistance, usually associated with increases in cardiac output. It has been found that resting ejec-tion fractions also rise with nifedipine therapy. Reflex increases in heart rate have been reported, but most investigators have found heart rate to remain the same and, in isolated cases, to decrease. Left ventricular filling pressures usu-ally decrease or do not change significantly, but there are instances when pul-monary capillary wedge pressures rise with the use of nifedipine in heart failure. Patients with left ventricular dysfunction and nearly normal levels of left ventricular afterload, i.e., disproportionately low wall stress, and those with intrinsic fixed mechanical interference to forward flow, such as aortic stenosis, appear most likely to have unfavorable hemodynamic responses to nifedipine therapy. Most of the published data have dealt only with the acute hemody-namic effects of the agent after single sublingual dosing, with little work done on the use of nifedipine as chronic oral therapy for left ventricular failure.

There is a promising experience in clinical trials with the newer dihy-dropyridine calcium blockers amlodipine and felodipine in patients with congestive cardiomyopathy. One study has demonstrated the efficacy and safety of diltiazem in patients with idiopathic cardiomyopathy.

Although evidence is incomplete, there are indications that a cardiac tis-sue renin-angiotensin system may counteract the actions of calcium channel blockers, especially in patients with heart failure. However, because calcium channel blocking drugs are potent vasodilators, particularly on the arterial circulation, the combination of an ACE inhibitor and a calcium channel blocker might appear to be useful in further augmenting vasodilation, thus improving myocardial perfusion and ejection fraction. Hence, the Third Vasodilator-Heart Failure Trial was conducted to test the efficacy of the combination of felodipine, enalapril, digoxin, and a diuretic in patients with congestive heart failure. The end points evaluated were exercise tolerance, quality of life, left ventricular function, levels of plasma norepinephrine and atrial natriuretic factor, and reductions in the occurrence of arrhythmias and mortality. A similar pilot multicenter, placebo-controlled study investigated using amlodipine in addition to ACE inhibitors, digoxin, and diuretics. This study, known as the Prospective Randomized Amlodipine Survival Evaluation (PRAISE), indicated no clear overall mortality or harm from the use of the drug in patients with severe congestive heart failure. Contrary to the prior experiences of the investigators, there appeared to be little beneficial effect in the large subgroup of patients who had coronary artery disease and a barely significant reduction in morbidity and mortality in the minority of patients who did not have coronary artery disease.

The investigation was followed up in a study comparing amlodipine with placebo in a study of 1800 patients having cardiomyopathy without coronary artery disease who were receiving digoxin, diuretics, and ACE inhibitors (PRAISE II), with no additional benefit from the calcium blocker being observed (data were presented at the 51st Annual Scientific Sessions of the American College of Cardiology, Atlanta, GA, March 17 to 20, 2002). Mibefradil, a nondihydropyridine calcium blocker with little negative inotropic activity, was evaluated in a double-blind, placebo-controlled trial of 2000 patients with class II to III heart failure (New York Heart Association) who were already receiving standard heart failure therapies (First Mortality Assessment in Congestive Heart Failure).The study demonstrated no benefit of mibefradil. The potential interaction with antiarrhythmic drugs, especially amiodarone, and drugs associated with torsades may have contributed to poor outcomes early in the study.

In a retrospective analysis of the Studies of Left Ventricular Dysfunction, in which enalapril was compared with placebo in patients with class I to III heart failure, it was observed that those patients who were receiving concomitant immediate-release calcium channel blocker treatment had a higher mortality than did subjects who were receiving concomitant beta-blocker therapy.

Use of long-acting dihydropyridine calcium blockers as adjunctive vasodilator therapy in patients with left ventricular failure should be considered only if additional clinical reasons for their administration exist, i.e., angina pectoris, systemic hypertension, and aortic regurgitation, particularly if these conditions play important contributory roles in the development or exacerbation of left ventricular dysfunction. Some investigators now propose that calcium antagonists may provide some benefit to patients with predominant diastolic ventricular dysfunction, but more clinical data are needed to substantiate this claim.

Aortic Regurgitation

Dihydropyridine calcium blockers have been used successfully as arterial vasodilators in patients with chronic asymptomatic aortic and mitral regurgitation. These beneficial hemodynamic effects may postpone the need for valve replacement.

Primary Pulmonary Hypertension

Primary pulmonary hypertension is an entity characterized by excessive pulmonary vasoconstriction and increased pulmonary vascular resistance induced by unknown stimuli. Recently, it was suggested that endothelial cell dysfunction and injury may be responsible for the disease process. Typically, the affected patient is a young to middle-age woman presenting with fatigue, dyspnea, chest discomfort, or syncope. Despite many attempts to develop effective therapy, the results of drug treatment have been generally unsatisfactory, and the syndrome continues to bear a poor prognosis.

Based on the currently available data, it may be concluded that some calcium channel antagonists provide beneficial responses in selected patients with pulmonary hypertension. In general, patients with less severe pulmonary hypertension appear to respond better than do those with more advanced disease. Further, early treatment may serve to attenuate progression of the disease.

In patients with chronic hypoxia-induced pulmonary vasoconstriction, the use of calcium channel blockers may be associated with a worsening of ventilation or perfusion mismatching secondary to inhibition of hypoxic pulmonary vasoconstriction.

Cerebral Arterial Spasm and Stroke

A major complication of subarachnoid hemorrhage is cerebral arterial spasm, which may occur several days after the initial event. Such a spasm may be a focal or diffuse narrowing of one or more of the larger cerebral vessels, which may cause additional ischemic neurologic deficits. Although the exact etiology of this spasm is unknown, a combination of various blood constituents and neurotransmitters has been postulated to produce a milieu that enhances the reactivity of the cerebral vasculature. The final pathway for the vasoconstriction, however, involves an increase in the free intracellular calcium concentration. Accordingly, it is reasonable to postulate that the calcium channel antagonists may have a beneficial effect in reducing cerebral spasm.

Although verapamil and nifedipine have been shown to prevent cerebral arterial spasm in experimental studies, nimodipine and nicardipine, both nifedipine analogues, have demonstrated a preferential cerebrovascular action in this disorder. The lipid solubility of nimodipine enables it to cross the blood–brain barrier; this may account for its more potent cerebrovascular effects. A multicenter placebo-controlled study involving 125 patients demonstrated that nimodipine significantly reduces the occurrence of severe neurologic deficits after angiographically demonstrated cerebral arterial spasm. All patients had a documented subarachnoid hemorrhage and a normal neurologic status within 96 h of entry into the study. Although 8 of the 60 placebo-treated patients developed a severe neurologic deficit, only 1 of 55 nimodipine-treated patients had such an outcome. Nimodipine is now approved for the improvement of neurologic outcome by reducing the incidence and severity of ischemic deficits in patients with subarachnoid hemorrhage from ruptured congenital aneurysms who are in good neurologic condition after ictus. The recommended dose is 60 mg by mouth every 4 h for 21 consecutive days.

Subsequent investigations have suggested that increased cellular calcium concentration may be implicated in neuronal death after ischemia. Nimodipine administered to laboratory animals after global cerebral ischemia had a more favorable effect on neurologic outcome than did placebo. The results of a prospective double-blind, placebo-controlled trial of oral nimodipine administered to 186 patients within 24 h of an acute ischemic stroke showed a reductions in mortality and neurologic deficit with active treatment. The benefit was confined predominantly to men. However, subsequent studies in which nimodipine therapy was begun up to 48 h after the onset of symptoms reported no benefit of therapy.

Migraine and Dementia

Classic migraine is characterized by prodromal symptoms with transient neurologic deficits. Cerebral blood flow is reduced during these prodromes and then is increased during the subsequent vasodilatory phase, causing severe headache. Because the entry of calcium ions into the smooth muscle cells is the final common pathway that controls vasomotor tone, calcium antagonists may prevent or ameliorate the initial focal cerebral vasoconstriction.

Results from controlled studies have demonstrated that 80% to 90% of patients with vascular headaches benefit from nimodipine, thus confirming the selectivity of this agent for the cerebral blood vessels. Verapamil and nifedipine also have been reported to be effective in the prophylaxis of migraine but are less selective for the cephalic blood vessels and thus cause more systemic side effects. Relief from the migraine prodrome usually began 10 to 14 days after initiation of the drugs but could be delayed 2 to 4 weeks. Cerebral vascular resistance was decreased by all three established calcium antagonists, but only nimodipine reduced the cerebral vasoconstriction induced by inhalation of 100% oxygen. None of the calcium entry blocking drugs are effective against muscle contraction or tension headaches.

Multiple clinical trials are currently examining the effects of calcium entry blockers on the progression of dementing illness, both vascular and Alzheimer types. Preliminary results have shown equivocal benefit from treatment. However, the SYST-EUR trial showed a reduction in the incidence of cognitive decline in elderly patients receiving nitrendipine for isolated systolic hypertension compared to placebo.

Other Vascular Uses

Amaurosis Fugax

Hypoperfusion of the retinal circulation may lead to a brief loss of vision in one eye, a syndrome known as *amaurosis fugax*. This brief loss of sight has been attributed to embolism from the heart or great vessels or to carotid occlusive disease. In a small group of patients with amaurosis but no signs of emboli or carotid hypoperfusion, administration of aspirin or warfarin did not relieve symptoms. However, oral doses of verapamil or nifedipine abolished attacks. In several patients, the attacks returned when the calcium-blocking agent was discontinued.

High-Altitude Pulmonary Edema

Hypoxic pulmonary hypertension appears to play a role in the pathogenesis of high-altitude pulmonary edema. Nifedipine has been used for the emergency treatment of this condition, with its benefit coming from its ability to reduce pulmonary artery pressure.

Raynaud's Phenomenon

Raynaud's phenomenon is characterized by well-demarcated ischemia of the digits, with pallor or cyanosis ending abruptly at one level on the digits. Nifedipine has been shown to decrease the frequency, duration, and intensity of vasospastic attacks in approximately 66% of patients with primary or secondary Raynaud's phenomenon. Patients with primary Raynaud's phenomenon usually demonstrate the most improvement; digital ulcers have been reported to heal in patients with scleroderma. Doses of 10 to 20 mg of nifedipine thrice daily have been used (see Chapter 50). Felodipine and isradipine are as effective as nifedipine. Diltiazem, 60 to 360 mg daily, was also useful in patients with primary or secondary Raynaud's phenomenon in multiple placebo-controlled trials.

Atherosclerosis

Atherosclerosis develops through numerous and interrelated processes involving the accumulation of cholesterol, calcium, and matrix materials in the major arteries and at lesion sites. Many of the intracellular and extracellular processes involved in atherosclerotic plaque formation require calcium, and it has been suggested that large deposits of cholesterol may trigger physiologic changes in membranes that favor uptake of calcium into the vascular smooth muscle.

The results of controlled studies using angiography have suggested that some calcium channel blockers may retard the progression of atherosclerosis in humans. In the International Nifedipine Trial on Atherosclerosis Coronary Therapy study, it was shown that nifedipine reduces the formation of new lesions when compared with placebo. However, nifedipine had no effect on the progression or regression of already existing coronary lesions, and an increased mortality as compared with placebo was observed.

There is a suggestion from available experimental and clinical data that calcium blockers have an atherosclerotic plaque–stabilizing action. However, a recent study with amlodipine showed that the drug has no demonstrable effects on the progression of coronary atherosclerosis or the risk of major cardiovascular events.

The administration of nicardipine for 24 months also had no effect on the progression or retardation of advanced stenoses in patients with coronary atherosclerosis as confirmed by arteriography. However, the drug did appear to retard the progression of small lesions. Diltiazem was shown to retard the development of coronary artery disease in heart transplant recipients, an action independent of the drug's blood pressure–lowering effect.

In the Multicenter Isradipine Diuretic Atherosclerosis Study (MIDAS), which was a 3-year, double-blind, randomized trial designed to compare the effectiveness of isradipine and hydrochlorothiazide in retarding the progression of atherosclerotic lesions in the carotid arteries, no apparent benefit was seen with either treatment. A study similar to MIDAS is now being carried out with lacidipine, a new dihydropyridine calcium antagonist, in the 4-year European Lacidipine Study on Atherosclerosis.

Calcium blockers also have been used to treat patients with intermittent claudication and mesenteric insufficiency.

Other Cardiovascular Uses

Diltiazem has been used as part of an ice-cold cardioplegia solution in patients undergoing coronary surgical procedures. The addition of diltiazem appeared to preserve high-energy phosphate levels, with an improvement in hemodynamics in the postoperative period. Concomitant use of nifedipine appears to reduce the incidence of myocardial infarction and transient ischemia in patients undergoing bypass surgery.

Intracoronary diltiazem has been used to reduce the severity and delay the onset of ischemic pain in patients undergoing percutaneous transluminal angioplasty. Calcium blockers also have been used as a long-term treatment to prevent restenosis after balloon angioplasty, with questionable results. They also have been used to prolong graft patency in patients with radial artery coronary bypass grafts with no benefit seen.

It has been shown that coronary artery vasospasm may be an important pathophysiologic mechanism in explaining some types of experimental cardiomyopathy. Experimentally, verapamil has been shown to preserve the functioning of human renal transplants. The drugs dilate the preglomerular afferent arterioles and appear to possess inherent immunosuppressive properties and the ability to ameliorate the nephrotoxic effects of cyclosporine.

ADVERSE EFFECTS

In addition to their widely different effects on cardiovascular function, these agents have different spectra of adverse effects (Table 4-7). Immediate-release nifedipine is associated with a very high incidence of minor adverse effects (approximately 40%), but serious adverse effects are uncommon. The most frequent adverse effects reported with nifedipine and other dihydropyridines include headache, pedal edema, flushing, paresthesias, gingival hyperplasia, and dizziness; the most serious adverse effects of this drug include exacerbation of angina, which may occur in up to 10% of patients, and occasional hypotension. These side effects are reduced in number with the new long-acting formulation of nifedipine and may be fewer in number with some of the new dihydropyridine calcium antagonists. The side effect of pedal edema is often reduced when dihydropyridines are combined with ACE inhibitors.

Diltiazem and verapamil can exacerbate sinus node dysfunction and impair AV nodal conduction, particularly in patients with underlying conduction system disease. The most frequent adverse effect of verapamil is constipation. The drug also may worsen congestive heart failure, particularly when used in combination with beta blockers or disopyramide. There have been recent reports of verapamil-induced parkinsonism. Most of the adverse effects noted with diltiazem have been cardiovascular, with occasional headache and gastrointestinal complaints. The side effects of calcium blockers may increase considerably when these agents are used in combination.

An increased risk of gastrointestinal hemorrhage in older patients has been reported with calcium channel blockers, as has intraoperative bleeding during coronary artery bypass surgery. An increased risk of developing cancer in older subjects also has been reported. These findings have not been confirmed by subsequent prospective studies.

Bepridil, which has class I antiarrhythmic properties, has the potential to induce malignant ventricular arrhythmias. In addition, because of its ability to prolong the QT interval, bepridil can cause torsades de pointes–type ventricular tachycardia. Because of these properties, bepridil should be reserved for patients in whom other antianginal agents do not offer a satisfactory effect.

TABLE 4-7 Adverse Effects of Calcium Channel Blockers

	Overall	Headache	Dizziness	GI	Flushing	Paresthesia	Decreased SA and/or AV conduction	CHF	Hypotension	Pedal edema	Worsening of angina
Diltiazem	5	+	+	+	+	0	3+	+	+	+	0
Diltiazem SR	5	+	+	+	+	0	3+	+	+	+	0
Verapamil	8	+	+	3+	0	0	3+	2+	+	+	0
Verapamil SR	8	+	+	3+	0	0	3+	2+	+	0	0
Bepridil	15	0	2+	3+	0	0	+	+	0	0	0
Amlodipine	15	2+	+	+	+	+	0	0	+	2+	0
Isradipine	15	2+	2+	+	+	+	0	0	+	2+	0
Nifedipine	20	3+	3+	+	3+	+	0	+	+	2+	+
Nifedipine GITS	10	+	+	+	+	+	0	+	+	+	0
Nicardipine	20	3+	3+	+	3+	+	0	0	+	2+	+
Nimodipine	15	+	+	+	+	0	0	+	+	+	0
Nisoldipine	15	2+	+	+	0	0	2+	0	+	2+	0
Felodipine	20	2+	2+	+	2+	+	0	0	+	2+	0

Key: +, rare; 0, no report; 2+, occasional; 3+, frequent; AV, atrioventricular node; CHF, congestive heart failure; GI, gastrointestinal; GITS, gastrointestinal therapeutic system; SA, sinoatrial node; SR, sustained release.
Source: Adapted with permission from Frishman WH, Stroh JA, Greenberg SM, et al: Calcium channel blockers in systemic hypertension. Med Clin North Am 71 449, 1988.

Drug Withdrawal

Serious problems that appear to be related to heightened adrenergic activity have been reported with abrupt withdrawal of long-term beta-blocker therapy in patients with angina. Clinical experiences with the withdrawal of calcium entry blockers suggest that, although patients with angina get worse after treatment when a calcium entry blocker is stopped abruptly, there is no evidence of an overshoot in anginal symptoms.

Drug Overdose

Calcium entry blocker overdosage is being reported with increasing frequency and is now the second leading cause of death from toxic exposure to cardiovascular medications. The cardiovascular problems associated with this condition are hypotension, left ventricular conduction, bradycardia, nodal blocks, and asystole. Treatment approaches are described in Table 4-8.

Drug–Drug Interactions

There are few data on the interactions of diltiazem with other drugs. Rifampin severely reduces the bioavailability of oral verapamil by enhancing the first-pass liver metabolism of the drug. Nifedipine and verapamil increase serum digoxin levels, an observation not made with diltiazem (see Chapter 21). Verapamil has been reported to increase serum digoxin levels by approximately 70%, apparently by decreasing renal clearance, nonrenal clearance, and the volume of distribution. Studies of the time course of this effect have shown that it begins with the first dose and reaches steady state within 1 to 4 weeks. Nifedipine also has been reported to increase serum digoxin concentrations in patients, but to a lesser extent (about 45%). The mechanism for this interaction is not clear. Verapamil and diltiazem have additive effects on AV conduction in combination with digitalis. They can be

TABLE 4-8 Cardiovascular Toxicity with Calcium Channel Blockers and Recommendations for Treatment

Effects*	Suggested treatment
Profound hypotension	10% calcium gluconate or calcium chloride; norepinephrine or dopamine
Severe LV dysfunction	10% calcium gluconate or calcium chloride; isoproterenol or dobutamine; glucagon; milrinone, norepinephrine, or dopamine; hyperinsulinemia euglycemic therapy
Profound bradycardia	Atropine sulfate (not always effective)
Sinus bradycardia	10% calcium gluconate or calcium chloride
SA and AV nodal blocks	Isoproterenol or dobutamine
Asystole	External cardiac massage and cardiac pacing (if above measures fail)

* These effects are seen more frequently in patients who have underlying myocardial dysfunction and/or cardiac conduction abnormalities and who are receiving concomitant β-adrenergic blocker treatment.
Key: AV, atrioventricular; LV, left ventricular; SA, sinoatrial.
Source: Reproduced with permission from Frishman WH, Klein NA, Charlap S, et al: Recognition and management of verapamil poisoning, in Pack M, Frishman WH (eds): *Calcium Channel Antagonists in Cardiovascular Disease*. Norwalk, Appleton-Century-Crofts, 1984, p 365.

used to cause further decreases in heart rate as compared with digitalis alone when patients are in atrial fibrillation.

Combinations of propranolol with nifedipine or verapamil have been studied extensively for the therapy of angina pectoris. Several studies have shown improved efficacy for the combination of atenolol and nifedipine as compared with any of the drugs used alone. Hemodynamic studies have shown mild negative inotropic effects of verapamil in patients on a beta blocker. There are also slight decreases in heart rate, cardiac output, and left ventricular ejection fraction. Combinations of nifedipine and propranolol or metoprolol and of verapamil and propranolol are well tolerated by patients with normal left ventricular function, but there may be a greater potential for hemodynamic compromise in patients with impaired left ventricular function with combined verapamil and propranolol treatment. Combinations of diltiazem, nifedipine, or verapamil with nitrates are well tolerated and clinically useful. When diltiazem is combined with nifedipine, blood levels of nifedipine increase significantly, which may contribute to an increased frequency of adverse reactions with this combination. The combination of verapamil and nifedipine is less effective in lowering pressure than is diltiazem plus nifedipine, perhaps related to the pharmacokinetic interaction between diltiazem and nifedipine.

CONCLUSION

Each of the calcium antagonists exerts its effects through inhibition of slow channel–mediated calcium ion transport. However, many of the drugs appear to accomplish this by different mechanisms and with different effects on various target organs. These differences allow the clinician to select the particular drug most suitable for the specific needs of the patient. In addition, the side effect profiles of these drugs (with little overlap between them) ensure that most patients will tolerate at least one of these agents.

ADDITIONAL READINGS

Abrams J, Frishman WH, Bates SM, et al: Pharmacologic options for treatment of ischemic disease, in Antman EM (ed): *Cardiovascular Therapeutics*, 2nd ed. Philadelphia, Saunders, 2002, p 97.

ACC/AHA Task Force on Practice Guidelines (Committee on Management of Patients with Unstable Angina): ACC/AHA Guideline update for the management of patients with unstable angina and non-ST-segment elevation myocardial infarction. Available at: www.acc.org/clinical/ guidelines/unstable.pdf. 2002.

ALLHAT Officers and Coordinators: Major outcomes in high-risk hypertensive patients randomized to angiotensin converting enzyme inhibitor therapy or calcium channel blocker vs diuretic: The Antihypertensive and Lipid-Lowering Treatment to Prevent Heart Attack Trial (ALLHAT). *JAMA* 288:2981, 2002.

Black HR, Elliott WJ, Grandits G, et al: CONVINCE Research Group. Principal results of the Controlled Onset Verapamil Investigation of Cardiovascular End Points (CONVINCE) trial. *JAMA* 289:2073, 2003.

Black HR, Elliott WJ, Weber MA, et al: for the Stage I Systolic Hypertension (SISH) Study Group: One-year study of felodipine or placebo for stage 1 isolated systolic hypertension. *Hypertension* 38:1118, 2001.

Frishman WH, Cheng-Lai A, Chen J (eds): *Current Cardiovascular Drugs*, 3rd ed. Philadelphia, Current Medicine, 2000.

Frishman WH, Katz B: Controlled-release drug delivery systems in cardiovascular disease treatment, in Frishman WH, Sonnenblick EH (eds): *Cardiovascular Pharmacotherapeutics*. New York, McGraw-Hill, 1997, p 1347.

Frishman WH, Landzberg BR, Weiss M: Pharmacologic therapies for the prevention of restenosis following percutaneous coronary artery interventions, in Frishman WH, Sonnenblick EH, Sica DA (eds): *Cardiovascular Pharmacotherapeutics,* 2nd ed. New York, McGraw-Hill, 2003, p 741.

Frishman WH, Qureshi A: Calcium antagonists in elderly patients with systemic hypertension, in Epstein M (ed): *Calcium Antagonists in Clinical Medicine*, 3rd ed. Philadelphia, Hanley and Belfus, 2002, p 48.

Frishman WH, Sica DA: Calcium channel blockers, in Frishman WH, Sonnenblick EH, Sica DA (eds): *Cardiovascular Pharmacotherapeutics,* 2nd ed. New York, McGraw-Hill, 2003, p 105.

Frishman WH, Skolnick AE: Secondary prevention post-infarction: the role of β-adrenergic blockers, calcium-channel blockers and aspirin, in Gersh BJ, Rahimtoola SH (eds): *Acute Myocardial Infarction,* 2nd ed. New York, Chapman & Hall, 1997, p 766.

Frishman WH, Sonnenblick EH: Beta-adrenergic blocking drugs and calcium channel blockers, in Alexander RW, Schlant RC, Fuster V (eds): *Hurst's the Heart,* 9th ed. New York, McGraw-Hill, 1998, p 1583.

Hachamovitch R, Strom JA, Sonnenblick EH, Frishman WH: Left ventricular hypertrophy in hypertension and the effects of antihypertensive drug therapy. *Curr Probl Cardiol* 13:371, 1988.

Mancini GBJ: Antiatherosclerotic effects of calcium channel blockers. *Prog Cardiovasc Dis* 45:1, 2002.

Mason RP: Atheroprotective effects of long-acting dihydropyridine-type calcium channel blockers: Evidence from clinical trials and basic scientific research. *Cerebrovasc Dis* 16:(suppl 3):11, 2003.

Opie LH: Calcium channel antagonists in the treatment of coronary artery disease: Fundamental pharmacological properties relevant to clinical use. *Prog Cardiovasc Dis* 38:273, 1996.

Opie LH, Schall R: Evidence-based evaluation of calcium channel blockers for hypertension. *J Am Coll Cardiol* 39:315, 2002.

Opie LH, Yusuf S, Kubler W: Current status of safety and efficacy of calcium channel blockers in cardiovascular diseases: A critical analysis based on 100 studies. *Prog Cardiovasc Dis* 43:171, 2000.

Packer M, Frishman WH (eds): *Calcium Channel Antagonists in Cardiovascular Disease.* Norwalk, Appleton-Century-Crofts, 1984.

Pahor M, Psaty BM, Alderman MH, et al: Health outcomes associated with calcium antagonists compared with other first-line antihypertensive therapies: A meta-analysis of randomised controlled trials. *Lancet* 356:1949, 2000.

Psaty BM, Lumley T, Furberg CD, et al: Health outcomes associated with various antihypertensive therapies used as first-line agents: A network meta-analysis. *JAMA* 289:2534, 2003.

Scognamiglio R, Rahimtoola S, Fasoli G, et al: Nifedipine in symptomatic patients with severe aortic regurgitation and normal left ventricular function. *N Engl J Med* 331:689, 1994.

Sica DA: Combination calcium channel blocker therapy in the treatment of hypertension. *J Clin Hypertens* 3:322, 2001.

Sica DA, Douglas JG: The African American Study of Kidney Disease and Hypertension (AASK): New findings. *J Clin Hypertens* 3:244, 2001.

Sica DA, Gehr TWB: Calcium-channel blockers and end-stage renal disease, in Epstein M (ed): *Calcium Antagonists in Clinical Medicine,* 3rd ed. Philadelphia, Hanley and Belfus, 2002, p 701.

Smith RF, Germanson T, Judd D, et al: Plasma norepinephrine and atrial natriuretic peptide in heart failure: Influence of felodipine in the Third Vasodilator Heart Failure Trial. V-HeFT III Investigators. *J Card Fail* 6:97, 2000.

Weinberger J, Frishman WH, Terashita D: Drug therapy of neurovascular disease. *Cardiol Rev* 11:122, 2003.

Weinberger J, Terashita D: Drug therapy of neurovascular disease. *Heart Dis* 1:163, 1999.

5 | The Renin–Angiotensin Axis: Angiotensin-Converting Enzyme Inhibitors and Angiotensin-Receptor Blockers

Domenic A. Sica   Todd W. B. Gehr
William H. Frishman

Over the past two decades, the renin–angiotensin–aldosterone (RAA) axis has been increasingly viewed as an important effector system for hypertension, cardiovascular disease, and cardiorenal disease; thus, it has become an important target for pharmacologic intervention. Of those drugs known to interrupt the RAA axis, by far the greatest treatment experience exists for angiotensin-converting enzyme (ACE) inhibitors.

ACE inhibitors have earned an important place in medical therapy since captopril, the initial compound in this class, was released in 1981. This compound proved to be an extremely effective blood pressure (BP)–lowering agent as demonstrated in a wide range of renin-dependent models of hypertension. The ACE inhibitor field thereafter quickly mushroomed so that there are currently 10 ACE inhibitors available in the United States. Losartan, the first angiotensin-receptor blocker (ARB), was released in 1995, and there currently are seven ARBs on the U.S. market. In addition to their vasodepressor properties, ACE inhibitors and, in sequence, ARBs, were quickly recognized for their ability to slow progressive renal, cardiac, and/or vascular disease processes. Thus, it was a logical step in their development to seek additional indications in the areas of congestive heart failure (CHF), post–myocardial

TABLE 5-1 FDA-Approved Indications for ACE Inhibitors

Drug	HTN	CHF	Diabetic nephropathy	High-risk patients without LVD
Captopril	•	• (post-MI)*	•	
Benazepril	•			
Enalapril	•	•†		
Fosinopril	•	•		
Lisinopril	•	• (post-MI)*		
Moexipril	•			
Perindopril	•			
Quinapril	•	•		
Ramipril	•	• (post-MI)		•
Trandolapril	•	• (post-MI)		•

*Captopril and lisinopril are indicated for CHF treatment both post-MI and as adjunctive therapy in general heart failure therapy.
†Enalapril is indicated for asymptomatic LVD.
Key: ACE, angiotensin-converting enzyme; CHF, congestive heart failure; FDA, U.S. Food and Drug Administration; HTN, hypertension; LVD, left ventricular dysfunction; MI, myocardial infarction.

96

TABLE 5-2 FDA-Approved Indications for ARBs

Drug	HTN	CHF	Diabetic nephropathy	Post-MI*	High-risk patients without LVD*	Stroke prevention
Candesartan	•					
Eprosartan	•					
Irbesartan	•		•			
Losartan	•		•			•
Olmesartan	•					
Telmisartan	•					
Valsartan	•	•				

*FDA-approved indications for ARB therapy in these disease states are anticipated in the near future.
Key: ARB, angiotensin-receptor blocker; CHF, congestive heart failure; FDA, U.S. Food and Drug Administration; HTN, hypertension; LVD, left ventricular dysfunction; MI, myocardial infarction.

infarction (post-MI), and diabetic nephropathy (Tables 5-1 and 5-2). More recently, a therapeutic indication for the treatment of the high-risk vascular disease in patients without discernible left ventricular dysfunction has emerged for the ACE inhibitor ramipril. A full description of the tissue-protective properties of ACE inhibitors and ARBs exceeds the scope of this chapter. The reader is referred to a number of comprehensive thematic reviews on this topic.

MECHANISM OF ACTION

An understanding of how ACE inhibitors and ARBs work requires an appreciation of how each class interacts with the RAA axis and how they differ from other compounds, such as beta blockers, that diminish RAA axis activity. For example, ACE inhibitors alter RAA axis activity by decreasing plasma angiotensin II production, as do beta blockers; beta blockers decrease plasma renin activity (PRA), whereas ARBs curb angiotensin II effects by blocking the type I angiotensin receptor (AT_1-R).

The locus of activity of ACE inhibitors within the RAA axis is at ACE. ACE is pluripotent in that it catalyzes the conversion of angiotensin I to angiotensin II and facilitates the degradation of bradykinin and a range of other vasoactive peptides.

Although ACE inhibitors effectively curb the generation of angiotensin II from angiotensin I, they do not prevent the generation of angiotensin II by non–ACE-dependent pathways. These alternate pathways depend on chymase and other tissue-based proteases to produce angiotensin II, a process that to a large extent represents the dominant mode of angiotensin II generation in myocardial and vascular tissue. The long-term administration of ACE inhibitors is frequently marked by a gradual rise in angiotensin II levels, termed *angiotensin escape*, presumably due to an upregulation in the productive capacity of these alternative pathways. In this regard, another facet of angiotensin II effect is important. Within the RAA axis a negative feedback loop exists wherein downstream components of this cascade act to suppress upstream activity; thus, by its presence, angiotensin II operationally shuts this system down. When an ACE inhibitor is administered, by virtue of its temporarily diminishing angiotensin II, there is a disinhibition of renin secretion from the juxtaglomerular apparatus. As this controlling influence dissipates, the concentrations of PRA and angiotensin I increase. These increases in PRA and angiotensin I thus emerge as potential sources of substrate for alternative pathway action and, hence, angiotensin II escape. The rise in angiotensin I, which accompanies ACE inhibition, seems to derive from an enhanced release of active renin rather than an accumulation of angiotensin I and is effectively blunted by β-adrenergic antagonism.

Because ACE inhibitors reduce angiotensin II levels transiently (days to weeks), other mechanisms for their BP-lowering effect need to be considered, particularly if the pattern of BP response to ACE inhibition is probed. When first administered, ACE inhibitors transiently reduce BP in parallel with the degree of RAA axis activation. With long-term therapy, any relation between the fall in BP and the pretreatment levels of angiotensin II fades. This latter observation makes renin profiling of little practical value in predicting the degree to which an ACE inhibitor will reduce BP in a particular patient; instead, the BP response achieved shortly after beginning an ACE inhibitor appears to provide a better indication of any long-term response. This pattern of response and limited predictive value of pretherapy PRA values are similar to those of ARBs.

The persistence of the antihypertensive effect of ACE inhibitors despite angiotensin II escape argues for an active BP-reducing role of alternative vasodepressor systems, such as bradykinin, although most such studies with bradykinin have evaluated only the short-term BP contribution of its effect. How ACE inhibitors interact with the kallikrein–kinin system is a matter of considerable interest. ACE processes several vasoactive peptides other than angiotensin II, one of which is bradykinin. Therefore, in theory, ACE inhibitor administration should elevate tissue and or circulating bradykinin levels, although the reproducibility of such measurements has proven methodologically complex. Bradykinin also appears to increase with ARB administration, although by a different mechanism. ARBs, although they block the AT_1-R, conversely lead to stimulation of the AT_2-R because their administration is followed by a reactive rise in angiotensin II levels. AT_2-R stimulation thus appears to be associated with increased bradykinin, nitric oxide, and cyclic guanosine monophosphate levels at least in renal interstitial fluid, although the significance of these changes is unclear.

The rise in bradykinin, which accompanies ACE inhibitor administration, also stimulates the production of endothelium-derived relaxing factor and the release of prostacyclin (PGI_2), although the exact contribution of prostaglandins to the antihypertensive effect of ACE inhibitors is still unknown. ARBs have been studied in a rather limited fashion relative to their having any effect on components of the prostaglandin axis. Although circulating levels of prostaglandin E_2 and PGI_2 metabolites are not significantly changed after ACE inhibitor administration, it has been recognized for some time that nonsteroidal anti-inflammatory drugs (NSAIDs) blunt the BP-lowering effect of ACE inhibitors (see "Class and Agent-Specific Drug Interactions" later in this chapter). Low-dose aspirin (<100 mg/day) has no significant effect on ACE inhibitor or ARB-induced BP reduction. Higher doses, generally above 236 mg/day, can occasionally blunt the antihypertensive response to ACE inhibitors.

A percentage of ACE inhibitor and ARB effect is also considered to be due to their reducing activity in the sympathetic nervous system (SNS). This is attributable to a change in central and peripheral SNS activities and to an attenuation of sympathetically mediated vasoconstriction, although these have not been consistent findings. ACE inhibitors are poorly differentiable as to their individual effects on the SNS, which may relate to differences among the various class members in tissue compartmentalization and/or penetration through the blood–brain barrier. In the instance of ARBs, there is little to distinguish one compound from the other in their central nervous system effects. Where differences are noted between the various compounds in this class, confounding variables such as route of administration, dose amount, duration of dosing, and a compound's ability to cross the blood–brain barrier have limited the generalizability of the findings. Alternatively, there is emerging evidence suggesting a differential effect of the ARB eprosartan on reducing SNS activity; however, this requires additional study. ACE inhibitors and ARBs also do not alter circulatory reflexes and/or baroreceptor function; thus, they do not increase heart rate when BP is lowered. This latter property explains why both of these drug classes are seldom accompanied by postural hypotension.

ACE inhibitors and ARBs also improve endothelial function, facilitate vascular remodeling, and favorably alter the viscoelastic properties of blood vessels. These additional properties of ACE inhibitors and ARBs may provide an explanation for the observation that the long-term BP reduction with these drug classes generally exceeds that observed in the short term. In addition, the heptapeptide angiotensin 1-7, which can be formed directly from angiotensin I by at least three endopeptidases, is a bioactive component of the RAA axis that may offset the actions of angiotensin II. ACE hydrolyzes angiotensin 1-7 to inactive peptide fragments, a process that is blocked by ACE inhibition. The counterregulatory role of angiotensin 1-7 to the pressor and proliferative actions of angiotensin II relates in part to its interaction with kinins.

PHARMACOLOGY

ACE Inhibitors

The first orally active ACE inhibitor was the drug captopril, which was released in 1981. Captopril is a sulfhydryl-containing compound, with a rapid and not particularly prolonged duration of action. Subsequently, the more long-acting compound enalapril maleate became available. Enalapril is a prodrug requiring in vivo hepatic and intestinal wall esterolysis to yield the active diacid inhibitor enalaprilat. All ACE inhibitors are administered as prodrugs with the exception of lisinopril and captopril. It was originally believed that the formation of the active diacid metabolite of an ACE inhibitor, such as enalapril, could be inhibited in the presence of hepatic impairment, such as in advanced CHF, but this has proven not to be the case. The extent of absorption, the degree of hydrolysis, and the bioavailability of enalapril in CHF patients appear to be similar to those values observed in normal subjects with the exception of the rates of absorption and hydrolysis being slightly slower in CHF.

ACE inhibitors are structurally heterogeneous. All ACE inhibitors reduce the activity of ACE but do so by binding different chemical side groups to ACE. The chemical structure of this ligand serves as a criterion for dividing the ACE inhibitors into three classes. For example, the active chemical side group, or ACE ligand, for captopril is a sulfhydryl moiety and that for fosinopril it is a phosphinyl group; each of the remaining ACE inhibitors contains a carboxyl group. The side group on an ACE inhibitor is one factor, which has been suggested as being responsible for different pharmacologic responses among these compounds. Thus, the sulfhydryl group on captopril is purported to act as a recyclable free-radical scavenger, and for this reason captopril has been suggested to differentially retard the process of atherogenesis and/or protect against MI and diabetes; however, this has not been clinically substantiated. In addition, captopril directly stimulates prostaglandin synthesis, whereas other ACE inhibitors accomplish this indirectly by increasing bradykinin activity. Alternatively, the sulfhydryl side group found on captopril is believed to lead to a higher rate of skin rash—usually in the form of maculopapular rashes—and dysgeusia. The presence of a phosphinyl group on fosinopril has been offered as the reason for its low incidence of cough and its ability to improve diastolic dysfunction. In the instance of the latter, the phosphinyl group may facilitate the myocardial penetration and/or retention of fosinopril and thereby improve myocardial energetics.

Although ACE inhibitors can be distinguished by differences in absorption, protein binding, half-life, and metabolic disposition, they behave quite similarly in how they lower BP (Table 5-3). Rarely, beyond the issue of frequency of dosing, should these pharmacologic subtleties govern selection of an agent. This being said, two pharmacologic considerations for the ACE inhibitors— route of systemic elimination and tissue binding—have generated considerable recent debate and warrant specific discussion.

Pharmacokinetics

There is no evidence for accumulation of the prodrugs ramipril, enalapril, fosinopril, trandolapril, and benazepril in chronic renal failure (CRF), which suggests that they undergo intact biliary clearance or that the metabolic conversion of these drugs to their active diacid is unaffected by renal failure. These findings have been offered by some as evidence for a dual–route of elimination for these compounds. Technically, this is true, but it is irrelevant to dosing of ACE inhibitors in CRF because these prodrug forms are marginally active. True dual–route-of-elimination ACE inhibitors are those whose active diacid is hepatically and renally cleared. Only the active diacids of the ACE inhibitors, fosinopril and trandolapril, undergo any significant degree of hepatic clearance. For all other ACE inhibitors, elimination is almost exclusively renal with different degrees of filtration and tubular secretion occurring. Tubular secretion as a mode of elimination for ACE inhibitors is compound specific and occurs via the organic anion secretory pathway. This property of combined renal and hepatic elimination minimizes accumulation of these compounds in CRF once dosing to steady state has occurred. To date, a direct adverse effect from ACE inhibitor accumulation has not been identified, although cough has been suggested but not proven to be an ACE inhibitor concentration-dependent side effect. It is probable, however, that the longer drug concentrations remain elevated—once a response occurs—the more likely BP will remain reduced. Thus, the major adverse consequence of drug accumulation may be that of prolonged hypotension and its organ-specific sequelae.

Tissue Binding

The second controversial pharmacologic feature of the ACE inhibitors relates to the concept of tissue binding. The physicochemical differences among ACE inhibitors, including binding affinity, potency, lipophilicity, and depot effect, allow for the arbitrary classification of ACE inhibitors according to tissue ACE affinity. The degree of functional in vivo inhibition of tissue ACE

TABLE 5-3 Pharmacokinetic Parameters of ACE Inhibitors

Drug	Onset/duration (h)	Peak hypotensive effect (h)	Protein binding (%)*	Effect of food on absorption	Serum half-life	Elimination†
Benazepril	1/24	2–4	>95	None	10–11	Renal/some biliary
Captopril	0.25/dose related	1–1.5	25–30	Reduced	<2	Renal, as disulfides
Enalapril	1/24	4–6	50	None	11	Renal
Fosinopril	1/24	2–6	95	None	11	Renal = hepatic
Lisinopril	1/24	6	10	None	13	Renal
Moexipril	1/24	4–6	50	Reduced	2–9	Renal/some biliary
Perindopril	1/24	3–7	10–20	Reduced	3–10	Renal
Quinapril	1/24	2	97	Reduced	2	Renal > hepatic
Ramipril	1–2/24	3–6	73	Reduced	13–17	Renal
Trandolapril	2–4/24	6–8	80–94	None	16–24	Renal > hepatic

*Protein binding may vary for the prodrug and the active diacid of an ACE inhibitor.
†The concept of renal elimination of an ACE inhibitor takes into account prodrug elimination and that of the active diacid when such is applicable.
Key: ACE, angiotension-converting enzyme.

produced by an ACE inhibitor parallels two compound properties: the inhibitor's binding affinity and the free inhibitor concentration within the tissue under survey. The free inhibitor concentration in turn represents the dynamic equilibrium state, which arises from the shuttling of ACE inhibitor to the tissue and its subsequent washout and return into the blood. Free inhibitor tissue concentrations are driven by traditional pharmacologic variables, including dose frequency and amount, absolute bioavailability, plasma half-life, tissue penetration, and subsequent retention at the tissue level. Bioavailability and half-life in blood can easily be determined and are important in the initial choice of an ACE inhibitor dose. When blood levels of an ACE inhibitor are high—typically in the first third to half of the dosing period—tissue retention of an ACE inhibitor is unlikely to significantly affect functional ACE inhibition. However, as ACE inhibitor blood levels drop toward the end of the dosing period, two factors appear to be crucial in prolonging functional ACE inhibition, inhibitor-binding affinity and tissue retention, which will directly influence the concentration of the free inhibitor in tissue.

The rank order of potency for several ACE inhibitors has been determined by using competition analyses and direct binding of tritium-labeled ACE inhibitors to tissue ACE (Table 5-4). The potency is quinaprilat = benazeprilat > ramiprilat > perindoprilat > lisinopril > enalaprilat > fosinopril > captopril. The process of tissue retention of ACE inhibitors also has been studied. Isolated organ bath studies examining the duration of ACE inhibition after the removal of ACE inhibitor from the external milieu have shown that functional inhibition of ACE lasts well beyond (two to five times longer) the time predicted solely on the basis of inhibitor dissociation rates or binding affinity. The rank order of tissue retention is quinaprilat > lisinopril > enalaprilat > captopril and reflects the binding affinity and lipophilicity of these inhibitors.

The question arises as to whether the degree of tissue ACE inhibition may extend to differences in efficacy among various ACE inhibitors. This is a very different question than whether an ACE inhibitor displays tissue-protective effects independent of the degree to which it lowers BP, as suggested by the HOPE Study. Clearly, a reduction in angiotensin II and increased nitric oxide bioavailability may represent mechanisms by which ACE inhibitors confer vascular protection. Consequently, endothelial function may be regarded as a surrogate marker for vascular protection. The effects of ACE inhibitors on endothelium-dependent relaxation appear to differ among several reports and appear to be dependent on the agents used and the construct of the experimental design. It should be noted that consistent improvement in endothelial function is reported with those ACE inhibitors with higher tissue ACE affinity, such as quinapril and ramipril. Despite the appealing nature of these relations, there have been few direct head-to-head trials between ACE inhibitors, which are highly tissue bound, and those ACE inhibitors with more limited tissue binding. In situations where such comparisons have occurred, the results do not convincingly support the claim of overall superiority for lipophilic ACE inhibitors.

Application of Pharmacologic Differences

Because there is very little that truly separates one ACE inhibitor from another in the treatment of hypertension, the cost of an ACE inhibitor has become a dominant issue. Allowing pricing to be a major factor behind the selection of an ACE inhibitor ignores the fact that only a small number of

TABLE 5-4 Pharmacologic Properties of Various ACE Inhibitors in Plasma and Tissue

Tissue potency	ACE inhibitor potencies $(\text{mmol/L} \times 10^{-9}$, ID$)$	Enzymatic (IC_{50})† — Inhibition	Radioligand (DD_{50})* — Displacement	Plasma half-life‡	Relative lipid solubility#
High					
Quinaprilat	0.07	5.5×10^{-11}	4.5×10^{-11}	25	++
Benazeprilat	NA	1.3×10^{-9}	4.8×10^{-11}	11	+
Ramiprilat	0.08	1.9×10^{-9}	7.0×10^{-11}	>50	++
Perindoprilat	0.40	NA	NA	10	++
Lisinopril	NA	4.5×10^{-9}	1.7×10^{-10}	12	NA
Enalaprilat	1.00	4.5×10^{-9}	1.1×10^{-9}	11	+
Fosinoprilat	NA	1.6×10^{-8}	5.1×10^{-10}	11.5	+++
Low					
Captopril	15.00	NA	NA	2	+

*Radioligand binding studies using the active drug moiety.

†Comparison of IC_{50} with DD_{50} from human plasma ACE.

‡Values cited for quinaprilat and ramiprilat are for dissociation from tissue ACE, i.e., terminal half-life.

#Lipid solubility based on log-P logarithm of the octanol/water partition coefficient of the active drug moiety, except for captopril.

Key: ACE, angiotensin-converting enzyme; DD_{50}, 50% displacement of ^{125}I-351A from human plasma ACE; IC_{50}, 50% inhibition of enzymatic activity; ID_{50}, inhibitor concentration required to displace 50% of ^{125}I-5311A bound to human plasma; NA, not available; + signs represent increased lipid solubility.

Source: Adapted with permission from Dzau VJ, Bernstein K, Celermajer D, et al: The relevance of tissue angiotensin converting enzyme: manifestations in mechanistic and endpoint data. Am J Cardiol 88(suppl 9):20L, 2001.

ACE inhibitors has been studied specifically for their ability to protect end organs. *Class effect* is a phrase often invoked to legitimatize use of a less costly ACE inhibitor when a higher priced agent in the class was the one specifically studied in a disease state, such as CHF or diabetic nephropathy. The concept of class effect may be best suited for application to the use of ACE inhibitors in the treatment of hypertension. Therein, little appears to distinguish one ACE inhibitor from another. Alternatively, it is less certain as to what represents true dose equivalence among ACE inhibitors when they are being used to treat proteinuric renal disease or CHF. In the treatment of proteinuric renal disease, the dose–response relationship for an ACE inhibitor and proteinuria reduction has been poorly explored, a situation made more complex by the observation that the antiproteinuric effects of ACE inhibitors are greater in patients with higher than the baseline urine protein excretion. Because there are very few hard end-point studies in nephropathic patients with ACE inhibitors, it seems reasonable, at least for now, to use cost as a criterion for selection of an ACE inhibitor.

Alternatively, in the case of CHF, BP normalization and reduction in urine protein excretion are not specific treatment goals. Rather, dose titration is attempted to a presumed maximal tissue effect dose because improvement in the morbidity and mortality of CHF with ACE inhibitors is dose dependent, although the differences are relatively modest between different doses of a specific ACE inhibitor. Thus, the success of an ACE inhibitor in CHF may derive from many neurohumoral and tissue-based changes and not just from changes in angiotensin II consequent to inhibition of ACE. Because not all ACE inhibitors have been thoroughly studied in CHF or, for that matter, clinically approved for CHF use (see Table 5-1), in particular relative to secondary neurohumoral response parameters, it is less likely that specific doses of different ACE inhibitors are truly interchangeable in the treatment of CHF.

Angiotensin-Receptor Blockers

The ARBs are a relatively new class of drugs employed in the treatment of hypertension. These agents work selectively at the AT_1-R subtype, the receptor that mediates all of the known physiologic effects of angiotensin II that are believed to be relevant to cardiovascular and cardiorenal homeostasis. Similar to ACE inhibitors, the ARBs each have a unique pharmacologic profile. The pharmacologic differentiation of the various ARBs is a topic of growing relevance in that the ability to reduce BP may differ among the individual drugs comprising this class. Since the release of the first ARB losartan (Cozaar) in 1995, six other compounds have been developed and are now marketed in the United States. These compounds include candesartan (Atacand), eprosartan (Teveten), irbesartan (Avapro), olmesartan (Benicar), telmisartan (Micardis), and valsartan (Diovan). These compounds are now commonly given together with hydrochlorothiazide (HCTZ) as fixed-dose combination antihypertensive products. Currently available information does not suggest that any specific pharmacologic differences exist for an ARB if it were to be administered alone or with HCTZ in a fixed-dose combination product.

Pharmacokinetics

Bioavailability The bioavailabilities of the individual ARBs are quite variable (Table 5-5). Three of the ARBs are administered in a prodrug form— losartan, candesartan cilexetil, and olmesartan medoxomil—although, technic-

TABLE 5-5 Bioavailability of the ARBs

Drug	Bioavailability (%)	Food effect
Candesartan cilexetil	15	No
Eprosartan	6–29	AUC ↓ ≈25%
Irbesartan	60–80	No
Losartan	33	AUC ↓ ≈10%
Olmesartan	29	No
Telmisartan	42–58	AUC ↓ ≈6–24%
Valsartan	25	AUC ↓ ≈50%

Key: AUC, area under the curve.

ally speaking, losartan is an active compound, albeit one ultimately converted to its more potent E-3174 metabolite. The bioavailability of eprosartan is low (≈13%), a phenomenon that is not due to high first-pass elimination. Eprosartan absorption is to a degree saturable over the dose range of 100 to 800 mg, most likely due to the physicochemical properties of the drug. Irbesartan demonstrates a bioavailability profile with an absorption range between 60% and 80% and is without a food effect. Losartan has a moderate bioavailability (≈33%), with 14% of an administered dose being transformed to the E-3174 metabolite. Telmisartan appears to have a saturable first-pass effect for its absorption; thus, the higher the dose the greater the absolute bioavailability. Unfortunately, the most pertinent absorption characteristic of individual AT_1-RAs, day-to-day variability in bioavailability, is not routinely reported.

Dose proportionality   The concept of dose proportionality is important in any consideration of dose escalation for an antihypertensive agent to obtain BP control. One pattern of dose proportionality is displayed by irbesartan. In this regard, the results of two double-blind, placebo-controlled studies involving 88 healthy subjects showed irbesartan to display, linear, dose-related pharmacokinetics for its area under the curve (AUC) with escalating doses over a dose range from 10 to 600 mg. The maximum plasma concentration (C_{max}) over this same dose range was related to the dose in a linear but less than dose-proportional manner. Increases in plasma AUC and C_{max} in subjects receiving 900 mg of irbesartan were smaller than predicted from dose proportionality. Possible explanations for this phenomenon are that intestinal absorption is dose limited, perhaps due to saturation of a carrier system at high drug concentrations, or that the dissolution characteristics of a compound are dose dependent. In the instance of irbesartan, that the terminal half-life of irbesartan is unchanged with higher irbesartan doses suggests that the intestinal absorption of irbesartan may saturate with increasing doses but that its metabolism and excretion are not so dose limited. Each of these proposed mechanisms may explain the absence of dose proportionality at doses above 400 mg that is observed with the ARB eprosartan. It should be noted that the absence of dose proportionality for various of the ARBs, at doses, which are rarely employed clinically, has little, if any, relevance to the use of these compounds in the treatment of hypertension.

Volume of distribution   The ARBs typically have a volume of distribution (V_D), which approximates extracellular fluid volume, in part, in relation to the extensive protein binding of these compounds. For example, the V_D for losartan and its E-3174 metabolite are 34 L and 12 L, respectively, whereas the V_D for candesartan, olmesartan, valsartan, and eprosartan are approximately 10 (0.13 L/kg body weight), 30 L, 17 L, and 13 L, respectively. Alternatively, telmisartan and irbesartan have the highest V_D of any of the ARBs, with values of 500 and 53 to 93/L (data on file, Bristol-Myers Squibb), respectively. That telmisartan has a V_D that is so high likely relates to a loose binding relation with its predominant protein carrier, albumin. To date, the clinical significance of ARBs having a high V_D remains unclear. Moreover, the V_D of the ARBs in disease states, such as renal failure, is unreported. Parenthetically, it has been suggested that the greater the V_D for an ARB, the more likely it is that extravascular AT_1-Rs can be accessed and, therefore, at least in theory, the more profound the vasodepressor response.

Protein binding The protein binding of the ARBs is typically well in excess of 90%. The exception to this pharmacologic characteristic is the ARB irbesartan, which has the highest plasma-free fraction (4% to 5%; data on file, Bristol-Myers Squibb). In general, none of the ARBs binds to red blood cells in a pharmacokinetically significant fashion. Further, the extent of protein binding for the ARBs remains fairly constant over a wide concentration range. Typically, protein binding dictates the V_D for a compound, and, in fact, irbesartan demonstrates a V_D somewhat higher than that of the other ARBs, with the exception of telmisartan. The significance of high protein binding for any ARB remains to be determined.

Metabolism and active metabolite generation There are two ways to view metabolic conversion of an ARB. It may be a step required to produce an active metabolite; such is the case with losartan, candesartan cilexetil, and olmesartan medoxomil. Alternatively, metabolic conversion may factor into the conversion of a compound to a physiologically inactive metabolite, as in the case of irbesartan. Losartan, an active substrate molecule, is converted via the P450 isozyme system (2C9 and 3A4) to its more active metabolite, E-3174, whereas candesartan cilexetil, a prodrug, is hydrolyzed to the active compound candesartan in the course of absorption from the gastrointestinal tract.

The metabolic conversion of candesartan cilexetil, an ester prodrug, seems not to be affected to any degree by disease state, genetic variation in metabolism, or chronic dosing. The metabolic conversion of losartan to E-3174 has been evaluated. Variants of cytochrome CYP2C9 have been identified. The presence of certain of these variants decreases the conversion of losartan to its active E-3174 metabolite. To date, fewer than 1% of the population of patients exposed to therapy with losartan have this abnormal genetic profile for the metabolism of losartan. Thus, it is unlikely that a metabolic polymorphism for losartan breakdown will ever be found in sufficient numbers of patients to matter clinically.

It has also been suggested that known inhibitors of the P450 system and, more specifically, inhibitors of the P450 2C9 and 3A4 isozymes, such as fluconazole and ketoconazole, might interfere with the conversion of losartan to its E-3174 metabolite. In theory, such drugs might interfere with the rate and the extent of metabolism of losartan to its active E-3174 metabolite. Consequently, BP control might become more difficult to achieve and/or maintain if losartan-treated patients were simultaneously treated with such enzyme inhibitors. Although this hypothesis seemed attractive initially, the available data do not support it. Drug–drug interactions of this nature are difficult to predict in broad population bases; thus, if a losartan-treated patient is simultaneously treated with inhibitors of the P450 2C9 and/or 3A4 isozymes,

BP should be closely monitored. A final consideration with losartan is its degree of interaction with grapefruit juice. Although not formally tested as to its influencing the BP-lowering effect of losartan, grapefruit juice given with losartan will reduce its conversion to E3174 and will activate P-glycoprotein, which in sum significantly increases the $AUC_{losartan}/AUC_{E-3174}$ ratio.

Telmisartan is exclusively metabolized by conjugation to glucuronic acid. This lack of CYP450-dependent metabolism distinguishes telmisartan from other ARBs. Irbesartan undergoes metabolism to several glucuronidated or oxidated metabolites via the P450 2C9 pathway, with metabolism by the P450 3A4 pathway being negligible. The primary circulating metabolite is irbesartan glucuronide, which represents approximately 6% of circulating metabolites. These metabolites do not possess relevant pharmacologic activity.

Route of elimination It is well recognized that the systemic clearance of a compound is dependent on the integrity of renal and hepatic functions. As a result, if renal and/or hepatic dysfunction exists in a patient, repeated dosing of an antihypertensive compound inevitably will lead to drug accumulation and the occasional need to adjust the dose to lessen concentration-related side effects. The ARBs have been studied only recently as to their renal and/or hepatic handling (Table 5-6). All these drugs undergo a significant degree of hepatic elimination with the exception of olmesartan, candesartan, and the E-3174 metabolite of losartan, which are 40%, 60%, and 50% hepatically cleared, respectively. Among the ARBs, irbesartan and telmisartan undergo the greatest degree of hepatic elimination, with each having greater than 95% of their systemic clearance to be hepatic. Valsartan and eprosartan each undergo about 70% hepatic clearance. On the surface, the mode of elimination for an ARB may seem like a trivial issue. In reality, it proves to be an important variable in the renally compromised patient and may in fact dictate various elements of the change in renal function that occasionally occurs in the renal failure patient. In those who develop acute renal failure after receipt of a hepatically cleared ARB, the duration of any renal failure episode is tempered by the quick hepatic disposition of the compound, a process that does not occur when the compound in question is mainly renally cleared.

To date, very few studies have assessed the BP-lowering effect of ARBs in the renally compromised patient. In the studies reported to date, the BP-lowering effect of these compounds is evident in the renal failure patient and, in certain instances, may be quite significant. Dose adjustment, or more so, cautious use in CRF is advocated with some ARBs—such as valsartan and olmesartan—that are partly renally cleared. This is more likely because of presumed heightened sensitivity to this drug class rather than compound-

TABLE 5-6 Mode of Elimination for ARBs

Drug	Renal (%)	Hepatic (%)
Candesartan	60	40
Eprosartan	30	70
Irbesartan	1	99
Losartan	10	90
E-3174	50	50
Olmesartan	40	60
Telmisartan	1	99
Valsartan	30	70

specific adverse effects. A final consideration with the ARBs is that they are not dialyzable. Additional experience is needed with the ARBs before definitive statements can be made concerning their efficacy in the renal failure population and whether relevant drug accumulation occurs with those ARBs, which undergo significant renal clearance, as is the case with the E-3174 metabolite of losartan, candesartan, and olmesartan.

Receptor binding and half-life The half-life ($t_{1/2}$) of a compound is a purely pharmacokinetic term that often correlates poorly with the duration of effect of a compound. This has typically been the case with antihypertensive compounds, including ACE inhibitors and the ARBs. The discrepancy between the pharmacokinetic and pharmacodynamic $t_{1/2}$ of a compound derives from the fact that the predominant site of drug action for many compounds is to be found somewhere other than the vascular compartment. Because of the inability to sample at these extravascular sites of action for many drugs, the more meaningful tissue-based $t_{1/2}$ cannot be determined. This is particularly the case for the ARBs, because AT_1-Rs are found in multiple locations outside the vascular compartment, and blocking AT_1-Rs at these alternative locations may, in an as of yet undefined fashion, influence the manner in which BP is reduced.

With these observations in mind, the pharmacokinetic $t_{1/2}$ of an ARB will roughly approximate its duration of effect. Several of the ARBs, such as candesartan, olmesartan, telmisartan, and irbesartan, are observed to be once-daily compounds in pharmacokinetic terms. The true impact of pharmacologic $t_{1/2}$ for these compounds probably lies more so in the fact that the drug is available for a longer period and thereby binds to additional AT_1-Rs as they are formed during a dosing interval. This phenomenon becomes obvious if the pressor response to angiotensin II is evaluated. For example, a 300-mg dose of irbesartan maintains almost 60% inhibition of the pressor response to angiotensin II 24 h after the dose is administered. This observation, although interpretable in several ways, suggests that drug half-life has a role in duration of response. Such data at best provide guidelines for therapy because patient responses are typically highly individualized.

Application of pharmacologic differences/receptor affinity Receptor affinity is just one of several factors that determine the action of an ARB. An ARB demonstrates *insurmountable* or *noncompetitive* blockade if incrementally higher concentrations of angiotensin II can not overcome receptor blockade. The terms *surmountable*, *competitive*, *insurmountable*, and *noncompetitive* often are used interchangeably and often in an inconsistent fashion. *Surmountable antagonism* implies that receptor blockade eventually can be overcome if high enough concentrations of angiotensin II are made available. *Surmountable* antagonists shift concentration–response curves parallel one to the other and rightward without diminishing the maximal response to an agonist. Losartan behaves as a surmountable antagonist. In the case of *competitive* antagonism, mass action kinetics exists, and agonists and antagonists individually compete for receptor binding. Eprosartan functions as a *competitive* antagonist. *Noncompetitive*, irreversible antagonism is a phenomenon of loss of receptor numbers occurring by a process of chemical modification.

Insurmountable antagonism mimics *noncompetitive* antagonism. *Insurmountable* antagonists bind to their receptors in a semi-irreversible fashion, which differs from the permanent binding that occurs with *noncompetitive* antagonists. An *insurmountable* antagonist releases from its receptor slowly;

thus, its drug-receptor dissociation constant can be quite prolonged. *Insurmountable* antagonists elicit a parallel shift of the agonist concentration-response curves, with a depression in the maximal agonist response that is not overcome by increasing concentrations of the agonist. Valsartan, irbesartan, telmisartan, and the E-3174 metabolite of losartan exhibit this form of antagonism.

Insurmountable antagonists also can elicit nonparallel shifts of the agonist concentration–response curves, thus depressing the maximal response to the agonist, a process that is not overcome by increasing concentrations of the agonist. Candesartan demonstrates this form of *insurmountable* antagonism. To date, the specific mode of receptor occupancy and/or differential pharmacokinetic features of an ARB have not been clearly linked with the different BP responses to these drugs; thus, the actual basis for the superior efficacy of drugs, such as candesartan and irbesartan, as compared with losartan in terms of reduction in BP and maintenance of antihypertensive efficacy between doses is not clear. Instead, compound-specific differences in angiotensin II receptor blockade, a surrogate for the BP-lowering response of these drugs, can be explained by differences in dosing, as was recently shown, wherein the effects of 160-mg or 320-mg doses of valsartan hardly differed from those obtained with recommended doses of irbesartan and candesartan.

HEMODYNAMIC EFFECTS

Many well-described hemodynamic effects occur with the administration of an ACE inhibitor (Table 5-7). Although not comprehensively examined in a head-to-head fashion with ACE inhibitors, ARBs seem to exhibit quite similar hemodynamic profiles with the occasional difference, which may depend on the study design. The underlying disease being treated frequently dictates the magnitude change in many of these hemodynamic parameters. This is particularly evident in the treatment of CHF and/or renal failure, in which hemodynamic responses may be exaggerated and linked to the degree to which BP drops. In addition, many of these hemodynamic changes are accentuated in the presence of an activated RAA axis, as may occur with diuretic therapy and/or a low-salt diet. The latter is a well-established risk factor for the occurrence of *first-dose hypotension* with an ACE inhibitor and/or an ARB.

In the treatment of hypertension, the observed reduction in BP with an ACE inhibitor or an ARB is not accompanied by a decrease in cardiac output or an increase in heart rate. Occasionally, cardiac output increases with ACE inhibitor therapy, particularly if cardiac output is reduced before therapy has begun. The fall in peripheral vascular resistance that accompanies ACE inhibitor therapy is occasionally accompanied by a decrease in cardiac filling pressures. Angiotensin II can actively modulate coronary vascular tone and blood flow, particularly if the RAA axis is activated. In turn, treatment with an ACE inhibitor can correct angiotensin II–mediated reductions in coronary blood flow. Several small trials, which have typically been of short duration, have assessed the effects of ACE inhibitors on the severity of angina and/or on objective measures of myocardial ischemia and have generated conflicting results.

In addition, ACE inhibitors lower BP without diminishing cerebral blood flow. This phenomenon is believed to represent a favorable effect of ACE inhibition on cerebral autoregulatory ability and is potentially of relevance to the treatment of hypertension in the elderly. Further, ACE inhibitors decrease capacitance vessel tone, which may explain why ACE inhibitors can alleviate the peripheral edema associated with calcium-channel blocker (CCB) ther-

TABLE 5-7 Predominant Hemodynamic Effects of ACE Inhibitors and ARBs

Hemodynamic parameter	Effect	Clinical significance
Cardiovascular		
Total peripheral resistance	Decreased	
Mean arterial pressure	Decreased	
Cardiac output	Increased or no change	These parameters contribute to a general decrease in systemic blood pressure
Stroke volume	Increased	
Preload and afterload	Decreased	
Pulmonary artery pressure	Decreased	
Right atrial pressure	Decreased	
Diastolic dysfunction	Improved	
Renal		
Renal blood flow	Usually increased	Contributes to the renoprotective effect of these agents
Glomerular filtration rate	Variable, usually unchanged but may decrease in renal failure	
Efferent arteriolar resistance	Decreased	
Filtration fraction	Decreased	
Peripheral nervous system		
Biosynthesis of noradrenaline	Decreased	Enhances blood pressure–lowering effect and resets baroreceptor function
Reuptake of adrenaline	Inhibited	
Circulating catecholamines	Decreased	

apy. ACE inhibitors do not limit the peak heart rate response to exercise, although they do effectively reduce the peak BP response. The addition of a diuretic to an ACE inhibitor does not alter the hemodynamic profile of ACE inhibition except in the instance of exercise, when the exercise-related increase in cardiac output may be blunted.

ACE inhibitors and ARBs routinely increase effective renal plasma flow (ERPF) and maintain glomerular filtration rate (GFR). The rise in ERPF evoked by these two drug classes is characterized by a preferential vasodilatation of the post-glomerular or efferent arteriolar vascular bed. The functional consequence of these renal hemodynamic changes is a drop in the filtration fraction (GFR/ERPF), a well-accepted marker for a reduction in angiotensin II effect on the kidney. When glomerular filtration is strongly reliant on efferent arteriolar tone, as in CHF, dehydration, and/or renal artery stenosis, and an ACE inhibitor or an ARB is administered, the GFR may suddenly and precipitously fall.

BLOOD PRESSURE–LOWERING EFFECT

Diuretics and beta blockers are commonly employed as first-step therapy for hypertension, although ACE inhibitors and, more recently, ARBs are increasingly viewed as a suitable first-step alternative. The enthusiasm for the use of

ACE inhibitors is not purely a matter of efficacy because they have a pattern of efficacy comparable to (and no better than) most other drug classes, with response rates from 40% to 70% in stage I or II hypertension. A similar range of response rates has been reported with ARBs. In head-to-head BP trials comparing ACE inhibitors with ARBs, there appears to be scant difference between the two drug classes. Clinical trial results obviously do not reflect conditions in actual practice in which the favorable side effect profile of ACE inhibitors and ARBs and their highly touted end-organ protection features seem to dominate the thinking of many practitioners. In this regard, ACE inhibitors are extensively used because they are well tolerated and patients will continue to take these drugs over a long period. The same can be said for ARBs, a drug class with a tolerability profile that is superior to that of the ACE inhibitors.

The enthusiasm for these two drug classes must be put in proper perspective because, in uncomplicated nondiabetic hypertensive patients, a number of drug classes given at low doses can prove effective and are well tolerated at a fraction of the cost of ACE inhibitors and ARBs. Alternatively, increasing evidence supports the preferential use of ACE inhibitors and, more recently, ARBs in the diabetic and/or at-risk cardiac or renal patient with established atherosclerotic disease or proteinuria and offers a positive view of these drugs that is not available from prior comparator trials with ACE inhibitors. For many of these at-risk cardiac or renal patients, the recommendations for ACE inhibitor use are not based on the BP-lowering ability of these drugs, but rather on proposed tissue-based anti-inflammatory and antiproliferative effects, which likely are specific to the class and not to the agent.

There are very few predictors of the BP response to ACE inhibitors or ARBs. When hypertension is accompanied by significant activation of the RAA axis, as in renal artery stenosis, the response to an ACE inhibitor or an ARB can be immediate and profound. In most other cases, there is a limited relation between the pre- and posttreatment PRA value, which is used as a marker of RAA axis activity, and the vasodepressor response to an ACE inhibitor or an ARB. Certain patient types demonstrate lower response rates to ACE inhibitor and ARB monotherapy, including low-renin, salt-sensitive individuals such as the diabetic and African American or elderly hypertensive. The low-renin state, characteristic of the elderly hypertensive, differs from other low-renin forms of hypertension in that it develops not as a response to volume expansion, but because of senescence-related changes in the activity of the axis. The elderly generally respond well to ACE inhibitors at conventional doses, although senescence-related renal failure, which slows the elimination of these drugs, complicates interpretation of dose-specific treatment successes. The elderly hypertensive, with systolic-predominant hypertension, also responds well to ARBs. African American hypertensives, who as a group tend to have reduced activity in the RAA axis, are perceived as being poorly responsive to ACE inhibitor monotherapy when compared with Caucasians; nevertheless, in many instances, if careful dose titration occurs, BP eventually will be reduced with monotherapy or an appropriately constructed multidrug regimen based on ACE inhibitor therapy. This response pattern suggests that eliminating even small amounts of activity in the RAA axis is important to BP control.

All 10 ACE inhibitors are currently approved by the U.S. Food and Drug Administration (FDA) for the treatment of hypertension. The Joint National Committee (JNC) on the Detection, Evaluation, and Treatment of High Blood Pressure and the World Health Organization/International Society of Hypertension now recognize ACE inhibitors as an option for first-line therapy in patients with essential hypertension, especially in those with diabetes who also have renal disease or proteinuria and in those with CHF. The advisory position for ACE inhibitor use is currently in a state of flux. The results of the Antihypertensive and Lipid Lowering Treatment to Prevent Heart Attack Trial showed that the ACE inhibitor lisinopril is similar in its effects on a composite end point of fatal coronary heart disease and nonfatal MI when compared with chlorthalidone. In contrast, the results of a smaller comparative trial in older hypertensive patients showed the superiority of ACE inhibitors over HCTZ with regard to cardiovascular outcomes. Considerable dosing flexibility exists with the available ACE inhibitors. Enalaprilat is the sole ACE inhibitor available in an intravenous form (Table 5-8). The dosing frequency for ACE inhibitors is somewhat arbitrary and should consider the fact that these drugs may begin to lose their effect at the end of the dosing interval and necessitate a second dose. Likewise, in the treatment of CHF, ACE inhibitors indicated for once-daily dosing might require split dosing if BP drops excessively with a single administered dose.

Results from a number of head-to-head trials have supported the comparable antihypertensive efficacy and tolerability of the various ACE inhibitors. However, there are differences among the ACE inhibitors as to the time to onset of effect and/or the time to maximum BP reduction, which may relate to the absorption characteristics of the various compounds. These differences, however, do not translate into different response rates *if* comparable doses of the individual ACE inhibitors are given. Typical confounding variables, which confuse the interpretation of the findings in BP studies with ACE inhibitors, have included differences in study design and methodology and in dose frequency and amount. ACE inhibitors labeled as "once-daily" differ in their ability to reduce BP for a full 24 h, as defined by a trough:peak ratio greater than 50%. Unfortunately, the trough:peak ratio, as an index of duration of BP control, is oftentimes prone to misrepresent the true BP reduction seen with a compound. As stated previously, dosing instructions for many of these compounds include the proviso to administer a second-daily dose if the antihypertensive effect has dissipated by the end of the dosing interval.

The question is often raised as to what to do if an ACE inhibitor fails to normalize BP. One approach is simply to raise the dose; however, the dose–response curve for ACE inhibitors, like most antihypertensive agents, is fairly steep at the beginning doses and thereafter shallow to flat. Responders to ACE inhibitors typically do so at doses well below those necessary for prolonged 24-h suppression of ACE. In addition, the maximal vasodepressor response to an ACE inhibitor does not occur until several weeks after therapy is begun and may involve factors, such as vascular remodeling, above and beyond inhibition of ACE. Thus, only with complete failure to respond to an ACE inhibitor should an alternative drug class be substituted. If a partial response has occurred, then therapy with an ACE inhibitor can be continued in anticipation of an additional drop in BP over the next several weeks. Alternatively, an additional compound such as a diuretic, CCB, or peripheral alpha blocker can be combined with an ACE inhibitor to effect better BP control (see Chapter 16).

Virtually all of the previous comments directed to the pharmacotherapeutic response to ACE inhibitors apply to the ARB class of drugs (Table 5-9). These include considerations of predictors of response, onset and duration of response, the structure of their dose–response curves, and their capacity to have a late onset additional BP response. Several head-to-head studies have

TABLE 5-8 ACE Inhibitors: Dosage Strengths and Treatment Guidelines

Drug	Trade name	Usual total dose (frequency/d)		Comment	Fixed-dose combination*
		Hypertension	Heart failure		
Benazepril	Lotensin	20–40 (1)	Not FDA approved for heart failure		Lotensin-HCT, Lotrel
Captopril	Capoten	12.5–100 (2–3)	18.75–150 (3)	Generically available	Capozide†
Enalapril	Vasotec	5–40 (1–2)	5–40 (2)	Generic and intravenous	Vaseretic
Fosinopril	Monopril	10–40 (1)	10–40 (1)	Renal and hepatic elimination	Monopril-HCT
Lisinopril	Prinivil, Zestril	2.5–40 (1)	5–20 (1)	Generically available	Prinizide, Zestoretic, Uniretic
Moexipril	Univasc	7.5–30 (1)	Not FDA approved for heart failure		
Perindopril	Aceon	2–16 (1)	Not FDA approved for heart failure		
Quinapril	Accupril	5–80 (1)	10–40 (1–2)		Accuretic
Ramipril	Altace	2.5–20 (1)	10 (2)	Indicated in high-risk vascular patients	
Trandolapril	Mavik	1–8 (1)	1–4 (1)	Renal and hepatic elimination	Tarka

*Fixed-dose combinations in this class typically contain a thiazide-like diuretic or a calcium-channel blocker.
†Capozide is indicated for first-step treatment of hypertension.
Key: FDA, U.S. Food and Drug Administration; HCT, hydrochlorothiazide.

113

TABLE 5-9 ARBs: Dosage Strengths and Treatment Guidelines

Drug	Trade name	Usual total dose range (frequency/d)	Comment	Fixed-dose combinations
Candesartan	Atacand	2–32 (1)	Superior to losartan for BP control	Atacand-HCT
Eprosartan	Teveten	400–800 (1)	Possibly decreases SNS	
Irbesartan	Avapro	75–300 (1)	Indicated in diabetic nephropathy	Avalide
Losartan	Cozaar	25–100 (1)	Indicated in diabetic nephropathy; uricosuric	Hyzaar
Olmesartan	Benicar	10–40 (1)		
Telmesartan	Micardis	20–80 (1)		Micardis-HCT
Valsartan	Diovan	80–320 (1)	Indicated in congestive heart failure	Diovan-HCT

Key: BP, blood pressure; HCT, hydrochlorothiazide; SNS, sympathetic nervous system.

been conducted between different ARBs. The results of these comparisons have suggested that candesartan cilexetil, irbesartan, and olmesartan may be more effective than the prototype ARB, losartan. Moreover, studies mimicking the common event of a missed or delayed dose of antihypertensive medication have shown that the antihypertensive effect of candesartan cilexetil extends well beyond the 24-h dosing interval, whereas the effect of losartan declines rapidly over this period.

Few studies have directly compared more than two ARBs. Exceptions to this include a meta-analysis of randomized controlled trials by Conlin et al. and a crossover study by Fogari et al. Both studies compared the efficacy of losartan, valsartan, irbesartan, and candesartan at low doses (50, 80, 150, and 8 mg, respectively) and after titration to double these doses. The meta-analysis revealed no differences among these drugs in their ability to reduce BP at the starting dose or after forced or elective titration. In the crossover study, valsartan and irbesartan reduced BP more effectively than losartan when the drugs were used at their respective starting doses, although the difference was not maintained after elective dose titration. In attempting to evaluate real or perceived differences among the ARBs, a meta-analysis can be useful in determining dose–response relations for individual drugs, but randomized, prospective, double-blind, head-to-head comparative studies remain the most accurate way to compare efficacy between drugs and seem to favor several of the more recent additions to the ARB class over losartan. The FDA recently allowed an additional labeling claim for candesartan as being superior to losartan in its antihypertensive efficacy.

ACE INHIBITORS AND ARBS IN COMBINATION WITH OTHER AGENTS

To date, there appears to be little difference in the BP-lowering effects between ACE inhibitors and ARBs given in combination with other drug classes including diuretics and CCBs. Because of the paucity of published information for ARBs given in combination with other antihypertensive medication classes—with the exception of diuretic therapy—this section emphasizes the available combination therapies with ACE inhibitors. The BP-lowering effect of an ACE inhibitor is enhanced by the simultaneous administration of a diuretic, particularly in the African American hypertensive. This pattern of response has spurred the development of a number of fixed-dose combination products comprised of an ACE inhibitor and low to moderate doses of thiazide-type diuretics. The rationale for combining these two drug classes derives from the observation that the sodium depletion produced by a diuretic increases activity in the RAA axis. Consequently, BP shifts to an angiotensin II–dependent mode, which is the optimal circumstance for an ACE inhibitor to reduce BP. Even very low-dose diuretic therapy, such as 12.5 mg of HCTZ, can evoke this synergistic response, suggesting that even subtle alterations in sodium balance are sufficient to bolster the effect of an ACE inhibitor (see Chapters 6 and 16). Noteworthy is the observation that the addition of a diuretic to an ACE inhibitor or an ARB eliminates the racial disparity in response to ACE inhibitors and ARBs.

ACE inhibitors have been given with beta blockers. The rationale behind this combination is that the beta blocker presumably aborts the rise in PRA induced by an ACE inhibitor. It was presumed that, by preventing this hyper-reninemic response, the ACE inhibitor response might be more robust. Although this hypothesis originally seemed attractive, in practice only a modest additional vasodepressor response occurs when these two drug classes are combined. When BP substantively falls after addition of a beta blocker to an ACE inhibitor, it is generally because pulse rate has been reduced in a patient whose BP is pulse rate dependent. Alternatively, the addition of a peripheral α-antagonist, such as doxazosin, to an ACE inhibitor can be followed by a significant additional BP response. The mechanism behind this additive response remains to be more fully elucidated. Further, the BP-lowering effect of an ACE inhibitor is considerably enhanced by the coadministration of a CCB.

This additive response occurs whether the CCB being given is a dihydropyridine (e.g., felodipine or amlodipine) or a nondihydropyridine, such as verapamil. The potency of this combination has provided the practical basis for the development of a number of fixed-dose combination products comprised of an ACE inhibitor and a CCB. Adding an ACE inhibitor to a CCB is also useful because the ACE inhibitor component of the combination attenuates the peripheral edema that accompanies CCB therapy.

The efficacy of using ACE inhibitors and ARBs as antihypertensive agents is well documented. Quite logically, this has led to the belief that these two drug classes in combination may reduce BP better than if either were to be given alone. In contradistinction to the wealth of information on monotherapy with these drugs, there is strikingly little information about the efficacy of combined ACE inhibitor and ARB therapy. Moreover, the trials currently published are not generalizable because, in many instances, they involve a small number of patients and employ study designs with inherent limitations. For example, in one clinical trial, 20 patients received monotherapy with benazepril for 6 weeks. If average awake ambulatory diastolic BPs remained above 85 mm Hg, subjects were randomized to valsartan, 80 mg/day, or matching placebo in a blinded manner for 5 weeks while continuing to receive background benazepril. The patients then crossed over to the alternative regimen for a second 5-week period. Valsartan added to benazepril reduced BP by 6.5 ± 12.6/4.5 ± 8.0 mm Hg (systolic/diastolic) over placebo for average awake ambulatory BP. Nocturnal systolic and diastolic BPs were similarly reduced by 7.1 ± 9.4/5.6 ± 6.5 mm Hg. Until more substantive supporting information is forthcoming, the combination of an ACE inhibitor and an ARB should have a limited role in the treatment of hypertension.

Many studies have demonstrated the utility of ACE inhibitors in the management of hypertensive patients otherwise unresponsive to multidrug combinations. Typically, such combinations have included a diuretic and minoxidil, a CCB, and/or a peripheral alpha blocker. The key to this approach, as with two-drug combination therapy with ACE inhibitors, is to combine agents with different mechanisms of action. In addition, if an acute reduction in BP is desired, it can be achieved with oral or sublingual captopril because its onset of action occurs as soon as 15 min after its administration. An additional option for the management of hypertensive emergencies is that of parenteral therapy with enalaprilat. Compounds that interrupt RAA axis activity, such as ACE inhibitors, should be administered cautiously in patients with suspected marked activation of the RAA axis (e.g., prior treatment with diuretics). In such subjects, sudden and extreme drops in BP have occasionally been observed with the first dose of an ACE inhibitor.

ACE INHIBITORS AND ARBS IN HYPERTENSION ASSOCIATED WITH OTHER DISORDERS

ACE inhibitors effectively regress left ventricular hypertrophy (LVH) in the face of prolonged lowering of BP. ARBs seem to have a similar effect on LVH, although fewer studies of a long-term nature have been conducted with compounds in this drug class. This is an important feature because the presence of LVH portends a significant future risk of sudden death or MI. The question of whether LVH regression is associated with a positive outcome has been answered with the completion of the Losartan Intervention for End-Point Reduction in Hypertension (LIFE) study. The main LIFE study randomized 9193 patients aged 55 to 80 years with essential hypertension (baseline casual blood pressure 160 to 200/95 to 115 mm Hg) and electrocardiographic LVH (according to Cornell voltage-duration or Sokolow-Lyon voltage criteria) to a longer than 4-year, double-blind treatment with losartan versus atenolol. This study showed a substantially reduced rate of stroke in the losartan-treated group despite comparably reduced BP readings in the losartan and atenolol treatment groups.

A primary composite outcome of death, stroke, and cardiovascular morbidity showed a significant benefit in favor of losartan primarily due to a difference in stroke rate. There was also a greater effect on LVH regression with losartan than with atenolol.

ACE inhibitors and ARBs can be safely used in patients with coronary artery disease. Although they do not specifically vasodilate coronary arteries, they do improve hemodynamic factors that dictate myocardial oxygen consumption and thereby reduce the risk of ischemia (see Table 5-7). For example, ACE inhibitors do not reflexly increase myocardial sympathetic tone in hypertensive patients with angina, as can occur with other antihypertensives.

ACE inhibitors and ARBs are also useful in the treatment of isolated systolic hypertension or systolic-predominant forms of hypertension, which relates in part to their ability to improve arteriolar compliance. In addition,

ACE inhibitors are useful in the treatment of patients with cerebrovascular disease because they maintain cerebral autoregulatory ability despite reducing BP. This is particularly important in the treatment of the elderly hypertensive. ACE inhibitors dilate small and large arteries, can be used safely in patients with peripheral vascular disease, and on occasion may lessen intermittent claudication symptomatology. As an example, of the 9297 patients in the HOPE study, 4051 had peripheral arterial disease defined by a history of peripheral arterial disease, claudication, or an ankle brachial index of less than 0.90. These patients had similar reductions in the primary end point when compared with those without peripheral arterial disease, thus demonstrating that the ACE inhibitor ramipril is effective in lowering the risk of fatal and nonfatal ischemic events among patients with peripheral arterial disease.

ACE inhibitors and ARBs are also touted as agents of choice in the diabetic hypertensive patient, whether or not they have diabetic renal disease. Such enthusiasm needs to be tempered by the realization that these compounds, when administered as monotherapy, do not effectively reduce BP in many diabetics. This effect may relate to the fact that many diabetics have a low-renin, volume-expanded form of hypertension, which is generally less responsive to an ACE inhibitor or an ARB. This efficacy hurdle can be overcome by addition of a diuretic to the treatment regimen, or a different antihypertensive drug class may be considered for use. This rationale for therapy changes when the diabetic demonstrates evidence for diabetic nephropathy. The final results of the African American Study of Kidney Disease and Hypertension demonstrated an advantage of the ACE inhibitor ramipril over the beta blocker metoprolol and the calcium antagonist amlodipine in preventing adverse renal outcomes in black patients with hypertension. The data are now very impressive in support of ACE inhibitors and even more so with ARBs being a major element of the treatment regimen, although many times they must be given in conjunction with other antihypertensive medications to effect BP control in this typically difficult to manage population. A final consideration with ACE inhibitors in the hypertensive diabetic relates to their effect on hyperlipidemia and/or insulin resistance. In this regard, ACE inhibitors and ARBs have failed to demonstrate an unambiguous effect on serum lipids and/or insulin resistance, although in the Captopril Prevention Project (CAPPP) and the HOPE studies, the ACE inhibitors captopril and ramipril, respectively, were found to decrease the incidence of new-onset type 2 diabetes mellitus. Similarly, the incidence of new-onset type 2 diabetes was decreased with losartan in the LIFE trial.

END-ORGAN EFFECTS

Stroke

Given the significant public health impact of stroke and the identification of non-modifiable (age, sex, race/ethnicity) and modifiable (BP, diabetes, lipid profile, and lifestyle) risk factors, early prevention strategies are increasingly considered. When a patient and, in particular, a diabetic suffers a stroke, the focus of care becomes the prevention of secondary events. This can be accomplished with antiplatelet and lipid-lowering therapy and by reducing BP. Despite the clear risk reduction with effective implementation of these preventative strategies, new approaches are needed. In particular, it is unclear whether the benefit gained from BP reduction is unique to the agent employed or a simple consequence of improvement in the hemodynamic profile.

The Perindopril Protection Against Recurrent Stroke (PROGRESS) study reported for the first time that antihypertensive therapy with a combination of the ACE inhibitor perindopril and the thiazide diuretic indapamide reduces the recurrence of stroke even in patients with normal BP. In this study, 6105 hypertensive and non-hypertensive patients who had stroke and no major disability within the previous 5 years were randomized to a 4-mg dose of perindopril with or without a 2.5-mg dose of indapamide. After 4 years of follow-up (40% received perindopril alone and 60% received combination therapy), there was a considerable disparity in the BP findings between these two treatment groups. In the subgroup of patients receiving perindopril and indapamide, BP was reduced by 12/5 mm Hg, and the risk of stroke was reduced by 43%. Perindopril monotherapy reduced BP by 5/3 mm Hg and produced no significant reduction in the risk of stroke. Based on the degree of BP reduction in the perindopril group, a 20% reduction in stroke risk would have been anticipated; thus, the findings in PROGRESS are somewhat enigmatic. A similar observation was made in the CAPPP trial, where—despite its design problems—fatal or nonfatal stroke was 1.25 times more common in patients randomized to captopril than in those assigned to conventional therapy with diuretics and/or beta blockers. Nevertheless, the beneficial effect of combination therapy with perindopril and indapamide is consistent with results of prior studies showing a positive effect of diuretics on recurrent stroke rate.

In contradistinction to the PROGRESS study, the HOPE study provided compelling evidence that treatment with the ACE inhibitor ramipril can further reduce the risk of stroke in high-risk patients without left ventricular dysfunction by mechanisms above and beyond reduction in BP. Ramipril at a dose of 10 mg/day achieved a significant 32% reduction in total stroke, and recurrent strokes were reduced by 33%. In a sub-analysis of this trial, nonfatal stroke was reduced by 24% and fatal stroke by 61%. Interestingly, in the HOPE study, ramipril was given at night, so its peak effect, hemodynamic or otherwise, occurred in the morning hours, a time when strokes occur more frequently. Based on the HOPE study, the recently published American Heart Association guidelines for the primary prevention of stroke recommend ramipril to prevent stroke in high-risk patients and in patients with diabetes and hypertension. Thus, it would appear that ACE inhibitor therapy—and in ACE inhibitor-intolerant patients, ARB treatment—is warranted if primary prevention is contemplated in a high-risk patient or secondary prevention is being considered in a patient with a previous cerebrovascular event. The positive results with losartan in the LIFE trial as related to stroke adds a different layer of complexity to the selection process of an antihypertensive agent. Based on the findings of the LIFE study, the FDA recently granted losartan a unique stroke prevention approval. There is evidence that this benefit does not apply to black hypertensive patients with left ventricular hypertrophy. Recently, the Study on Cognition and Progress in the Elderly found a significant (28%) reduction in nonfatal strokes in elderly subjects with mild hypertension when treated with candesartan. Lowering BP in this study did not interfere with cognitive function.

Renal

The JNC VII recommends the use of ACE inhibitors and ARBs in patients with hypertension and chronic renal disease to control hypertension and to slow the rate of progression of CRF. With the growing amount of data supporting the renal protective effects of ARBs, it is likely that ACE inhibitors and ARBs will be used interchangeably for this purpose. Irrespective of the drug class being used to lower BP, the most important element in the management of the patient with hypertension and CRF remains tight BP control. The JNC VII recommendations advise a goal BP of 130/85 mm Hg, with even a lower value of 125/75 mm Hg being recommended for patients with proteinuria in excess of 1 g/day. Because of the volume dependency of the hypertension in this group of patients, ACE inhibitor and ARB therapy alone do not always provide the desired level of BP control. For example, in the Reduction of Endpoints in Non–Insulin-Dependent Diabetes Mellitus with the Angiotensin II Antagonist Losartan study (RENAAL) and the Irbesartan Diabetic Nephropathy Trial (IDNT), the average number of medications required to achieve BP control, which were 140/90 and 135/85 mm Hg, respectively, in these studies, was three plus the study medication. Thus, it is not uncommon in the treatment of these patients that diuretics and/or other drugs, such as CCBs, are needed to achieve goal BP.

Proteinuria has emerged as a robust marker for renal disease in diabetes and as an independent risk factor for cardiovascular disease. Microalbuminuria typically augurs the development of progressive diabetic nephropathy, and it is now routinely measured in all diabetics. Not only is screening for microalbuminuria recommended in diabetes, but it is also suggested for others at increased risk for renal or CVR disease. The National Kidney Foundation's PARADE task force recently reviewed the evidence relating proteinuria and renal and cardiovascular risks and recommended that therapies used to treat hypertension should also target reductions in proteinuria. Therapies directed at proteinuria reduction in nondiabetic renal disease are also recommended. ACE inhibitors and ARBs have a number of renal effects that culminate in substantial reductions in proteinuria and are obvious first choices for hypertensive patients with micro- or macroalbuminuria.

ACE inhibitors have proven useful in the setting of established type 1 insulin-dependent diabetes mellitus nephropathy, non–insulin-dependent diabetic nephropathy, normotensive type 1 insulin-dependent diabetes mellitus with microalbuminuria, and a variety of nondiabetic renal diseases. However, not all studies have demonstrated beneficial effects of ACE inhibitors. The Ramipril Efficacy in Nephropathy study did not detect a renoprotective effect in patients with type 2 diabetic nephropathy treated with ramipril. Interestingly, those patients treated with ramipril lost renal function at a significantly faster rate than did patients treated with a conventional non-ACE inhibitor–based regimen. ACE inhibitor regimens shown to slow the rate of CRF progression include captopril 25 mg twice daily, enalapril 5 to 10 mg daily, benazepril 10 mg daily, and ramipril 2.5 to 5 mg daily. It is presumed that renal failure increases the pharmacologic effect of these doses by reducing the renal clearance of the ACE inhibitor.

ARBs have also been found in recently published clinical trials to be useful in the setting of type 2 diabetes in established diabetic nephropathy with proteinuria and in microalbuminuric diabetes. Results of these trials are quite reminiscent of results observed in type 1 diabetic nephropathy patients treated with captopril. ARB regimens used in these trials included irbesartan 150 to 300 mg/day, losartan 50 to 100 mg/day, and valsartan 80 to 160 mg/day (Table 5-10). Therapies directed at reducing the production or effects of angiotensin II have a variety of potentially beneficial effects on the kidney. ACE inhibitors transiently reduce GFR secondary to their ability to reduce

TABLE 5-10 Studies with ARBs in Diabetic Nephropathy

	IDNT	IRMA 2	RENAAL	MARVAL
Study design	IRB 300 mg vs.AML 10 mg vs. PLA	IRB 150 mg vs. 300 mg vs. PLA	LOS 50–100 mg vs. AML	VAL 80 mg vs. AML
N	1715	590	1513	332
Patient type	HT/type 2 diabetes/nephropathy	HT/type 2 diabetes/micro-albuminuria	Type 2 diabetes/nephropathy	Type 2 diabetes/microalbuminuria/ SBP< 180 and/or DBP<105 mm Hg
Duration	Mean 2.6 y	2 y	Mean 3.4 y	24 wk
End points	Primary composite: doubling of serum creatinine, ESRD, death	Time to onset of nephropathy with UAER >200 µg/min, 30% greater than baseline	Primary composite: doubling of serum creatinine, ESRD, death	≡UAER
Results	Risk of primary end point 20% lower with IRB vs. PLA; 23% lower vs. AML; lower doubling of serum creatinine; ESRD with IRB; no difference in death rate	IRB was renoprotective: 5.2% reached end point in 300-mg groups; 9.7% reached end point in 150-mg group vs. 14.9% in PLA group ($P = 0.08$)	Risk of primary end point lowered by 15% ($P = 0.02$) with LOS, lower doubling of serum creatinine and ESRD with LOS; no difference in death rate	VAL significantly lowered UAER (44%) vs. AML (17%; $P<0.001$)

Key: AML, amlodipine; DBP, diastolic blood pressure; ESRD, end-stage renal disease; HT, hypertension; IDNT, Irbesartan Diabetic Nephropathy Trial; IRB, irbesartan; IRMA, study of irbesartan in hypertensive patients with type 2 diabetes and microalbuminuria; LOS, losartan; MARVAL, Microalbuminuria reduction with valsartan; PLA, placebo; RENAAL, reduction of endpoints in non–insulin-dependent diabetes melitus with the angiotensin II antagonist losartan; SBP, systolic blood pressure; UAER, urinary albumin excretion rate; VAL, valsartan.

glomerular capillary pressures. Such decrements in GFR, ordinarily in the order of a 10% to 15% drop, are readily reversible and actually predictive of the degree of long-term renal protection. Current practice considerations suggest that there is no specific level of renal function at which an ACE inhibitor or an ARB cannot be started; rather, significant hyperkalemia accompanying the use of these drugs may be the basis for their being discontinued at least temporarily, pending resolution of the hyperkalemia.

Reduction in proteinuria has been employed as a marker for the beneficial effects of these therapies. Reducing proteinuria in and of itself also may favorably affect the progression rate of the renal failure process. The renoprotective effect of ACE inhibitors is most evident in patients with heavy proteinuria (>3 g/day) who, if left untreated, generally progress quite rapidly. ACE inhibitors and ARBs also modify tissue-based growth factors, such as transforming growth factor β, which are activated by prior or ongoing renal disease and are stimulated by the presence of angiotensin II. Inhibition of these tissue-based processes may further slow the progression of renal disease. There may be differences in the tissue-based effects of ACE inhibitors and ARBs, because the effect of ACE inhibitors on renal hemodynamics might be limited by the non–ACE-dependent generation of angiotensin II.

Three factors are potential modifiers of the renal response to ACE inhibitors. First, a low sodium intake enhances the antiproteinuric effect of ACE inhibitors. Second, short-term studies have suggested that dietary protein restriction complements the ACE inhibitor effect on protein excretion in nephrotic patients. This possibly implies that combining ACE inhibitors and protein restriction might prove more effective than an ACE inhibitor alone in slowing the progression of renal failure. A third factor is that of inherited variation in ACE activity. Two common forms of ACE gene I (insertion) and D (deletion) give rise to three potential genotypes: II, ID, and DD. The DD phenotype is associated with higher circulating ACE levels and a greater pressor response to the infusion of angiotensin I as compared with the II phenotype, with the ID phenotype displaying intermediate characteristics. These phenotypic characteristics can be expected to be relevant to the response to ACE inhibition. The finding that DD patients are at increased risk for MI and ischemic cardiomyopathy first established the clinical significance of the inherited variation in ACE activity. In this regard, recent work has suggested that GFR declines more rapidly in DD than in II patients and that such patients do not demonstrate significant reductions in proteinuria or slowing in the rate of progression of renal failure when administered ACE inhibitors. These three factors, which clearly modify the response to an ACE inhibitor, may also modify the response to ARBs, although ACE gene polymorphism should, in theory, not influence the effect of ARBs.

Cardiac

Data from placebo-controlled and open trials have suggested that ACE inhibitors substantially reduce the risk of death and hospitalization for CHF and improve its symptomatology, making ACE inhibitors first-line therapy for the treatment of CHF. By modifying production of angiotensin II, these agents interrupt the neurohumoral activation characteristic of CHF. Although statistically significant reductions in mortality have been observed with enalapril, similar trends have been observed with other ACE inhibitors, including captopril, ramipril, quinapril, trandolapril, and lisinopril. Further, these agents have demonstrated efficacy and tolerability in the treatment of CHF based on the end points of improved exercise tolerance and symptomatology. Although ACE inhibitors are almost universally recommended as a cost-effective strategy for the treatment of CHF, physician-prescribing practice is such that only approximately 50% of those patients eligible for treatment with ACE inhibitors actually receive them. Moreover, the dosages used in "real-world practice" are substantially lower than those proven efficacious in randomized, controlled trials, with evaluations reporting only a minority of patients achieving target doses and/or an overall mean dose achieved to be less than one-half the target dose. Factors predicting the use and optimal dose administration of ACE inhibitors include variables relating to the setting (previous hospitalization, specialty clinic follow-up), the physician (cardiology specialty versus family practitioner or general internist), the patient (increased severity of symptoms, male, younger), and the drug (lower frequency of administration).

Enalapril, captopril, lisinopril, and trandolapril significantly reduce morbidity and mortality rates in patients with MI over a wide range of ventricular function. There are presently insufficient data to establish whether clinically significant differences exist among the ACE inhibitors in the post-MI setting, given the paucity of head-to-head trials among these agents and the fact that the studies discussed above differ in length and duration. Currently, only captopril, lisinopril, ramipril, and trandolapril are approved specifically in post-MI left ventricular dysfunction, although enalapril is approved in asymptomatic left ventricular dysfunction. However, as in patients with CHF, numerous ACE inhibitors have demonstrated benefits in patients after MI, suggesting, to a certain degree, a class effect. Thus, ACE inhibitors are indicated in all patients with acute MI who can tolerate them. In a hemodynamically stable patient after an MI, an oral ACE inhibitor should be initiated, generally within 24 h of the event, particularly if the MI is anterior and associated with depressed left ventricular function. The hemodynamic effects and overall benefit of ACE inhibition are seen early, with 40% of the 30-day increase in survival observed in days 0 to 1, 45% in days 2 to 7, and approximately 15% after day 7. The benefits of ACE inhibitor therapy in the post-MI period appear not to be the result of a substantial decline in arrhythmic mortality. ARBs have been studied in CHF (Table 5-11) and are currently under study in the postmyocardial infarction patient. In the double-blind Optimal Trial in Myocardial Infarction with the Angiotensin II Antagonist Losartan (OPTIMAAL), losartan was compared with captopril and a nonsignificant difference in total mortality in favor of captopril was observed. A similar study is in progress where valsartan is being compared to captopril in postinfarction patients having ejection fractions above 40% (VALIANT). The ARBs do not appear to differ substantially from ACE inhibitors in symptomatic relief, improvement in exercise tolerance, and/or favorably influencing morbidity and mortality. The combination of an ACE inhibitor and an ARB, as occurred in the Valsartan-Heart Failure Trial (Val-HeFT), improved morbidity but not mortality, though the exact best way to combine an ACE inhibitor with another ACE inhibitor in the management of CHF remains to be determined. Concomitant use of valsartan with an ACE inhibitor and a beta blocker is not recommended based on the Val-HeFT findings; valsartan is now indicated for the treatment of heart failure (New York Heart Association classes II to IV) in patients who are intolerant of ACE inhibitors. A recently completed study assessed the effects of candesartan in patients with heart failure who were intolerant of ACE inhibitors (CHARM-ALTERNATIVE). Also

TABLE 5-11 Effect of ARBs on Mortality Rates in Heart Failure

Study	Agent	End point	ARB	ACEI or placebo	Risk reduction	P
ELITE	Losartan	Combined mortality/ HF hospitalization	33/352	49/370	0.32 (−0.04–0.55)	0.075
ELITE II	Losartan	All-cause mortality	280/1578	250/1574	1.13	(0.95–1.35) 0.16
Val-HeFT	Valsartan	All-cause mortality	495/2511	484/2499*	1.02 (0.9–1.15)	0.800
Val-HeFT	Valsartan	Combined morbidity and mortality	723/2511	801/2459*	0.87 (0.79–0.96)	0.035

Key: ACEI, angiotensin-converting enzyme inhibitor; ARB, angiotensin-receptor blocker; ELITE, evaluation of losartan in the elderly; HF, heart failure; Val-HeFT, Valsartan-Heart Failure Trial.

Hazards ratio.

*Placebo results.

assessed were the effects of candesartan in patients with systolic heart failure already receiving ACE inhibition (CHARM-ADDED). A study was also done evaluating the effects of candesartan in patients with diastolic dysfunction (CHARM-PRESERVED). Overall benefit was observed in all three studies.

Several dosing strategies are effective in reducing morbidity and mortality in patients with systolic left ventricular dysfunction. Most importantly, a systematic effort must be made to reach target doses shown to be effective in the randomized trials having used ACE inhibitors in CHF. Emerging data seem to suggest that the doses of ACE inhibitors used in clinical practice are less effective than the relatively high doses used in the randomized trials. Dose ranges used in community practice are typically 50 and 10 mg/day for captopril and enalapril, respectively; whereas randomized trials have associated successful treatment with captopril and enalapril doses approaching 150 and 40 mg/day, respectively. Until convincing evidence otherwise becomes available, the treatment of CHF should include sequential dose titration of the ACE inhibitor used. Such titration should strive to reach those doses shown to be successful in the randomized clinical trials. The ability to reach these doses in the CHF patient can sometimes be a vexing issue because a major deterrent is the development of systemic hypotension and/or a decline in GFR. Thus, reaching goal ACE inhibitor doses necessitates a keen understanding of the critical relation between volume status, BP, and the desired ACE inhibitor dose. Probably the single most important variable, which allows effective dose titration, is this understanding of the relation between volume status and BP.

OTHER CLINICAL USES

ACE inhibitors have been used in the diagnosis of renal artery stenosis (captopril-stimulated renography) and primary hyperaldosteronism. Patients with suspected renovascular occlusive disease by clinical criteria are administered a dose of a rapid-acting ACE inhibitor, such as oral captopril or intravenous enalaprilat 1 to 2 h before injection of a nuclear imaging tracer. Subtle differences in intraglomerular pressure between the two kidneys are amplified by the sudden decline in local and circulatory angiotensin II levels that result from the administration of the ACE inhibitor. It has been reported that the diagnostic sensitivity of captopril-stimulated nuclear renography is 90% to 100%. With regard to hyperaldosteronism, it has been shown that patients with adrenal adenomas do not show a decline in aldosterone levels with an ACE inhibitor, in contrast to patients with adrenal hyperplasia whose aldosterone levels usually decline by approximately 50%.

ACE inhibitors also have been used to treat altitude polycythemia and another form of secondary polycythemia that follows renal transplantation. The drugs have been used as treatment to prevent postangioplasty restenosis, but with little or no benefit being demonstrated in multiple clinical trials.

CANCER AND ACE INHIBITORS

It went largely unnoticed in the prospective Studies of Left Ventricular Dysfunction (SOLVD) study that patients with left ventricular dysfunction treated with enalapril showed a slightly higher incidence of malignancy than did those patients receiving placebo (odds ratio, 1.59; confidence interval, 0.90 to 2.82). In this study, there were 38 gastrointestinal malignancies in the enalapril group versus 22 in the placebo group (odds ratio, 1.7). Since the SOLVD study, several case reports have linked ACE inhibitors to the development of malignancies. For example, pemphigus vulgaris, which can be seen in association with internal malignancies, is a known adverse effect of captopril. One case report linked enalapril for the first time to pemphigus vegetans with a simultaneously occurring internal malignancy. In another case report, Kaposi's sarcoma appeared in a 70-year-old woman 8 months after starting captopril. After stopping the captopril, there was a marked reduction in the cutaneous and gastric lesions of this disease, suggesting a cause-and-effect relation between the captopril and the malignancy.

A subsequent study disputed these findings by reporting that captopril inhibits angiogenesis in Kaposi's sarcoma. These limited data are in contrast to a greater body of evidence supporting the lack of a cancer risk with ACE inhibitors. In the recent large-scale HOPE trial, 9297 high-risk patients treated with ramipril or placebo for a mean of 5 years had similar numbers of deaths from non-cardiovascular causes in both groups. In addition, several other retrospective studies investigating the possible association between various antihypertensives and cancer risk did not detect such a relation with the use of ACE inhibitors. The Scottish retrospective cohort study by Lever et al. who compared 1599 patients taking ACE inhibitors with 3648 patients on other antihypertensive drugs found a risk reduction for female-specific and lung cancers. Thus, the overall evidence available to date suggests that ACE inhibitors have a neutral cancer risk in hypertension and might conceivably decrease the risk. There is a limited number of long-term trials with ARBs; accordingly, no statement can be made about the risk of malignancy with this drug class.

SIDE EFFECTS OF ACE INHIBITORS AND ARBS

Soon after their release, a syndrome of "functional renal insufficiency" was observed as a class effect with ACE inhibitors, a process little different than what is occasionally seen with the ARBs. This phenomenon was initially recognized in patients with a solitary kidney and renal artery stenosis or in the setting of bilateral renal artery stenosis. Since these original reports, this phenomenon has been repeatedly observed. Predisposing conditions to this process include dehydration, CHF, and/or microvascular renal disease, and the aforementioned macrovascular renal disease. The mechanistic theme common to all of these conditions is a fall in afferent arteriolar flow. When this occurs, glomerular filtration temporarily drops. In response to this reduction in glomerular flow, local release of angiotensin II occurs, which then preferentially constricts the efferent or postglomerular arteriole. When the efferent arteriole constricts, upstream hydrostatic pressures within the glomerular capillary bed are restored despite the initial and frequently continuing decline in afferent arteriolar flow. The abrupt removal of angiotensin II, as occurs with an ACE inhibitor or an ARB, dilates the efferent arteriole. An offshoot of these hemodynamic changes is a sudden drop in glomerular hemodynamic pressures and a plummeting of glomerular filtration.

This phenomenon of "functional renal insufficiency" is best treated by discontinuation of the offending agent, whether an ACE inhibitor or an ARB, careful volume repletion if intravascular volume contraction exists, and, if strongly suspected, investigation for the presence of renal artery stenosis. An additional side effect with ACE inhibitors is that of hyperkalemia. Relevant degrees of hyperkalemia with ACE inhibitors occur in predisposed patients, such as diabetic or CHF patients with renal failure receiving potassium-sparing diuretics or potassium supplements. Typically, however, hyperkalemia is not that common with ACE inhibitors and is even less common with the ARBs. Alternatively, ACE inhibitors and ARBs are known to lessen the degree of hypokalemia produced by diuretic therapy.

A dry, irritating, nonproductive cough is a common complication with ACE inhibitors, with its incidence variously estimated at between 0% and 44%. Cough is a class phenomenon with ACE inhibitors and ostensibly has been attributed to increased bradykinin levels or other vasoactive peptides such as substance P, which may play a second-messenger role in triggering the cough reflex. Although numerous therapies have been tried, few have eliminated ACE inhibitor–induced cough with any lasting success. Most times the cough gradually disappears within 2 weeks after the offending agent is stopped. Alternatively, ARBs have been infrequently associated with cough, whether the cough incidence is determined in preselected patients having previously experienced ACE inhibitor-related cough or in parallel-limb treatment studies directly comparing an ACE inhibitor with an ARB. ACE inhibitor–related nonspecific side effects are generally uncommon, with the exception of taste disturbances, leukopenia, skin rash, and dysgeusia, which are almost exclusively seen in captopril-treated patients. The sulfhydryl-group found on captopril has been implicated in these abnormalities. Alternatively, the ARBs have demonstrated favorable safety and tolerability profiles, that appear to be equivalent to those observed with placebo. To date, no clear class-specific adverse effect has been attributed to the ARBs. In fact, certain side effects, such as headache, may occur less frequently with ARBs than with placebo, which is probably a consequence of greater BP reduction with an ARB than with placebo.

Angioneurotic edema is a potentially life-threatening complication of ACE inhibitors that is more common in blacks. The incidence rate ranges from 0.1% to 0.5% among ACE inhibitor users and it can occur quite unpredictably. Among all-cause factors for angioedema, ACE inhibitors are causal 20% of the time. Typically, it is not a first-dose phenomenon. It is easily recognized because of its characteristic involvement of the mouth, tongue, and upper airway. ACE inhibitor–induced angioedema of the intestine also can occur. This typically presents with acute abdominal symptoms with or without facial and/or oropharyngeal swelling and is more common in females. Angioedema also occurs with ARBs, but much less frequently. The mechanism of angioedema with ARBs is unknown, although in ARB-treated patients who develop angioedema, up to one-third had previously developed angioedema on an ACE inhibitor. Because patients with previous ACE inhibitor–induced angioedema are at increased risk for recurrent angioedema with an ARB, these drugs should not be considered an absolutely safe substitute in patients with previous ACE inhibitor–induced angioedema. ARB use can be considered in a patient with previously experience angioedema, but only if compelling indications exist, such as progressive CHF and/or proteinuric renal disease, and only with appropriate patient instruction.

A final issue with ACE inhibitors and ARBs is their capacity to cause birth defects. These drugs are not teratogenic; rather, their use during the second and third trimesters of pregnancy can cause oligoamnios, neonatal anuria, hypocalvaria, pulmonary hypoplasia, and/or fetal or neonatal death because the maturing fetus is heavily reliant on angiotensin II for proper development. Unintended pregnancy remains common in young women; thus, in women of gestational age, a clinician must be alert to this possibility when the treatment of hypertension is contemplated and an agent is to be selected. This is particularly so with ACE inhibitors and/or ARBs. If ACE inhibitors or ARBs are required or are being incidentally used when a women is nursing, there is minimal entry of these compounds into breast milk. Although not all ACE inhibitors or ARBs have been submitted to formal study, in most cases, breast milk selectively restricts the entry of these drugs.

CLASS AND AGENT-SPECIFIC DRUG INTERACTIONS

Several class-specific drug interactions occur with drugs in these two classes (see Chapter 21). For example, the concurrent administration of lithium with an ACE inhibitor or an ARB is associated with a greater likelihood of lithium toxicity. Potassium supplements or potassium-sparing diuretics, when given with ACE inhibitors or ARBs, increase the probability of developing hyperkalemia. In this regard, NSAIDs, such as indomethacin, also reduce the antihypertensive effects of ACE inhibitors and ARBs, although ARBs have been less well studied. NSAIDs also attenuate the natriuretic response seen with ACE inhibitors and ARBs. ACE inhibitors and NSAIDs can lead to functional renal insufficiency, particularly in those taking diuretics. This combination of drugs should be administered with extreme care to patients, such as the elderly, who are highly vulnerable to such interactions.

The issue of whether aspirin attenuates the effects of an ACE inhibitor in hypertension and/or CHF has been a matter of some controversy. To whatever extent the improvement in symptoms and survival rendered by treatment with ACE inhibitors is attributable to their effects on the circulation and the kidneys, this benefit can be rescinded by concomitant administration of aspirin. There is a wealth of data suggesting an important interaction between aspirin and ACE inhibitors in patients with chronic stable cardiovascular disease. An interaction is biologically plausible because there is considerable evidence that ACE inhibitors exert important effects through increasing the production of vasodilator prostaglandins, whereas aspirin blocks their production through inhibition of cyclooxygenase, even at low doses. There is some evidence that low-dose aspirin may also raise systolic and diastolic BPs. There is also considerable evidence that aspirin may entirely neutralize the clinical benefits of ACE inhibitors in patients with CHF, possibly by blocking endogenous vasodilator prostaglandin production and/or enhancing the vasoconstrictor potential of endothelin. In patients requiring treatment for CHF, if possible, aspirin should be avoided and the integrity of prostaglandin metabolism respected; the more severe the CHF, the more compelling the argument. As an alternative in these patients, antiplatelet therapy should be considered with agents that do not block the cyclooxygenase system.

Combining an ACE inhibitor with allopurinol is associated with a higher risk of hypersensitivity reactions, with several reports of the Stevens-Johnson syndrome described with the combination of captopril and allopurinol. Quinapril reduces the absorption of tetracycline by approximately 35%, which may be due to the high magnesium content of quinapril tablets. To date, no drug–drug interactions have been described with regard to the absorption of ARBs.

CONCLUSION

ACE inhibitors and ARBs are commonly used in the treatment of hypertension and of an increasing number of end-organ diseases. These compounds reduce

BP by mechanisms involving change in the quantity and/or effect of angiotensin II and by increasing bradykinin. Moreover, there is increasing evidence that these compounds alter sympathetic outflow, albeit in a compound-specific manner. Early belief held that these drugs were minimally effective in low-renin forms of hypertension, such as in the case of African American hypertensives. More recently, it has become clear that the African American hypertensive can respond well to these drugs, although with some interindividual variability in the pattern of response. Several ACE inhibitors and ARBs are available, with distinctions between individual members of each drug class sometimes being quite subtle. Pharmacologic properties proposed as distinguishing features for ACE inhibitors and ARBs include their tissue and receptor-binding potentials and whether their mode of elimination is renal or renal and hepatic. ACE inhibitors and, more recently, ARBs are of clearly proven benefit in slowing the progression of CRF, and both drug classes have a major influence on the morbidity and mortality that attend progressive CHF. ACE inhibitors are generally without significant side effects other than cough, which, unfortunately, can occur in a significant number of patients receiving these drugs. Alternatively, ARBs are virtually free of side effects, which is a substantial advantage supporting the expanding use of drugs in this class.

ADDITIONAL READINGS

Agodoa LY, Appel L, Bakris GL, et al: Effect of ramipril vs amlodipine on renal outcomes in hypertensive nephrosclerosis: A randomized controlled trial. *JAMA* 285:2719, 2001.

ACC/AHA: Guidelines for the evaluation and management of chronic heart failure in the adult: Executive summary. *Circulation* 104:2996, 2001.

ALLHAT Officers and Coordinators: Major outcomes in high-risk hypertensive patients randomized to angiotensin converting enzyme inhibitor therapy or calcium channel blocker vs diuretic: The Antihypertensive and Lipid-Lowering Treatment to Prevent Heart Attack Trial (ALLHAT). *JAMA* 288:2981, 2002.

Brenner BM, Cooper ME, de Zeeuw D, et al: Effects of losartan on renal and cardiovascular outcomes in patients with type 2 diabetes and nephropathy. *N Engl J Med* 345:861, 2001.

Burnier M: Angiotensin II type 1-receptor blockers. *Circulation* 103:904, 2001.

Carswell CI, Goa KL: Losartan in diabetic nephropathy. *Drugs* 63:407, 2003.

Chobanian AV, Bakris GL, Black HR, et al: Seventh Report of the Joint National Committee on Prevention, Detection, Evaluation, and Treatment of High Blood Pressure. *JAMA* 289:2560, 2003.

Cohn JN, Tognoni G: A randomized trial of the angiotensin-receptor blocker valsartan in chronic heart failure. *N Engl J Med* 345:1667, 2001.

Conlin PR, Spence JD, Williams B, et al: Angiotensin II antagonists for hypertension: Are there differences in efficacy? *Am J Hypertens* 13:418, 2000.

Dahlof B, Devereux RB, Kjeldsen SE, et al: Cardiovascular morbidity and mortality in the Losartan Intervention for Endpoint reduction in hypertension study (LIFE): A randomised trial against atenolol. *Lancet* 359:995, 2002.

Devereux RB, Dahlof B, Kjeldsen SE, et al: Effects of losartan or atenolol in hypertensive patients without clinically evident vascular disease: A substudy of the LIFE randomized trial. *Ann Intern Med* 139:169, 2003.

Fogari R, Mugellini A, Zoppi A, et al: A double-blind crossover study of the antihypertensive efficacy of angiotensin II-receptor antagonists and their activation of the renin-angiotensin system. *Curr Ther Res Clin Exp* 61:669, 2000.

Frishman WH, Cheng-Lai A, Chen J: Angiotensin converting enzyme inhibitors, in Frishman WH, Cheng-Lai A, Chen J (eds): *Current Cardiovascular Drugs,* 3rd ed. Philadelphia, Current Medicine, 2000, p 18.

Frishman WH, Cheng-Lai A, Chen J: Angiotensin II receptor blockers, in Frishman WH, Cheng-Lai A, Chen J (eds): *Current Cardiovascular Drugs,* 3rd ed. Philadelphia, Current Medicine, 2000, p 45.

Frishman WH, Chiu R, Landzberg BR, Weiss M: Medical therapies for the prevention of restenosis after percutaneous coronary interventions. *Curr Probl Cardiol* 23:533, 1998.

Gradman AH, Lewin A, Bowling BT, et al: Comparative effects of candesartan cilexetil and losartan in patients with systemic hypertension. Candesartan Versus Losartan Efficacy Comparison (CANDLE) Study Group. *Heart Dis* 1:52, 1999.

Granger CB, McMurray JJV, Yusuf S, et al: Effects of candesartan in patients with chronic heart failure and reduced left ventricular systolic function intolerant to angiotensin converting enzyme inhibitors: The CHARM Alternative trial. *Lancet* 362: September 6, 2003.

Jackson EK, Garrison JC: Renin and angiotensin, in: Hardman JG, Limbird L (eds): *Goodman & Gilman's the Pharmacological Basis of Therapeutics.* New York, McGraw-Hill, 1999, p 743.

Jafar TH, Schmid CH, Landa M, et al: Angiotensin-converting enzyme inhibitors and progression of nondiabetic renal disease. A meta-analysis of patient-level data. *Ann Intern Med* 135:73, 2001.

Jamali AH, Tang WH, Khot UN, Fowler MB: The role of angiotensin receptor blockers in the management of chronic heart failure. *Arch Intern Med* 161:667, 2001.

Lewis EJ, Hunsicker LG, Bain RP, Rohde RD: The effect of angiotensin-converting-enzyme inhibition on diabetic nephropathy: The Collaborative Study Group. *N Engl J Med* 329:1456, 1993.

Lewis EJ, Hunsicker LG, Clarke WR, et al: Renoprotective effect of the angiotensin-receptor antagonist irbesartan in patients with nephropathy due to type 2 diabetes. *N Engl J Med* 345:851, 2001.

McMurray JJV, Ostergren J, Swedberg K, et al: Effects of candesartan in patients with chronic heart failure and reduced left-ventricular systolic function taking angiotensin converting enzyme inhibitors: The CHARM-Added trial. *Lancet* 362: September 6, 2003.

Nawarskas JJ, Spinler SA: Does aspirin interfere with the therapeutic efficacy of angiotensin-converting enzyme inhibitors in hypertension or congestive heart failure. *Pharmacotherapy* 18:1041, 1998.

Packer M, Poole-Wilson PA, Armstrong PW, et al: Comparative effects of low and high doses of the angiotensin-converting enzyme inhibitor, lisinopril, on morbidity and mortality in chronic heart failure. ATLAS Study Group. *Circulation* 100:2312, 1999.

Pfeffer MA, Braunwald E, Moye LA, et al on behalf of the SAVE Investigators: Effect of captopril on mortality and morbidity in patients with left ventricular dysfunction after myocardial infarction: results of the SURVIVAL and Ventricular Enlargement Trial. *N Engl J Med* 327:669, 1992.

Pfeffer MA, Swedberg K, Granger CB, et al: Effects of candesartan on mortality and morbidity in patients with chronic heart failure: The CHARM-OVERALL PROGRAMME. *Lancet* 2003, in press.

Pitt B: The role of ACE-inhibitors in patients with coronary artery disease. *Cardiovasc Drugs Ther* 15:103, 2001.

Pitt B, Poole-Wilson PA, Segal R, et al: Effect of losartan compared with captopril on mortality in patients with symptomatic heart failure: Randomised trial—The Losartan Heart Failure Survival Study ELITE II. *Lancet* 355:1582, 2000.

Sica DA: Pharmacology and clinical efficacy of angiotensin-receptor blockers. *Am J Hypertens* 14:242SS, 2001.

Sica DA: Rationale for fixed-dose combinations in the treatment of hypertension: The cycle repeats. *Drugs* 62:443, 2002.

Sica DA: Doxazosin and congestive heart failure. *Congest Heart Fail* 8:178, 2002.

Sica DA: Renal handling of angiotensin receptor blockers: Clinical relevance. *Curr Hypertens Rep* 5:337, 2003.

Sica DA, Gehr TWB: Angiotensin-converting enzyme inhibitors, in Izzo JL Jr, Black HR (eds): *Hypertension Primer,* 3rd ed. Dallas, American Heart Association, 2003, p. 426.

Sica DA, Gehr TWB, Frishman WH: The renin-angiotensin axis: angiotensin converting enzyme inhibitors and angiotensin receptor blockers, in Frishman WH, Sonnenblick EH, Sica DA (eds): *Cardiovascular Pharmacotherapeutics,* 2nd ed. New York, McGraw-Hill, 2003, p 131.

SOLVD Investigators: Effect of enalapril on survival in patients with reduced left ventricular ejection fractions and congestive heart failure. *N Engl J Med* 325:293, 1991.

SOLVD Investigators: Effect of enalapril on mortality and the development of heart failure in asymptomatic patients with reduced left ventricular ejection fraction. *N Engl J Med* 327:685, 1992.

The European Trial on Reduction of Cardiac Events with Perindopril in Stable Coronary Artery Disease Investigators: Efficacy of perindopril in reduction of cardiovascular events among patients with stable coronary artery disease: Randomized, double-blind, placebo-controlled, multicentre trial (the EUROPA study). *Lancet* 362: September 6, 2003.

Weber MA: Angiotensin II receptors blockers, in Izzo JL Jr, Black HR (eds): *Hypertension Primer*, 3rd ed. Dallas; American Heart Association, 2003, p. 430.

Wing LMH, Reid CM, Ryan P, et al, for the Second Australian National Blood Pressure Study Group: A comparison of outcomes with angiotensin converting enzyme inhibitors and diuretics for hypertension in the elderly. *N Engl J Med* 348:583, 2003.

Yusuf S, Pfeffer MA, Swedberg K, et al: Effects of candesartan in patients with chronic heart failure and preserved left ventricular ejection fraction: The CHARM Preserved trial. *Lancet* 362: September 6, 2003.

Yusuf S, Sleight P, Pogue J, et al: Effects of an angiotensin-converting enzyme inhibitor, ramipril, on cardiovascular events in high-risk patients. The Heart Outcomes Prevention Evaluation Study Investigators. *N Engl J Med* 342:145, 2000.

6 | Diuretic Therapy in Cardiovascular Disease

Todd W. B. Gehr   Domenic A. Sica
William H. Frishman

Modern diuretic therapy grew out of two apparently unrelated endeavors in the 1930s: the development of sulfanilamide, the first effective antibacterial drug, and the identification of the enzyme carbonic anhydrase. Clinical experience with sulfanilamide showed that this drug increased urine flow in addition to sodium (Na^+) and potassium (K^+) excretion. The recognition that sulfanilamide inhibited carbonic anhydrase fueled attempts to synthesize compounds that might be more specific inhibitors of carbonic anhydrase. One such compound was acetazolamide. Unfortunately, the diuretic effect of acetazolamide was self-limited, lasting no more than a few days. One consequence of the search for inhibitors of carbonic anhydrase was the discovery of a series of potent diuretic compounds with greater long-term effectiveness. The prototype of these diuretics was chlorothiazide, which became available in 1958 and ushered in the modern era of diuretic therapy.

Diuretics remain important therapeutic tools. First, they are capable of reducing blood pressure (BP) and simultaneously decreasing the morbidity and mortality that attends the hypertensive state. Diuretics are currently recommended as first-line therapy for the treatment of hypertension by the Joint National Commission on Detection, Evaluation, and Treatment of Hypertension of the National High Blood Pressure Education Program (JNC). In addition, they remain an important element of the treatment regimen for congestive heart failure (CHF) because they improve the congestive symptomatology, which characterizes the more advanced stages of CHF. This chapter reviews the mechanism of action of the various diuretic classes and the physiologic adaptations that accompany their use and establishes the basis for their use in the treatment of hypertension and CHF. In addition, commonly encountered side effects with diuretics are elaborated on.

INDIVIDUAL CLASSES OF DIURETICS

The predominant sites of action of various diuretic classes along the nephron are depicted in Fig. 6-1. The range of diuretic classes available have different pharmacokinetics and, in many instances, pharmacodynamic responses dependent on the nature and the extent of underlying disease (Table 6-1).

Carbonic Anhydrase Inhibitors

The administration of a carbonic anhydrase inhibitor ordinarily produces a brisk alkaline diuresis. By inhibiting carbonic anhydrase, these compounds decrease the generation of intracellular H^+, which is a necessary prerequisite for the absorption of Na^+; therein lies their primary diuretic effect. Although carbonic anhydrase inhibitors work at the proximal tubule level, where the bulk of Na^+ reabsorption occurs, their final diuretic effect is typically rather modest being blunted by reabsorption more distally in other nephron seg-

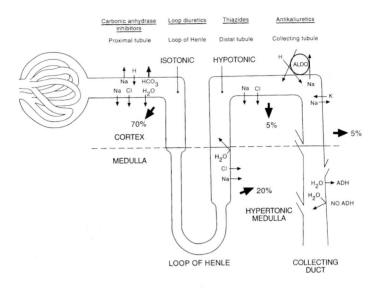

FIG. 6-1 Schematic of the nephron illustrating the handling of water and electrolytes by the different segments and the major nephron sites of diuretic action. Arrows represent the approximate percentage of sodium reabsorbed by the various nephron segments.

TABLE 6-1 Pharmacokinetics of Diuretics

Diuretic	Oral bioavailability (%)	Normal subjects	Half-life in renal insufficiency (h)	CHF
Loop				
Furosemide	10–100	1.5–2	2.8	2.7
Bumetanide	80–100	1	1.6	1.3
Torsemide	80–100	3–4	4–5	6
Thiazide				
Bendroflumethiazide	ND	2–5	ND	ND
Chlorthalidone	64	24–55	ND	ND
Chlorothiazide	30–50	1.5	ND	ND
Hydrochlorothiazide	65–75	2.5	Increased	ND
Hydroflumethiazide	73	6–25	ND	6–28
Indapamide	93	15–25	ND	ND
Polythiazide	ND	26	ND	ND
Trichlormethiazide	ND	1–4	5–10	ND
Distal				
Amiloride	?	17–26	100	ND
Triamterene	>80	2–5	Prolonged	ND
Spironolactone	?	1.5	No change	ND
Active metabolites	?	>15	ND	ND

Key: CHF, congestive heart failure; ND, not determined.
Source: Adapted with permission from Brater DC: Diuretic therapy. *N Engl J Med* 339:387, 1998.

ments. Acetazolamide is currently the only carbonic anhydrase inhibitor employed primarily for its diuretic action. It is readily absorbed and is eliminated by tubular secretion. Its use is limited by its transient action and because prolonged use causes metabolic acidosis, among other side effects. Acetazolamide (250 to 500 mg daily) can be carefully used in patients with CHF who have developed metabolic alkalosis from thiazide or loop diuretic use and who cannot tolerate the volume load associated with the Cl^- repletion required for correction of the alkalemic state. Topiramate, a recently released anticonvulsant, inhibits carbonic anhydrase and is associated with the development of metabolic acidosis.

Osmotic Diuretics

Mannitol is a polysaccharide diuretic given intravenously that is freely eliminated by glomerular filtration. Mannitol is poorly reabsorbed along the length of the nephron and thereby exerts a dose-dependent osmotic effect. This osmotic effect traps water and solutes in the tubular fluid, thus increasing Na^+ and water excretion. The half-life for plasma clearance of mannitol depends on the level of renal function but usually is between 30 and 60 min; thus, its diuretic properties are quite transient. Because mannitol also expands extracellular volume and can precipitate pulmonary edema in patients with CHF, it is contraindicated in these patients. Moreover, excessive mannitol administration, particularly when the glomerular filtration rate (GFR) is reduced, can cause dilutional hyponatremia and/or acute renal failure. The latter seems to be dose dependent and typically corrects with elimination of mannitol, as may be accomplished with hemodialysis.

Loop Diuretics

Loop diuretics act predominately at the apical membrane in the thick ascending limb of the loop of Henle, where they compete with chloride for binding to the $Na^+/K^+/2Cl^-$ cotransporter, thereby inhibiting Na^+ and Cl^- reabsorption. Besides this primary action, loop diuretics have a variety of other effects on other nephron segments. Loop diuretics reduce Na^+ reabsorption in the proximal tubule by weakly inhibiting carbonic anhydrase and through poorly defined mechanisms independent of carbonic anhydrase inhibition. Loop diuretics also have effects in the distal tubule, descending limb of the loop of Henle, and collecting duct. Although the action of loop diuretics in these other nephron segments is quantitatively minor, as compared with their effects in the thick ascending limb, these actions serve to blunt the expected increase in more distal reabsorption, which is triggered with the use of these potent diuretics. Other clinically important effects of loop diuretics include an impairment in free water excretion during water loading and free water absorption during dehydration, a 30% increase in fractional calcium excretion, a substantial increase in magnesium excretion, and a transient increase followed by a decrease in urate excretion.

In addition to their effects on water and electrolyte excretion, loop diuretics modulate renal prostaglandin synthesis, particularly that of prostaglandin E_2. The increased angiotensin II generation after the administration of loop diuretics coupled with the increased synthesis of vasodilatory prostaglandin E_2 likely accounts for the marked redistribution of renal blood flow from the inner to the outer cortex of the kidney. Despite these alterations in renal blood flow distribution, total renal blood flow and GFR are preserved after loop diuretic administration to normal subjects.

Loop diuretics in clinical use include furosemide, bumetanide, and torsemide. Ethacrynic acid is no longer available. The loop diuretics are highly protein bound and therefore are minimally filtered by the glomerulus. They typically access the tubular lumen by secretion via an organic anion transporter localized to the proximal tubule. The urinary diuretic concentration best represents the fraction of drug delivered to the medullary thick ascending limb and significantly correlates with the natriuretic response after diuretic administration.

Furosemide is the most widely used diuretic in this class. Furosemide is somewhat erratically absorbed, with a bioavailability of 49% ± 17% and a range of 12% to 112%. The coefficients of variation for absorption for different furosemide products varies from 25% to 43%; thus, switching from one formulation to another likely will not result in any predictable change in the patient's response to furosemide. Furosemide is an organic anion compound that is highly bound to albumin in plasma, which gains entry to the tubular lumen through a probenecid-sensitive proximal tubular secretory mechanism. Furosemide protein binding may be influenced by accumulated uremic toxins and/or fatty acids, although this is of poorly defined clinical significance. Secretion of furosemide and other loop diuretics may be impaired by the presence of elevated levels of endogenous organic acids, such as those seen in chronic renal failure (CRF), and by other drugs that share the same transporter such as salicylates and nonsteroidal anti-inflammatory drugs (NSAIDs). After an oral dose of furosemide to normal subjects, the onset of action is within 30 to 60 min, peak effect occurs within 2 h, and its duration of action is approximately 6 h. The relation between renal furosemide excretion and its natriuretic effect is best described by a sigmoidal dose–response curve (Fig. 6-2). This same pharmacokinetic-pharmacodynamic relation

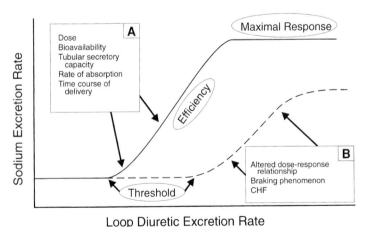

Loop Diuretic Excretion Rate

FIG. 6-2   Pharmacokinetic (*A*) and pharmacodynamic (*B*) determinants of the loop diuretic response. The broken line represents an altered dose-response relation as observed in a typical diuretic resistant state. Diuretic delivery necessary to achieve a threshold response can vary substantially in diuretic resistance.

based on urinary diuretic delivery applies to the other loop diuretics. Alterations in this normal dose–response relation can occur in a variety of pathophysiologic states such as CHF and volume depletion. The NSAID indomethacin also alters this relation through its inhibition of prostaglandin synthesis. This relation appears not to be perturbed by increased amounts of urinary protein, as is seen in the nephrotic syndrome; thus, urinary protein binding of loop diuretics is not a major mechanism for the diuretic resistance of the nephrotic syndrome. Bumetanide is 40 times more potent than furosemide and, like the other loop diuretics, is available in oral and intravenous forms. In normal subjects, the bioavailability of bumetanide is 80% and the onset of diuretic effect occurs within 30 min, with a peak effect within 1 h. The duration of action of oral bumetanide is between 3 and 6 h and its half-life is between 1 and 3.5 h. In healthy subjects, 60% of bumetanide is excreted unchanged in the urine, and the remaining drug is hepatically metabolized via the cytochrome P450 pathway. Because of this extrarenal metabolism, bumetanide does not accumulate in renal failure, although renal disease does impair tubular delivery. In contrast, in patients with hepatic disease, the plasma half-life of bumetanide is prolonged and more drug ultimately reaches the tubular fluid.

Torsemide is the newest member of the loop diuretic class. It is rapidly absorbed and is 80% to 90% bioavailable. Maximal sodium excretion occurs within the first 2 h after intravenous or oral administration. Only 20% of the drug is excreted unchanged in the urine and the remaining 80% undergoes hepatic metabolism. In healthy subjects, the half-life of torsemide is 3.3 h but is prolonged to 8 h in cirrhotic patients. When selecting an oral agent in patients with CHF, oral torsemide may be particularly advantageous because its absorption is not reduced and is much less variable than is the case with oral furosemide. In fact, torsemide disposition in CHF patients is comparable to that of normal subjects. Compared with furosemide-treated patients, torsemide-treated patients are less likely to be readmitted for CHF and for all cardiovascular and renal causes and are less fatigued. As with furosemide, however, torsemide pharmacodynamics in CHF patients is typical for this group of patients, with a shift of the dose–response relation downward and to the right.

Thiazides

The major site of action of the thiazide diuretics is the early distal convoluted tubule, where they inhibit the coupled reabsorption of Na^+ and Cl^-. The water-soluble thiazides such as hydrochlorothiazide (HCTZ) also inhibit carbonic anhydrase and, at high doses, further increase Na^+ excretion by this mechanism. Thiazides also inhibit NaCl and fluid reabsorption in the medullary collecting duct. Aside from these effects on Na^+ excretion, the thiazides impair urinary diluting capacity without affecting urinary concentrating mechanisms, reduce Ca^{2+} and urate excretion, and increase Mg^{2+} excretion.

HCTZ is the most widely prescribed drug in this diuretic class. It is well absorbed, with a bioavailability of 71%. The onset of diuresis with HCTZ generally occurs within 2 h, peaks between 3 and 6 h, and continues for as long as 12 h. The half-life of HCTZ is prolonged in patients with decompensated CHF and/or renal insufficiency. Large doses of thiazide diuretics in the order of 100 to 200 mg/day will initiate a diuresis in patients with CRF, however the magnitude of the diuretic response will be a function of the GFR and, hence, the filtered load and the site at which these drugs work.

Metolazone is a quinazoline diuretic and is similar to the thiazides in structure and locus of action. Although its major site of action is in the distal tubule, metolazone has a minor inhibitory effect on proximal Na^+ reabsorption through a carbonic anhydrase–independent mechanism. Metolazone is also lipid soluble, has a longer duration of action, and thereby more readily accesses the tubular lumen during states of renal insufficiency, unlike the thiazides. These unique properties in combination likely account for the enhanced natriuretic efficacy of metolazone and its effectiveness in diuretic-resistant states when given with a loop diuretic. Metolazone is available in different formulations, with some being very poorly and slowly absorbed. If the unpredictability of metolazone absorption is not recognized, its failure to elicit a diuretic response may incorrectly be attributed to the severity of the underlying illness.

Distal Potassium-Sparing Diuretics

Potassium-sparing diuretics can be divided into two distinct classes: competitive antagonists of aldosterone, such as spironolactone and eplerenone, and those that do not interact with aldosterone receptors, such as amiloride and triamterene. These agents act on the principal cells in the late distal convoluted tubule, the initial connecting tubule, and the cortical collecting duct, where they inhibit active Na^+ reabsorption. The inhibition of Na^+ entry into the cell causes a reduction in the activity of the basolateral Na^+, K^+-ATPase, which in turn reduces intracellular K^+ concentration. The resulting fall in the electrochemical gradient for K^+ and H^+ reduces the subsequent secretion of each of these cations. Because these drugs are capable of producing only a modest natriuresis, their clinical utility lies elsewhere in their ability to reduce the excretion of K^+ and net acid, especially when distal fluid delivery is enhanced by more proximally acting diuretics or in states of hyperaldosteronism. These agents reduce Ca^{2+} and Mg^{2+} excretion.

Spironolactone is a lipid-soluble K^+-sparing diuretic that is readily absorbed and highly protein bound. It has a 20-h half-life for elimination and takes 10 to 48 h to become maximally effective. It is also metabolized to active metabolites. Spironolactone is particularly useful during states of reduced renal function because access to its site of action is not dependent on GFR, although its tendency to cause hyperkalemia in renal failure patients limits its use in these situations.

Eplerenone is a new aldosterone receptor antagonist that selectively binds to the aldosterone receptor. However, as compared with spironolactone, it has a lower affinity for the androgen and progesterone receptors. The molecular structure of eplerenone replaces the 17-α-thioacetal group of spironolactone with a carbomethyl group, thereby conferring excellent selectivity for the aldosterone receptor over steroid receptors. The drug has been evaluated against placebo and other antihypertensive drugs in more than 4000 patients with mild to moderate hypertension and has a favorable efficacy and safety profile. Similarly, the drug has been used in patients with heart failure after an acute myocardial infarction with attendant decrease in CHF-related morbidity and mortality. The drug soon will be available for clinical use in the United States.

Amiloride is poorly absorbed and is actively secreted into the tubular lumen, where it works at the apical membrane. It has a duration of action of about 18 h. Conversely, triamterene is well absorbed and is hydroxylated to active metabolites. The half-life of triamterene and its metabolites ranges from 3 to 5 h. It also depends on active secretion to gain access to its site of action. Triamterene accumulates in cirrhotic patients owing to a reduction in hydroxylation and biliary secretion. Triamterene and amiloride accumulate in renal failure patients and are associated with worsening of renal function, particularly when given with NSAIDs.

DIURETICS IN HYPERTENSION

Hypertension is loosely defined by a systolic BP (SBP) of at least 140 mm Hg and/or a diastolic BP (DBP) of at least 90 mm Hg and is one of the most common disorders in the United States, with more than 58 million people affected. Hypertension is definition dependent and, if one adds to this figure those patients with borderline hypertension, this number grows larger. Cardiovascular and cerebrovascular events, renal disease, and all-cause mortality increase in a continuous fashion with increases in SBP and DBP. SBP is more predictive of morbidity and mortality than is DBP. In its most recent report, JNC VII advocated the use of diuretics as preferred first-line therapy for uncomplicated hypertension. This position was adopted based on a number of outcome studies that used diuretics and that reported therapy-related reductions in stroke and cardiovascular end points. All JNC documents dating to the original JNC I—published in 1977—have advocated a similar position favoring the early use of diuretics in the management of hypertension.

Mechanism of Action

The exact means by which diuretics lower BP is not known, although these agents have been used for longer than 40 years. The effect of diuretics on BP may be separated into three sequential phases, acute, subacute, and chronic (Fig. 6-3), that correspond to periods of roughly 1 to 2 weeks, several weeks, and several months, respectively. In the acute phase of response to diuretics, the major hypotensive effect of these agents is to reduce extracellular fluid (ECF) volume and thereby decrease cardiac output. The initial response to diuretic therapy in a patient receiving a "no added salt" diet (100 to 150 mmol/day) is a negative Na^+ balance of 100 to 300 mmol, which occurs in the first 2 to 4 days of treatment. Plasma Na^+ concentrations remain normal, and the loss of body Na^+ translates into a 1 to 2 L decrease in ECF volume. Direct measurements of hypertensive patients treated with diuretics show a 12% decrease in ECF. There is a similar reduction in plasma volume, which suggests that the acute volume loss arises proportionally from the plasma and the interstitial compartments. The decrease in plasma volume reduces venous return and diminishes cardiac output, thereby producing the initial vasodepressor response. The change in plasma volume variably stimulates the sympathetic nervous system (SNS) and the renin–angiotensin–aldosterone (RAA) axis. The degree to which these systems are activated may govern the magnitude of the acute BP decrease observed with diuretics. It also has been shown in hypertensive patients that diuretics can restore nocturnal BP decline in a manner similar to Na^+ restriction, which suggests that the kidneys and sodium metabolism play a role in the circadian rhythm of BP.

Over time, these effects on volume and cardiac output lessen in importance, although BP remains lowered. During the first few weeks of treatment, plasma volume returns to slightly less than pretreatment levels, despite the

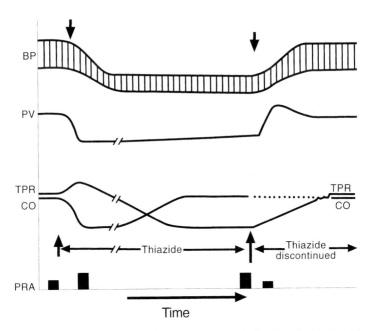

FIG. 6-3 Effects of thiazide administration in an "idealized" patient. BP, blood pressure; CO, cardiac output; PRA, plasma renin activity; PV, plasma volume; TPR, total peripheral resistance. (*Modified with permission from Moser M: Diuretics in the management of hypertension. Med Clin North Am 71:935, 1987.*)

continued administration of a diuretic. Thus, the chronic vasodepressor effect of diuretics is less an issue of volume reduction than it is a process coupled to a persistent reduction in total peripheral resistance (TPR). The subacute phase of BP reduction with diuretics seems to be a transitional period during which both of these factors prevail. There is no simple explanation for the drop in TPR that accompanies long-term diuretic use. The decrease in TPR during prolonged therapy has been attributed to several factors, including changes in the ionic content of vascular smooth-muscle cells, altered ion gradients across smooth muscle cells, and changes in membrane-bound ATPase activity. The ability of diuretics to reduce BP seems to be critically linked to the presence of functioning renal tissue; thus, a thiazide diuretic does not reduce BP in patients undergoing maintenance hemodialysis.

Understanding these mechanistic aspects of diuretic actions is important to the practical treatment of hypertension. The early action of diuretics to reduce ECF volume is optimized if dietary Na^+ is restricted at the beginning of therapy. This restriction limits the repercussions of the breaking phenomenon, which inevitably occurs with continued diuretic use. Some limitation of dietary Na^+ intake may also be relevant to how diuretics maintain reduced TPR over the long term. It is believed that changes in Na^+/Ca^{2+} balance in vascular smooth muscle cells arise from the short-term volume contraction seen during the first several days of thiazide diuretic therapy. How this phenomenon of volume contraction actually translates into a reduction in TPR is very poorly understood. Whatever the mechanism, it can be very long-lived, because a residual BP-reduction can be seen several weeks after the withdrawal of thiazide diuretics.

Another consideration in the ability of a diuretic to reduce BP over the long term relates to the natriuretic pattern of diuretics. For example, when long-term therapeutic responses to HCTZ and furosemide are compared in hypertensive patients, SBP and DBP are more consistently reduced with HCTZ. One explanation offered for this difference is the diuretic pattern of each agent. The natriuresis produced by a thiazide diuretic can be fairly prolonged but is generally modest at best, whereas a loop diuretic produces a brisk early diuretic response that rapidly falls off. The latter pattern of diuretic response is often accompanied by a significant post-diuretic period of Na^+ and water retention. When these two processes are summed, the result may be that the loop diuretic produces minimal volume loss despite its greater immediate potency. This period of antinatriuresis is of less consequence with the relatively less potent thiazide diuretic. In the end, a thiazide diuretic may be able to maintain a mild state of volume contraction more efficiently than a loop diuretic. An exception to this may be found with the response to the loop diuretic torsemide. Small doses of this compound may cause significant BP reduction, a vasodepressor process that seems to be independent of the observed degree of diuresis.

Diuretics in Clinical Trials

By the mid 1990s, evidence about the effects of BP-lowering regimens mainly based on diuretics and β blockers was available from a series of randomized controlled clinical trials involving more than 47,000 hypertensive patients. Systematic overviews and/or meta-analyses of these trials showed that reductions in BP of about 10 to 12 mm Hg systolic and 5 to 6 mm Hg diastolic confer relative reductions in stroke risk of 38% and a risk of coronary heart disease of 16% within just a few years of beginning therapy. The sizes of these effects were similar in major subgroups of trials and patients and seemed to be largely independent of differences in disease event rates among study patients. The few studies that directly compared diuretics and β blockers detected no clear differences in the risk of stroke or coronary artery disease. However, in elderly patients with hypertension, first-line diuretic therapy was shown to reduce cerebrovascular events, coronary artery disease, and stroke and cardiovascular and all-cause mortality, in contrast to first-line β blockers therapy that only reduced cerebrovascular events.

In 1995, many studies of BP-lowering drugs were identified as planned or ongoing. Most of these trials had been designed to detect large differences in relative risk and had insufficient power to detect small to moderate differences between the studied regimens. To maximize the information acquired by these and future trials, a collaborative program of prospectively designed overviews was developed. The first publication of these overviews occurred in 2000. Overviews of trials comparing angiotensin-converting enzyme (ACE) inhibitor–based regimens with diuretic or β blocker–based regimens in hypertensive patients provided no evidence that the benefits of ACE inhibitors were any different from those conferred by diuretics or β blockers. Overviews of trials comparing calcium antagonists with diuretic- or β blocker–based regimens provided some evidence of differences in the effects of the two regimens on cause-specific outcomes, with the risk for stroke being significantly less with calcium antagonists than with diuretics. There was no evidence of differences between the treatment effects of calcium antagonists regimens based on dihydropyridine versus nondihydropyridine agents.

The Antihypertensive and Lipid-Lowering Treatment to Prevent Heart Attack Trial (ALLHAT) was a randomized clinical outcome trial of antihypertensive and lipid-lowering therapy in a diverse population (including substantial numbers of women and minorities) of 33,357 high-risk hypertensives 55 years of age or older, with a mean follow-up of 4.9 years. The trial compared three classes of antihypertensive therapy, the α-blocker doxazosin, the calcium-channel blocker amlodipine, and the ACE inhibitor lisinopril, to the thiazide-type diuretic chlorthalidone. The study was terminated for the doxazosin arm of the study approximately 2 years early because of its inferiority to chlorthalidone with regard to two combined end points—coronary revascularization and angina—and more importantly, CHF. The final results of ALLHAT did not show any difference in the primary outcome, which was comprised of fatal CHD or nonfatal myocardial infarction. Secondary outcome results, such as stroke rate, found chlorthalidone to be better than lisinopril. New-incident CHF was also less frequent with chlorthalidone when compared with amlodipine and lisinopril. Interpretation of these secondary outcome results were confounded by between-group blood pressure differences favoring chlorthalidone, particularly in the black hypertensives.

Regression of Left Ventricular Hypertrophy with Diuretic Therapy

Left ventricular (LV) mass has been recognized as a powerful independent risk factor for cardiovascular morbidity. Antihypertensive therapy, with the exception of direct vasodilators, is effective in regressing LV hypertrophy (LVH). In 1991, Moser and Setaro compiled an overview of all studies evaluating LVH regression in diuretic-treated hypertensive patients, which supported the efficacy of diuretics in regressing LV mass. Two meta-analyses were undertaken specifically to examine LVH regression with different antihypertensive agents. Using echocardiography, Dahlof and colleagues analyzed 109 studies comprising 2357 patients. Diuretics were associated with an 11.3% reduction in LV mass; however, this was primarily due to a reduction in LV volume. Alternatively, the reductions of LV mass were 15% for ACE inhibitors, 8% for β blockers, and 8.5% for CCBs, with structural changes largely reflected by a reversal of posterior and intraventricular septal thicknesses. Another analysis of 39 trials of diuretics, β blockers, CCBs, and ACE inhibitors showed that LV mass is related to the treatment-induced decline in BP and, in particular, SBP. Reductions in LV mass of 13%, 9%, 6%, and 7% occurred with ACE inhibitors, CCBs, β blockers, and diuretics, respectively. Accordingly, diuretics are comparable to most other drug classes in their ability to regress LV mass. Significant reductions in LVH with antihypertensive therapy have not been shown in prospective randomized trials to be related to reduced cardiovascular morbidity and mortality. These trials are sorely needed.

Responsive Patient Populations

When used alone in the non-edematous patient, thiazide diuretics are as efficacious as most other classes of drugs. Although it is imprudent to offer universal recommendations about antihypertensive care on the basis of race alone, this is done routinely. That said, black and elderly hypertensives typically respond better to diuretics than do non-black and younger patients. The same can be said for other salt-sensitive forms of hypertension, such as that seen in diabetic patients.

Elderly

Five studies were performed specifically in the elderly hypertensive (age > 60 years): the Systolic Hypertension in Elderly Program (SHEP), the Swedish Trial in Old Patients (STOP), the Medical Research Council Trial in the treatment of older adults (MRC-2), the European Working Party on High Blood Pressure in the Elderly, and the trial of Coope and Warrender. Significant reductions in stroke similar to those observed in younger patients and greater benefits in terms of protection from myocardial infarction and CHF were demonstrated in these older patients. In addition, diuretics were shown to improve the quality of life as assessed by exercise capacity.

Four clinical trials, with a total of 34,676 patients, compared diuretics with β blockers: the International Prospective Primary Prevention Study in Hypertension, Heart Attack Primary Prevention in Hypertension Research Group, the Medical Research Council (MRC), and MRC-2. These two drug classes were comparable with regard to the incidence of stroke. With regard to myocardial infarction, two studies favored diuretics or β blockers over the other, although differences between these classes were quite small.

Three multicenter prospective clinical trials were performed specifically in the elderly: SHEP, STOP, and MRC-2. All three trials found significant reductions in cerebrocardiovascular morbidity and mortality associated with diuretic and/or β-blocker therapy. Just to highlight one of these trials, the SHEP trial was a double-blind, placebo-controlled trial comprised of 4736 men and women with isolated systolic hypertension who were older than 60 years. Patients were randomized to receive a low dose of the diuretic chlorthalidone as initial therapy; β blockers were then added as needed to reach the goal BP. At the end of the 5-year follow-up period, 46% of the subjects had adequate BP control when using only a low dose of chlorthalidone. Another 23% of patients had controlled BP with the addition of a β blocker. Outcome included a statistically significant reduction in strokes (36%) and statistically nonsignificant reductions in myocardial infarction (27%) and overall mortality (13%). Results of these trials have clearly established the benefit of low-dose diuretics and/or β blockers for the treatment of isolated systolic hypertension in the elderly and have been the basis for current treatment recommendations advocating diuretic therapy in uncomplicated forms of hypertension.

Blacks

In black patients, hypertension is more prevalent at a younger age, is usually more severe, and is associated with a greater incidence of cardiac, central nervous system, and renal complications than in white patients. Although the pathogenesis of hypertension has not been clearly defined, the majority of blacks fall into the low-renin category. This low-renin status cannot be explained by volume expansion alone, because no consistent relation between these two factors has been found in this population. In addition, the INTERSALT (International Study of Salt and Blood Pressure), a multicenter, cross-sectional study that evaluated the relation between electrolytes and BP, did not correlate excessive salt intake as a contributing factor to the development of hypertension in blacks. Although not fully resolved, there appears to be an important emerging role for potassium intake in the BP patterns expressed in normotensive and hypertensive blacks.

Nonetheless, black patients respond very well to diuretics. It has been reported that between 40% and 67% of young black patients and between 58% and 80% of elderly blacks respond to monotherapy with diuretics. As a rule, diuretics are more effective than β blockers, ACE inhibitors, or angiotensin-receptor blockers in blacks. However, when diuretics are added to any of these antihypertensive drug classes in black patients, their efficacy is substantially improved.

Diuretic therapy has been associated with reductions in morbidity and mortality in blacks. Black patients made up approximately half of the study participants in the Veterans Administration Cooperative Study and the Hypertension Detection and Follow-Up Program (HDFP), both of which were diuretic-based studies, and 35% of the ALLHAT population. In the Veterans Administration study, diuretic treatment was associated with a reduction in morbid events, from 26% to 10%, in black patients. In the HDFP study, there was an 18.5% mortality reduction for black men and a 27.8% mortality reduction for black women. In ALLHAT, diuretic therapy reduced BP more so than did lisinopril in blacks. This BP difference likely accounted for a portion of the difference in new-incident cases of CHF and stroke in blacks. However, the ability of diuretics to delay or prevent renal dysfunction in hypertensive blacks was put into question by the Multiple Risk Factor Intervention Trial (MRFIT), which did not show a benefit in this regard.

General Considerations

Diuretics are likely to find their greatest future use as "sensitizing" agents. Their primary modes of sensitization derive from volume depletion-related neurohumoral activation. In this regard, even subtle degrees of volume contraction or RAA axis activation, as produced by low-dose thiazide-type diuretics, can enhance the effect of coadministered antihypertensive compounds. This additive effect has rekindled interest in the use of fixed-dose combination antihypertensive therapy in the primary management of essential hypertension (see Chapter 16). The concept of using two drugs at low doses for BP control is not necessarily of recent vintage but has gained new support because it is increasingly evident that most patients who receive such treatment not only achieve their target BPs but do so with a minimum of side effects.

The dose–response relation for the antihypertensive effect of diuretics has been fully characterized over the past decade. In the process, many of the supposed negative attributes of diuretics have been shown not to exist. In the early days of diuretic use, doses were unnecessarily high. At that time, the concept of "if a little is good, a lot is better" was a routine part of practice. It was soon recognized that the dose–response relation for a thiazide-type diuretic, such as HCTZ, was extremely flat beyond a dosage of 25 mg/day. Much of the early negative biochemical and metabolic experiences with diuretics occurred with the very high dosages (100 to 200 mg/day) routinely used in the early days. When it was found that the BP reduction with HCTZ was similar whether the dosage was 12.5 or 25 to 100 mg/day, diuretics were "back in the game."

As practice patterns shifted to a low-dose strategy for thiazide-type diuretics, it was soon apparent that the frequency of the metabolically negative side effects had dramatically diminished; thus, such entities as hypokalemia, hypomagnesemia, glucose intolerance, and hypercholesterolemia are much less common with low-dose diuretics. When the strong end-organ protection data for diuretics are combined with the fact that these agents produce few side effects at low doses, a compelling argument can be made for the use of diuretics as initial therapy for many persons with uncomplicated mild to moderate hypertension.

DIURETICS IN CONGESTIVE HEART FAILURE

Diuretic use remains a vital part of the treatment of CHF. CHF is extremely common, with an estimated 500,000 new cases diagnosed each year in the United States. The prevalence of heart failure is increasing as the population ages and patients with CHF survive longer. CHF is the leading discharge diagnosis in persons older than 65 years, thus having an enormous economic impact. Up to the middle 1970s, the treatment of CHF was limited to dietary salt restriction, diuretics, and digitalis. Since then, the therapeutic options have grown dramatically and therapy has had a beneficial impact on survival in these patients. Use of diuretics depends on the circumstances causing the CHF, but they prove to be most efficacious in patients with chronic CHF. Unfortunately, the pharmacokinetics and pharmacodynamics of diuretics are altered in the setting of CHF, which may limit their overall efficacy. Such diuretic resistance often can be overcome with the judicious use of loop diuretics or combinations of diuretic classes. The following section briefly reviews the pathophysiology of CHF and highlights mechanisms of diuretic resistance and strategies to overcome this resistance.

Diuretics in CHF

Diuretics are useful in the long-term management of chronic stable CHF patients who have continuing salt and water retention despite dietary Na^+ restriction. They are also useful in patients who experience acute decompensation of CHF. Intravenous diuretics can improve the hemodynamic profile of decompensated CHF rapidly, but they also can be associated with further deterioration. In a study of 15 patients with severe acutely decompensated CHF, intravenous furosemide led to an abrupt increase in systemic vascular resistance and BP and to a decrease in cardiac performance parameters. This deleterious effect reversed itself over 2 h, coinciding with, but not necessarily relating to, the onset of diuresis. This phenomenon of acute decompensation is likely dose dependent; thus, caution needs to be exercised in acutely decompensated CHF as to the amount of furosemide administered. In patients with compensated CHF and severe edema, loop diuretics can be important add-on therapy to ACE inhibitors. In a study of 13 patients with severe edema secondary to CHF, furosemide therapy increased stroke volume owing to a reduction in systemic vascular resistance and afterload. In a double-blind study comparing a loop diuretic or cardiac glycoside with placebo, symptoms and pulmonary capillary wedge pressure were improved to a similar extent by both drug classes. However, patients treated with diuretics were more likely to develop a decreased effective blood volume and symptoms such as orthostatic hypotension, weakness, and prerenal azotemia.

Therefore, salt-depleting therapy requires a continual assessment of effective blood volume and adjustments in dietary salt intake and/or diuretic dose to optimize cardiac performance.

Mild CHF often responds to dietary salt restriction (100 to 150 mmol/day) and/or low doses of a thiazide diuretic. As CHF worsens, the GFR also decreases and patients become less responsive to thiazide diuretics. This usually occurs as the GFR falls below 30 mL/min (plasma creatinine concentration of 2 to 4 mg/dL). Larger, more frequent doses of loop diuretics and tighter control of dietary salt intake may then be required as the disease progresses.

Factors Influencing Diuretic Efficacy

Alterations in Pharmacokinetics

CHF modifies diuretic disposition. Although diuretic pharmacokinetics are usually unaltered in mild CHF, major abnormalities occur with severe CHF. Although the absolute absorptions of furosemide and bumetanide are normal in CHF patients, the time required to reach peak serum diuretic concentrations after oral dosing is significantly delayed. The delayed absorption can reduce the peak diuretic concentrations in plasma and urine, thus diminishing diuretic tubular delivery and thereby efficacy. Impaired drug absorption is thought to be related to reduced gastric and intestinal motility, edematous bowel wall, and/or decreased splanchnic blood flow.

As renal plasma flow declines in CHF, so does the delivery of furosemide or other loop diuretics to their site of action in the loop of Henle. The secretion of furosemide is reduced when the GFR falls below 30 mL/min because of the accumulation of endogenous organic acids that compete with furosemide for secretion by the organic anion transporter. At this level of renal insufficiency, loop diuretics must be administered in higher doses to circumvent factors that limit tubular secretion.

Alterations in Pharmacodynamics

The relation between natriuresis and excretion of loop diuretics is not altered in mild CHF, but the dose–response curve is shifted rightward in more advanced CHF (Fig. 6-4). The factors behind this shift in diuretic responsiveness are numerous, including structural adaptations that occur in the distal nephron and excessive activation of the renin–angiotensin system and SNS. ACE inhibitors sometimes can reestablish a diuresis in resistant CHF patients by inhibiting the generation of angiotensin II and thereby favorably alter afterload and/or renal blood flow. Conversely, if the BP drop is excessive with an ACE inhibitor, the diuretic response can be attenuated.

Diuretic Dosing in CHF

Because of alterations in diuretic pharmacokinetics and pharmacodynamics, patients with CHF often appear to be resistant to diuretics. The first step in evaluating a CHF patient for diuretic resistance is to assess the level of dietary salt and fluid intake. At steady state, dietary salt intake can be assessed from the measurement of 24-h Na^+ excretion. Patients ingesting a high-salt diet will overwhelm the capacity of the diuretic to produce a net diuresis and weight loss. If this is the case, a dietitian may be necessary to suitably reduce daily Na^+ intake to 100 mmol/day or less. Before labeling the

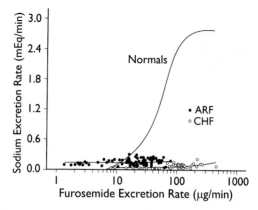

FIG. 6-4 Sodium excretory response after furosemide infusions in acute renal failure (ARF) or congestive heart failure (CHF) patients. Despite the flatness of the dose-response curves, most patients responded with an increment in urine volume and sodium excretion after having failed prior bolus therapy.

patient as truly diuretic resistant, it is important to ensure that the patient is compliant with the diuretic dosing (usually twice a day dosing is necessary) and that the patient is not taking medication that interferes with the action of diuretics, such as NSAIDs. Once these factors are eliminated from consideration, changes in diuretic doses or route of administration and diuretic combinations should be considered.

In CHF patients refractory to standard furosemide doses, high-dose therapy may prove efficacious. Daily doses between 500 and 2000 mg of intravenous furosemide were administered to 20 patients with CHF and refractory edema. With this regimen, a diuresis was established, body weight was reduced, and the CHF class was improved. Similar studies have reported improved furosemide efficacy in refractory CHF when high-doses of oral furosemide were employed. When moderate to severe renal impairment is present in decompensated CHF, a brief trial of high-dose furosemide is reasonable. Gerlag and Van Meijel treated patients with renal insufficiency (mean GFR, 32 mL/min) and refractory CHF with high-dose oral and intravenous furosemide over a 4-week period. Patients experienced a mean reduction in weight of 11.1 kg and an improvement in New York Heart Association (NYHA) classification.

Continuous intravenous administration of loop diuretics is another effective method of overcoming diuretic resistance in CHF patients. In a randomized crossover study comparing continuous infusion with bolus bumetanide in patients with severe renal insufficiency (mean GFR, 17 mL/min), Rudy and associates observed a greater net Na^+ excretion during continuous infusion despite comparable total 14-h drug excretion. The rate of urinary bumetanide excretion remained constant when infused. With intermittent administration, peak bumetanide excretion was observed within the first 2 h and tapered thereafter. In a similar study employing furosemide, a continuous intravenous infusion of furosemide (loading dose of 30 to 40 mg followed by infusion at a rate of 2.5 to 3.3 mg/h for 48 h) was compared with intermittent intravenous bolus administration (30 to 40 mg every 8 h for 48 h) in NYHA class III and class IV heart failure. A significantly greater diuresis and natriuresis was observed when using continuous furosemide infusion as compared with intermittent administration; this was accomplished at a lower peak furosemide concentration. When continuously infused, the pattern of furosemide delivery produced more efficient drug use. In a recent study examining the cost of care for 17 elderly patients with class IV CHF, continuous intravenous furosemide infusion resulted in a successful diuresis between 9 and 20 L over an average of 3.5 days. The length of stay for these patients was an average of 2.3 days shorter when compared with a contemporary group of class III and class IV CHF patients who were managed with conventional dosing of furosemide, and resulted in significant cost savings.

Combinations of diuretic classes have been used frequently in CHF patients refractory to loop diuretics alone. Because of structural adaptation occurring in the distal nephron with prolonged loop diuretic therapy, the combination of a distal diuretic and a loop diuretic is particularly effective in these patients. The combination of bumetanide and metolazone (a thiazide) produces a synergistic diuretic effect. During prolonged furosemide therapy, the responsiveness to a thiazide is augmented. Numerous reports have demonstrated a profound diuresis (several L daily) accompanied by clinical improvement after the addition of metolazone to furosemide in CHF patients previously resistant to furosemide therapy alone. Metolazone is particularly effective because its duration of action is prolonged, it is lipophilic, and it remains effective in states of renal impairment. However, in a study comparing metolazone with a short-acting thiazide, both used in combination with a loop diuretic, no significant difference in sodium excretion or urine output was observed between the two drugs.

Spironolactone also has been used in combination with loop diuretics and has been associated with an improvement in diuretic response in CHF patients. Above and beyond the known diuretic properties of spironolactone, it was recently shown that, as an aldosterone-receptor antagonist, spironolactone blocks a wide range of deleterious tissue-based effects attributable to aldosterone, which include augmentation of vascular and myocardial fibrosis. Accordingly, spironolactone is increasingly advocated as adjunct therapy in CHF. The basis for this therapeutic recommendation is the Randomized Aldactone Evaluation Study (RALES). In the RALES trial, spironolactone was shown to reduce the risk of all-cause mortality in NYHA class IV CHF patients treated with standard ACE inhibitor and diuretic therapy. It was recently demonstrated that aldosterone levels may often be elevated in CHF patients despite the use of ACE inhibitors. The future appears bright for aldosterone-receptor antagonist therapy, and the approval of eplerenone provides an additional and better tolerated option in this drug class. Moreover, the proof of concept heart failure study, Eplerenone's Neurohormonal Efficacy and Survival Study (EPHESUS) has succeeded in meeting both of its primary end points, which were death from any cause and death or hospitalization from cardiovascular causes. Based on the results of Eplerenone Post-Acute Myocardial Infarction Heart Failure Efficacy and Survival Study (EPHESUS) an additional labeled indication is being sought for eplerenone in the post-myocardial infarction patient with CHF. In the future, diuretic combinations, including loop and distal tubular diuretics and the aldosterone receptor inhibitors, will be more routinely used in patients with CHF.

Other Pharmacologic Approaches to Diuresis

Other approaches to diuresis include the use of dopamine agonists (see Chapter 17) and natriuretic peptides (see Chapter 19).

ADVERSE EFFECTS OF DIURETICS

Hyponatremia

Severe diuretic-induced hyponatremia is a serious complication of diuretic therapy. Elderly women treated with thiazide diuretics are most commonly affected, and the condition is usually seen within the first 2 weeks of therapy. Elderly women seem to exhibit an exaggerated natriuretic response to a thiazide diuretic but have a diminished capacity to excrete free water. These individuals also may have a low solute intake, which further diminishes their capacity for free water elimination.

Thiazide diuretics are more likely than loop diuretics to cause hyponatremia because they increase Na^+ excretion, prevent maximal urine dilution, and preserve the kidney's concentrating capacity. Loop diuretics inhibit salt transport in the renal medulla, prevent the generation of a maximal osmotic gradient, and actually can be used in hyponatremic subjects to increase free water clearance. CHF-related hyponatremia is more often a consequence of neurohumoral activation than a consequence of diuretic use, although diuretic use undoubtedly contributes to its development.

Mild asymptomatic hyponatremia can be treated by withholding diuretics, restricting free water intake, and restoring K^+ losses. Severe, symptomatic hyponatremia complicated by seizures is an emergency requiring intensive therapy, although steps should be taken to avoid rapid or overcorrection of the hyponatremia, because central pontine myelinolysis has occurred under these circumstances. The risks of ongoing hyponatremia must be weighed against those of too rapid a correction, and current recommendations are that plasma Na^+ should be corrected by no more than 12 to 20 mmol in the first 24 h. Controversy continues, however, in this area of therapy.

Hypokalemia and Hyperkalemia

Hypokalemia is a common finding in patients treated with loop and/or thiazide diuretics. During the first week of therapy with a thiazide diuretic, plasma K^+ in subjects not taking K^+ supplements fell by an average of 0.6 mmol/L as compared with 0.3 mmol/L in those taking furosemide. Mechanisms that contribute to hypokalemia during thiazide or loop diuretic use include augmented flow-dependent K^+ secretion in the distal nephron, a fall in luminal Cl^- concentration in the distal tubule, metabolic alkalosis, and/or stimulation of aldosterone and/or vasopressin release, both of which promote distal K^+ secretion (Fig. 6-5).

The clinical significance of diuretic-induced hypokalemia remains controversial, although mild degrees of diuretic-induced hypokalemia can be associated with increased ventricular ectopy. The MRFIT trial found a significant inverse relation between serum K^+ concentration and the frequency of ventricular premature contractions (VPCs). This relation, however, has not been observed in all trials, possibly because of the short duration of many of these trials. In the MRC study involving 324 patients with mild hypertension, 287 of whom underwent ambulatory electrocardiogram monitoring, after 8 weeks

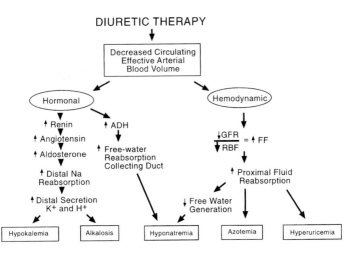

FIG. 6-5 Adaptive changes to conserve salt and water in states of extracellular volume depletion resulting in side effects related to diuretic use.

of therapy, diuretic use was not associated with an increased frequency of VPCs, whereas after 24 months, there was a significant difference in VPCs in those patients receiving diuretics as compared with those patients receiving placebo (20% versus 9%). These VPCs were significantly correlated with the serum K^+ concentration. Patients with LVH, CHF, or myocardial ischemia are at a particularly high risk of developing lethal ventricular arrhythmias in the setting of K^+ depletion.

Despite a concern about diuretic-related increases in cardiac risk due in part to electrolyte abnormalities, recent clinical trials, including SHEP, STOP, and MRC, have shown that low-dose diuretic therapy is actually associated with a 20% to 25% reduction in cardiovascular events. Perhaps the use of lower doses of thiazides or combination therapy with a K^+-sparing diuretic explains these favorable results as compared with earlier trials, such as MRFIT, in which higher doses of diuretics were employed and VPCs were more frequent. However, in the SHEP trial, patients with hypokalemia did not achieve the benefit of treatment seen in normokalemic patients.

Comparative effects on sudden cardiac death of different doses and combinations of diuretics have been reported. The risk of cardiac arrest among patients receiving combined thiazide and K^+-sparing diuretic therapy was lower than that found in patients treated with thiazides alone (odds ratio, 0.3:1). Compared with low-dose thiazide therapy (25 mg/day), intermediate-dose thiazide therapy (50 mg/day) was associated with a moderate increase in the risk of cardiac arrest (odds ratio, 1.7:1) and high-dose (100 mg/day) therapy was associated with an even greater increase in risk (odds ratio, 3.6:1). In contrast with K^+-sparing diuretics, the addition of K^+ supplements to thiazide therapy had little effect on the risk of sudden cardiac death (odds ratio, 0.9:1). Among patients receiving one antihypertensive medication, the risk of cardiac arrest was not higher with diuretic treatment than with β blockers (odds ratio, 1:1). Serum K^+ concentrations below 3 mmol/L occur infrequently with thiazide diuretics and, when found, are more common with loop diuretics or carbonic anhydrase inhibitors. Profound hypokalemia with serum K^+ concentrations below 2.5 mmol/L can lead to diffuse muscle weakness, including diaphragmatic paralysis, rhabdomyolysis, and acute renal failure

Distal K^+-sparing diuretics and spironolactone can cause dangerous hyperkalemia. Hyperkalemia is usually encountered in patients predisposed to this complication, those with a reduction in the GFR (especially the elderly or those given potassium chloride supplements or salt substitutes), those on an ACE inhibitor or an NSAID, or in other situations that predispose to hyperkalemia such as acidosis, hyporeninemic hypoaldosteronism, or heparin therapy.

Hypomagnesemia

Loop diuretics inhibit magnesium (Mg) reabsorption in the loop of Henle, a site where approximately 30% of the filtered load of Mg is reabsorbed. Potassium-sparing diuretics, including spironolactone, diminish the increase in Mg excretion that accompanies thiazide or loop diuretic use. Prolonged therapy with thiazides and loop diuretics reduces plasma Mg concentration by an average of 5% to 10%, although patients occasionally develop severe hypomagnesemia. Cellular Mg depletion occurs in 20% to 50% of patients during thiazide therapy and can be present despite a normal serum Mg concentration. This complication is more common in the elderly and in those patients receiving prolonged, high-dose diuretic therapy. Hypomagnesemia often coexists with diuretic-induced hyponatremia and hypokalemia disorders that cannot be fully reversed until the underlying Mg deficit is corrected. In one study, 41% of patients with hypokalemia were found to also have low serum Mg concentrations. Two studies have reported hypomagnesemia in 19% to 37% of CHF patients treated with loop diuretics. The data regarding the association of hypomagnesemia with an increased prevalence of VPCs, sudden death, and overall cardiovascular survival are conflicting, and a definite causal relation is lacking. Associated symptoms of hypomagnesemia include depression, muscle weakness, refractory hypokalemia, hypocalcemia, and atrial fibrillation. Many of these abnormalities and, in particular, refractory hypokalemia and hypocalcemia correct promptly with Mg administration.

Acid–Base Changes

Thiazides and loop diuretics can cause a metabolic alkalosis. The generation of this metabolic alkalosis is due primarily to a contraction of the ECF space caused by urinary loss of a relatively HCO_3-free fluid. The maintenance of the alkalosis probably involves increased net acid excretion in response to hypokalemia, mineralocorticoid excess, and continued Na^+ delivery to the distal nephron sites of H^+ secretion. Diuretic-induced metabolic alkalosis is best managed by administration of potassium and/or sodium chloride, although sodium chloride administration may not be feasible in the CHF patient who is already volume overloaded. In these cases, a potassium-sparing diuretic or, on rare occasions, a carbonic anhydrase inhibitor, such as acetazolamide, may be considered. Metabolic alkalosis also impairs the natriuretic response to loop diuretics and may contribute to diuretic resistance in the CHF patient.

Spironolactone, amiloride, and triamterene can cause hyperkalemic metabolic acidosis that, in elderly patients or in those patients with renal impairment or CHF, can occasionally be severe and of a life-threatening nature.

METABOLIC ABNORMALITIES

Hyperglycemia

Prolonged thiazide diuretic therapy impairs glucose tolerance and occasionally may precipitate diabetes mellitus. Hyperglycemia and carbohydrate intolerance have been linked to diuretic-induced hypokalemia, which inhibits insulin secretion by β cells and reduces ECF volume and cardiac output. These aberrations are compounded by increases in SNS activity, which decreases peripheral glucose use. Short-term metabolic studies, epidemiologic studies, and a variety of clinical trials have suggested a causal link between the use of thiazide diuretics and subsequent development of type 2 diabetes. However, these studies were compromised by small numbers of patients, relatively limited follow-up periods, different definitions of new-onset diabetes, inadequate comparison groups, selection criteria that limited the generalizability of the findings, and study designs that precluded inter-class comparisons among antihypertensive drug classes.

For example, in one study non–insulin-dependent diabetics given HCTZ for only 3 weeks increased their fasting serum glucose concentration by 31%; when combined with propranolol, the increase was 53%.

Diuretic-associated glucose intolerance appears to be dose related, less common with loop diuretics, and reversible on withdrawal of the agent, although the data on reversibility in HCTZ-treated patients appear conflicting. Ramsay and colleagues reviewed this issue and found several studies that support unaltered glucose homeostasis by using low-dose HCTZ therapy (25 to 50 mg/day). However, they also reported three long-term trials noting abnormalities in glucose homeostasis with HCTZ doses between 12.5 and 50 mg/day. Recently, Gress and coworkers conducted a large, prospective, cohort study that included 12,250 adults who did not have diabetes and that was designed to examine the independent relation between the use of antihypertensive medications and the subsequent development of type 2 diabetes. After appropriate adjustment for confounders, patients with hypertension who were taking thiazide diuretics were found not to be at greater risk for subsequent diabetes development than patients who were not receiving antihypertensive therapy. The doses of thiazide diuretic given in the cohort study by Gress and colleagues were not reported; thus, because of the perceived variability of this effect, blood glucose should be monitored during thiazide therapy, particularly in obese or diabetic patients. Consequently, long-term thiazide therapy can be viewed as causing only small, if any, changes in fasting serum glucose concentration, an effect that might be reversed with the concomitant use of potassium-sparing diuretics.

Hyperlipidemia

The short-term administration of loop diuretics or thiazides increases the plasma cholesterol concentrations by 4% to 14% and raises the levels of low-density and very–low-density lipoproteins and triglycerides, an effect that may be simply related to mild volume depletion. Long-term clinical trials have reported unchanged cholesterol levels after 1 year of diuretic therapy. Moreover, data from the HDFP study have indicated that hypertensive subjects with baseline cholesterol values above 250 mg/dL and treated with diuretics experience a decline in cholesterol levels from the second to the fifth years of treatment.

Hyperuricemia

Thiazide therapy increases serum urate concentrations by approximately 35%, an effect related to decreased urate clearance. Decreased urate clearance may be related to increased reabsorption secondary to diuretic-related ECF volume depletion. Hyperuricemia is dose related and does not usually precipitate a gouty attack unless the patient has an underlying gouty tendency or serum urate concentrations exceeding 12 to 14 mg/dL. In the MRC trial, patients receiving thiazide diuretics had significantly more withdrawals for gout than did placebo-treated patients (4.4 versus 0.1 per 1000 patient years). If a gouty attack occurs, diuretic therapy should be discontinued. If this is not feasible, then the lowest clinically effective dose should be given and the degree of volume contraction limited. An additional alternative in the gouty patient requiring diuretic therapy is that of allopurinol. However, allopurinol should be used cautiously in patients receiving HCTZ because the incidence of hypersensitivity reactions is higher with this combination.

Other Adverse Effects

Impotence

In the MRC trial, in which 15,000 hypertensive subjects received placebo, thiazide, or a β blocker for 5 years, impotence rates were 22-fold and 4-fold higher in those receiving a thiazide than in those receiving placebo or a β blocker, respectively. Another smaller trial by Chang and associates confirmed the higher frequency of decreased libido, difficulty in gaining and sustaining an erection, and difficulty in ejaculating in patients receiving a thiazide. Multivariate analysis has suggested that these findings are not mediated by low serum potassium levels or by low BP. The exact mechanism of diuretic-related impotence is not known. Patients on diuretics with impotence can respond favorably to sildenafil.

Ototoxicity

The association between ototoxicity and loop diuretics is well established. Loop diuretics are direct inhibitors of the $Na^+/K^+/2Cl^-$ cotransport system, which also exists in the marginal and dark cells of the stria vascularis, which are responsible for endolymph secretion; thus, the ototoxicity of these agents may be indirect due to changes in ionic composition and fluid volume within the endolymph.

Loop diuretic-induced ototoxicity usually occurs within 20 min of infusion and is typically reversible, although permanent deafness has been reported. Ototoxicity has been seen with ethacrynic acid, furosemide, and bumetanide with intravenous and oral administrations. The frequency appears to be higher with furosemide than with bumetanide. Patients with renal failure and those receiving concomitant aminoglycoside therapy are at greatest risk of developing ototoxicity.

Ototoxicity is clearly related to the rate of infusion and to peak serum concentrations. Heidland and Wigand conducted audiometric studies during the infusion of furosemide at a constant rate of 25 mg/min and reported reversible hearing loss in two-thirds of patients. Fries and colleagues found no hearing loss in renal failure patients receiving 500 to 1000 mg over 6 h. Plasma levels of furosemide higher that 50 μg/mL are associated with a greater incidence of auditory disturbances, and Brown and colleagues found patients with levels higher than 100 μg/mL to be at risk for permanent deafness. In general, the rate of furosemide infusion should not exceed 4 mg/min and serum concentrations should be maintained below 40 μg/mL.

Drug Allergy

Photosensitivity dermatitis occurs rarely during thiazide or furosemide therapy. HCTZ more commonly causes photosensitivity than do the other thiazides. Diuretics occasionally may cause a more serious generalized dermatitis and, at times, even a necrotizing vasculitis. Cross-sensitivity with sulfonamide drugs may occur with all diuretics, with the exception of ethacrynic acid. Severe necrotizing pancreatitis is an additional serious, life-threatening complication of thiazide therapy. Acute allergic interstitial nephritis with fever, rash, and eosinophilia, although an uncommon complication of diuretics, is one that may result in permanent renal failure if the drug exposure is prolonged. It may develop abruptly or some months after therapy is begun with a thiazide diuretic or, less commonly, with furosemide. Ethacrynic acid is chemically dissimilar from the other loop diuretics and can be safely substituted in diuretic-treated patients who experience a number of these allergic complications.

Carcinogenesis

Two reports have suggested an increased risk of renal cell carcinoma and colon cancer with long-term diuretic therapy, but further confirmation is necessary.

ADVERSE DRUG INTERACTIONS

Aside from those interactions already reviewed, other drug–diuretic interactions may occur with diuretics (see Chapter 21). Loop diuretics are known to potentiate aminoglycoside nephrotoxicity. By causing hypokalemia, diuretics increase digitalis toxicity. Plasma lithium concentrations can increase with thiazide therapy if significant volume contraction occurs; this is due to increased reabsorption of fluid and lithium in the proximal tubule. However, some diuretics, such as chlorothiazide or furosemide, with significant carbonic anhydrase inhibitory effect decrease proximal fluid reabsorption and increase lithium clearance, thus leading to a fall in lithium levels. Whole-blood lithium should be closely monitored in all patients being administered lithium in conjunction with diuretics. Furosemide can potentiate the myotoxic effects of clofibrate through the displacement of clofibrate from plasma protein-binding sites.

NSAIDs can antagonize the effects of diuretics and predispose diuretic-treated patients to renal insufficiency. The combination of indomethacin and triamterene may be particularly dangerous because acute renal failure can be precipitated. A reversible form of renal insufficiency may also develop when excessive diuresis occurs in ACE inhibitor–treated CHF patients. Risk factors for this form of functional renal insufficiency include hyponatremia, diabetes, and the use of long-acting ACE inhibitors. This response may be exaggerated if NSAIDs are added to the mix of medications. Na^+ balance plays an important role in modulating the BP response to ACE inhibitors in CHF. Patients with Na^+ and volume depletion before ACE inhibitors are started are at greater risk of developing first-dose hypotension.

ADDITIONAL READINGS

ALLHAT Collaborative Research Group: Major cardiovascular events in hypertensive patients randomized to doxazosin vs chlorthalidone: The antihypertensive and lipid-lowering treatment to prevent heart attack trial (ALLHAT). *JAMA* 283:1967, 2000.

ALLHAT Officers and Co-ordinators for the ALLHAT Collaborative Group: Major outcomes in high-risk hypertensive patients randomized to angiotensin converting enzyme inhibitor or calcium channel blocker vs diuretic. The Antihypertensive and Lipid-Lowering Treatment to Prevent Heart Attack Trial (ALLHAT). *JAMA* 288: 2981, 2002.

Blood Pressure Lowering Treatment Trialists Collaboration: Effects of ACE inhibitors, calcium antagonists, and other blood-pressure-lowering drugs: Results of prospectively designed overviews of randomised trials. *Lancet* 355:1955, 2000.

Brater DC: Diuretic therapy. *N Engl J Med* 339:387, 1998.

Chobanian AV, Bakris GL, Black HR, et al, and the National High Blood Pressure Education Program Coordinating Committee: The seventh report of the Joint National Committee on Prevention, Detection, Evaluation, and Treatment of High Blood Pressure. The JNC 7 report. *JAMA* 289:3560. 2003.

Cooper HW, Dries DL, Davis CE, et al: Diuretics and risk of arrhythmic death in patients with left ventricular dysfunction. *Circulation* 100:1311, 1999.

Epstein M: Aldosterone blockers and potassium-sparing diuretics, in Izzo JL Jr, Black HR (eds): *Hypertension Primer*, 3rd ed. Dallas, American Heart Association, 2003, p 414.

Frishman WH, Bryzinski BS, Coulson LR, et al: A multifactorial trial design to assess combination therapy in hypertension: Treatment with bisoprolol and hydrochlorothiazide. *Arch Intern Med* 154:1461, 1994.

Gress TW, Nieto FJ, Shahar E, et al: Hypertension and antihypertensive therapy as risk factors for type 2 diabetes mellitus. *N Engl J Med* 342:905, 2000.

Hajjar I, Kotchen TA: Trends in prevalence, awareness, treatment, and control of hypertension in the United States, 1988–2000. *JAMA* 290:199, 2003.

Jessup M: Aldosterone blockade and heart failure. *N Engl J Med* 348:1380, 2003.

Jorde UP, Vittorio T, Katz SD, et al: Elevated plasma aldosterone levels despite complete inhibition of the vascular angiotensin-converting enzyme in chronic heart failure. *Circulation* 106:1055, 2002.

Kramer BK, Schweda F, Riegger GAJ: Diuretic treatment and diuretic resistance in heart failure. *Am J Med* 106:90, 1999.

Lakshman MR, Reda DJ, Materson BJ, et al: Diuretics and β blockers do not have adverse effects at 1 year on plasma lipid and lipoprotein profiles in men with hypertension. *Arch Intern Med* 159:551, 1999.

LeJemtel TH, Sonnenblick EH, Frishman WH: Diagnosis and medical management of heart failure, in Fuster V, Alexander RW, O'Rourke RA (eds): *Hurst's the Heart*, 11th ed. New York, McGraw-Hill, in press.

Papademetriou V, Sica DA, Izzo JL Jr: Thiazide and loop diuretics, in Izzo JL Jr, Black HR (eds): *Hypertension Primer*, 3rd ed. Dallas, American Heart Association, 2003, p 411.

Pitt B, Remme W, Zannad F, et al: Eplerenone, a selective aldosterone blocker, in patients with left ventricular dysfunction after myocardial infarction. *N Engl J Med* 348:1309, 2003.

Pitt B, Zannad F, Rime WJ, et al: The effect of spironolactone on morbidity and mortality in patients with severe heart failure. *N Engl J Med* 341:709, 1999.

Rocha R, Williams GH: Rationale for the use of aldosterone antagonists in congestive heart failure. *Drugs* 62:723, 2002.

Schuller D, Lynch JP, Find D: Protocol-guided diuretic management: comparison of furosemide by continuous infusion and intermittent bolus. *Crit Care Med* 25:1969, 1997.

Sica DA: Pharmacotherapy in congestive heart failure: Metolazone and its role in edema management. *Congest Heart Failure* 9:100, 2003.

Sica DA: ALLHAT—Is the final answer in? (editorial). *Heart Dis* 5:171, 2003.

Sica DA: Aldosterone receptor blockade: A therapy resurrected (editorial). *Heart Dis* 5:85, 2003.

Stier CT Jr, Koenig S, Lee DY, et al: Aldosterone and aldosterone antagonism in cardiovascular disease. Focus on eplerenone (Inspra). *Heart Dis* 5:102, 2003.

Weber KT: Aldosterone in congestive heart failure. *N Engl J Med* 345:1689, 2001.

7 | Magnesium, Potassium, and Calcium as Potential Cardiovascular Disease Therapies

Domenic A. Sica   William H. Frishman
Erdal Cavusoglu

Deficiency states and abnormalities in the metabolism of the electrolytes magnesium (Mg^{2+}), potassium (K^+), and calcium (Ca^{2+}) have been considered as etiologic factors in systemic hypertension, ischemic heart disease, congestive heart failure (CHF), stroke, atherosclerosis, diabetes mellitus, asthma, and a variety of arrhythmias. In experimental animals, deficit replacement or simple supplementation of these cationic substances has been shown to prevent and treat these cardiovascular maladies. In this chapter, Mg^{2+}, K^+, and Ca^{2+} are discussed as potential cardiovascular disease therapies.

MAGNESIUM

Magnesium is the second most common intracellular cation in the human body, second only to K^+, with a free cytosolic concentration of approximately 0.5 mmol/L. Magnesium is also the fourth most abundant cation in the body. It is distributed in three major body compartments: approximately 65% in the mineral phase of bone, about 34% in muscle, and 1% in plasma and interstitial fluid. Unlike plasma Ca^{2+}, which is 40% protein bound, only approximately 20% of plasma Mg^{2+} is protein bound. Consequently, changes in plasma protein concentrations have less effect on plasma Mg^{2+} than on plasma Ca^{2+}. Magnesium is a cofactor in well over 300 different enzymatic reactions in the body and is of particular importance for those enzymes that use nucleotides as cofactors or substrates, because, as a rule, it is not the free nucleotide but its Mg^{2+} complex that is the actual cofactor or substrate. Magnesium is important in many cell membrane functions, including the gating of Ca^{2+} ion channels, in mimicking many of the effects of Ca^{2+}-channel blockade. Magnesium is a necessary cofactor for any biochemical reaction involving ATP and is essential for the proper functioning of the Na^+/K^+ and Ca^{2+} ATPase pumps, which are critical to the maintenance of a normal resting membrane potential. Intracellular Mg^{2+} ion deficiency can lead to abnormalities in myocardial membrane potential, which then serves as a trigger for cardiac arrhythmias. Deficiency states or abnormalities in Mg metabolism also play important roles in ischemic heart disease, CHF, sudden cardiac death, diabetes mellitus, preeclampsia–eclampsia, and/or hypertension.

Cardiovascular Effects of Magnesium

The Mg^{2+} ion has numerous properties that theoretically can benefit the cardiovascular system. Magnesium modulates the contraction and tone of vascular smooth muscle cells, thus reducing systemic vascular resistance and

155

thereby decreasing blood pressure. Magnesium also dilates coronary and cerebral arteries and is effective in the relief of coronary vasospasm. Magnesium slows heart rate, preserves mitochondrial function and high-energy phosphate levels, and serves as an antiarrhythmic. In addition, Mg^{2+} possesses antiplatelet and anticoagulant properties and anti-atherosclerotic properties, the ability to improve endothelial function, and the capacity to protect against the formation of oxygen free radicals. Magnesium deficiencies or metabolic abnormalities can cause abnormalities in cardiovascular function.

Role of Magnesium in Ischemic Heart Disease and Myocardial Infarction

For many years Mg^{2+} deficiency has been loosely tied to ischemic heart disease and myocardial infarction (MI). Although innumerable animal and human studies have attempted to establish a definitive role for Mg^{2+} deficiency in the incidence and limitations in the management of ischemic heart disease, much confusion remains in this regard. Epidemiologic studies comparing death rates from ischemic heart disease from geographically diverse areas have attempted to link low Mg^{2+} concentrations in soil and water with a higher cardiovascular mortality. Several autopsy series dating back to the 1970s have also suggested that patients dying of acute MI tend to have reduced myocardial Mg^{2+} concentrations compared with those dying from noncardiac causes. A series of basic science studies have since demonstrated that acute ischemia is, in fact, associated with a dramatic increase in the efflux of Mg^{2+} from the injured myocyte and with an increase in cellular Ca^{2+} and Na^+ content. Moreover, low myocardial Mg^{2+} concentrations have been demonstrated in chronic ischemic heart disease. In addition, Mg^{2+} deficiency has been etiologically involved with many of the known risk factors for coronary artery disease, such as diabetes mellitus, hypertension, and hyperlipidemia.

Studies in animal models of ischemia and infarction have suggested a beneficial role for Mg^{2+}. It has been theorized that Mg^{2+} protects against reperfusion injury by limiting cellular Ca^{2+} overload. Reports of the use of Mg^{2+} in acute MI in humans date back to the 1950s. Magnesium administration was found to have beneficial effects in patients with MI in several small studies, and an early overview on this topic suggested that the morbidity and mortality rates were lower with Mg^{2+} therapy.

The beneficial effects of intravenous (IV) Mg^{2+} sulfate ($MgSO_4$; 8 mmol over 5 min followed by 65 mmol over 24 h) given immediately to patients with suspected acute MI were initially documented in a large prospective double-blind trial, the Leicester Intravenous Mg Intervention Trial (LIMIT-2). In this study the mortality rate was 7.8% in the $MgSO_4$ treatment arm versus 10.3% in the placebo group. The side effects of Mg^{2+} treatment in this study were minimal and included transient flushing related to the speed of injection of the loading dose and an increased incidence of sinus bradycardia. However, the routine administration of Mg^{2+} during acute MI has been discontinued largely on the basis of the Fourth International Study of Infarct Survival (ISIS-4), which included 58,050 patients and found that Mg^{2+} administration does not decrease 35-day mortality when compared with controls. The timing of the Mg^{2+} loading dose in relation to thrombolytic therapy or spontaneous reperfusion has been offered as an explanation for the opposing results in LIMIT-2 and ISIS-4. Early treatment appears essential because serum Mg^{2+} concentrations must be raised by the time of reperfusion to avoid immediate injury. This observation agrees with the 25% reduction in early left ventricular failure in the Mg^{2+} group of LIMIT-2. Other studies using an earlier IV Mg^{2+} loading dose (8 mmol $MgSO_4$ over 5 min plus 65 mmol over the next 24 h) have also failed to demonstrate a significant difference in cardiac arrhythmias compared with control therapy.

Magnesium administration may have a greater therapeutic role in those patients experiencing an acute MI who are unable to receive thrombolytic therapy, a population with an inherently high in-hospital mortality rate. A 48-h infusion of $MgSO_4$ in this group of patients has been shown to significantly reduce the incidence of arrhythmias, CHF, and conduction disturbances compared with placebo. Left ventricular ejection fraction 72 h and 1 to 2 months after admission and in-house survival rates were higher in patients who received $MgSO_4$. Similarly, a beneficial effect of Mg^{2+} therapy has been reported in patients with unstable angina undergoing bypass grafting.

The use of Mg^{2+} in the preoperative and early postoperative periods is also highly effective in reducing the incidence of atrial fibrillation after elective coronary artery bypass grafting; however, other studies have not confirmed these cardioprotective effects. For example, $MgSO_4$ given intravenously before, during, and after reperfusion did not decrease myocardial damage and did not improve short-term clinical outcome in patients with acute MI treated with direct angioplasty.

The discrepancy in the results of these studies has dampened the enthusiasm for routine use of Mg^{2+} in the management of patients with acute MI. The disparate results between these two large clinical trials (LIMIT-2 and ISIS-4) remain puzzling. However, the ISIS-4 trial was not specifically designed to test the hypothesis that Mg^{2+} might limit reperfusion injury, and the time factor when Mg^{2+} is given needs to be further clarified. It is also important to determine whether those patients with Mg^{2+} deficiency are the ones who benefit or whether Mg^{2+} should be used as a true cardioplexic agent in the non–Mg^{2+}-deficient individual. At this time, Mg^{2+} therapy cannot be recommended as routine treatment in the management of acute MI. The current American College of Cardiology/American Heart Association guidelines for the treatment of patients with acute MI currently recommend IV Mg^{2+} only for correction of documented Mg^{2+} deficiency and for the treatment of the torsades de pointes–type of ventricular tachycardia. Ongoing studies, such as the Magnesium in Coronaries study, may help define a future role for Mg^{2+} in ischemic heart syndromes.

Magnesium in Diabetes and Congestive Heart Failure

Magnesium deficiency occurs in association with various medical disorders but is particularly common in diabetes mellitus, CHF, and after diuretic use. Recognition of K^+ deficiency and/or its correction follows fairly standard guidelines in these conditions; alternatively, the circumstances are much different for Mg^{2+}, because serum Mg^{2+} values poorly reflect total body stores. Potassium repletion in a hypokalemic patient can prove difficult unless underlying Mg^{2+} deficiency is first corrected. Hypocalcemia is another common sequela to hypomagnesemia and can prove resistant to treatment owing to hypomagnesemia-related defects in parathyroid release and/or action. This form of hypocalcemia responds to small amounts of supplemental Mg^{2+} but can redevelop unless the underlying Mg^{2+} deficit is fully repleted.

The incidence of diuretic-related hypokalemia and/or hypomagnesemia in CHF or hypertension can be considerably lessened by using K^+-sparing diuretics, angiotensin converting enzyme inhibitors, or angiotensin-receptor blockers.

Excessive glycosuria is the main cause of Mg^{2+} deficiency in diabetes mellitus, and its severity is inversely correlated with the level of glycemic control. Fat and protein mobilization during acute hyperglycemia-associated metabolic decompensation in addition to other factors also play roles in diabetes-related hypomagnesemia. Hypomagnesemia can be a cause and an effect of hyperglycemia and is associated with insulin resistance. The prevalence and severity of Mg^{2+} deficiency can be influenced by other conditions, in particular CHF and diuretic use. In these cases, multiple electrolyte imbalances can develop simultaneously, predicting poor patient survival. Hyponatremia is closely associated with a poor prognosis, hypokalemia with increased ventricular dysrhythmias, and hypomagnesemia with arrhythmias and the aforementioned refractory hypokalemia and/or hypocalcemia. However, Mg^{2+} deficiency has yet to be established as an independent cardiovascular mortality risk factor in such conditions.

Magnesium in Arrhythmias

There is an inverse correlation between myocardial irritability and serum Mg^{2+} concentrations, which is well illustrated in CHF. For example, 0.2 mEq/kg of $MgSO_4$ given over 1 h to CHF patients reduced ectopic beats in a 6-h postdosing monitoring period, and MgCl given as a 10-min bolus (0.3 mEq/kg) followed by a 24-h maintenance infusion (0.08 mEq/kg/h) also succeeded in reducing hourly ectopic beats. Noteworthy was the fact that Mg^{2+} concentrations 30 min and 24 h after the bolus were 3.6 ± 0.1 and 4.2 ± 0.1 mg/dL, respectively. Oral Mg^{2+} replacement (15.8 mmol MgCl/day for 6 weeks) also reduced ventricular irritability during the chronic phase of CHF treatment despite the fact that serum Mg^{2+} changed insignificantly (0.87 ± 0.07 to 0.92 ± 0.05 mmol/L). The risk of hypomagnesemia is particularly high in individuals concurrently receiving digitalis because this association has an additive effect on arrhythmia development.

Magnesium is an essential cofactor for the Na^+, K^+-ATPase enzyme. Magnesium deficiency impairs the function of this enzyme, which in turn lowers intracellular K^+ concentrations. As a consequence, the resting membrane potential becomes less negative, thereby lowering its threshold for the development of arrhythmias. In addition to its effect on the Na^+, K^+-ATPase pump, Mg^{2+} has been shown to have profound effects on the several different types of K^+ channels that are known to exist within cardiac cells. Studies in animals appear to support the theory that Mg^{2+} increases cellular resistance to the development of arrhythmias. For example, Mg^{2+} infusion has been shown to raise the threshold for ventricular premature contractions and the induction of ventricular fibrillation in normal denervated (heart and lung preparations) and whole-animal digitalis-treated hearts. Moreover, considerable evidence links Mg^{2+} deficiency with an increased incidence of supraventricular and ventricular arrhythmias.

Evidence of the salutary effects of IV Mg^{2+} in treating supraventricular and ventricular tachyarrhythmias has been available for many years. In addition, numerous anecdotal reports have been published attesting to the utility of Mg^{2+} in cases of refractory ventricular arrhythmias, although most of these cases probably were associated with Mg^{2+} deficiency. Interestingly, K^+-sparing diuretics, compounds that also exhibit Mg^{2+}-sparing effects, do not carry the same increased risk for sudden cardiac death observed with non–K^+-sparing diuretics. Despite these observations and the theoretical benefits of Mg^{2+} with regard to the development of arrhythmias, there has been no controlled study designed to evaluate the specific efficacy of Mg^{2+} as an antiarrhythmic agent in the treatment of ventricular arrhythmias. Further, it is unclear whether the potential effectiveness of Mg^{2+} in these situations represents a pharmacologic effect of Mg^{2+} or merely reflects repletion of an underling deficiency state. Whatever its potential role in the management of ventricular fibrillation, supraventricular arrhythmias, and "run-of-the-mill" ventricular arrhythmias, Mg^{2+} clearly does have a time-honored and proven place in the treatment of ventricular arrhythmias associated with digoxin toxicity.

Magnesium in Hypertension

Many studies have observed some form of hypomagnesemia (in serum and/or tissue) in hypertensive patients, with significant inverse correlations between Mg^{2+} concentration and blood pressure. Dietary Mg^{2+} appears to be of some importance to this relation. Epidemiologic studies have linked hypertension, hypertensive heart diseases, and ischemic heart disease with "soft water," low in Mg^{2+}, and protection from cardiovascular disease with "hard water," high in Mg^{2+}, with an inverse relation between dietary Mg^{2+} and the level of blood pressure. This reduction in serum or tissue Mg^{2+} might be enough to induce peripheral vasoconstriction and thereby raise blood pressure, although the exact mechanism triggering this change in vascular tone is not known.

The therapeutic value of Mg^{2+} in the treatment of hypertension was suggested as early as 1925, when Mg^{2+} infusions were found to be effective in treating malignant hypertension. Considering the inexpensive nature of the agent and the fact that it is easy to handle, Mg^{2+} is theoretically a useful adjunctive, if not primary, treatment modality for hypertension. However, this has not proven to be the case in most patients, although successful drug therapy of hypertension appears to be associated with elevations in the levels of intracellular free Mg^{2+} in erythrocytes. Ingestion of foodstuffs with a high content of Mg^{2+} may have an effect on blood pressure, although Mg^{2+}-enriched diets also typically contain higher amounts of the vasodepressor cations K^+ and Ca^{2+}. However, Mg^{2+} supplementation has not been found to affect blood pressure in a primary prevention of hypertension study in 698 patients treated for 6 months with 360 mg of Mg^{2+} diglycine.

However, the results of studies in which Mg^{2+} was used to treat hypertension have demonstrated conflicting results with regard to blood pressure reduction. Methodologic issues and heterogeneity of study populations likely explain the inconsistency in treatment results. Nevertheless, Mg^{2+} supplementation may be of benefit more consistently in certain patient subsets, including blacks, obese patients, those with insulin resistance, patients with hypertriglyceridemia, those with severe or malignant forms of hypertension, situations in which Mg^{2+} is supplemented long term, and hypertensive patients receiving thiazide diuretics. Also, in many forms of secondary hypertension and in preeclampsia, Mg^{2+} is effective in reducing blood pressure. Together these data suggest that Mg^{2+} is at best weakly hypotensive. The use of Mg^{2+} supplementation with diuretics, especially thiazide diuretics, is advisable to prevent intracellular Mg^{2+} and K^+ depletion.

Magnesium in Stroke

Magnesium exhibits a range of neuronal and vascular actions that may ameliorate ischemic central nervous system insults, including stroke. Significant neuroprotection with Mg^{2+} has been observed in different models of focal cerebral ischemia, with infarct volume reduction from 25% to 61%. Maximal neuroprotection is evident at readily attainable serum concentrations, and neuroprotection is still seen when administration is delayed up to 6 h and in some cases 24 h after the onset of ischemia. Several small trials have reported a reduced incidence of death or dependence with administration of Mg^{2+}, but confidence intervals are wide, and more definitive data from ongoing large trials are needed before specific recommendations can be made for the use of Mg^{2+} in the victim of acute stroke.

Clinical Use of Magnesium

There is a high incidence of Mg^{2+} deficiency in hospitalized patients, particularly in those with other conditions that may aggravate Mg^{2+} deficiency, such as poor nutrition and multisystem disorders. This is particularly important in patients receiving treatment with a myriad of medications—such as diuretics and aminoglycoside antibiotics—that increase urinary losses of Mg^{2+}.

Difficulty in establishing the diagnosis of Mg^{2+} deficiency is due to the lack of reliable laboratory tests and the minimal or often absent clinical manifestations accompanying this disturbance. When present, clinical manifestations are nonspecific and confined to mental changes or neuromuscular irritability. Tetany, one of the most striking and better known manifestations, is only rarely found; instead, less specific signs such as tremor, muscle twitching, bizarre movements, focal seizures, generalized convulsions, delirium, or coma are more common findings. Magnesium deficiency should be suspected when other electrolyte abnormalities coexist because it tends to cluster with abnormalities such as hypocalcemia and hypokalemia. Electrocardiographic (ECG) changes—such as prolongation of the QT and PR intervals, widening of the QRS complex, ST-segment depression, low T waves, and supraventricular and ventricular tachyarrhythmias—should also raise the index of suspicion for Mg^{2+} deficiency.

Once hypomagnesemia is suspected, the measurement of serum Mg^{2+} concentration continues to be the routine test for detection of hypomagnesemia. Although a low level is helpful and typically indicative of low intracellular stores, normal serum Mg^{2+} values can still be observed in the face of significant body deficiencies of Mg^{2+}; thus, serum Mg^{2+} determinations are an unreliable measure of total body Mg^{2+} balance. Intracellular Mg^{2+} measurements and other technologies are available but remain clinically impractical. A more practical measure of Mg^{2+} balance is the "Mg^{2+} loading test," which is at once therapeutic and diagnostic. This test consists of the parenteral administration of $MgSO_4$ and a time-wise assessment of urinary Mg^{2+} retention, which can be accomplished on an outpatient basis in as short a time as 1 h. Individuals in a state of normal Mg^{2+} balance eliminate at least 75% of an administered load.

This approach is recommended in all patients with a high index of suspicion for hypomagnesemia, particularly in those with ischemic heart disease or cardiac arrhythmias. Repletion of a Mg^{2+} deficit should occur cautiously in anuric individuals and in those with significant renal impairment. In mild deficiency states, Mg^{2+} balance often can be reestablished by simply eliminating the causative factors and allowing the Mg^{2+} content in a normal diet to repair the

TABLE 7-1 Available Forms of Magnesium

Salt	Chemical formula	Molecular weight	Mg (%)	Mg (mEq/g)	Mg (mmol/g)
Sulfate	$MgSO_4 \cdot 7H_2O$	246.5	10	8.1	4
Chloride	$MgCl_2 \cdot 6H_2O$	203.23	12	9.8	4.9
Oxide	MgO	40.3	60	49.6	25
Lactate	$C_6H_{10}MgO_6$	202.45	12	9.8	4.9
Citrate	$C_{12}H_{10}Mg_3O_{14}$	451	16	4.4	2.2
Hydroxide	$Mg(OH)_2$	58.3	42	34	17
Gluconate	$C_{12}H_{22}MGO_{14} \cdot {}_xH_2O$	414.6	5.8	4.8	2.4

deficit. Parenteral Mg^{2+} administration, however, is the most effective way to correct a hypomagnesemic state and should be the route used when replacement is necessary during medical emergencies. Total body deficits of Mg^{2+} in the depleted patient are typically 1 to 2 mEq/kg of body weight. A recommended regimen is 2 g of $MgSO_4$ (16.3 mEq) given intravenously over 30 min, followed by a constant infusion rate providing between 32 and 64 mEq/day until the deficit is presumed corrected. A variety of oral Mg^{2+} salts is available for clinical use (Table 7-1). Magnesium oxide is commonly employed, but this salt form is poorly soluble on a formulation basis, and acts as a cathartic, thereby decreasing absorption. Magnesium gluconate is the preferred salt form for oral therapy because this agent possesses a high degree of solubility and does not cause diarrhea. Magnesium carbonate is poorly soluble and does not appear to be as effective in reversing hypomagnesemia as the gluconate salt. Oral Mg^{2+} is not recommended for therapy during acute situations because the high doses necessary almost always cause significant diarrhea. The intramuscular route for Mg^{2+} administration is a useful but painful means of delivery and should be avoided as long as IV access is available.

Conclusion

Deficiency states or abnormalities in Mg^{2+} metabolism also play important roles in ischemic heart disease, CHF, sudden cardiac death, diabetes mellitus, preeclampsia–eclampsia, and hypertension. How best to use Mg^{2+} in these conditions, individually or collectively, remains to be determined. Of similar importance is the effect of diuretic therapy on Mg^{2+} balance and the difficulty in accurately identifying the presence and degree of a deficiency state. Therefore, presumptive therapy in patients at risk for Mg^{2+} deficiency-related complications should be considered.

POTASSIUM

Potassium (K^+) has a diverse relation to cardiovascular disease, including issues as varied as its dietary intake, such deficiency states as may occur with diuretic therapy, and the consideration of specific K^+ membrane channels, which have an important cardiovascular role. For example, a relation between a high dietary intake of K^+ and a reduced risk of cardiovascular disease has been suggested by animal experiments and clinical investigations. Conversely, diuretic-induced hypokalemia carries with its development an increased cardiovascular risk.

Drugs affecting membrane K^+ channels also have been shown to favorably affect a variety of cardiovascular conditions.

Potassium in Systemic Hypertension

In experimental animals prone to cardiovascular events, high dietary K^+ appears to protect against the development of stroke, cardiac hypertrophy, and/or systemic hypertension.

Observational population studies have shown a direct correlation between arterial blood pressure levels and dietary and/or urinary Na^+:K^+ ratios and an inverse relation with urinary K^+. The urinary Na^+:K^+ is typically more strongly correlated with blood pressure than Na^+ or K^+ excretion alone. The negative relation between K^+ intake and blood pressure is more sharply defined for hypertensives than for normotensives and for those with a family history of hypertension. In particular, hypertension is more strongly associated with lower K^+ intake in black adults than in white adults with similar Na^+ intake.

Potassium has multiple potential vasodepressor effects in humans, which support its use as a blood pressure–lowering agent (Table 7-2). Potassium supplementation in humans has a natriuretic action even in the presence of elevated aldosterone and can decrease cardiac output. Potassium can increase kallikrein and augment nitric oxide production by the endothelium, both factors that could lower blood pressure. Potassium administration also has been shown to attenuate sympathetic activity and to decrease the amount and effect of several vasoactive hormones. Potassium may have a direct systemic vasodilatory action by enhancing Na^+, K^+-ATPase activity and improving the compliance of large arteries. In addition, K^+ intake may have a substantial influence on diurnal patterns of blood pressure responses. An increase in the intake of dietary K^+ converts nocturnal dipping status from non-dipping to dipping in salt-sensitive normotensive adolescent blacks.

In clinical trials, oral K^+ supplementation (as opposed to dietary K^+) has been shown to lower blood pressure in hypertensive patients on a normal or high Na^+ intake. The effect of oral K^+ supplementation on blood pressure is particularly prominent in patients with a low dietary intake of K^+. Similar observations have been made in elderly hypertensive subjects. Fotherby and Potter observed reductions in 24-h blood pressure of 6/3 mm Hg and clinic blood pressure of 10/6 mm Hg after 4 weeks of supplementation with 60 mmol of K^+. In patients on salt-restricted diets, K^+ supplementation is less effective in reducing elevated blood pressure, suggesting that this form of treatment is most effective in the management of salt-sensitive hypertension.

TABLE 7-2 Proposed Mechanisms of Blood Pressure Reduction with Potassium

1. Direct natriuretic effect and conversion of salt-sensitive hypertension to salt-resistant hypertension
2. Increased renal kallikrein and eicosanoid production
3. Increased nitric oxide (increased vasodilatory response to acetylcholine)
4. Attenuation of sympathetic activity
5. Decreased amount and effect of plasma renin activity and blunted rise in plasma renin activity after K^+-related natriuresis
6. Direct arterial effect—enhanced activity of Na^+, K^+-ATPase
7. Enhanced vascular compliance
8. Conversion of nocturnal non-dipping to dipping blood pressure status

Dietary K^+ (60 mEq/day) also has been examined as a blood pressure–lowering supplement in patients already receiving antihypertensive drugs, such as diuretics or beta blockers, thus providing additional effectiveness in reducing blood pressure.

In summary, there is good evidence to suggest that dietary K^+ supplementation can cause a mild reduction in blood pressure, especially in hypertensive patients on high Na^+ diets. It is still not known for how long the blood pressure–lowering effect of K^+ is maintained. In diuretic-treated patients who become hypokalemic, K^+ supplementation can correct the deficiency and at the same time further reduce blood pressure. Rather than recommending K^+ supplements for the entire population of hypertensive patients or, more particularly, for those patients at risk for developing hypertension, biological markers need to be identified that might predict a response to K^+ supplements. A recent Canadian consensus panel offered commentary on aspects of this issue. This panel advised that the daily dietary intake of K^+ should be 60 mmol or greater and that dietary K^+ supplementation above this amount is not indicated as a means of preventing an increase in blood pressure in normotensive subjects.

Potassium in Stroke

A protective effect of K^+ intake on risk of stroke has been recognized for a number of years, dating to the initial report by Khaw and Barrett-Connor. More recently, in the National Health Professionals Study, K^+ intake was shown to relate inversely to the risk of stroke. This finding was further corroborated in a review by Fang and associates of the first National Health and Nutrition Examination Survey (NHANES-I), although the inverse association between K^+ intake and stroke mortality was detected only among black men and hypertensive men in this study. The study by Fang and colleagues examined stroke mortality only and did not adjust for dietary factors that might confound the risk relation between K^+ and stroke—such as dietary intake of fiber, Ca^{2+}, or vitamin C—which may explain its ethnicity- and sex-related findings. With regard to the relation between K^+ intake and stroke, Bazzano and coworkers evaluated data from the NHANES-I Epidemiologic Follow-Up Study and also detected an independent association between low dietary K^+ intake and an increased hazard of stroke. The relation between decreased K^+ intake and stroke occurrence is not mechanistically resolved. It is possible, although not definitively proven, that the reduction in blood pressure that accompanies a high K^+ intake and/or a more primary effect in slowing the atherosclerotic process may contribute to the positive effects of this nutritional factor.

The U.S. Food and Drug Administration has approved a health claim that "diets containing foods that are good sources of K^+ and low in fat may reduce the risk of high blood pressure and stroke."

Potassium in the Prevention of Atherosclerosis

It is currently believed that the development of the atherosclerotic lesion is initiated by the oxidation of low-density lipoproteins within the intimal layer of arteries. Oxidized low-density lipoproteins are then phagocytized by macrophages and monocytes, leading to the development of the lipid-laden foam cell, which is the prototypic cell of atherosclerosis. These foam cells lead to the formation of the fatty streak, the first microscopically visible element of the atherosclerotic plaque. Fatty streaks are of no clinical significance. In fact, many of them disappear spontaneously. However, certain fatty streaks progress into true atherosclerotic, fibrofatty plaques. Then endothelial cell injury occurs, leading to endothelial cell dysfunction. Subsequently, hemodynamic stress or induction of an inflammatory state triggers the release of platelet-derived growth factor from platelets or macrophages, which determines the transition of a fatty streak to a fibrous plaque. Ultimately, the transformation, proliferation, and migration of subintimal smooth muscle cells lead to the development of the atherosclerotic lesion, with its well-described consequences.

Recent data have suggested that the protective effect of K^+ on the atherosclerotic process may relate to its effect on the function of those cells involved in lesion formation, as described above. Increases in K^+ have been shown in vitro to inhibit the formation of free radicals from vascular endothelial cells and macrophages. This inhibitory effect on free radical formation could lead to a significant reduction in lesion formation in individuals with a high K^+ intake. Indeed, studies in animals have demonstrated reduced cholesterol content in the aorta of rats given large amounts of K^+. In addition to its effect on free radical formation, elevation of K^+ has been shown to inhibit proliferation of vascular smooth muscle cells and to inhibit platelet aggregation and arterial thrombosis. Thus, through a variety of mechanisms, elevations in K^+ could, at least theoretically, slow the initiation and progression of the atherosclerotic lesion and the occurrence of thrombosis in the atherosclerotic vessel wall. By these actions, small elevations of K^+ related to high levels of dietary intake could account for the apparent protection against cardiovascular diseases of atherosclerotic origin observed in primitive cultures with diets rich in K^+ and low in Na^+.

Electrophysiologic Effects

Hypokalemia

Hypokalemia reduces the rate of repolarization of the cardiac cell, leading to a prolongation of the recovery time. In addition, hypokalemia causes the slope of phase 3 of the transmembrane action potential to become less steep. As a result, there is an increase in the interval during which the difference between the transmembrane potential and the threshold potential is small. Consequently, the period of increased excitability is prolonged and the appearance of ectopic atrial and/or ventricular beats is facilitated. A decrease in the extracellular K^+ concentration increases the difference in K^+ concentration across the cell membrane and tends to hyperpolarize the cell during diastole.

Electrocardiographically, hypokalemia produces a flattening or inversion of the T wave, with concomitant prominence of the U wave. This generally occurs without any significant change in the QT interval. Although, if the T wave fuses with the U wave, the QT interval may prove difficult to measure. When hypokalemia is severe, the QRS complex may widen slightly in a diffuse manner. The ECG pattern of hypokalemia is not specific, and a similar pattern may be seen after the administration of digitalis, antiarrhythmic agents, or phenothiazines or in patients with ventricular hypertrophy or bradycardia.

Potassium Supplementation

General Considerations

Potassium may be administered for multiple reasons. First, in diuretic-treated patients, it is given to replace a total body deficit, which may be as much as 300 to 400 mEq. Such replacement may be followed by a lower rate of cardiovascular events, as has been observed in a wide-range of diuretic-treated patients. Second, K^+ may be given in a temporizing fashion to patients with hypokalemia attributable to transcellular shifts of K^+, in whom there is no total body deficit but a perceived need to treat a low serum K^+ value. This is not uncommonly the case in patients with high endogenous levels of catecholamines and, in particular, the β_2 agonist epinephrine or in those receiving β_2 agonists, such as asthmatics or post-code patients. In addition, subjects with salt-sensitive hypertension may see a beneficial response to K^+ supplementation. Further, dietary K^+ may be as effective as supplementation, although the data in this regard are not as abundant. Some investigators have proposed that the small elevations of serum K^+ concentration related to high levels of dietary K^+ intake might be enough to inhibit free radical formation, smooth muscle proliferation, and thrombus formation. In this way, the rate of progression to atherosclerotic lesions may be slowed and thrombosis in atherosclerotic vessels diminished.

The issues surrounding K^+ replacement in clinical practice have recently been carefully articulated.

Oral Therapy

If a patient consumes a diet that is deficient in K^+-rich foods (i.e., fruits and vegetables), dietary alterations may be sufficient to correct hypokalemia. Such dietary modifications can provide 40 to 60 mEq/day of K^+, although generally in the form of K^+ citrate or acetate, which is somewhat less effective than K^+ chloride in correcting diuretic-induced hypokalemia. Salt substitutes provide another economical alternative to prescription K^+ supplements, although their bitter taste may dissuade patients from continuous use. They contain 7 to 14 mEq K^+/g (5 g equals approximately 1 teaspoon). Potassium supplements are usually given as K^+ chloride, available in liquid or tablet formulations, although there are other forms (Table 7-3). The most common side effect of K^+ supplements is gastric irritation. The non–chloride-containing K^+ supplements provide an alternative for those unable to tolerate the K^+ chloride preparations or in whom K^+ depletion occurs in the setting of metabolic acidosis. Because severe hyperkalemia can occur as a consequence of oral supplementation, serum K^+ levels should always be monitored during therapy. This is particularly relevant to the patient also receiving angiotensin-converting enzyme inhibitors, angiotensin receptor blockers, or spironolactone.

Intravenous Therapy

Potassium can be administered intravenously in patients with severe hypokalemia and in those unable to tolerate oral preparations. A detailed discussion of the approximation of a K^+ deficit is beyond the scope of this chapter, although in the absence of an independent factor causing transcellular K^+ shifts, the magnitude of the deficit in body stores of K^+ correlates with the degree of hypokalemia. However, in the absence of ECG changes and with a K^+ level greater than 2.5 mEq/L, K^+ can generally be safely administered at a rate of up to 10 mEq/h in concentrations as high as 200 mEq/L. However, higher concentrations (200 mEq/L) and faster rates of delivery (20 mEq/h) have been shown to be well tolerated. Maximum daily administration should rarely exceed 100 to 200 mEq. If the serum K^+ level is under 2 mEq/L and is associated with ECG changes or neuromuscular symptoms, K^+ can be administered intravenously at a rate of 40 mEq/h and at concentrations as high as 200 mEq/L. This should be accompanied by continuous ECG monitoring and measurement of serum K^+ levels every several hours. In cases of life-

TABLE 7-3 Oral Potassium Formulations*

Supplements	Attributes
Controlled-release microencapsulated	Disintegrate better in the stomach than encapsulated tablets microparticles; less adherent and less cohesive
Encapsulated controlled-release microencapsulated particles	Fewer erosions than with wax matrix tablets
K+ chloride elixir	Inexpensive, tastes bad, poor compliance; few erosions, immediate effect
K+ chloride (effervescent tablets) for solution	Convenient, more expensive than elixir, immediate effect
Wax-matrix extended-release tablets	Easier to swallow, more gastrointestinal tract erosions than with micro-encapsulated formulations

*Other K+ formulations: K+ gluconate, K+ citrate, K+ acetate, and K+ carbonate, for use in hyperchloremia and hypokalemia. All K+ formulations are readily absorbed.
Source: Adapted with permission from Cohn JN, Kowey PR, Whelton PK, Prisant LM: New guidelines for potassium replacement in clinical practice: A contemporary review by the National Council on Potassium in Clinical Practice. *Arch Intern Med* 160:2429, 2000.

threatening hypokalemia, K+ should be given initially in glucose-free solutions because glucose may further lower K+.

Conclusion

Potassium has traditionally been used as a replacement in hypokalemia related to systemic illness and drug use. Magnesium often must be given with K+ to successfully correct hypokalemia. Recent evidence is mounting that K+ could be used to prevent or treat a range of cardiovascular diseases, such as hypertension and atherosclerosis, with favorable effects on morbidity and mortality.

CALCIUM

Abnormalities in Ca^{2+} homeostasis, like those in Mg^{2+} and K+, appear to play important roles in the pathogenesis of cardiovascular disease.

Cardiovascular Effects of Calcium

Calcium in Systemic Hypertension

Calcium metabolism is linked closely to the regulation of systemic blood pressure, and Ca^{2+} supplementation has been proposed as a treatment for systemic hypertension, even though data on the association between dietary Ca^{2+} intake and blood pressure have been inconsistent. Increased cytosolic concentrations of free Ca^{2+} within vascular smooth muscle cells are thought to be responsible for the increased contractility of vessels characteristic of hypertension. In animal models, acute intracellular Ca^{2+} overload of vascular smooth muscle cells can spark hypercontractility. Hypertension can then develop if a general increase in systemic arteriolar tone ushers in a rise in peripheral resistance. Further, with progressive elevation of intracellular

Ca^{2+}, the structural integrity of arterial and arteriolar walls is compromised. Thus, in various animal models, Ca^{2+} overload initiates lesions of an arteriosclerotic character. The increased concentrations of free Ca^{2+} within vascular smooth muscle cells could be secondary to alterations in Ca^{2+} entry, binding, or extrusion from the cells. Studies on human cells have shown changes related to all three of these potential mechanisms.

Beyond the probability that an increased intracellular Ca^{2+} is involved in the pathogenesis of hypertension, there are other recognized relations between Ca^{2+} and hypertension. These include the relation between serum Ca^{2+} levels and blood pressure, the effect of dietary and supplemental Ca^{2+} on blood pressure, obesity, and the renal excretion of Ca^{2+} or endogenous parathyroid hormone (PTH) in patients with hypertension.

Serum Calcium and Hypertension

Hypertension is more common in the presence of hypercalcemia and, in many but not all studies, there appears to be a direct relation between the total serum Ca^{2+} level and blood pressure. However, the relation between serum ionized Ca^{2+} and blood pressure does not appear to be as strong. Nevertheless, there are sufficient data to suggest a vasoconstrictive effect of increasing extracellular Ca^{2+} levels, presumably by a stimulation of catecholamine release or a direct vascular effect.

Increased Renal Excretion of Calcium

Compared with normotensive subjects, hypertensive individuals excrete more Ca^{2+} under basal circumstances and during Na^+ loading. This may be due to the increase in Ca^{2+} excretion known to occur after intravascular volume expansion, with the resultant rise in Na^+ excretion. Alternatively, it may be secondary to a decreased binding of Ca^{2+} to kidney cells. Whatever the precise mechanism, patients with volume-expanded forms of hypertension excrete Ca^{2+} in excess.

Increased Levels of Parathyroid Hormone

Hypertensive patients tend to have increased levels of plasma PTH, most likely as a homeostatic response to their urinary Ca^{2+} leak. Although not nearly as high as those seen with primary hyperparathyroidism, these elevated PTH levels could exert a pressor effect and thereby cause or contribute to hypertension, a finding that is particularly prominent in women.

Observational Studies and Clinical Trials with Calcium Supplements

There have been more than 30 reports on observational studies of Ca^{2+} and hypertension, with most demonstrating an inverse relation between dietary Ca^{2+} intake and the level of blood pressure. However, clinical trials of Ca^{2+} supplementation (1 to 2 g/day for up to 4 years) have been less consistent in this regard, with only approximately two-thirds of such studies demonstrating any beneficial effect of supplemental Ca^{2+} on blood pressure. The rationale for supplemental Ca^{2+} therapy is based on the assumption that PTH levels are elevated in response to low levels of ionized Ca^{2+} resulting from the hypercalciuria seen in some forms of volume-expanded hypertension. Additional Ca^{2+}, by raising plasma calcium, would tend to suppress PTH and thereby lower blood pressure. Indeed, in selected populations of hypertensives characterized by increased urinary Ca^{2+} excretion, low ionized Ca^{2+}, or increased PTH levels, Ca^{2+} supplements often have caused a significant fall in blood pressure. In addition, increased Ca^{2+} intake acts to increase Na^+ excretion in the urine and may lower blood pressure by this mechanism. However, in unselected populations of hypertensives, most clinical studies have shown little or no effect of Ca^{2+} supplementation on blood pressure. Further, even those patients with lower serum Ca^{2+} and higher PTH levels, who may benefit from calcium supplementation, may do so with the potential risk of developing kidney stones in a dose-dependent manner, although the risk of calcium oxalate stone formation does not increase significantly in postmenopausal women with osteoporosis given calcium carbonate. In contrast, studies in pregnant women have shown that Ca^{2+} supplementation can provide important reductions in systolic and diastolic blood pressures and can reduce their risk of developing preeclampsia.

In summary, based on the available data, Ca^{2+} supplementation or an increased intake of Ca^{2+} through enriched foods cannot be recommended as a treatment for the general hypertensive population or for the prevention of hypertension. Individual patients, such as pregnant women, may benefit from this approach, but there are currently no screening methods for identifying those patients in the general population who would benefit from Ca^{2+} supplementation.

Calcium and Myocardial Contractility

Calcium is of fundamental importance to the process of myocardial contraction. The initial event is activation of Na^+ channels resulting in rapid Na^+ influx and membrane depolarization. As a consequence, voltage-gated, dihydropyridine-sensitive sarcolemmal Ca^{2+} channels are opened, allowing an influx of Ca^{2+} into the myocyte. There is a close proximity between sarcolemmal Ca^{2+} channels and Ca^{2+} channels of the sarcoplasmic reticulum, which is pertinent because Ca^{2+} then stimulates the junctional sarcoplasmic reticulum to release Ca^{2+} via a tryanodine-sensitive Ca^{2+}-release channel. The sum of the released Ca^{2+} represents a substantial increase in the free intracellular Ca^{2+}, which then diffuses into the myofibrils to combine with troponin. Troponin, in its Ca^{2+}-free state, inhibits the interaction of myosin and actin. With the rise in intracellular Ca^{2+}, troponin is bound to Ca^{2+}, and this inhibition disappears. Actin then combines with myosin, leading to the split of ATP by a Ca^{2+}-dependent ATPase. The energy that is released from this process is then transformed into mechanical work leading to the interaction of actin and myosin filaments and the resultant shortening of myofibrils.

Recently, there has been much interest in the cellular abnormalities of Ca^{2+} homeostasis in the failing human heart. Studies of animal models and myocardia from patients with heart failure have demonstrated abnormalities of cytosolic Ca^{2+} handling, myofilament Ca^{2+} sensitivity, and myocyte energetics. Many of these metabolic abnormalities have been shown to be the result of alterations in the activity or number of myocyte enzymes and transport channels that are important in excitation and contraction coupling. Although a great deal of research work remains to be done in this area, it is becoming evident that cardiac dysfunction is intimately associated with Ca^{2+} handling abnormalities in cardiac cells. A discussion of agents used to increase Ca^{2+} at the myosin–actin interaction sites and Ca^{2+} sensitivity at those sites for the treatment of CHF is provided in Chapter 8. Calcium supplementation itself has been poorly studied as a possible treatment for CHF.

Calcium Use in Cardiac Arrest

Calcium plays an essential role in excitation and contraction coupling, and for many years intravenous calcium chloride was administered in cardiac resuscitation efforts in patients with bradyasystolic arrest. It is no longer used for this indication because no survival benefit was observed, and there is evidence that Ca^{2+} may induce cerebral vasospasm and affect the extent of reperfusion injury in the heart and brain.

Calcium Use in Arrhythmia

Intravenous Ca^{2+} can slow the heart rate and has been used to treat tachycardias. The drug must be used cautiously in patients receiving digoxin because it can precipitate digitalis toxicity and ventricular arrhythmias related to after-depolarization. After-depolarizations are membrane potential voltage oscillations that are dependent on a preceding action potential. There are two types of after-depolarizations. Early after-depolarizations occur during phase 2 or 3 of the action potential, whereas delayed after-depolarizations (DADs) occur after the resting membrane potential has been reestablished (phase 4). DADs have been shown in vitro to occur in the setting of digitalis toxicity, catecholamine excess, hypertrophied myocardium, and Purkinje cells after myocardial infarction. DADs appear to result from the oscillatory release of Ca^{2+} ions from sarcoplasmic reticulum during conditions of Ca^{2+} overload. The clinical significance of DADs and triggered activity is not completely clear, but this mechanism has been etiologically invoked to explain at least some ventricular arrhythmias. Although much remains to be learned, it seems likely that DADs will emerge as an important mechanism of human arrhythmia.

Decreases in extracellular Ca^{2+} concentration can increase the action potential duration resulting from an increase in duration and a decrease in amplitude of phase 2 of the cardiac action potential. Hypocalcemia may cause a clinically insignificant decrease in the QRS duration; cardiac arrhythmias are uncommon. Intravenous calcium has been used to treat intoxications from Ca^{2+}-channel blockers (see Chapter 4) complicated by bradyarrhythmia and hypotension.

Clinical Use of Calcium

A number of Ca^{2+} salts are available (Table 7-4). Each has a different amount of elemental Ca^{2+} per administered gram. These supplements are generally administered in conjunction with meals two to three times daily. The solubilities of the various Ca^{2+} salts differ. For example, calcium carbonate, although attractive as a therapy because it is 40% elemental Ca^{2+} by weight, is poorly absorbed, which limits its utility. In contrast, Ca^{2+} citrate and glubionate tend to be better absorbed.

In cases in which hypocalcemia persists despite adequate Ca^{2+} supplementation, a vitamin D supplement may be required to enhance Ca^{2+} absorption. Intravenous Ca^{2+} is available as several different salts including calcium chloride (27.2 mg/mL), Ca^{2+} gluceptate (18 mg/mL), and Ca^{2+} gluconate (9 mg/mL). Calcium chloride is the preferred formulation because it produces more predictable levels of ionized Ca^{2+} in plasma, although it can be quite venotoxic and should be used carefully whenever adequate vascular access is in question.

Conclusion

Except for specific situations, such as calcium entry blocker overdose, pregnancy, and hypocalcemia, treatment with Ca^{2+} is not recommended for the

TABLE 7-4 Available Forms of Calcium

Calcium salt	Calcium (%)	Calcium (mEq/g)
Calcium acetate	25	12.5
Calcium carbonate	40	20
Calcium citrate	21	10.5
Calcium glubionate	6.5	3.3
Calcium gluconate	9	4.5
Calcium lactate	13	6.5
Calcium phosphate, dibasic	23	11.5
Calcium phosphate, tribasic	39	19.5

prevention and treatment of cardiovascular disease. Dietary Ca^{2+}, however, should be maintained for the purpose of general health maintenance.

ADDITIONAL READINGS

Akita S, Sacks FM, Svetkey LP, et al: Effects of the dietary approaches to stop hypertension (DASH) diet on the pressure-natriuresis relationship. *Hypertension* 42:8, 2003.

Al-Delaimy WK, Rimm E, Willett WC, et al: A prospective study of calcium intake from diet and supplements and risk of ischemic heart disease among men. *Am J Clin Nutr* 88:814, 2003.

Altura BM, Altura BT: Role of magnesium in the pathogenesis of hypertension updated: Relationship to its actions on cardiac, vascular smooth muscle, and endothelial cells, in Laragh JN, Brenner BM (eds): *Hypertension: Pathophysiology, Diagnosis and Management*. New York, Raven Press, 1995, p 1213.

Bazzano LA, he J, Ogden LG, et al: Dietary potassium intake and risk of stroke in US men and women. National Health and Nutrition Examination Survey I Epidemiologic Follow-Up Study. *Stroke* 32:1473, 2001.

Booth JV, Phillips-Bute B, McCants CB, et al: Low serum magnesium level predicts major adverse cardiac events after coronary artery bypass graft surgery. *Am Heart J* 145:1108, 2003.

Cermuzynski L, Gebalska J, Wolk R, Makowska E: Hypomagnesemia in heart failure with ventricular arrhythmias. Beneficial effects of magnesium supplementation. *J Intern Med* 247:78, 2000.

Cohen HW, Madhavan S, Alderman MH: High and low serum potassium associated with cardiovascular events in diuretic-treated patients. *J Hypertens* 19:1315, 2001.

Cohn JN, Kowey PR, Whelton PK, Prisant LM: New guidelines for potassium replacement in clinical practice: A contemporary review by the National Council on Potassium in Clinical Practice. *Arch Intern Med* 160:2429, 2000.

Franse LV, Pahor M, DiBari M, et al: Hypokalemia associated with diuretic use and cardiovascular events in the Systolic Hypertension in the Elderly Program. *Hypertension* 35:1025, 2000.

Hajjar IM, Grim CE, Kotchen TA: Dietary calcium lowers the age-related rise in blood pressure in the United States: The NHANES III Survey. *J Clin Hypertens* 5:122, 2003.

Harlan WR, Harlan LC: Blood pressure and calcium and magnesium intake, in Laragh JH, Brenner BM (eds): *Hypertension: Pathophysiology, Diagnosis and Management*. New York, Raven Press, 1995, p 1143.

Hatton DC, Young EW, Bukoski RD, McCarron DA: Calcium metabolism in experimental genetic hypertension, in Laragh JH, Brenner BM (eds): *Hypertension: Pathophysiology, Diagnosis and Management*, 2nd ed. New York, Raven Press, 1995, p 1193.

ISIS-4: A randomized factorial trial assessing early oral captopril, oral mononitrate, and intravenous magnesium sulphate in 58,050 patients with suspected acute myocardial infarction. ISIS-4 (Fourth International Study of Infarct Survival) Collaborative Group. *Lancet* 345:669, 1995.

Jorde R, Sundsfjord J, Haug E, Bønaa KH: Relation between low calcium intake, parathyroid hormone, and blood pressure. *Hypertension* 35:1154, 2000.

Kelsch T, Kikuchi K, Vahdat S, Frishman WH: Innovative pharmacologic approaches to cardiopulmonary resuscitation. *Heart Dis* 3:46, 2001.

Laurant P, Touyz RM: Physiological and pathophysiological role of magnesium in the cardiovascular system: Implications in hypertension. *J Hypertens* 18:1177, 2000.

Magnesium in Coronaries (MAGIC) Trial Investigators: Early administration of intravenous magnesium to high-risk patients with acute myocardial infarction in the Magnesium in Coronaries (MAGIC) Trial: A randomised controlled trial. *Lancet* 360:1189, 2002.

Moore TJ, Conlin PR, Ard J, Svetkey LP: DASH (dietary approaches to stop hypertension) diet is effective treatment for stage 1 isolated systolic hypertension. *Hypertension* 38:155, 2001.

Morris RC Jr, Sebastian A: Potassium-responsive hypertension, in Laragh JH, Brenner BM (eds): *Hypertension: Pathophysiology, Diagnosis and Management,* 2nd ed. New York, Raven Press, 1995, p 2715.

Oparil S: Diet-micronutrients—Special foods, in Oparil S, Weber M (eds): *Hypertension: A Companion to the Kidney.* Philadelphia, Saunders, 2000, p 433.

Rardon DP, Fisch C: Electrolytes and the heart, in Schlant RC, Alexander RW (eds): *Hurst's the Heart,* 8th ed. New York, McGraw-Hill, 1994, p 768.

Ryan TJ, Antman EM, Brooks NH, et al: ACC/AHA guidelines for the management of patients with acute myocardial infarction. A report of the American College of Cardiology/American Heart Association Task Force on Practice Guidelines (Committee on Management of Acute Myocardial Infarction). *Circulation* 100:1016, 1999.

Sacks FM, Svetkey LP, Vollmer WM, et al: Effects on blood pressure of reduced dietary sodium and the Dietary Approaches to Stop Hypertension (DASH) diet. DASH-Sodium Collaborative Research Group. *N Engl J Med* 344:3, 2001.

Shechter M, Bairey Merz CN, Stuehlinger HG, et al: Effects of oral magnesium therapy on exercise tolerance, exercise-induced chest pain, and quality of life in patients with coronary artery disease. *Am J Cardiol* 91:517, 2003.

Shechter M, Sharir M, Labrador MJ, et al: Oral magnesium therapy improves endothelial function in patients with coronary artery disease. *Circulation* 102:2353, 2000.

Siani A, Strazzullo P: Relevance of dietary potassium intake to antihypertensive drug treatment, in Laragh JH, Brenner BM (eds): *Hypertension: Pathophysiology, Diagnosis and Management,* 2nd ed. New York, Raven Press, 1995, p 2727.

Sica DA, Frishman WH, Cavusoglu E: Magnesium, potassium, and calcium as potential cardiovascular disease therapies, in Frishman WH, Sonnenblick EH, Sica DA (eds): *Cardiovascular Pharmacotherapeutics,* 2nd ed. New York, McGraw-Hill 2003, p 177.

Sica DA, Struthers AD, Cushman WC, et al: Importance of potassium in cardiovascular disease. *J Clin Hypertens* (Greenwich) 4:1, 2002.

Svetkey LP, Simons-Morton D, Vollmer WM, et al: Effects of dietary patterns on blood pressure: Subgroup analysis of the Dietary Approaches to Stop Hypertension (DASH) randomized clinical trial. *Arch Intern Med* 159:285, 1999.

Tobian L: The protective effects of high-potassium diets in hypertension, and the mechanisms by which high-NaCl diets produce hypertension—A personal view, in Laragh JH, Brenner BM (eds): *Hypertension: Pathophysiology, Diagnosis and Management,* 2nd ed. New York, Raven Press, 1995, p 299.

Whelton PK, He J, Cutler JA, et al: Effects of oral potassium on blood pressure. Meta-analysis of randomized controlled clinical trials. *JAMA* 277:1624, 1997.

Woods KL, Abrams K: The importance of effect mechanism in the design and interpretation of clinical trials: The role magnesium in acute myocardial infarction. *Prog Cardiovasc Dis* 44:267, 2002.

Woods KL, Fletcher S: Long-term outcome after intravenous magnesium sulphate in suspected acute myocardial infarction: The second Leicester Intravenous Magnesium Intervention Trial (LIMIT-2). *Lancet* 343:816, 1994.

Ziegelstein RC, Hilbe JM, French WJ, et al: Magnesium use in the treatment of acute myocardial infarction in the United States (observations from the Second National Registry of Myocardial Infarction). *Am J Cardiol* 87:7, 2001.

8 | Inotropic Agents

Edmund H. Sonnenblick   Thierry H. LeJemtel
William H. Frishman

DIGITALIS GLYCOSIDES

Digitalis glycosides have had a long and venerable history in the treatment of congestive heart failure (CHF). In 1785, William Withering reported on his use of the digitalis leaf as a purported diuretic agent to treat anasarca, presumably due to CHF (see Chapter 6). Indeed, the major effects of digitalis were thought to be on the kidneys, although important effects on heart rate were noted. Only in the latter part of the 19th century did it become apparent that there was a direct action of digitalis glycosides to increase cardiac contractility; in the earlier part of the 20th century, its effects on the peripheral circulation and the autonomic nervous system were noted.

Pharmacologic Action

Digitalis glycosides have important effects on multiple systems in addition to augmenting myocardial contractility. Electrophysiologically, digitalis glycosides speed conduction in the atrium and inhibit conduction through the atrioventricular (AV) node. In the normal circulation, digitalis glycosides also produce generalized arteriolar vasoconstriction; they also affect the central nervous system by enhancing parasympathetic and reducing sympathetic nervous system activation. Digitalis sensitizes baroreflexes to decrease efferent sympathetic activity, which acts to reduce sinus node activity and thus reduce heart rate. The increase in baroreflex sensitization also increases parasympathetic tone, and central vagal nuclei are also stimulated. The broad enhancement of parasympathetic activity with digitalis glycosides contributes to slow the heart rate and to control supraventricular arrhythmias. As discussed below, in the failing state, the effects of sympathetic withdrawal may be dominant, so as to reduce arterial vascular resistance, whereas in the normal circulation, arterial vasoconstriction may be dominant. Integration of these various actions adds to the inotropic activity of digitalis glycosides and their therapeutic usefulness.

The action of digitalis glycosides to increase contractility and alter the electrophysiology of heart muscle occurs through inhibition of the enzyme Na^+, K^+-ATPase on the surface membrane of myocardial cells, which results in an increase in the amount of Ca^{2+} to activate contraction. The Na^+, K^+-ATPase is an energy-requiring "sodium pump" that extrudes three Na^+ ions that enter the cell during depolarization in exchange for two potassium ions, thus creating an electrical current and a negative resting potential. Contraction is brought about by an action potential that depolarizes the surface membrane of the cell. This action potential is created by a rapid inward current of Na^+ into the cell that opens Ca^{2+} channels, thereby permitting Ca^{2+} to enter the cell. This in turn releases substantially more Ca^{2+} from stores in the sarcoplasmic reticulum within the cell and thereby activates the contractile mechanism by binding to a component of the troponin-tropomyosin system, which had been maintaining the resting state. With Ca^{2+} bound to troponin, actin and myosin can interact to produce force and shortening. The greater the amount of activating Ca^{2+}, the greater the force and shortening. When Ca^{2+} is released from troponin and taken up by the sarcoplasmic reticulum, relaxation occurs. The relatively small amount of Ca^{2+} that enters the cell with activation is ultimately removed by an electrogenic Na^+–Ca^{2+} exchange that extrudes one Ca^{2+} ion for three Na^+ ions. When intracellular Na^+ is increased, less exchange occurs, and the net amount of intracellular Ca^{2+} is increased. Thus, by inhibiting the Na^+, K^+-ATPase, digitalis glycosides produce a decrease in intracellular K^+ and an increase in intracellular Na^+, which increases intracellular Ca^{2+}.

In general, the main pathway by which all inotropic agents, including digitalis glycosides, increase contractility is by increasing the amount of Ca^{2+} available for activation. This is the case in normal and failing myocardia. In the failing heart, there appears to be a decrease in the Ca^{2+} released into the cytosol with activation. The inotropic effects of digitalis glycosides are apparently due to an increase in intracellular Ca^{2+} that augments Ca^{2+} stores in the sarcoplasmic reticulum, resulting in a subsequent increase in the extent of myocyte activation.

The electrophysiologic actions of digitalis glycosides are complex because they are intimately related to autonomic actions, K^+ effects, and the type of cardiac tissue affected. In pacemaker cells in the atria, there is little effect except for increased automaticity at toxic levels. In the sinoatrial node and AV conduction system, the refractory period is prolonged. At toxic levels, conduction block can be produced through decreasing resting potential, which results in slowed conduction. At toxic levels of glycoside, the Purkinje system may become autonomous due to decreased resting potentials. These effects are magnified by decreased extracellular K^+, so that toxicity is enhanced by a low serum K^+ and reduced by an increased K^+.

At therapeutic levels, the effects of digitalis glycosides reflect the direct electrophysiologic actions of the drug and the indirect actions of neurohormonal stimuli. In the atria, increased parasympathetic tone decreases the refractory period, which overrides the direct digitalis effect to prolong the refractory period. Increased parasympathetic stimulation may reduce automaticity through hyperpolarization of pacemaker cells, and sinus node activity, which is not affected directly by digitalis, is reduced through increased parasympathetic and decreased sympathetic tone.

Toxic levels of digitalis glycosides tend to exaggerate the parasympathetic augmentation, which may actually lead to atrial arrhythmias. Sympathetic activity may increase at toxic levels, which, added to the direct actions of digitalis glycosides, can potentially result in life-threatening ventricular tachyarrhythmias.

In addition to effects on heart muscle to increase contractility and on vascular smooth muscle to increase contraction, digitalis glycosides exert significant actions on the autonomic nervous system, and these effects may provide a major part of purported beneficial actions. These effects include stimulation and inhibition and may vary with dose of drug and underlying state of disease. In addition, short- and long-term effects may differ and alter ultimate efficacy. Relatively low doses of digitalis glycosides increase parasympathetic tone through apparent increased sensitivity of the efferent limb of ventricular and arterial baroreceptors. Increased sensitivity of arterial baroreceptors enhances efferent parasympathetic activity and leads to withdrawal of reflex sympathetic tone, resulting in sinus bradycardia and arterial and venous dilatations. This indirect effect is opposite to the direct effect of glycosides to produce smooth muscle vasoconstriction. Added effects of this sympathetic withdrawal include increased renal blood flow, renin release inhibition, and decreased antidiuretic hormone release. Release of acetylcholine by vagal fibers is also thought to inhibit norepinephrine release from nerve endings and to reduce β-receptor responses.

The overall effects of digitalis glycoside in the healthy individual are the result of the sum of its actions on the heart, the circulation, and the central nervous system, so that it is difficult to differentiate direct from indirect effects of glycosides in many instances. Digitalis glycosides increase myocardial contractility directly in the normal and failing heart, although the effects are relatively greater in the latter situation. However, hemodynamic results differ. In the absence of CHF, where sympathetic and parasympathetic tones are minimal, digitalis glycosides increase peripheral arterial resistance directly, with a concomitant modest increase in arterial pressure accompanied by a shift in blood volume to the splanchnic bed, with a decline in venous return and cardiac output. In contrast, with CHF, with withdrawal of elevated sympathetic nerve activity and increased parasympathetic tone, a fall in peripheral arterial resistance occurs with an increase in cardiac output. In terms of the heart, a decrease in ventricular filling pressure also occurs and stroke volume increases. These effects are increased by enhancing parasympathetic tone in the failing circulation, which may mimic some of the beneficial effects of beta blockers and unloading agents, as noted elsewhere.

Whether the effects of digitalis glycosides are always beneficial, and if so, at what dose, remains controversial. Studies in the elderly and in patients with myocardial infarction have demonstrated an increased threat of digitalis toxicity without careful monitoring. However, in the presence of severe failure [New York Heart Association (NYHA) class III], withdrawal of digoxin has resulted in substantial and rapid clinical deterioration despite concomitant therapy, including angiotensin-converting enzyme (ACE) inhibitors and diuretics. When used in mild CHF, digitalis glycosides increase ejection fraction, whereas ACE inhibitors are largely effective only in increasing exercise performance. These beneficial effects are observed whether the patients are in atrial fibrillation or in sinus rhythm. The placebo-controlled multicenter Digitalis Investigation Group study, comprising more than 7000 patients with CHF, showed that digoxin does not affect mortality but reduces hospitalization for heart failure when compared with control. Digoxin therapy was also shown to improve ventricular function and patients' symptoms.

Digitalis Preparations: Structure, Pharmacokinetics, and Metabolism

All cardiac glycosides contain a ring structure termed an *aglycone*, to which are attached up to four sugar molecules at the C3 position. The aglycone itself is formed by a steroid nucleus to which a β-unsaturated lactone ring is attached at the C17 position. Hydroxyl groups are generally found at C3 and C14, whereas a glucose moiety is generally attached through the C3 hydroxyl group. At present, digoxin and digitoxin are the glycosides that are used clinically; they differ structurally only by the presence in digoxin of a hydroxyl group in the C12 position. Cardiac activity, which correlates with the binding of drug to Na^+, K^+-ATPase on the cell surface sarcolemma, depends on the unsaturated lactone ring, the hydroxyl at C14, and a cis configuration in C8 to C17 in the aglycone ring. As the number of sugars on C3 is reduced, water solubility increases, and hepatic metabolism rather than renal excretion is favored. Thus, digoxin is excreted primarily by the kidneys while digitoxin is metabolized in the liver. Digitoxin is 90% bioavailable, as compared with 60% for digoxin. A major difference between these agents is that digoxin is 25% protein bound, whereas digitoxin is 93% bound; hence, the half-life of digoxin is 1.7 days and that of digitoxin is quite long at 7.0 days.

At present, digoxin and digitoxin are the only glycosides readily available in the United States, and digoxin is used in most instances. Digoxin has an onset of action from 30 min to 2 h when given orally and from 5 to 30 min when given intravenously. Peak action occurs in 6 to 8 h when given orally and in 1 to 4 h when given intravenously. The plasma half-life of digoxin is 32 to 48 h, and 50% to 70% is renally cleared as an intact molecule. Renal impairment may delay excretion of digoxin, which may lead to its accumulation and the development of toxicity. Digitoxin has a much longer half-life of several days and is metabolized largely by the liver.

Clinical Use

A loading dose for digoxin and for digitoxin is necessary to reach a steady state rapidly, although with digoxin this is attained in 5 to 7 days with only a maintenance dose. Although intravenous digoxin is available, the oral dosage is generally adequate except in urgent settings. The average loading dose of digoxin is 1.0 to 1.5 mg given in divided doses over 24 h, with a maintenance dose of 0.125 to 0.25 mg/day. These doses are commonly halved in the elderly or in patients with renal insufficiency. The maintenance dose commonly needs adjustment to regulate resting heart rate in atrial fibrillation (between 55 and 70 beats/min). In sinus rhythm, the dose is more uncertain, and a desired serum level near 1.0 ng/mL should be sought.

The beneficial effects of augmented parasympathetic tone and sympathetic withdrawal may be obtained with relatively small doses of digitalis without encountering the potential for toxicity. Thus, the issue of dosage of digoxin remains unsettled relative to the benefit sought.

Digitoxin requires a loading dose because steady state on maintenance dosing is attained only after several weeks. The loading dose is about 1.0 mg in divided doses, with maintenance of 0.1 to 0.15 mg/day. The advantage of digitoxin is its hepatic excretion in the presence of renal insufficiency and the lessened impact of poor patient compliance due to its much longer duration of action. Its disadvantage is the long time required for washout should toxicity occur or be suspected.

The serum level of digoxin can be affected by several other drugs. Cholestyramine, kaolin-pectin, neomycin, and bran can decrease digoxin absorption. Erythromycin, omeprazole, and tetracycline can increase digoxin absorption. Thyroxine can increase the volume of distribution of digoxin and enhance renal clearance. Quinidine increases serum digoxin levels, doubling levels in most patients over 1 to 2 days. The mechanism remains unclear, but if digoxin intake is not reduced, toxicity can occur. Verapamil reduces renal excretion and can increase serum digoxin levels by as much as 50% over a period of time. Amiodarone and propafenone appear to have a similar effect. With concurrent verapamil, amiodarone, and propafenone use, digoxin doses should be halved. Other antiarrhythmic agents do not exhibit interactions with digoxin.

Thiazides and loop diuretics may lead to K^+ depletion, which augments myocardial sensitivity to digitalis glycosides and leads to arrhythmias, often requiring oral K^+ replacement or the use of K^+-sparing diuretics such as amiloride. This may lead to arrhythmias of digoxin toxicity at even relatively low serum digoxin levels. Spironolactone, which inhibits the effects of aldosterone and thus serves to save K^+, may also have an opposing effect to reduce renal clearance of digoxin, thus raising its serum level.

In general, digoxin is used most commonly and thus is the focus of the remaining discussion.

Digoxin in the Treatment of Congestive Heart Failure

Digoxin has its most beneficial hemodynamic actions when substantial ventricular depression is evident in addition to CHF. In this circumstance, it augments myocardial performance and reflexly reduces peripheral resistance. Slowing of the heart rate—whether via enhanced parasympathetic tone and reduced sympathetic activity to reduce sinus rate or via control of heart rate in atrial fibrillation (as discussed below)—will greatly benefit ventricular filling and reduce pulmonary congestion. Thus, the actions of digitalis glycosides not only affect the performance of the depressed myocardium but also have a central action to favorably alter the neurohumoral milieu that may adversely affect the heart and circulation. In the treatment of CHF, digoxin is generally employed with diuretics, beta blockers, and vasodilator agents. By reducing peripheral resistance, digoxin and peripheral vasodilators act in a complementary manner.

In acute heart failure—characterized by acute pulmonary edema, severe limitations of cardiac output, and perhaps hypotension—more rapidly acting inotropic agents such as intravenous dobutamine or milrinone may be required in addition to loop diuretics, natriuretic peptides, and vasodilators. This situation may occur in the setting of rapid deterioration of the patient with CHF or after a large myocardial infarction. In this circumstance, the main aim is to increase cardiac output and reduce filling pressure as a means to longer-term stabilization.

While rapidly acting inotropic agents are being used, digitalization may be begun cautiously for its longer-term effects. In the setting of myocardial infarction, the situation is more complex. Due to a fear that arrhythmias may be induced or oxygen consumption increased, which may be detrimental, digoxin is generally avoided in the first few days after the infarction; in the longer term, however, digitalization, especially if dosing is carefully controlled, may be of value in addition to other agents, especially ACE inhibitors. In the absence of clear CHF with only lower ejection fraction (NYHA classes I and II), digitalis has had an apparent adverse effect on long-term mortality and should be avoided. For chronic CHF, digoxin is useful over the long term when administered in association with loop diuretics and ACE inhibitors. Benefits are most evident in patients with NYHA class III or IV CHF. In this circumstance, the response of the circulation is characterized by decreases in venous pressure and ventricular filling pressure and an increase in cardiac output. Heart rate is slowed and ejection fraction tends to rise, whereas peripheral resistance falls with little or no change in arterial pressure. These salutary effects are attributed to a combination of augmented myocardial contractility and restoration of baroreceptor sensitivity, which results in enhanced parasympathetic and decreased sympathetic tone. Myocardial oxygen consumption tends to be reduced in heart failure due to a decrease in heart size, and thus ventricular wall tension, and a slowing of heart rate. Earlier concepts supported the view that digoxin is of greatest benefit when atrial fibrillation is present and controlled. It is now clear that efficacy is also present when the patient with heart failure is in sinus rhythm. Withdrawal of digoxin from such patients has led to rapid deterioration even when diuretics and ACE inhibitors were used. Although digoxin has been associated with an increase in ejection fraction, vasodilators have shown more significant increments in exercise performance. These considerations would justify the combined use of these agents. However, whereas the use of ACE inhibitors may well be indicated when the ejection is reduced but symptoms are limited (classes I and II), digoxin probably should be reserved for use with more overt symptoms (classes III and IV).

Although digoxin can be given once a day without tolerance or tachyphylaxis, the dose is a matter of issue. In general, a serum level of 0.5 to 0.8 ng/dL is felt to be therapeutic. This level may vary from patient to patient, and a clear dose–response relation has not been established. Indeed, some of the greatest benefits may be gained from lower doses (e.g., 0.125 mg/day) that result in serum digoxin concentrations in the 0.5 to 0.8 ng/dL range. There appear to be no adverse effects from digoxin usage in terms of mortality in patients with CHF, and substantially increased morbidity is noted when the drug is withdrawn. Effects on mortality with digoxin are complicated by the fact that the nature and progression of the underlying process, which has led to failure in the first place, may well be the ultimate determinant of mortality. If morbidity is reduced substantially with digoxin, a neutral effect on ultimate mortality would be acceptable. This was demonstrated in the Digitalis Investigation Group Study, a controlled trial in patients with CHF sponsored by the National Institutes of Health, which showed no effect on survival when compared with placebo, a reduction in hospitalizations, and a low incidence of digoxin toxicity.

Digoxin has been of limited value in the treatment of right-sided heart failure, as may occur in cor pulmonale or left-to-right shunts. Digoxin also has limited value in the face of acute left ventricular (LV) failure due to acute myocardial infarction. After the first few days of an infarction have passed, longer-term digoxin use has been employed, as it would be in any form of chronic failure, but its effects on mortality have remained controversial. Nevertheless, because mortality may be increased by giving digoxin postinfarction, especially when clear evidence of heart failure is absent, its use is best reserved for those with overt CHF.

Digitalis Toxicity

Digoxin levels can be readily measured in the serum by immunologic techniques, and the therapeutic level is thought to be 1.0 to 2.0 ng/mL. Administration of other drugs may change the serum level by altering absorption or elimination and may contribute to toxicity. For example, verapamil, clarithromycin, and quinidine may increase plasma levels. Drugs such as spironolactone and canrenone can also falsely lower the measured concentration of digoxin.

The signs and symptoms of digitalis toxicity have been amply described, although some may be very subtle. These include nausea and anorexia, which may lead to weight loss, fatigue, and visual disturbances. Psychiatric disturbances may occur less commonly; they may include delirium, hallucinations, or even seizures. Electrocardiographic alterations occur with variable degrees of AV block and ventricular ectopy. Sinus bradycardia, junctional rhythm, paroxysmal tachycardia with variable AV block, Wenckebach AV block, and ventricular tachycardia leading to ventricular fibrillation may be seen. Such arrhythmias are potentiated by hypokalemia and digitalis-mediated enhanced parasympathetic tone. They may be life-threatening in the presence of severe heart failure and should be avoided or controlled as much as possible.

The diagnosis of digitalis toxicity is suggested by signs and symptoms and electrocardiographic alterations and is supported by an elevated serum digoxin level. Certainty of the diagnosis may be made only with drug withdrawal accompanied by subsidence of these findings. With the therapeutic level of digoxin between 1.0 and 2.0 ng/mL, digitalis toxicity levels would be unlikely but should not excluded; levels above 3.0 ng/mL suggest toxicity, whereas levels below 1.5 ng/mL, when not complicated by hypokalemia, suggest other problems. It is important to note that only steady-state serum drug concentrations show any relation to cardiac glycoside toxicity. Thus, for example, in monitoring serum digoxin concentration, the samples should be collected at least 6 to 8 h after drug administration. Nevertheless, there is considerable crossover between patients reflecting variable sensitivity, such that withdrawal of digoxin on suspicion is always advisable for treatment and diagnosis. This is especially true because some patients experience profound vagal responses with relatively small amounts of digoxin.

Although withdrawal of digoxin and correction of hypokalemia as a potentiating cause may be adequate treatment of digitalis toxicity in most instances, a temporary pacemaker may be required for severe bradycardia or complete heart block. Lidocaine is useful to treat ventricular ectopy or ventricular tachycardia. Dilantin also has been used, and quinidine, which may displace digoxin from binding sites and thus raise serum digoxin levels further, should be avoided. Amiodarone and intravenous magnesium also have been used successfully for this purpose.

In the presence of massive digoxin overdosage, most commonly associated with suicide attempts, digitalis-specific antibodies (digoxin-specific Fab fragments) have been remarkably effective. In general, such an approach in the usual therapeutic setting is unnecessary but provides a backup to more conservative approaches, if they are not proceeding well, such as normalizing serum K^+ and withholding digoxin.

Digoxin reduction should be considered and individualized in the elderly patient with renal insufficiency. Because electrical conversion is accompanied by ventricular arrhythmias, reduction of dosage 1 to 2 days before the procedure is advisable.

CATECHOLAMINES

In general, positive inotropism is based on enhancing the delivery of Ca^{2+} to the contractile system to increase force and shortening. Increasing Ca^{2+} in the serum will effect this transiently, whereas digitalis glycosides will increase Ca^{2+} for activation by inhibiting sarcolemmal Na^+, K^+-ATPase. Catecholamines increase activating Ca^{2+} via β-adrenergic receptors and the adenylate cyclase system.

β-Receptors are located in the sarcolemma and comprise a complex structure that spans the membrane. The β receptor is connected with G proteins that activate (Gs) or inhibit (Gi) a secondary system, adenylate cyclase, which, when activated by Gs, induces the formation of cyclic $3'-5'$ adenosine monophosphate (cAMP). Cyclic AMP in turn activates certain protein kinases, which lead to intracellular phosphorylation of proteins that enhance the entry and removal of intracellular Ca^{2+}. When more Ca^{2+} is provided to the troponin tropomyosin system, a greater interaction between actin and myosin occurs, thereby increasing force and shortening. Increasing the rate of Ca^{2+} removal from the cytoplasm speeds the rate of relaxation.

In the normal heart, norepinephrine is synthesized and stored in sympathetic nerve endings that invest the entire heart, atria, conduction system, and ventricle. When activated, these nerve endings are depolarized and norepinephrine is released from granules in nerve endings into myocardial clefts containing β-adrenergic receptors, which, when activated, turn on the sequence of events noted above. This not only enhances Ca^{2+} entry into the myocyte to augment contraction but also phosphorylates phospholamban, which enhances relaxation. Subsequently, most of the released norepinephrine is taken back up and re-stored in the sympathetic nerve endings. Released norepinephrine is also inactivated by two enzymes, catechol-O-methyltransferase and monoamine oxidase, and the products are excreted largely by the kidneys.

In very severe heart failure, stores of norepinephrine in the ventricle are largely depleted and the sympathetic nerve endings fail to take up norepinephrine normally. At the same time, circulating norepinephrine released from peripheral sympathetic nerve endings may be increased, especially in severe failure. In less severe heart failure, the decreased norepinephrine levels may reflect enhanced release due to increased sympathetic nerve activity.

In the normal and failing myocardia, activation of the adenylate cyclase system can augment contractility. Agents that do this may be divided into two categories. The first comprises the catecholamines (e.g., norepinephrine, epinephrine) and their synthetic derivatives (e.g., dobutamine, isoproterenol), which act via cell-surface adrenergic receptors. The second includes agents that inhibit the breakdown of cAMP by inhibition of phosphodiesterase (PDE) type III (PDE III; e.g., amrinone, milrinone, and enoximone). Other agents, such as levosimendan, increase myofibrillar sensitivity to calcium and then further augment contraction.

Catecholamines constitute an endogenous hormonal system exerting reflex control of the heart and circulation. Their effects depend on localized controlled neural release and receptor specificity in terms of action.

Dopamine is the naturally occurring precursor of norepinephrine and epinephrine. Whereas epinephrine is released from the adrenal medulla, norepinephrine is the primary mediator in the heart and peripheral circulation.

The actions of endogenous and exogenous catecholamines depend on their activation of specific α- and β-adrenergic receptors (Table 8-1). α Receptors include $α_1$ receptors, which are postsynaptic and located in vascular smooth muscle and in the myocardium. In smooth muscle, they mediate vasoconstriction; in the heart, they have weak positive inotropic and negative chronotropic effects. $α_2$ Receptors are presynaptic; when stimulated, they decrease norepinephrine release from peripheral nerve endings and sympathetic outflow from the central nervous system. α Receptors also may mediate vasoconstriction in specific peripheral vascular beds.

β-Adrenergic receptors can be divided into two types: $β_1$ and $β_2$. $β_1$ Receptors are located in the myocardium, where they mediate positive inotropic, chronotropic, and dromotropic effects. They are activated primarily

TABLE 8-1 Adrenergic Receptor Activity of Sympathomimetic Amines

	α_1	β_1	β_2	Dopaminergic	Dose
Dopamine	+++	++	+	++++	<2 μg—μg/kg/min vasodilation effects on peripheral dopaminergic receptors 2–10 μg/kg/min— inotropic effects, β_1-receptor activation 5–20 μg/kg/min— peripheral vasoconstriction, α effects
Norepinephrine	++++	++++	0	0	Initiate with 8–12 μg/min; maintain 2–4 μg/min
Epinephrine	+++	++++	++	0	
Isoproterenol	0	++++	++++	0	0.5–5 μg/min
Dobutamine	+++	++++	++	0	Start at 2–3 μg/kg/min and titrate upward

by norepinephrine released from neurons in the heart. β_2 Receptors are located in vascular smooth muscle, where they mediate vasodilatation, and in the sinoatrial node, where they are chronotropic. In general, β_2 receptors are activated by circulating catecholamines released from peripheral sites, such as the adrenal medulla.

Another type of receptor has been termed the *dopaminergic receptor*, which is localized to the mesenteric and renal circulations and mediates arterial vasodilatation (drugs that act on peripheral dopaminergic receptors are discussed in Chapter 17). The physiologic and pharmacologic actions of various catecholamines depend on which receptor they activate in the heart and in the periphery (Table 8-2).

Norepinephrine has potent α_1 and β_1 activities. When norepinephrine is released from cardiac nerve endings, as occurs in normal exercise, myocardial contractility and heart rate are augmented. When norepinephrine is administered exogenously, its major action is to stimulate α_1 receptors, leading to marked peripheral arterial vasoconstriction. Thus, norepinephrine has been used to reverse severe hypotension to preserve blood flow to vital

TABLE 8-2 Physiologic and Pharmacologic Actions of Catecholamine Receptors

Receptor	Receptor activity	Primary location
β_1	Positive inotropic and chronotropic action; increased AV conduction	Heart (atria, ventricle AV node)
β_2	Peripheral vasodilation	Arterioles, arteries, veins, bronchioles
α_1	Arteriolar vasoconstriction	Arterioles
α_2	Presynaptic inhibition of norepinephrine release	Sympathetic nerve endings, CNS
Dopaminergic	Renal and mesenteric vasodilation, natriuresis, diuresis	Kidneys

Key: AV, atrioventricular; CNS, central nervous system.

organs. Continued administration of norepinephrine may produce ischemic renal damage due to sustained renal vasoconstriction. For the failing heart, this peripheral vasoconstriction also provides an undesirable added pressure load (afterload) and altered oxygen consumption, which tends to vitiate the potential benefits of β_1 stimulation.

Dopamine has α_1 and β_1 activities but also stimulates dopaminergic receptors in the renal vasculature to produce arterial dilation and increased renal blood flow. Its β_1 effects in the heart occur largely through the release of endogenous norepinephrine, which may be largely depleted in the failing heart. As doses of dopamine are increased, conversion to norepinephrine also occurs, which tends to produce relatively more pressor effects than myocardial inotropic stimulation. Dopamine also can depress minute ventilation in patients with heart failure. As such, the benefits of dopamine administration, if any, are at low doses (e.g., 2 μg/kg per minute), at which they may induce renal arterial vasodilatation in association with administration of other more potent inotropic agents (e.g., dobutamine). Low-dose dopamine also can be used in combination with norepinephrine to blunt norepinephrine-induced renal vasoconstriction.

A recent randomized, placebo-controlled study showed that the administration of low-dose dopamine by continuous infusion to critically ill patients provides no significant protection from renal dysfunction.

Dobutamine is a synthetic variant of the catecholamines whose structure has been altered to optimize hemodynamic response in the dog, characterized by an increase in cardiac output and a decrease in ventricular filling pressure with little change in heart rate. Because arterial pressure also rises modestly, peripheral vascular resistance must of necessity fall. The positive inotropic activity of dobutamine is mediated by direct stimulation of β_1-adrenergic receptors in the myocardium (see Tables 8-1 and 8-2). It is unclear why heart rate does not increase concomitantly. The increased arterial pressure resulting from enhanced cardiac output may increase baroreceptor activity and thereby offset the rise in heart rate induced by β-adrenergic stimulation. Given the capacity of dobutamine to increase cardiac output and reduce filling pressure without substantial heart rate change, dobutamine has been widely used to treat severe acute LV failure in the absence of profound hypotension, which is poorly responsive to diuretics, natriuretic peptides, and vasodilators, as may be seen after a very large myocardial infarction or in acute decompensation in the course of chronic CHF. In the presence of severe hypotension, the β_2 stimulation of dobutamine may be harmful, and administration of an α_1-stimulating vasoconstrictor such as norepinephrine or a higher dose of dopamine may also be necessary to increase arterial peripheral resistance.

Dobutamine infusion is generally begun at 2 μg/kg per minute and titrated to optimize cardiac output and reduce LV filling pressure. Tachycardia is carefully avoided so as not to increase ischemia. The effects on myocardial oxygen consumption (MVO_2) are complex. Enhanced contractility increases MVO_2, whereas the resulting decrease in LV wall tension tends to reduce it. The net result is most often an increase in MVO_2. However, a rise in systolic arterial pressure coupled to a reduction in LV filling pressure may enhance myocardial perfusion in the absence of tachycardia. The major side effects of dobutamine are an excessive increase in heart rate with high rates of infusion and ventricular arrhythmias, both of which may mandate dose reduction and even drug discontinuation. Tachyphylaxis also may occur to a variable degree.

In general, once hemodynamic benefits are attained, dobutamine is slowly withdrawn. In some cases, this is not possible and sustained administration becomes necessary, which may require portable pumps for outpatient administration. The outcome in this circumstance is generally dire.

In chronic CHF, the patient is commonly maintained on vasodilators such as ACE inhibitors, loop diuretics, and digoxin. Nevertheless, episodes of acute decompensation may intervene, characterized by increased pulmonary congestion, edema, and reduced renal function with increasing fluid accumulation. Intermittent infusion of dobutamine in conjunction with amiodarone may stabilize clinical benefits in patients with heart failure refractory to standard medical treatment.

PDE INHIBITORS

The adenylate cyclase cAMP system also can be activated beyond the β receptor. Hormones such as glucagon activate the system and can increase myocardial contractility acutely despite β_1 blockade. Although useful in overcoming β-adrenergic blockade, if necessary, glucagon may induce gastric atony and nausea, which has limited its more generalized use.

Amrinone and milrinone are prototypes of a class of cardiotonic agents that activates the adenylate cyclase system through inhibition of the enzyme that breaks down cAMP: PDE III. PDE III inhibitors decrease the breakdown of cAMP in the myocardium and increase cyclic guanidine monophosphate in vascular smooth muscle, resulting in an increase in myocardial contractility and arterial and venous vasodilations. Another member of this class of drugs is enoximone. At present, only amrinone and milrinone have been approved by the U.S. Food and Drug Administration (FDA) for treatment of acute heart failure. The mechanisms by which vasodilation occurs is not completely understood. Increased cAMP induces phosphorylation of myosin light-chain kinase, which decreases sensitivity to calcium and calmodulin. In the heart, inotropism may relate not only to increased cAMP-mediated calcium availability for contraction and increased rates of its removal for relaxation but also to increased sensitivity of the contractile system for calcium. Amrinone and milrinone, which are available as intravenous agents, have substantial ability to augment cardiac output and reduce right ventricular and LV filling pressures. The lowering of filling pressures is greater than that seen with dobutamine. Dilatation of the pulmonary vasculature is also a very useful therapeutic effect. Arterial pressure tends to be reduced, although an increase in heart rate may occur. Because dobutamine increases cAMP and milrinone reduces its breakdown, the combination of these agents is substantially more potent than either agent alone. When dobutamine or milrinone is used, ectopic activity may be increased, which requires careful supervision in their use.

PDE III inhibitors are also orally active and produce the same hemodynamic improvement as seen with intravenous use. However, in longer-term oral use, increased mortality was seen with the use of milrinone, especially in the presence of NYHA class IV heart failure. This increased mortality may have been due to the relatively short duration of action of this agent (30-min half-life), which leads to large peaks and valleys in dosing and concomitant arrhythmias. For the time being, this has vitiated clinical study of these agents, but more stringent control of the use of this class of agents as adjuncts to other agents ultimately may increase their value.

Milrinone

Intravenous milrinone therapy is commonly initiated with a bolus of 50 μg/kg and immediately followed by a continuous infusion at a rate of 0.375 to 0.75 μg/kg per minute. Initiation of milrinone therapy with a loading bolus has the advantage of producing immediate hemodynamic improvement. However, the loading bolus may precipitate ventricular arrhythmias and/or systemic hypotension. In clinical conditions that do not require immediate improvement of LV performance, as in patients with decompensated CHF, initiating milrinone therapy without a bolus is preferable to avoid the risk of precipitating ventricular arrhythmias or hypotension. Whether or not a bolus is administered, intravenous milrinone produces identical hemodynamic improvement 2 h after initiation of therapy. The intravenous bolus of milrinone is particularly useful to evaluate the reversibility of pulmonary hypertension in patients with severe CHF who are being screened for cardiac transplantation. The rapid onset of the direct relaxant effect of milrinone on the pulmonary vasculature is well suited to test pulmonary vascular reactivity. Milrinone decreases pulmonary vascular resistance by increasing cardiac output. In contrast to nitroprusside and nitric oxide, which also decrease pulmonary vascular resistance, milrinone does not affect the transpulmonary pressure gradient. The milrinone-induced increase in cardiac output presumably lowers pulmonary vascular resistance by recruiting accessory vessels in the pulmonary circulation and flow-mediated pulmonary vasodilatation.

In addition to its positive inotropic action, milrinone substantially increases Ca^{2+}-ATPase activity in the sarcoplasmic reticulum (SR) and thereby LV relaxation in the canine pacing model of heart failure. Increased SR Ca^{2+}-ATPase activity is due to a selective inhibition by milrinone of SR membrane-bound PDE III. Increased SR Ca^{2+}-ATPase activity mediates the well-documented lusitropic action of milrinone. Of note, whereas the positive inotropic action of milrinone is limited by reduced cAMP and PDE levels in the failing cardiac myocyte, the lusitropic effect is completely preserved due to a compartmentalized modulation of cAMP in the failing heart.

The clinical effects of intermittent or long-term administration of milrinone in patients with severe CHF are controversial. Uncontrolled reports have suggested its usefulness in reducing the use of mechanical LV devices in patients awaiting cardiac transplantation. A recent controlled trial of intermittent administration of milrinone failed to document any clinical benefits. It is clear that not every patient with severe CHF is improved by long-term administration of milrinone. However, most heart failure and cardiac transplantation specialists have seen patients who undoubtedly improve while receiving long-term milrinone therapy, especially those with non-ischemic cardiomyopathy. Attempts also have been made to use milrinone to increase the tolerability of beta-blocker initiation by counteracting the myocardial depressant action of catecholamine withdrawal. Thus, this mode of therapy should be tailored to the individual response of patients and initiated only when other FDA-approved therapeutic modalities at the appropriate dosages have failed.

CONCLUSION

Inotropic agents still play a role in the management of patients with acutely decompensated CHF that is refractory to optimal standard therapy. Their

TABLE 8-3 Relative Hemodynamic Effects of Agents in Heart Failure

	Ventricular filling pressure	Peripheral vascular resistance	Cardiac output	Blood pressure	Ejection fraction
Inotropic agents					
Digoxin	↓	↓	↑	—	↑
Dobutamine	↓/NC	↓↓	↑↑	↑	↑↑
Norepinephrine	↓/NC	↑↑	↑/NC	↑↑	↑/NC
Dopamine	↓/NC	↑	↑	↑	↑/NC
Inodilators					
Milrinone	↓↓	↓↓	↑↑	↓	↑
Diuretics	↓↓	↑/NC	↓/NC	↓/NC	—
Vasodilators					
NTG, oral	↓↓	↓↓	—	↓/NC	—
NTG, IV	↓↓↓	↓↓↓	—	↓/NC	—
Nitroprusside	↓↓	↓↓↓	↑	↓	—
Hydralazine	↓/NC	↓↓	↑	↓/NC	—
ACE inhibitors	↓↓	↓↓	↑/NC	↓	—
β blockers	↓	↓/NC	↑/NC	NC/↓	↑

Key: ↑, increase; ↓, decrease; ACE, angiotensin-converting enzyme; IV, intravenous; NC, no change; NTG, nitroglycerin.

hemodynamic effects are compared with other classes of drugs used to treat acute CHF in Table 8-3. Dobutamine and milrinone can be used in combination with vasodilator drugs and diuretics to maximize hemodynamic benefit. There is now strong evidence that, when used properly, digoxin is safe and effective when added to diuretics and ACE inhibitors.

ADDITIONAL READINGS

Adams KF Jr., Gheorghiade M, Uretsky BF, et al: Clinical benefits of low serum digoxin concentrations in heart failure. *J Am Coll Cardiol* 39:946, 2002.

American College of Cardiology/American Heart Association Task Force on Practice Guidelines (Committee to Revise the 1995 Guidelines for the Evaluation and Management of Heart Failure): ACC/AHA Guidelines for the evaluation and management of chronic heart failure in the adult: Executive summary). *J Am Coll Cardiol* 38:2101, 2001.

Australian and New Zealand Intensive Care Society (ANZICS) Clinical Trials Group: Low-dose dopamine in patients with early renal dysfunction: A placebo-controlled randomised trial. *Lancet* 356:2139, 2000.

Cuffe MS, Califf RM, Adams KF Jr, et al: Short-term intravenous milrinone for acute exacerbation of chronic heart failure. A randomized, controlled trial. *JAMA* 287: 1541, 2002.

Digitalis Investigation Group: The effect of digoxin on mortality and morbidity in patients with heart failure. *N Engl J Med* 336:525, 1997.

Eberhardt RT, Frishman WH, Landau A, et al: Increased mortality incidence in elderly individuals receiving digoxin therapy: Results of the Bronx Longitudinal Aging Study. *Cardiol Elderly* 3:177, 1995.

Felker GM, Benza RL, Chandler AB, et al: Heart failure etiology and response to milrinone in decompensated heart failure. Results from the OPTIME-CHF Study. *J Am Coll Cardiol* 41:997, 2003.

Frishman WH, Cheng-Lai A, Chen J: Inotropic and vasopressor agents, in Frishman WH, Cheng-Lai A, Chen J (eds): *Current Cardiovascular Drugs*, 3rd ed. Philadelphia, Current Medicine, 2000, p 194.

Hoffman BB, Taylor P: Neurotransmission, in Hardman JG, Limbird LE (eds): *Goodman & Gilman's the Pharmacological Basis of Therapeutics*, 10th ed. New York, McGraw-Hill, 2001, p 115.

Juurlink DN, Mamdani M, Kopp A, et al: Drug-drug interactions among elderly patients hospitalized for drug toxicity. *JAMA* 289:1652, 2003.

LeJemtel TH, Sonnenblick EH, Frishman WH: Diagnosis and medical management of heart failure, in Fuster V, Alexander RW, O'Rourke RA (eds): *Hurst's the Heart*, 11th ed. New York, McGraw-Hill, in press.

McMurray J, Pfeffer MA: New therapeutic options in congestive heart failure, part II. *Circulation* 105:2223, 2002.

Milfred-LaForest SK, Shubert J, Mendoza B, et al: Tolerability of extended duration intravenous milrinone in patients hospitalized for advanced heart failure and the usefulness of uptitration of oral angiotensin-converting enzyme inhibitors. *Am J Cardiol* 84:894, 1999.

Nanas JN, Kontoyannis DA, Alexopoulos GP, et al: Long-term intermittent dobutamine infusion combined with oral amiodarone improves the survival of patients with severe congestive heart failure. *Chest* 119:1173, 2001.

Packer M, Carver JR, Rodeheffer RJ, et al: Effect of oral milrinone on mortality in severe chronic heart failure. *N Engl J Med* 325:1468, 1991.

Packer M, Gheorghiade M, Young JB, et al: Withdrawal of digoxin from patients with chronic heart failure treated with angiotensin-converting enzyme inhibitors. RADI-ANCE Study. *N Engl J Med* 329:1, 1993.

Patel MB, Kaplan IV, Patni RN, et al: Sustained improvement in flow mediated vasodilation after short-term administration of dobutamine in patients with severe congestive heart failure. *Circulation* 99:60, 1999.

Rathore SS, Curtis JP, Wang Y, et al: Association of serum digoxin concentration and outcomes in patients with heart failure. *JAMA* 289:871, 2003.

Smith TW, Antman EM, Friedman PL, et al: Digitalis glycosides: Mechanisms and manifestations of toxicity. Part I. *Prog Cardiovasc Dis* 26:413, 1984.

Smith TW, Antman EM, Friedman PL, et al: Digitalis glycosides: Mechanisms and manifestations of toxicity. Part II. *Prog Cardiovasc Dis* 26:495, 1984.

Smith TW, Antman EM, Friedman PL, et al: Digitalis glycosides: Mechanisms and manifestations of toxicity. Part III. *Prog Cardiovasc Dis* 27:21, 1984.

Sonnenblick EH, Frishman WH, LeJemtel TH: Dobutamine: A new synthetic cardioactive sympathetic amine. *N Engl J Med* 300:17, 1979.

Sonnenblick EH, LeJemtel TH, Frishman WH: Inotropic agents, in Frishman WH, Sonnenblick EH, Sica DA (eds): *Cardiovascular Pharmacotherapeutics*, 2nd ed. New York, McGraw-Hill 2003, p 191.

Tauke J, Goldstein S, Gheorghiade M: Digoxin for chronic heart failure: a review of the randomized controlled trials with special attention to the PROVED and RADIANCE trials. *Prog Cardiovasc Dis* 37:49, 1994.

Uretsky BF, Young JB, Shahidi FE, et al: Randomized study assessing the effect of digoxin withdrawal in patients with mild to moderate chronic congestive heart failure: Results of the PROVED Trial. *J Am Coll Cardiol* 22:955, 1995.

Warner Stevenson L: Inotropic therapy for heart failure. *N Engl J Med* 339:1848, 1998.

Williamson KM, Thrasher KA, Fulton KB, et al: Digoxin toxicity. An evaluation in current clinical practice. *Arch Intern Med* 158:2444, 1998.

9 | The Organic Nitrates and Nitroprusside

Jonathan Abrams   William H. Frishman

The organic nitrates and sodium nitroprusside (NP) make up a class of drugs known as *nitrovasodilators*. The common denominator of these agents is the production of nitric oxide (NO) within vascular smooth muscle cells and platelets (Fig. 9-1). NO activates the enzyme guanylate or guanylyl cyclase, which in turn results in an accumulation of intracellular cyclic guanosine 3', 5' monophosphate (cGMP). Cyclic GMP in turn activates a cGMP-dependent protein kinase, which has been shown to mediate vasorelaxation via phosphorylation of proteins that regulate intracellular Ca^{2+} levels. Smooth muscle cell relaxation is induced by cGMP through fluxes in intracellular calcium. In the platelet, increases in cGMP exert an anti-aggregatory action and thus decreased platelet activation, resulting in less thrombosis. The predominant actions of the nitrovasodilators are the hemodynamic perturbations resulting from vascular dilatation. In contrast to the majority of vasodilating

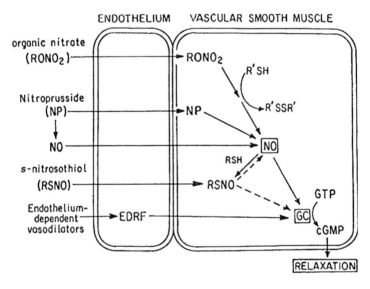

FIG. 9-1 Nitrovasodilators, endothelium-dependent vasodilators, and vascular smooth muscle relaxation. EDRF, endothelium-derived relaxing factor; GC, guanylate cyclase; NO, nitric oxide; R9SH and RSH, two distinct pools of intracellular sulfhydryl groups; R9SSR9, disulfide groups. (*Reproduced with permission from Kowaluk E, Fung H-L: Pharmacology and pharmacokinetics of nitrates, in Abrams J, Pepine C, Thadani U (eds): Medical Therapy of Ischemic Heart Disease: Nitrates, Beta Blockers, and Calcium Antagonists. Boston, Little Brown and Co 1992, p 152.*)

TABLE 9-1 Nitrate Formulations: Dosing Recommendations and Pharmacokinetics

	Usual dose (mg)*	Onset of action (min)	Effective duration of action
Sublingual NTG	0.3–0.6	2–5	20–30 min
Sublingual ISDN	2.5–10.0	5–20	45–120 min
Buccal NTG	1–3 bid tid	2–5	30–300 min[†]
Oral ISDN	10–60 bid tid	15–45	2–6 h
Oral ISDN-SR	80–120 qd	60–90	10–14 h
Oral ISMN	20 bid[‡]	30–60	3–6 h
Oral ISMN-SR	60–120 qd	60–90	10–14 h
NTG ointment	0.5–2.0 tid	15–60	3–8 h
NTG patch	0.4–0.8 mg/h[#]	30–60	8–12 h

*Higher doses often are required in heart failure.
[†]Effect persists only while the tablet is intact in the buccal cavity.
[‡]Two daily doses 7 h apart (e.g., 8 A.M., 2 P.M.).
[#]Patch should be removed daily for 10–12 h.
Key: bid, twice daily; ISDN, isosorbide dinitrate; ISMN, isosorbide mononitrate; qd, daily; SR, sustained release; NTG, glyceryl trinitrate (nitroglycerin); tid, thrice daily.

agents available to the clinician, the nitrates and NP relax the venous capacitance bed in addition to arteries and arterioles. The role of the antiplatelet and antithrombotic actions of these compounds remains somewhat controversial, although much recent evidence supports a true benefit for nitrate-induced decreases in platelet and thrombus activations.

Nitroglycerin (NTG) has been used in medicine for well over 100 years. This drug, initially employed for anginal chest pain, became a mainstay of the homeopathic tradition in the early part of the 20th century. For the past three decades or longer, NTG and the organic nitrates have been widely used for the acute and chronic therapy of ischemic chest pain. More recently, these compounds have been employed in patients with acute and post–myocardial infarction (MI) and, importantly, as adjunctive therapy in congestive heart failure. NP, available only as an intravenous agent, is effective in the treatment of severe or acute hypertension, acute or chronic congestive heart failure, and pulmonary edema. As a general rule, NP is not used to alleviate myocardial ischemia.

Attenuation of nitrate effects, or nitrate tolerance, is the major obstacle to successful utilization of these drugs in clinical practice. There does not appear to be a significant degree of tolerance to the actions of NP, however. In recent years, a wide variety of nitrate formulations and compounds has become available (Table 9-1), whereas some older nitrate compounds (e.g., pentaerythritol tetranitrate) are no longer in use.

THE ORGANIC NITRATES

Mechanisms of Action

Cellular

NTG, isosorbide dinitrate (ISDN), and 5-isosorbide mononitrate (ISMN) are metabolized by vascular tissue at or near the plasma membrane of smooth muscle cells of veins and arteries (see Fig. 9-1). It was previously believed that nitrates underwent a stepwise denitration process that resulted in S-nitrosothiol (SNO) via the production of nitrite ion (NO_2^-). However, it now appears that these compounds may form NO directly through an enzymatic process that does not necessarily involve nitrite production as an intermediary. Further, the obligatory role of SNOs remains controversial (see Fig. 9-1). Nitrates can be converted into SNO but are dominantly a direct precursor of SNO. NO and SNO can activate guanylate or guanylyl cyclase, leading to the production of cGMP, a second messenger that relaxes vascular smooth muscle cells.

The enzymatic conversion of the nitrovasodilators is not homogeneous; NP and SNO appear to require different enzymes or "receptors," which presumably accounts for some of the differences in the hemodynamic spectrum among these agents and also may relate to the different susceptibilities to tolerance among the organic nitrates, NP or SNO. Intracellular chemical processes also result in NO formation in a nonenzymatic manner; this is much less important for the organic nitrates than for NP. In the platelet, increases in cGMP have been correlated with the degree of vasodilation in the coronary arteries. Presumably, nitrate platelet activation is modulated via cGMP-induced processes.

Nitrate Tolerance

Although the precise mechanisms of tolerance remain the subject of intense investigation, it is now known that NO production and cGMP responses become attenuated in the setting of nitrate tolerance. Further, the obligatory role of thiols during nitrate activation remains controversial with regard to tolerance phenomena. Although it now seems clear that intracellular glutathione or cysteine stores remain adequate and that thiol deficiency per se is not a factor in tolerance development, thiol or sulfhydryl (−SH) groups are critical to SNO and thionitrate formation. Further, a thiol moiety is a component of the enzyme that converts nitrates to NO. Thus, tolerance development may in part be related to thiols within the vascular smooth muscle cell in relation to the production of SNO or the nitrate enzyme(s) responsible for NO formation. Fung hypothesized that nitrates may oxidize SH proteins, resulting in thionitrate production. This compound can act as a potent oxidant for intracellular proteins, perhaps initiating a cascade of events resulting in abnormalities of NO synthase (NOS), activation of vasoconstrictors, and interference with the conversion of L-arginine to NO (Fung H-L, personal communication). Munzel and coworkers documented endothelial cell production of free radicals and the subsequent activation of protein kinase leading to endothelin and angiotensin II production (see below). Nitrate tolerance recently was associated with increased activity of the cGMP phosphodiesterase, which decreases cGMP levels necessary for mediating vasorelaxation via phosphorylation of proteins that regulate intracellular Ca^{2+} levels. These phenomena contribute to a vasoconstrictor milieu, for which oxidant stress is the probable cause.

Nitrate Effects on the Regional Circulations

Administration of NTG or other nitrates in sufficient dosage results in dilatation of veins and large to moderate-size arteries, with a fall in vascular impedance. At high concentrations, nitrates dilate the smaller arteries; at very high doses, nitrates can relax arterioles and the microcirculation. Venodilatation is seen at low nitrate concentrations and is near maximal at a moderate dosage

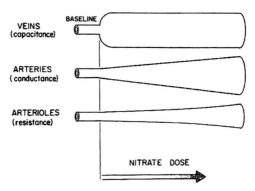

FIG. 9-2   Vasodilatory actions of organic nitrates in the major vascular beds. The venous or capacitance system dilates maximally with low doses of organic nitrates. Increasing the amount of drug does not cause appreciable additional venodilatation. Arterial dilatation and enhanced arterial conductance begin with low doses of nitrate. With further vasodilatation, appearing with increasing dosage at high plasma concentrations, the arteriolar or resistance vessels dilate, resulting in a decrease in systemic and regional vascular resistance. *(Reproduced with permission from Abrams J: Hemodynamic effects of nitroglycerin and long acting nitrates. Am Heart J 110:216, 1985.)*

(Fig. 9-2). Interesting studies by Harrison and associates have suggested that the enzymes responsible for nitrate conversion to NO apparently are not present in the coronary microvessels, thus limiting the degrees of increase in coronary blood flow and of decrease in coronary vascular resistance that can be achieved with NTG through dilatation of these small coronary vessels. Conversely, NP directly forms NO in the microcirculation and readily relaxes the resistance vessels; this can decrease distal coronary bed pressure and may allow for a coronary steal phenomenon in vessels beyond a coronary atherosclerotic obstruction (see below for discussion of NP).

Nitrates dilate the epicardial coronary arteries and, to a lesser degree, the smaller or distal coronary vessels. Coronary blood flow transiently increases and then declines below baseline as myocardial energy needs decrease. Systemic venous relaxation in the extremities and splanchnic circulation results in sequestration of the circulating blood volume away from the heart and lungs, with a decrease in cardiac output. Nitrates also relax the splanchnic and mesenteric arterial beds, possibly contributing to the decrease in blood flow returning to the heart. Renal blood flow is marginally affected by NTG; it may decrease to a modest degree. The cerebrovascular bed dilates with nitrates, and blood volume in the brain may increase. Thus, these agents are contraindicated when intracranial pressure is elevated.

An important clinical action of nitrates relates to the pulmonary circulation. These drugs consistently lower pulmonary venous and pulmonary capillary pressures, which contributes significantly to their efficacy in heart failure and myocardial ischemia. Relaxation of the pulmonary arterial bed is beneficial to subjects with secondary pulmonary hypertension; nitrates do not generally have a useful role in primary pulmonary hypertension.

Hemodynamic Correlates of Clinical Nitrate Efficacy

Table 9-2 lists the presumed mechanisms of action for the various clinical conditions for which these agents are prescribed. The traditional view has been that nitrate-induced reversal and prevention of myocardial ischemia are both due to reductions in myocardial oxygen consumption related to reduced cardiac chamber size and decreased systolic and diastolic pressures within the heart. These alterations are related predominantly to the venous and arterial vasodilating actions discussed above. The presumed paradigm is a major nitrate-induced decrease in cardiac work to match available coronary blood supply. However, in recent years, much evidence has contributed to the view that the organic nitrates have important actions in increasing regional or nutrient coronary blood flow, particularly to areas of myocardial ischemia. In addition to epicardial coronary artery dilatation, prevention or reversal of coronary artery vasoconstriction or spasm, increased coronary collateral size and flow, enhanced distal vessel and collateral caliber when constrictor forces predominate, coronary atherosclerotic stenosis enlargement, and improved coronary endothelial function are mechanisms that may interact in a favorable fashion to alleviate or prevent ischemia by directly enhancing coronary blood supply to myocardium downstream from a fixed or dynamic coronary obstruction (see Table 9-2).

In congestive heart failure, the beneficial effects and rationale for the nitrates are more obvious and are related to a predictable lowering of left and

TABLE 9-2 Mechanisms of Action of Nitrates: Relation to Clinical Indications

Acute attacks and prophylaxis of stable angina pectoris	Decreased myocardial oxygen consumption
	Decreased LV dimension
	Decreased LV filling pressure
	Decreased LV systolic pressure
	Decreased vascular impedance
	Increased coronary blood supply
	Epicardial coronary artery dilation
	Coronary stenosis enlargement
	Improved coronary endothelial function
	Dilation of coronary collaterals or small distal coronary vessels
Unstable angina	Same as above, plus antiplatelet, antithrombotic action
Acute myocardial infarction	Same as above, plus antiplatelet, antithrombotic action
CHF	Decreased LV and RV dimensions (few data on CHF)
Systolic dysfunction	Decreased LV and RV filling-pressures
	Decreased systemic vascular resistance
	Decreased arterial pressure
	Decreased PA and RA pressures
	Improved endothelial function
	CAD patients: increased coronary blood flow
	Decreased mitral regurgitation
Diastolic dysfunction	Decreased LV filling pressure
Hypertension	Decreased systolic blood pressure
	Decreased systemic vascular resistance
	Decreased LV preload—uncertain importance

Key: CAD, coronary artery disease; CHF, congestive heart failure; LV, left ventricular; PA, pulmonary artery; RA, right atrial; RV, right ventricular.

right ventricular filling pressures and the unloading actions that arise from decreased arterial pressure and impedance to left ventricular ejection. These afterload-reducing actions contribute to a modest increase in stroke volume and cardiac output in subjects with impaired left ventricular systolic function, in contradistinction to the typical nitrate-induced fall in forward cardiac output in the normal heart. In addition, NTG appears to improve impaired vascular endothelial function found in heart failure.

Nitroglycerin: The Exogenous Endothelium-Derived Relaxing Factor

Normal endothelial function is vasodilator and platelet anti-aggregatory. In the presence of even mild coronary atherosclerosis, the dilating actions of the endothelium are impaired in the coronary and systemic circulations. Thus, diminished vasodilation to physiologic stimuli (e.g., shear stress, platelet release products) and impaired platelet antiadhesion and aggregation responses are present in many to most individuals with clinically evident coronary artery disease (CAD). Abnormal vasoconstrictor responses to exercise, mental stress, cold pressor testing, and with the administration of endothelium-dependent dilator stimuli (e.g., acetylcholine, bradykinin) have been well documented in CAD subjects. Diminished availability of NO and prostacyclin in addition to increased endothelin and angiotensin II expression are common in such individuals; increased superoxide anions play a major role in inducing the endothelial dysfunction common to CAD. Stenotic constriction or collapse is an advanced manifestation of impaired endothelial function and may substantially contribute to the precipitation of myocardial ischemia in patients with angina or silent ischemia. NTG prevents or reverses this phenomenon, which has been documented with acetylcholine administration and exercise.

In congestive heart failure, disordered endothelial vasodilator activity is also common and contributes in an important way to the vasoconstrictor state common to heart failure. Enhanced sensitivity to catecholamines is part of the abnormal vascular physiology found in association with endothelial dysfunction; this phenomenon should be viewed as deleterious in heart failure and CAD.

Nitrates, as donors of NO, have been called exogenous endothelium-derived relaxing factor agents; these drugs improve responses to a variety of stimuli in the presence of endothelial dysfunction. Thus, in the patient with CAD, administration of organic nitrates may partly or completely normalize impaired endothelial-related vasodilation and, presumably but as yet unproved, restore endothelium-modulated antiplatelet activity toward normal. In fact, in some studies, vascular responses to administered NTG appear to be more robust in the setting of endothelial dysfunction than in the normal state. Nitrates also may improve endothelial function in heart failure. However, despite suggestive favorable data from studies in which nitrates were administered acutely, recent reports have suggested that, in the presence of unequivocal nitrate tolerance, endothelial dysfunction may actually be induced, perhaps due to impaired endothelial NOS activity and other intracellular perturbations of the NO cascade.

CLINICAL INDICATIONS FOR NITRATES

The major cardiovascular conditions for which nitrates are effective are listed in Table 9-2. The roles of NTG and the other organic nitrates in CAD are well established. Treatment and prophylaxis of anginal attacks and prevention of chest pain in chronic angina pectoris are the most important uses of these drugs. More problematic is the usefulness of nitrates in uncomplicated acute MI. Although sublingual or intravenous NTG are excellent drugs for recurrent ischemic chest pain, hypertension, or heart failure in the setting of an acute infarct, there is considerable uncertainty as to the benefits of routine 24- or 48-h infusions of NTG or the use of any nitrate when obvious indications are absent in the setting of acute infarction. Despite promising but limited animal and human data, the European mega-trials Gruppo Italiano per lo Studio della Supravivenza nell Infarcto Miocardico (GISSI-3) and Fourth International Study of Infarct Survival (ISIS-4) failed to show an important role for early administration of IV NTG immediately after an MI followed by 10 mg of transdermal glyceryl trinitrate for 6 weeks. More recently, the Delapril Remodeling after Acute Myocardial Infarction (DRAMI) trial showed that 3 months of ISMN together with an ACE inhibitor was safe and effective in reducing left ventricular dilation and dysfunction following an acute MI.

There is a suggestion that NTG pretreatment in patients undergoing angioplasty can protect the myocardium against ischemia. The mechanism proposed is a delayed preconditioning mimetic effect of NTG.

Nitrates are underused in congestive heart failure. These drugs are effective in improving symptoms and exercise tolerance and, in conjunction with the angiotensin-converting enzyme inhibitors, are useful for the treatment of symptomatic heart failure. Large doses are often required in these patients. Nitrate resistance and the necessity to use huge amounts of these drugs have been described in advanced heart failure. In the first Veterans Administration Cooperative Heart Failure Mortality study, the combination of ISDN, 40 mg four times daily, and hydralazine, 300 mg/day, reduced mortality. However, the combination of hydralazine and oral ISDN subsequently proved to be less effective in improving survival in heart failure patients than the ACE inhibitor enalapril.

Intravenous NTG is an effective formulation for lowering blood pressure in the setting of acute hypertension or for the control of mean arterial pressure during a variety of delicate surgical procedures. This agent has been used successfully for post–coronary bypass patients with elevated blood pressure. Oral nitrates, although used extensively in the early part of the 20th century for hypertension, are not part of contemporary conventional therapy of systemic hypertension, in part because of the appearance of tolerance to the systolic pressure–lowering effects of these drugs. However, a report from France has indicated a potential benefit for oral ISDN in systolic hypertension of the elderly.

There is also experimental evidence suggesting that NTG may be useful in reversing cerebral vasospasm in patients with subarachnoid hemorrhage.

NITRATE FORMULATIONS AND NITRATE PHARMACOKINETICS

Three organic nitrate compounds—NTG, ISDN, and ISMN—are currently used throughout the world and have been shown to provide benefits in angina pectoris and congestive heart failure. There does not appear to be any difference in clinical efficacy among these compounds. Choice of formulation, dosage, use of a tolerance–avoidance regimen, and the physician's experience and bias are major factors influencing which nitrate is prescribed for which patient. Tolerance is a problem for all nitrate formulations except for sublingual NTG and ISDN or transmucosal NTG, which are not designed to be

TABLE 9-3 Factors That Influence Nitrate Tolerance

Induce tolerance	Prevent tolerance
Continuous or prolonged nitrate exposure (e.g., transdermal patches, intravenous)	Intermittent dosing
	Small doses
Large doses	Infrequent dosing
Frequent dosing	Short-acting formulations
Sustained-action formulations	Provision of adequate
No or too brief nitrate-free interval	nitrate-free interval

administered continuously. Appropriately designed dosing regimens can prevent the appearance of significant nitrate tolerance, but limited available data suggest that attenuation of nitrate's hemodynamic action may begin to appear within hours of nitrate administration (see Tables 9-1 and 9-3).

Nitroglycerin

The classic prototype nitrate is NTG, which is available in many formulations (see Table 9-1). This molecule has a very short half-life of several minutes; cessation of an intravenous NTG infusion or removal of a transdermal patch results in a rapid fall in NTG plasma levels within 20 to 40 min. The metabolism of NTG occurs within the vascular wall (see Fig. 9-1). Veins take up NTG more avidly than arteries. It is not useful or practical to measure NTG plasma levels in clinical practice; this assay is technically difficult, and the relation between plasma NTG level and effect changes as tolerance develops. Early studies with sublingual NTG suggested that the therapeutic NTG level is at least 1 ng/mL; plasma concentrations with the NTG patch are substantially lower. The minimum recommended dose of the patch is 0.4 mg/h, with larger amounts often being more effective, particularly in heart failure. Several recent studies have confirmed a true anti-ischemic action of these agents, which must be administered in an on–off fashion. The patch should be applied continuously for only 12 to 14 h each day. Rebound angina and vasoconstriction are possible adverse effects of intermittent therapy. Several dosing systems for NTG have been available to physicians but are not widely used and may not be available in many pharmacies. These include the buccal or transmucosal formulation, NTG ointment, and oral sustained-release NTG capsules. Ointment and buccal NTG are effective but difficult for patients to use. NTG ointment is recommended for hospitalized or home-bound patients with nocturnal angina or symptomatic congestive heart failure. Oral NTG has virtually no reliable data supporting its effectiveness.

Isosorbide Dinitrate

ISDN is perhaps the most widely used long-acting nitrate in the world. It is available in short-acting and sustained-release formulations; most clinical studies in the literature have used short-acting oral ISDN. Table 9-4 outlines the relevant pharmacokinetic features of ISDN and ISMN. Sustained-release ISDN should be used only once daily. In Europe, intravenous ISDN is commercially available. Sublingual or chewable ISDN has long been used for acute attacks of chest pain or angina prophylaxis, but these formulations are infrequently prescribed in the United States.

TABLE 9-4 Pharmacokinetics of Isosorbide Dinitrate and 5-Mononitrate

	ISDN	5-ISMN
Bioavailability	20–25%*	100%
Half-life	30–60 min	4–5 h
Metabolites	2-ISMN, 5-ISMN	None
Plasma levels	Low	High
Formulations†	IV, SL, oral, oral sustained-release, ointment, spray	Oral, oral sustained release

*Extensive hepatic first-pass effect.
†Only oral and sublingual compounds are available in the United States.
Key: ISDN, isosorbide dinitrate; ISMN, isosorbide mononitrate; IV, intravenous; SL, sublingual.

When ISDN is administered, the parent compound is converted into two active metabolites, 2- and 5-isosorbide mononitrates. The latter is a pharmacologically active molecule that is commercially synthesized and is available in short-acting and sustained-release formulations. A dose of the parent compound ISDN results in plasma concentrations of all three molecules. ISDN has a short half-life of 50 to 60 min and rapidly disappears from the circulation. ISMN has a much longer half-life of 4 to 6 h and accounts for the protracted nitrate effects after administration of ISDN. Approximately 50% to 60% of ISDN is converted to 5-ISMN. Thus, although only 20% to 25% of ISDN itself is bioavailable when taken orally, a substantial component of the administered dose becomes pharmacologically active as 5-ISMN (Table 9-4).

Isosorbide 5-Mononitrate

The 5-mononitrate is the most recent nitrate formulation released in the United States. It was initially available only in the short-acting form; to avoid tolerance, short-acting 5-ISMN is recommended to be taken in a twice-daily regimen, with 7 to 8 h between doses (see Table 9-1). Earlier Scandinavian and European experience suggested that a 12-h regimen is satisfactory to avoid tolerance, but U.S. trials with this compound indicated that a longer overnight interval is necessary to avoid attenuation of clinical effectiveness. Sustained-release 5-ISMN is effective on a once-daily basis. A minimum of 60 mg/day is recommended; a large U.S. multicenter trial suggested that higher doses, such as 120 or 240 mg daily, may be necessary for sustained antianginal efficacy without tolerance. A 50-mg, once-daily, immediate-release and sustained-release ISMN formulation is now available, which appears to maintain antianginal efficacy without tolerance.

SUGGESTIONS FOR NITRATE DOSING

It is important to start nitrate therapy with small doses and to carefully increase to a predetermined end point or maximally tolerated amount over time. Headache and dizziness are the limiting symptoms with nitrate administration. Some individuals are extremely sensitive to organic nitrates; others experience few to no side effects. Many, if not most, patients are underdosed with long-acting nitrates, at least with respect to clinical trial data. For instance, 10 mg of oral ISDN, 30 or 60 mg of ISMN-SR, or 0.2 to 0.4 mg/h of the NTG patch are less likely to be clinically effective doses. If the angina is well controlled with these relatively low doses, it is satisfactory to continue such a regimen. However, the physician should recognize that if the desirable clinical response has not been achieved, larger doses of the nitrate should be tried. In congestive heart failure, the dosage of nitrates to achieve a significant hemodynamic effect is usually considerably higher than in patients with normal left ventricular function. Often patients who are troubled with nitrate headaches with initial nitrate dosing can be effectively treated with analgesics (aspirin, acetaminophen) to control the headache symptoms, which usually decrease or disappear over time. Nitrate hypotension is best handled by reducing the dose; concomitant therapy with calcium-channel antagonists, ACE inhibitors, or hypovolemia increase the likelihood of dizziness and/or syncope owing to low blood pressure after nitrate administration.

ADVERSE EFFECTS

In addition to headache and hypotension-related dizziness, nitrates can occasionally cause nausea. Patients with congestive heart failure tolerate large doses of nitrates surprisingly well. Rare cases of nitrate syncope have been reported, as have marked vasovagal responses and even atrioventricular block. Nitrates should be given with great care in the setting of right ventricular infarction complicating inferior MI because these drugs lower right ventricular filling pressure and can further depress cardiac output. Nitrates also should not be used with sildenafil because of a major hypotensive effect with this combination. Intravenous NTG may interfere with the actions of heparin, resulting in increased heparin requirements to achieve the desired prolongation of the activated clotting time. This interaction remains controversial. One report has suggested that NTG impairs tissue plasminogen activator activity during thrombolysis, and another recent report has suggested that NTG has adverse effects on atherosclerotic plaque irritability by activating matrix metalloproteinase activity. These effects may explain the lack of a positive association between NTG therapy and beneficial effects on plaque progression or coronary event rates, despite NTG's vasodilator activity. In general, the organic nitrates are well-tolerated drugs with little serious adverse sequelae. Headache, the most problematic symptom related to nitrate therapy, can be controlled in many patients. However, upward of 20% to 30% of individuals cannot tolerate long-acting nitrate therapy.

NITRATE TOLERANCE

Clearly, the most vexing issue regarding nitrate therapy is the attenuation of nitrate efficacy with repeated dosing. This subject has an enormous literature devoted to it and continues to engender considerable controversy. However, almost all experts agree that tolerance will predictably appear when protolerant dosing regimens are used. Dozens of high-quality clinical and basic research studies have underscored the magnitude of this problem. The rapid onset of tolerance can be substantiated after several repeated doses of oral nitrate given with too short an interdose interval. Major attenuation of nitrate action in angina has been repeatedly demonstrated with continuous 24-h application of transdermal NTG; in fact, an antianginal effect can no longer be detected by the second day of continuous patch therapy, even when very large doses are used. Similar findings have been demonstrated for intravenous NTG and for the oral agents ISDN and ISMN when these drugs are not

TABLE 9-5 Proposed Mechanisms of Nitrate Tolerance

Sulfhydryl depletion: inadequate generation of reduced –SH or cysteine groups required for organic nitrate biotransformation to NO

Desensitization of soluble guanylate cyclase; impaired activity of the enzyme guanylate cyclase

Counterregulatory neurohormonal activation: nitrate-induced increases in catecholamines, arginine vasopressin, plasma renin, aldosterone, and angiotensin II activity, with resultant vasoconstriction and fluid retention

Plasma volume shifts: increased intravascular blood volume related to decreased capillary pressure

Oxygen free radical destruction of NO with production of peroxynitrates resulting in enhanced sensitivity to vasoconstrictors, especially angiotensin II

Upregulation of PDE 1A1 expression resulting in decreased formation of cGMP

Key: cGMP, cyclic guanidine monophosphate; NO, nitric oxide; PDE, phosphodiesterase; SH, sulfhydryl.

administered in a tolerance–avoidance regimen. Table 9-3 lists the cardinal principles for avoiding nitrate tolerance. Table 9-1 outlines the recommended dosing schedules for the available nitrates. Intravenous NTG administered for the acute ischemic syndromes of unstable angina pectoris or acute MI should not be abruptly terminated to avoid tolerance; rebound phenomena are well known, and sudden withdrawal of intravenous NTG may be dangerous in this setting, even if some degree of hemodynamic tolerance is present.

The mechanisms of nitrate tolerance are not discussed here. Table 9-5 lists some current theories about tolerance mechanisms. Recent but preliminary studies have suggested that ACE inhibitor therapy, angiotensin II receptor blockade, diuretics, folic acid, vitamin C, or hydralazine may limit the appearance of nitrate tolerance.

Clinical Implications of Nitrate Tolerance

In addition to the loss of the desired actions of nitrates for specific cardiovascular disorders, nitrate tolerance may be associated with other adverse disturbances in vascular function, including withdrawal chest pain and/or ischemia and reflex vasoconstriction of coronary arteries or atherosclerotic stenoses. Several recent reports have suggested that long-term nitrate use may result in adverse clinical outcomes in patients with CAD. At the very least, the disappointing results of the large ISIS-4 and GISSI-3 postinfarction trials could be related in part to heretofore unsuspected abnormalities of vascular endothelial function induced by conventional nitrate dosing. Intermittent dosing strategies may reduce or attenuate the likelihood of nitrate tolerance, but it is possible or even likely that even shorter periods of nitrate exposure (e.g., <12 to 14 h) may initiate intracellular and endothelial mechanisms leading to unwanted alterations in endothelial NOS function and endothelial function modulated by a reduced availability of NO. There may be decreased NO synthesis and enhanced NO degradation induced by a variety of mechanisms. Thus, as some have suggested, chronic nitrate therapy for angina or heart failure may sow the seeds for unwanted outcomes with respect to long-term morbidity and even mortality. This would be a remarkable reversal of our concepts about these drugs and their utility in clinical cardiovascular disease; randomized clinical trial data are required to truly validate these concepts but are unlikely to become available in the future.

NITROPRUSSIDE

NP is an inorganic nitrovasodilator that results in abundant NO availability in vascular smooth muscle cells. It is likely that NP has antiplatelet activity, but there are limited data in this regard. NP is a ferrocyanide compound with a nitroso moiety. Cyanide molecules are released as the molecule undergoes metabolism to NO, but, in general, plasma cyanide and thiocyanate concentrations at clinically used dosages are too low to cause toxicity in subjects with normal renal function. NP provides NO throughout the vasculature; metabolic conversion to NO does not depend on enzymatic conversion to NO to any significant degree. Thus, NO is abundantly available in the microcirculation after NP infusion; these distal small vessels have a decreased capacity to metabolize the NTG molecule. This is an important dissimilarity between the two compounds because their spectra of vasodilatation differ significantly. Because NP has a potent effect on the small resistance vessels of the heart, there is a greater possibility for a coronary steal phenomenon than with NTG. NP induces relaxation of the microcirculation throughout the myocardium, potentially allowing for diversion of nutrient coronary blood flow away from regions of ischemia distal to a coronary obstruction. NP appears to dilate collateral vessels to a lesser degree than NTG, which could exacerbate a potentially deleterious diversion of blood from ischemic zones (see below). NP is a potent venodilator. On the arterial side, it is more hemodynamically active than NTG, particularly with regard to the smaller arterioles and resistance vessels. In general, there is a more equivalent degree of venous and arterial vasodilatations with NP than with NTG, which has a more dominant venodilator than arterial action, particularly at lower doses.

Indications for Nitroprusside

NP is a drug used exclusively in critical care settings and operating rooms. It is a highly effective vasodilator of great potency. NP was investigated extensively in the early days of vasodilator therapy for acute MI and congestive heart failure. Its balanced venous and arterial actions make it an ideal drug for the immediate therapy of acute and/or severe heart failure associated with high ventricular filling pressure and low stroke volume. It was recently shown to rapidly and markedly improve cardiac function in patients with decompensated heart failure due to severe LV systolic dysfunction and severe aortic stenosis, providing a safe and effective bridge to aortic valve replacement or oral vasodilator therapy. The drug is also a first-line choice for treatment of severe hypertension and is probably preferable to intravenous NTG in this capacity because of its greater arterial dilator potency. At very high NTG concentrations, the hemodynamic activity of intravenous NTG is quite similar to that of NP.

A series of animal and human investigations have suggested a potential hazard with the use of NP in nonhypertensive ischemic states, such as acute MI and unstable angina pectoris. Decreases in regional myocardial blood flow and collateral flow, associated with increased ischemia, have been demonstrated in human and canine studies when NP was compared with intravenous NTG. One early animal investigation suggested a more potent

TABLE 9-6 Indications for Nitroprusside
Severe hypertension
Acute pulmonary edema
Severe congestive heart failure
Acute and/or severe mitral or aortic regurgitation; aortic stenosis
Acute myocardial infarction complications: heart failure or uncontrolled hypertension
Use extreme caution
Hypotension or borderline systolic blood pressure
Acute myocardial ischemia in the absence of heart failure
Renal insufficiency

vasodilating action on the smaller coronary vessels than with NTG, which was more active in the larger coronary arteries. Another trial successfully treated patients with immediate post–coronary bypass grafting hypertension with NP or intravenous NTG. Two conflicting trials of NP in the setting of acute MI were published in 1982. In the Veterans Administration cooperative study, NP offered no advantage to patients given a 48-h infusion of NP as opposed to placebo when the infusion was instituted a mean of 17 h after onset of chest pain. However, a retrospective analysis suggested that patients treated early (within 9 h of onset of symptoms) fared less well with NP than with placebo, whereas subjects treated later had a decreased mortality. It was speculated that the former group may have had lower left ventricular filling pressures during the first 1 or 2 days, and thus may have been exposed to an NP-induced risk of hypoperfusion of the coronary bed or a coronary steal phenomenon; the late-treated cohort presumably had more patients with left ventricular dysfunction and elevated filling pressures, and in these subjects NP would have been of benefit when compared with placebo. However, another study from the Netherlands demonstrated a decrease in mortality in acute MI patients randomized to NP. The reasons for the different results are unknown, although the latter study may have included a number of hypertensive subjects who derived additional benefits from NP and may have affected the final outcome. In any case, this dilemma has not been resolved, and there have not been subsequent confirming studies. Warnings about the use of NP in acute MI are not new, and current guidelines for the therapy of MI include intravenous NTG but not NP. Tables 9-6 and 9-7 list the indications and precautions that should accompany the use of NP.

Dosage

The infusion of NP should begin at 0.5 to 1 µg/kg per minute, increasing to no more than 10 µg/kg per minute. Most experts recommend reducing the

TABLE 9-7 Precautions in the Use of Nitroprusside
Exposure of nitroprusside solution to light
Prolonged infusion (>48 h)
Renal insufficiency
Infusion rates greater than 10 µg/kg/min
Measure thiocyanate levels in high-risk subjects (prolonged infusion, azotemia)

mean or systolic arterial pressure by 10%, thereby avoiding central aortic hypotension. Meticulous care must be given to the patient with actual or potential myocardial ischemia to prevent an excessive central aortic pressure decrease. NP must be given with appropriate precautions, including protection from ambient light, to prevent an accelerated release of NO and cyanide. The infusion should be limited in duration to 48 h because NP toxicity can occur over time as the cumulative dose increases. Renal and hepatic insufficiency are risk factors for adverse reactions to NP, with excessive concentrations of cyanide and thiocyanate, the metabolic byproducts of NP metabolism. Thiocyanate toxicity should be suspected in patients receiving NP who develop abdominal pain, mental status changes, or convulsions. Cyanide toxicity can be manifest by a reduction in cardiac output and metabolic or lactic acidosis. Methemoglobinemia can be observed as a relatively pure manifestation of NP toxicity.

CONCLUSION

The available nitrovasodilators remain important cardiovascular drugs for the management of patients with ischemic heart disease, emergent hypertension, and congestive heart failure. Their actions appear to simulate many of the normal vascular physiologic processes involved in vasodilation and have provided tremendous insights into the pathophysiology of vascular disease. Nevertheless, nitrate tolerance remains a fascinating and complex subject, and recent work implicating tolerance-induced endothelial dysfunction has raised more questions than answers. Informed and judicious use of the nitrates and NP should provide benefit for many individuals with cardiovascular disease.

ADDITIONAL READINGS

Abrams J: The role of nitrates in coronary heart disease. *Arch Intern Med* 155:357, 1995.

Abrams J: Beneficial actions of nitrates in cardiovascular disease. *Am J Cardiol* 77:31C, 1996.

Abrams J, Frishman WH: The organic nitrates and nitroprusside, in Frishman WH, Sonnenblick EH, Sica DA (eds): *Cardiovascular Pharmacotherapeutics*, 2nd ed. New York, McGraw-Hill, 2003, p 203.

Abrams J, Frishman WH, Bates SM, et al: Pharmacologic options for treatment of ischemic disease, in Antman EM (ed): *Cardiovascular Therapeutics*, 2nd ed. Philadelphia, WB Saunders, 2002, p 97.

ACC/AHA Guidelines for the Management of Patients with Acute Myocardial Infarction: A report of the American College of Cardiology/American Heart Association Task Force on Practice Guidelines (Committee on Management of Acute Myocardial Infarction). *Circulation* 100:1016, 1999.

Beltrame JF, Stewart S, Leslie S, et al: Resolution of ST segment elevation following intravenous administration of nitroglycerin and verapamil. *Am J Cardiol* 89:452, 2002.

Berkenboom G, Fontaine D, Unger P, et al: Absence of nitrate tolerance after long-term treatment with ramipril: An endothelium-dependent mechanism. *J Cardiovasc Pharmacol* 34:517, 1999.

Cohn JN, Franciosa JA, Francis GS, et al: Effect of short-term infusion of sodium nitroprusside on mortality rate in acute myocardial infarction complicated by left ventricular failure. *N Engl J Med* 306:1129, 1982.

Darius H: Role of nitrates for the therapy of coronary artery disease patients in the years beyond 2000. *J Cardiovasc Pharmacol* 34(suppl 2):S15, 1999.

Death AK, Nakhla S, McGrath KCY, et al: Nitroglycerin upregulates matrix metallo-proteinase expression in human macrophages. *J Am Coll Cardiol* 39:1943, 2002.

Diodati J, Theroux P, Latour J-G, et al: Effects of nitroglycerin at therapeutic doses on platelet aggregation in unstable angina pectoris and acute myocardial infarction. *Am J Cardiol* 66:683, 1996.

Elkayam U, Johnson JV, Shotan A, et al: Double-blind, placebo-controlled study to evaluate the effect of organic nitrates in patients with chronic heart failure treated with angiotensin-converting enzyme inhibition. *Circulation* 99:2652, 1999.

Flaherty JT: Role of nitrates in acute myocardial infarction. *Am J Cardiol* 70:436, 1992.

Fourth International Study of Infarct Survival Collaborative Group (ISIS-4): A randomized factorial trial assessing early oral captopril, oral mononitrate, and intravenous magnesium sulphate in 58,050 patients with suspected acute myocardial infarction. *Lancet* 345:669, 1995.

Fung H-L, Chung S-J, Bauer JA, et al: Biochemical mechanism of organic nitrate action. *Am J Cardiol* 70:4B, 1992.

Glasser S: Prospects for therapy of nitrate tolerance. *Lancet* 353:1545, 1999.

Gori T, Burstein JM, Ahmed S, et al: Folic acid prevents nitroglycerin-induced nitric oxide synthase dysfunction and nitrate tolerance. *Circulation* 104:1119, 2001.

Gruppo Italiano per lo Studio della Supravivenza nell Infarto Miocardico (GISSI-3): Effects of lisinopril and transdermal glyceryl trinitrate singly and together on 6-week mortality and ventricular function after acute myocardial infarction. *Lancet* 343: 1115, 1994.

Gunasekara NS, Noble S: Isosorbide 5-mononitrate. A review of a sustained-release formulation (Imdur) in stable angina pectoris. *Drugs* 57:261, 1999.

Harrison DG, Bates JN: The nitrovasodilators: New ideas about old drugs. *Circulation* 87:1461, 1993.

Ito Y, Isotani E, Mizuno Y, et al: Effective improvement of the cerebral vasospasm after subarachnoid hemorrhage with low-dose nitroglycerin. *J Cardiovasc Pharmacol* 35:45, 2000.

Kim D, Rybalkin SD, Pi X, et al: Upregulation of phosphodiesterase 1A1 expression is associated with the development of nitrate tolerance. *Circulation* 104:2338, 2001.

Knot UN, Novaro GM, Popović ZB, et al: Nitroprusside in critically ill patients with left ventricular dysfunction and aortic stenosis. *N Engl J Med* 348:1756, 2003.

Kowaluk E, Fung H-L: Pharmacology and pharmacokinetics of nitrates, in Abrams J, Pepine C, Thadani U (eds): *Medical Therapy of Ischemic Heart Disease: Nitrates, Beta Blockers and Calcium Antagonists.* Boston, Little Brown and Co, 1992, p 152.

Latini R, Staszewsky L, Maggioni AP, et al: Beneficial effects of angiotensin-converting enzyme inhibitor and nitrate association on left ventricular remodeling in patients with large acute myocardial infarction: The Delapril Remodeling after Acute Myocardial Infarction (DRAMI) trial. *Am Heart J* 146:133, 2003.

Münzel T, Bassenge E: Long-term angiotensin converting enzyme inhibition with high-dose enalapril retards nitrate tolerance in large epicardial arteries and prevents rebound coronary vasoconstriction in vivo. *Circulation* 93: 2052, 1996.

Parker JD, Gori T: Tolerance to the organic nitrates: New ideas, new mechanisms, continued mystery. *Circulation* 104:2263, 2001.

Prakash A, Markham A: Long-acting isosorbide mononitrate. *Drugs* 57:93, 1999.

Sage PR, de la Lande IS, Stafford I: Nitroglycerin tolerance in human vessels. Evidence for impaired nitroglycerin bioconversion. *Circulation* 102:2810, 2000.

Steering Committee, Transdermal Nitroglycerin Cooperative Study: Acute and chronic antianginal efficacy in continuous twenty-four hour application of transdermal nitroglycerin. *Am J Cardiol* 68:1263, 1991.

Webb DJ, Muirhead GJ, Wulff M, et al: Sildenafil citrate potentiates the hypotensive effect of nitric oxide donor drugs in male patients with stable angina. *J Am Coll Cardiol* 36:25, 2000.

Zile MR, Gaasch WH: Heart failure in aortic stenosis—Improving diagnosis and treatment. *N Engl J Med* 348:1735, 2003.

10 | Antiadrenergic Drugs with Central Action and Neuron Depletors

Lawrence R. Krakoff   *William H. Frishman*

Drugs that reduce arterial pressure by interrupting the sympathetic nervous system are among the oldest antihypertensive agents. One of the first such agents to be shown effective in clinical trials was reserpine, derived from *Rauwolfia serpentina*, i.e., of herbal origin. Medicinal chemistry and pharmacology led to the discovery of the autonomic ganglion blockers and guanethidine, all introduced before 1965. Methyldopa became available and widely prescribed in the 1960s. Clonidine, an α_2-receptor agonist, emerged in the 1970s; several similar drugs were then developed (guanabenz and guanfacine). Guanethidine was the first peripheral adrenergic neuron depletor. New neuron depletors were developed during the past few decades: bethanidine and guanadrel. Most of these drugs remain available for use in cardiovascular therapy, primarily as antihypertensive agents. The ganglionic blockers, however, are no longer available.

This chapter focuses primarily on two groups of antiadrenergic drugs: (1) those whose actions lie primarily within the central nervous system and (2) peripheral adrenergic neuron depletors. These drugs have been used to treat hypertension, but some have been studied in congestive heart failure or have properties useful in cardiac arrhythmia management. The use of these agents for noncardiovascular indications (mainly anesthesia and pain management) is not included in this chapter.

CENTRALLY ACTING AGENTS: RESERPINE, METHYLDOPA, AND α_2 AGONISTS

The major pharmacologic features of the centrally acting agents covered in this chapter are listed in Table 10-1. Most of the therapeutic effects of these drugs can be explained by effects within the brain's cardiovascular regulatory centers. Likewise, the predominant adverse effects of these agents are best related to their central action. Some other drug classes have minor central effects (the β-receptor blockers and some α_1-receptor blockers). These agents are discussed in other chapters.

Reserpine

Reserpine is a distinct antihypertensive drug that has central and peripheral actions. Once absorbed, reserpine enters central and peripheral adrenergic and serotoninergic neurons, where it specifically eliminates amine storage granules. This action causes irreversible depletion of neurotransmitters through intraneuronal metabolism by monoamine oxidase. Blood pressure falls due to the sustained deficit in catecholamine release. Reserpine is rapidly eliminated from the circulation; its metabolism is poorly characterized. However, because of the time necessary for regeneration of new intraneuronal amine storage

TABLE 10-1 Major Features of the Centrally Acting Antiadrenergic Drugs

Drug name	Mechanism of action	Usual dose range and frequency	More frequent adverse effects
Reserpine	Aminergic neuron depletor Effective at low doses with diuretic	0.05–0.1 mg	Sedation, fatigue, nasal congestion, depression
α-Methyldopa	Mixed action: inhibits dopa decarboxylase, false transmitter, Use generally limited to hypertension during pregnancy	250–500 mg 2 or 3 times daily	Fatigue, dizziness, positive Coombs test, rare hepatitis
α-Methyldopa ester	Same as above	IV: 250–500 mg q 6–8 h	Sedation
Clonidine oral	α_2 Agonist Withdrawal overshoots hypertension	0.1–0.3 mg 2 to 3 times daily	Fatigue, dry mouth
Clonidine TTS*	α_2 Agonist May be useful for less compliant patients	1 patch/wk	Skin reactions
Guanabenz	α_2 Agonist Withdrawal overshoots hypertension	4–16 mg 1 or 2 times daily	Fatigue, dry mouth
Guanfacine	α_2 Agonist Withdrawal overshoots hypertension	1–3 mg daily	Fatigue, dry mouth

*Transdermal delivery system.
Key: IV, intravenous.

granules, there is a prolonged pharmacologic effect. After administration of reserpine is stopped, it may take weeks or even months for full adrenergic neuronal functional recovery.

Reserpine is an effective antihypertensive agent but has many adverse effects. Fatigue, depression, nasal congestion, and gastric hyperacidity often are observed. Depression may occur insidiously months after initiation of treatment and can be severe, even leading to suicide. Reserpine causes salt and water retention, thereby offsetting its antihypertensive effect (pseudotolerance) and then requiring the addition of a diuretic for control of pressure. Early retrospective studies implicated reserpine in breast cancer, but data from prospective studies have shown only a weak association between reserpine and breast cancer.

At present, reserpine is rarely used as monotherapy for hypertension. In combination with a thiazide-type diuretic, low-dose reserpine (0.1 mg daily) is highly effective for the reduction of pressure, with an acceptable side effect experience. Reserpine was used as additional therapy to low-dose chlorthalidone in a treatment subgroup of the Systolic Hypertension in the Elderly Program (SHEP) trial. This study demonstrated the benefit of antihypertensive drug treatment for prevention of fatal and nonfatal cardiovascular diseases in elderly patients with isolated systolic hypertension.

Reserpine (0.05 to 0.2 mg/day) also was used as a second-line antihypertensive drug in the Antihypertensive and Lipid-Lowering Treatment to

Prevent Heart Attack Trial (ALLHAT) in combination with chlorthalidone, doxazosin, lisinopril, or amlodipine for maximizing blood pressure control.

α-Methyldopa

α-Methyldopa is an antiadrenergic, antihypertensive agent with multiple actions at central and peripheral sites. Originally developed as an inhibitor of dopa-decarboxylase, α-methyldopa was conceived as a drug that would inhibit catecholamine synthesis (by preventing the enzymatic conversion of dihydroxyphenylalanine, dopa, to dopamine by dopa-decarboxylase). However, this effect was far too small to account for methyldopa's antihypertensive effect because dopa-decarboxylase is not a rate-limiting enzyme but is usually present in excess in a variety of tissues. Subsequent studies led to the recognition that α-methyldopa could be converted to α-methyldopamine, a false neurotransmitter but also an α_2 agonist, with the central and peripheral actions of the other members of this group. More recently, it has been proposed that conversion of α-methyldopa to α-methyl epinephrine (by *N*-methylation) may also participate in this drug's hypotensive action. α-Methyldopa is effective for only a portion of the day after administration of a single oral dose. It is usually prescribed as a twice-a-day agent.

α-Methyldopa is an effective antihypertensive agent when given orally or intravenously. Prolonged treatment with α-methyldopa is often associated with salt and water retention, thus reversing the antihypertensive effect (pseudotolerance), which then requires addition of a diuretic agent. The intravenous formulation is an ester of the parent drug and has been used for hypertensive emergencies, including toxemia during pregnancy.

Adverse effects related to α-methyldopa are fatigue, somnolence, possible memory impairment, and diminished sexual function (reduced libido and impotence). Several of these effects are common to other centrally active agents. Unique to α-methyldopa, however, are (1) a positive Coombs test (owing to the appearance of an antibody directed against red cell Rh determinants), which occasionally causes significant hemolysis; (2) a drug-induced hepatitis with fever, eosinophilia, and increased serum levels of hepatic enzymes; and (3) drug-induced lupus. The acute drug-induced hepatitis is self-limited once α-methyldopa is discontinued. There have been several case reports and small series of patients with chronic hepatitis and even cirrhosis found after many years of exposure to α-methyldopa. Whether these cases were truly drug induced or the consequence of undetected viral hepatitis (e.g., before the discovery of hepatitis C virus) is not certain. One drug surveillance study has reported an association of α-methyldopa with acute pancreatitis.

At present, α-methyldopa is used as monotherapy or with hydralazine for pregnancy-related hypertension. Treatment of essential hypertension with α-methyldopa as a single agent has become uncommon. Although the combination of a thiazide-type diuretic with α-methyldopa can reduce blood pressure, there are few recent studies evaluating this approach in comparison with other strategies or for outcomes. Thus, α-methyldopa has become a "niche" drug for hypertension during pregnancy.

α_2-Receptor Agonists: Clonidine and Related Drugs

The classic α_2-receptor agonists have been well studied for their various effects. They reduce sympathetic tone within the brain stem by stimulating α_2

receptors on neurons of vasomotor centers that inhibit outflow of impulses to spinal preganglionic neurons. In addition, they may achieve their effect by stimulating recently described imidazole receptors. In peripheral postganglionic noradrenergic neurons, stimulation of presynaptic α_2 receptors diminishes release of transmitter—a feedback system for control of intrasynaptic norepinephrine concentration. Thus, α_2 agonists reduce arterial pressure by central and peripheral effects. However, at post- or nonsynaptic sites on cardiac or smooth muscle cells, α_2 receptors may be stimulated by α_2 agonists, thereby causing an increase in pressure. Thus, a transient rise in pressure may occur within the first hour after administering a single dose of clonidine. Thereafter, blood pressure falls to well below pretreatment levels in parallel with a demonstrable decrement in sympathetic neural function. Clonidine's pressor effect accounts for occasional reports of hypertensive crises due to massive overdose of the drug when used in anesthesia.

The reduction of sympathetic (noradrenergic) function due to administration of α_2-receptor agonists has been the basis of a clinically useful assessment, the clonidine suppression test. In this test, normal subjects and those with essential hypertension have a greater than 40% reduction in plasma norepinephrine 2 to 3 h after clonidine is given. Patients with pheochromocytomas have little change in plasma norepinephrine concentration after clonidine is given, thus providing the rationale for the clonidine suppression test as a diagnostic assessment for these tumors. Several forms of suspected neurogenic hypertension have been evaluated by the clonidine suppression test. Those with hypertension and neurovascular compression of the ventrolateral medulla oblongata (by magnetic resonance imaging) tend to have high baseline plasma norepinephrine when compared with those without vascular compression, but responses to clonidine are similar. In a small series of four patients with hypertension associated with lumbosacral paraplegia, clonidine suppression of norepinephrine was greater than 35% in three but less than 5% in one.

Clonidine is the prototype α_2 agonist. Guanabenz and guanfacine are similar to clonidine but have longer durations of action. All the α_2 agonists are effective antihypertensive drugs as monotherapy or in combination with a thiazide-type diuretic. Resting and exercise-induced blood pressure are decreased by these agents. Clonidine (0.1 to 0.3 mg twice daily) was a second-line antihypertensive drug in the ALLHAT. The available α_2 agonists have a similar pattern of adverse effects: sedation, dry mouth, and a tendency to overshoot or produce rebound hypertension on withdrawal. In sleep studies, clonidine was found to reduce rapid-eye movement sleep, presumably a detrimental effect, when compared with the beta blocker atenolol. Clonidine also has been studied in sleep apnea, with inconsistent effects. However, a case report described severe somnolence with respiratory acidosis associated with clonidine treatment of a patient with known sleep apnea syndrome. Yohimbine, the α_2-receptor antagonist, was given and was thought to be beneficial in reversing the coma.

α_2 Agonists are active as oral preparations. Clonidine, in addition, is effective as a transdermal delivery system (TTS), which releases medication at a relatively constant rate over 7 days. Some studies have associated clonidine TTS with fewer adverse effects when compared with tablets. This preparation may be useful for selected noncompliant patients who do not like to take pills. For patients already taking clonidine tablets and who must have surgery with general anesthesia, the TTS formulation can be used to maintain control of blood pressure and avoid rebound hypertension during the perioperative period, when medications cannot be given by mouth. Prolonged use of the TTS patch can cause a skin reaction severe enough that a change to alternative therapy becomes necessary.

Clonidine has been studied in congestive heart failure as a strategy to reduce the sympathetic activation often found in this disorder. Short-term studies have suggested that reduction of sympathetic activity by clonidine may be beneficial in congestive heart failure. There is, however, evidence that presynaptic downregulation of norepinephrine release by α_2 agonists is impaired in congestive heart failure, which may limit the effectiveness of clonidine as treatment. Outcome studies evaluating α_2 agonists in congestive heart failure have not been reported as of this writing.

In addition, oral clonidine has been shown to be effective in controlling rapid ventricular rates in patients with new-onset atrial fibrillation, with an efficacy comparable to that of standard agents.

PERIPHERAL NEURON DEPLETORS

Guanethidine, bethanidine, and guanadrel enter peripheral noradrenergic nerve terminals via amine uptake channels, where these drugs bind to norepinephrine storage vesicles, thus inhibiting transsynaptic release of transmitter. In addition, norepinephrine stores are depleted by displacement from vesicles and intraneuronal metabolism by monoamine oxidase. Cardiac and vascular postganglionic sympathetic neurons are depleted by these drugs. Unlike reserpine, the peripheral neuron depletors do not damage or eliminate storage vesicles. As a consequence, sympathetic neurotransmission returns to normal as drug concentration decreases, with dissociation of the drug–vesicle complex. Duration of action is longest for guanethidine, about 24 h, and shorter for bethanidine and guanadrel, 6 to 10 h. Usual doses of these drugs are given below.

- Guanethidine: 10 to 50 mg daily
- Bethanidine: 25 to 50 mg once or twice daily
- Guanadrel: 10 to 50 mg twice daily

Reduction of sympathetic transmitter release during treatment with the neuron depletors affects basal or resting blood pressure but is much more prominent during standing or exercise, when sympathetic activity is normally increased. Orthostatic hypotension, exercise weakness, and even syncope have often been observed during treatment. It is therefore necessary to monitor supine and standing blood pressures when these agents are used as antihypertensive therapy. Bradycardia and possibly heart block may occur as a result of diminished cardiac adrenergic transmission. Other effects of reduced peripheral sympathetic function that may be observed during treatment with these agents are (1) retrograde ejaculation, (2) diarrhea-like change in bowel function, and (3) loss of normal adrenergic pupillary responses. Because the peripheral neuron depletors enter the nerve terminal via norepinephrine uptake, their action is prevented by drugs such as cocaine or tricyclic antidepressants (e.g., imipramine). This unique drug interaction accounts for the reversal of blood pressure control in patients receiving the peripheral neuron depletors when tricyclics are given concurrently.

The peripheral neuron depletors may be effective for treatment of hypertension as monotherapy or with low-dose diuretics. This drug class has not been studied in congestive heart failure. In general, because of their prominent adverse effects, the peripheral neuron depletors have nearly disappeared from clinical use in the United States.

EFFECTIVENESS OF CENTRALLY ACTING DRUGS AND PERIPHERAL NEURON DEPLETORS

Assessment of antihypertensive drugs includes, as a primary measure, whether they have been found to prevent cardiovascular mortality and morbidity in randomized clinical trials. In this context, reserpine and α-methyldopa deserve attention. Reserpine in combination with a thiazide diuretic and hydralazine as opposed to placebo reduced major trial end points in the Veterans Administration trial for severe and moderate hypertension. In the SHEP trial, reserpine was a second-step drug given in addition to chlorthalidone for the treatment of isolated systolic hypertension in the elderly. Methyldopa was used for active therapy in combination with a thiazide diuretic in several clinical trials of mild to moderate hypertension that are now considered pivotal in establishing the benefit of antihypertensive drug treatment. However, there is insufficient evidence to conclude that reserpine or α-methyldopa is beneficial as monotherapy or is superior to other drug classes when used in addition to a diuretic. The other available centrally acting agents, the α$_2$ agonists, have been used infrequently in the large, randomized clinical outcome trials.

The ganglionic blockers and guanethidine have been evaluated for treatment of severe or malignant hypertension. Observational studies have suggested that reduction of pressure in such patients is beneficial in comparison with historical controls or untreated patients by altering the rapidly fatal course of those with the highest blood pressure levels and evidence of extensive target-organ damage.

SPECIAL CONSIDERATIONS

Pregnancy

Few antihypertensive drugs have been thoroughly studied in pregnancy. The cumulative observations with α-methyldopa over the past decades suggest that it is a safe and effective agent for use in pregnancy-induced hypertension or for treatment of hypertensive women who become pregnant. In these settings, α-methyldopa has the legitimacy of an extensive but largely uncontrolled clinical experience. However, the value of drug treatment for mild to moderate hypertension in pregnancy has never been fully established by randomized clinical trials. Recent systematic reviews focusing on this issue have implied that this issue remains unresolved.

Alcohol Withdrawal

The cessation of alcohol intake in those who drink to excess, i.e., alcohol withdrawal syndrome, is a hyperadrenergic state in which tachycardia, cardiac arrhythmias, and hypertensive episodes may accompany the agitation and other signs and symptoms of the disorder. The cardiovascular features of the alcohol withdrawal syndrome are due to centrally mediated activation of the sympathetic nervous system. α_2 Receptors may be downregulated because the hypotensive response to clonidine during early alcohol withdrawal is less than that of age-matched controls. Nonetheless, clonidine may be effective for reducing blood pressure and heart rate, if needed, during treatment of alcohol withdrawal. The sedative effect of clonidine is also beneficial in this situation but of lesser magnitude than that of the benzodiazepines.

SUMMARY OF CURRENT AND RECOMMENDED USE

Most of the approved antihypertensive drugs reviewed in this chapter will have little or no role to play in the management of most patients with essential hypertension, having been largely replaced by more recently developed drug classes. However, the long-term safety record for these drugs cannot be discounted. If hypertensive patients are well controlled on these older agents and have no related adverse effects, there is no compelling rationale for changing medication.

ADDITIONAL READINGS

Aggarwal A, Esler MD, Socratous F, Kaye DM: Evidence for functional presynaptic alpha-2 adrenoceptors and their down-regulation in human heart failure. *J Am Coll Cardiol* 37:1246, 2001.

ALLHAT Officers and Coordinators: Major outcomes in high risk hypertensive patients randomized to angiotensin converting enzyme inhibitor therapy or calcium channel blockers versus diuretics. *JAMA* 288:2981, 2002.

Azevedo ER, Newton GE, Parker JD: Cardiac and systemic sympathetic activity in response to clonidine in human heart failure. *J Am Coll Cardiol* 33:186, 1999.

Gavras I, Manolis AJ, Gavras H: The alpha$_2$-adrenergic receptors in hypertension and heart failure: Experimental and clinical studies. *J Hypertens* 19:2115, 2001.

Grossman E, Goldstein DS, Hoffman A, Keiser HR: Glucogan and clonidine testing in the diagnosis of pheochromocytoma. *Hypertension* 17:733, 1991.

Hoffman BB, Taylor P: Neurotransmission: the autonomic and somatic motor nervous sytems, in Hardman JG, Limbird LE (eds): *Goodman & Gilman's the Pharmacological Basis of Therapeutics*, 10th ed. New York, McGraw-Hill, 2001, p 115.

Krakoff LR: Clinical trials, in *Management of the Hypertensive Patient*. New York, Churchill Livingstone, 1995, p 33.

Krakoff LR: Antiadrenergic drugs with central action and neuron depletors, in Frishman WH, Sonnenblick EH, Sica DA (eds): *Cardiovascular Pharmacotherapuetics*, 2nd ed. New York, McGraw-Hill, 2003, p 215.

Kronig B, Pittrow DB, Kirch W, et al: Different concepts in first-line treatment of essential hypertension. Comparison of a low-dose reserpine-thiazide combination with nitrendipine monotherapy. German Reserpine in Hypertension Study Group. *Hypertension* 29:651, 2001.

Lindheimer MD, Akbari A: Hypertension in pregnant women, in Oparil S, Weber MA (eds): *Hypertension: A Companion to Brenner and Rector's the Kidney*. Philadelphia, Saunders, 2000, p 688.

Mashour NH, Lin GI, Frishman WH: Herbal medicine for the treatment of cardiovascular disease. *Arch Intern Med* 158:2225, 1998.

Materson BJ: Central and peripheral sympatholytics, in Izzo JL, Black HR (eds): *Hypertension Primer*, 3rd ed. Dallas, American Heart Association, 2003, p 423.

Materson BJ, Reda DJ, Cushman WC, et al: Single-drug therapy for hypertension in men: A comparison of six antihypertensive agents with placebo. *N Engl J Med* 328:914, 1993.

Materson BJ, Reda DJ, Cushman WC, Henderson WG: Results of combination antihypertensive therapy after failure of each of the components. Department of Veterans

Affairs Cooperative Study Group on Anti-hypertensive Agents. *J Hum Hypertens* 9:791, 1995.

Oates JA, Brown NJ: Antihypertensive agents and the drug therapy of hypertension, in Hardman JG, Limbird LE (eds): *Goodman & Gilman's the Pharmacological Basis of Therapeutics*, 10th ed. New York, McGraw-Hill, 2001, p 871.

SHEP Cooperative Research Group: Prevention of stroke by antihypertensive drug treatment in older persons with isolated systolic hypertension: Final results of the Systolic Hypertension in the Elderly Program (SHEP). *JAMA* 265:3255, 1991.

Simpson CS, Ghali WA, Sanfilippo AJ, et al: Clinical assessment of clonidine in the treatment of new-onset rapid atrial fibrillation: A prospective, randomized clinical trial. *Am Heart J* 142:300, 2001.

Taler SJ: Treatment of pregnant hypertensive patients, in Izzo JL Jr, Black HR (eds): *Hypertension Primer*, 3rd ed. Dallas, American Heart Association. 2003, p 491.

Taylor P: Agents acting at the neuromuscular junction and autonomic ganglia, in Hardman JG, Limbird LE (eds): *Goodman & Gilman's the Pharmacological Basis of Therapeutics*, 10th ed. New York, McGraw-Hill, 2001, p 193.

11 | Nonspecific Antihypertensive Vasodilators

Lawrence R. Krakoff   William H. Frishman

Increased systemic vascular resistance has been considered a hemodynamic characteristic of arterial hypertension. In established essential hypertension and various forms of secondary hypertension, raised systemic vascular resistance is nearly always found when diastolic pressure is elevated. Nonetheless, reduced compliance of medium-size and large arteries may contribute to increased systolic pressure and wide pulse pressures in middle-aged and elderly hypertensives. Increased systemic vascular resistance and reduced arterial compliance (increased stiffness) may be due in part to activation of vascular smooth muscle. Thus, it is not surprising that drugs that relax vascular smooth muscle as a direct effect, i.e., vasodilators, specifically hydralazine, were among the first to be developed for treatment of hypertension. Other vasodilators, minoxidil and diazoxide, more recently defined as K(ATP) channel hyperpolarizers, have been developed and have found some use as antihypertensive agents.

It became evident during the initial assessment of vasodilators that their antihypertensive effect led to activation of sympathetic baroreflexes, with tachycardia and increased cardiac output, in compensation for the reduction in peripheral (systemic) vascular resistance. Further, fluid-volume retention and activation of the renin-angiotensin system were a consequence of unopposed nonspecific systemic arteriolar vasodilation. By the 1970s, the orally active nonselective vasodilators became recognized as third-line antihypertensive drugs to be used only in combination with diuretics and antiadrenergic agents, usually β-receptor blockers, as the triple-drug regimen for severe hypertension. With the availability of angiotensin-converting enzyme (ACE) inhibitors, angiotensin II type 1 receptor antagonists, and calcium-entry blockers, hydralazine and K(ATP) hyperpolarizers have become less used as third- to fourth-line drugs. There are, however, a few specific conditions when these vasodilators can play more specific or important therapeutic roles, as described in this chapter.

PHARMACOLOGY AND CLASSIFICATION OF THE NONSPECIFIC VASODILATORS

Hydralazine

1-Hydrazinophthalazine (hydralazine) was one of the first orally available active vasodilators. The hydrazine (HN-NH2) in position 1 of the double-ringed phthalazine confers activity as a vasodilator. Hydralazine is a direct arteriolar vasodilator, independent of any receptor blockade. Its mechanism of action remains somewhat unclear but seems to be dependent on endothelial cells and may be related to the formation of nitric oxide and/or hyperpolarization of vascular smooth muscle cells and interruption of intracellular calcium action.

Hydralazine lowers systemic vascular resistance with activation of sympathetic reflexes, which increases heart rate, and cardiac output on a neurogenic basis. The reflex-mediated changes in cardiac function after hydralazine treatment can be prevented by β-receptor antagonists. Chronic administration of hydralazine stimulates renin release, thereby raising plasma renin activity. Salt and water retention with gain in weight are also observed. Whereas the half-life of hydralazine, as reflected by plasma concentrations, is 1 to 2 h, the antihypertensive effect may last for 6 to 12 h. The drug should be taken two to three times daily at 8- to 12-h intervals.

After absorption from the gastrointestinal tract, hydralazine is acetylated in the liver to different degrees. Slow and fast acetylators are represented almost equally in the population of the United States. Hydralazine is relatively less bioavailable for slow acetylators, who require higher oral doses for an equal antihypertensive effect. Extrahepatic metabolism also occurs and accounts for the drug's elimination after reaching the circulation.

Adverse effects of hydralazine may be divided into two categories: (1) those related to the hemodynamic effect of the drug and (2) those specifically linked to its unique biochemical characteristics. Headaches, flushing, tachycardia, palpitations, angina-like chest discomfort or true angina of myocardial ischemia, dizziness, and orthostatic hypotension are the consequences of the vasodilating action of hydralazine and the significant sympathetic reflex activation as a physiologic response. In contrast, the hydralazine lupus syndrome, serum-sickness like reaction, hemolytic anemia, and glomerulonephritis syndromes seem best related to hydralazine itself and are more likely to occur in slow acetylators, often white women. Many patients treated with hydralazine who develop positive antinuclear antibodies do not proceed to symptomatic lupus. However, with so many alternative drugs, there is little basis for continuing antinuclear antibody-positive patients on hydralazine in most situations. Vitamin B_6 (pyridoxal-responsive)-dependent polyneuropathy is a rare adverse effect of sustained hydralazine administration, explainable by a direct chemical combination of the drug with pyridoxine, thereby reducing supply of the cofactor for many enzymes. Hydralazine lupus syndromes and polyneuropathy usually occur during treatment with doses higher than 50 mg daily.

Hydralazine is effective for essential hypertension, pregnancy-induced hypertension, and congestive heart failure.

For treatment of essential hypertension, hydralazine is a third- or fourth-line drug to be added when a diuretic and a beta blocker and/or ACE inhibitor have not achieved control. It was the third-line drug per protocol used in the Antihypertensive and Lipid-Lowering to Prevent Heart Attack Trial for blood pressure control in hypertensive patients. Although hydralazine must be given two to three times a day (thus hindering compliance), the drug is inexpensive and may be necessary for use in those health care systems that have limited financial resources. Otherwise, the once-a-day, long-acting calcium-channel blockers (nifedipine in controlled-release formulations, amlodipine, and isradipine) have largely replaced hydrala-zine in the multidrug combinations used to treat more severe or refractory hypertension.

Intramuscular or intravenous hydralazine remains useful for the treatment of hypertensive emergencies and severe pregnancy-induced hypertension, including toxemia. Its value for mild to moderate hypertension in pregnancy is not established. In studies of congestive heart failure, before the availability of the ACE inhibitors, hydralazine therapy used alone and in combination with isosorbide dinitrate was beneficial, especially when compared with the α_1-receptor blocker prazosin. The advent of the ACE inhibitors and other strategies for the treatment of heart failure has rendered the use of hydralazine somewhat obsolete. Studies need to be done to determine whether there is any additional benefit from giving hydralazine to patients with heart failure already receiving diuretics, digoxin, ACE inhibitors, or angiotensin-receptor blockers and beta blockers.

ATP-K1 Channel Openers: Minoxidil and Diazoxide

The powerful arteriolar vasodilators minoxidil and diazoxide were developed in the 1970s for use in the treatment of severe and refractory hypertension and hypertensive emergencies. Minoxidil became a part of the triple-drug regimen for treatment of severe hypertension, especially for patients who were unresponsive or had significant adverse reactions to hydralazine. Diazoxide, given as an intravenous bolus, was used for hypertensive emergencies as an alternative to sodium nitroprusside.

Minoxidil is a prodrug that becomes active with sulfation of an N-O site by a hepatic sulfotransferase. Minoxidil and diazoxide activate K(ATPase) channels, causing hyperpolarization of smooth muscle cell membranes with relaxation (vasodilation). Other K(ATPase) channel activators—nicorandil, cromokalim, aprikalim, bimakalim, and emakalim—have been assessed as coronary artery vasodilators. Some of the ATP-K1 channel activators inhibit release of insulin from pancreatic islet β cells (long recognized as an effect of diazoxide), thus antagonizing the effect of the sulfonylureas at the K1 channel. Experimental studies have suggested that diazoxide is the most potent agent for inhibition of hypoglycemia due to a sulfonylurea, with pinacidil having a detectable but lesser effect.

ATP-K1 channel openers cause a profound nonselective reduction in systemic vascular resistance. Sympathetic reflexes are activated, causing tachycardia, increased cardiac output, and an increase in plasma norepinephrine. β-Receptor blockade diminishes the degree of tachycardia and the increase in cardiac output. These drugs cause fluid retention in part by activation of the renin—angiotensin-aldosterone system (pseudotolerance) and by intrarenal proximal and distal tubular mechanisms. Sustained use of minoxidil may lead to increased pulmonary artery pressures, i.e., pulmonary hypertension, perhaps the result of the prolonged hyperdynamic state resulting from reduced precapillary vascular resistance and an arteriovenous shuntlike state. Other side effects of minoxidil include adverse effects on myocardial repolarization and idiosyncratic peripheral effusions.

The currently available ATP-K1 channel openers, minoxidil and diazoxide, are used only for severe hypertension when other agents are ineffective. At a dose of 5 to 20 mg once or twice daily, minoxidil in combination with a β-receptor blocker and a potent diuretic (most often, a loop-active agent such as furosemide) is almost always effective in reducing blood pressure. Weight gain, despite diuretic use, often occurs. Hair growth is inevitable and although cosmetically disfiguring to some, can be controlled with careful use of depilatories.

Diazoxide is given by bolus injection or rapid intravenous infusion for hypertensive emergencies at doses of 150 to 300 mg (or reduced doses in children). Hypotension can occur because the response to a given dose is unpredictable. Prolonged use of diazoxide often causes hyperglycemia due to inhibition of insulin release, an effect explained by activation of ATP-K1 channels.

SUMMARY: EFFECTIVENESS AND CURRENT USE OF VASODILATORS

Hydralazine remains an effective third- or fourth-line drug for treatment of some patients with refractory hypertension, pregnancy-related severe hypertension, and perhaps selected patients with congestive heart failure. Minoxidil's use as an antihypertensive is limited to those with the most refractory hypertension who are willing to deal with the burdensome adverse effect of hair growth. Diazoxide is seldom used for hypertensive emergencies, with more promising agents now available.

ADDITIONAL READINGS

ALLHAT Officers and Coordinators: Major outcomes in high-risk hypertensive patients randomized to angiotensin converting inhibitors or calcium channel blockers versus diuretics. The Antihypertensive and Lipid Lowering Treatment to Prevent Heart Attack Trial (ALLHAT). *JAMA* 288:2981, 2002.

Awad K, Ali P, Frishman WH, Tejani N: Pharmacologic approaches for the management of systemic hypertension in pregnancy. *Heart Dis* 2:124, 2000.

Cohn JN, Johnson G, Ziesche S, et al: A comparison of enalapril with hydralazine-isosorbide dinitrate in the treatment of chronic congestive heart failure. *N Engl J Med* 325:303, 1991.

Duley L, Henderson-Smart DJ: Drugs for rapid treatment of very high blood pressure during pregnancy. *Cochrane Database Syst Rev* 2000.

Frishman WH, Lee BY, Galandauer I, Phan AH: Potassium-channel openers and sodium/hydrogen—Channel effectors, in Frishman WH, Sonnenblick EH, Sica DA (eds): *Cardiovascular Pharmacotherapeutics*, 2nd ed. New York, McGraw-Hill, 2003, p 481.

Krakoff LR: Nonspecific antihypertensive vasodilators, in Frishman WH, Sonnenblick EH, Sica DA (eds): *Cardiovascular Pharmacotherapeutics*, 2nd ed. New York, McGraw-Hill, 2003, p 221.

McVeigh GE, Bratteli CW, Morgan DJ, et al: Age-related abnormalities in arterial compliance identified by pressure pulse contour analysis: Aging and arterial compliance. *Hypertension* 33:1392, 1999.

Oates JA, Brown NJ: Antihypertensive agents and the drug therapy of hypertension, in Hardman JG, Limbird LE, Gilman AG (eds): *Goodman & Gilman's the Pharmacological Basis of Therapeutics*, 10th ed. New York, McGraw-Hill, 2001, p 871.

Seedat YK: Hypertension in developing nations in Sub-Saharan Africa. *J Hum Hypertens* 14:739, 2001.

12 | Antiarrhythmic Drugs

Tatjana N. Sljapic   Peter R. Kowey
Eric L. Michelson

Cardiac arrhythmias form a spectrum from clinically insignificant rhythms to life-threatening and lethal arrhythmias. Effective pharmacologic treatment of arrhythmias requires an understanding of the underlying mechanism of arrhythmia in addition to the pharmacokinetics, pharmacodynamics, and electropharmacology of available antiarrhythmic medications. Whereas mechanisms have been established with some certainty for a number of arrhythmias, for many, the mechanisms remain to be elucidated. Interrelationships between cardiac anatomy, nature and extent of structural heart disease, severity of functional impairment, cellular electrophysiology, metabolic fluxes, and factors such as ischemia and autonomic state are only beginning to be understood. Moreover, a profound revolution in our understanding of electrophysiology and electropharmacology is just emerging, based on major advances in genomics and molecular cardiology. Moreover, the interface of advances in diagnostic techniques, interventional procedures, and devices must be integrated into any consideration of antiarrhythmic drugs in clinical practice. With these diverse factors acting within each patient, it should come as no surprise that antiarrhythmic drug action is often unpredictable and must be applied empirically to individual patients.

CLASSIFICATION

Several different classifications of antiarrhythmic drugs have been proposed. A useful classification scheme should relate drug class, cellular electrophysiologic effects, and utility of various antiarrhythmic agents in specific clinical situations. Currently, the most widely used classification system is a modification of the one proposed by Vaughn Williams (Table 12-1). It classifies drugs according to their effects on action potentials in individual cells. In this scheme, class I drugs block sodium channels responsible for the fast response in atrial, ventricular, and Purkinje tissues and depress conduction velocity. Class I drugs are further divided into three subclasses based on (1) the kinetics of association and dissociation of the drug with the sodium channel, (2) the strength of channel blockade, and (3) the effects on repolarization. Class II drugs are β-adrenergic receptor antagonists. Class III agents prolong cardiac repolarization, predominantly by blocking potassium channels during phases 2 and 3 of the action potential, thereby increasing tissue refractoriness. Class IV drugs block calcium channels and depress the slow response in sinus nodal, atrioventricular (AV) nodal, and perhaps other cells. Admittedly, such a classification is a considerable oversimplification and does not account for autonomic nervous system effects or the action of agents such as digoxin or adenosine, for example, all of which need to be considered in discussing antiarrhythmic drugs. In addition, it has become clear that one antiarrhythmic drug may have multiple effects on cardiac cells. For example, sotalol has β-blocking activity (class II) and significantly prolongs the action potential duration (class III). Amiodarone has been shown to have class I, II, III, and IV effects and perhaps other effects. Similarly, individual stereoisomers of

TABLE 12-1 Modified Vaughn Williams Classification of
Antiarrhythmic Drugs

Class	Main electrophysiologic properties	Examples
I		
Ia	Sodium channel blockade	Quinidine
	Intermediate channel kinetics	Procainamide
	Repolarization lengthened	Disopyramide
Ib	Sodium channel blockade	Lidocaine
	Rapid channel kinetics	Mexiletine
		Tocainide
Ic	Sodium channel blockade	Flecainide
	Slow channel kinetics	Propafenone
		Moricizine
II	β-Adrenergic blockade	Propranolol
		Esmolol
		Acebutolol
III	Potassium channel blockade	Sotalol*
	Sodium channel activation	Amiodarone
		Ibutilide
		Dofetilide
IV	Calcium channel blockade	Verapamil
		Diltiazem

*Also has major class II properties.

drugs may have diverse effects. For example, the dextro isomer of sotalol possesses class III activity with only minimal β-blocking activity, whereas the levo isomer possesses β-blocking and class III activities. Further, many drugs undergo metabolism to electrophysiologically active metabolites that may have electrophysiologic effects that differ from those of the parent compound. Procainamide, a class Ia drug, is metabolized in the liver to N-acetylpro-cainamide (NAPA), a drug with significant class III effects. A more recent classification scheme, called the Sicilian gambit, attempts to relate the various clinical effects of antiarrhythmic drugs to specific anatomic or physiologic weak points of target arrhythmias based on an understanding of ion channels and receptors and modulators of membrane activity. Although scientifically based and clinically oriented and therefore more appealing, it is not clear that this new classification will be more useful than the Vaughn Williams classification.

Successful clinical application of antiarrhythmic agents requires not only an understanding of the cellular electrophysiology of the drugs and a thorough understanding of their pharmacology but also knowledge of drug–drug interactions, hemodynamic effects, and the ancillary properties of these agents. Failure to consider these factors often results in drug inefficacy or toxicity. This chapter presents most antiarrhythmic drugs currently available in the United States. The pharmacology, electrophysiology, pharmacokinetics, antiarrhythmic effects, drug interactions, hemodynamic properties, side effects, indications, and dosing are presented. A complete discussion of these agents is beyond the scope of this chapter, and data for recently released drugs are often incomplete and based to a large measure on animal data and preliminary data from clinical studies. Adverse effects reported for new agents represent those effects seen in highly selected patient populations and are subject to investigator interpretation; they may not be representative of those effects seen in clinical practice. Moreover, virtually all antiarrhythmic drugs have the potential to depress automaticity, conduction, and contractility; all have potential proarrhythmic effects. One characteristic form of proarrhythmia is the occurrence of polymorphic ventricular tachycardia in association with QT prolongation, known as *torsades de pointes*. In addition, in many cases, there is relatively little information available on the effects of various drugs on abnormal myocardium or in patients with more advanced cardiac pathologies.

Antiarrhythmic drugs also must be considered potential cardiac toxins. A physician treating a patient with an arrhythmia hopes the drug is more toxic to tissue involved with the arrhythmia than to the rest of the heart or the patient. Often this is not the case, as the therapeutic index of these drugs can be quite low. In addition, noncardiac side effects are frequent. Achievement of therapeutic drug levels does not guarantee efficacy or eliminate the risk of toxicity. Further, agents effective for the acute management of arrhythmias may not be effective for chronic prophylaxis. The failure to reduce or paradoxically increase mortality also exists with antiarrhythmic drugs, as demonstrated by the Cardiac Arrhythmia Suppression Trial (CAST). Thus, antiarrhythmic therapy should be used cautiously and ideally should be reserved for those situations that significantly affect a patient's duration or quality of life. At the very least, it is incumbent upon practitioners to have a knowledge of the full prescribing information for drugs approved for use in the United States to maximize the chance of benefit and minimize the risk of harm. For most drugs, only limited information is available in special populations, such as pediatric and pregnant patients, and additional caution is warranted.

OVERVIEW OF OPTIMAL ANTIARRHYTHMIC MANAGEMENT

Although a complete discussion of the clinical use of antiarrhythmic drugs is beyond the scope of this chapter, the following generalizations for commonly occurring arrhythmias may be made.

Atrial Fibrillation

Atrial fibrillation (AF) is the most common sustained tachyarrhythmia encountered in clinical practice. Management goals include (1) prevention of thromboembolism and stroke, (2) control of ventricular rate, and (3) restoration and maintenance of sinus rhythm. Consensus guidelines have been published that provide a framework for the evidence-based management of patients with AF. Almost all patients with AF—paroxysmal, persistent, or permanent—should be anticoagulated with warfarin to reduce the risk of thromboembolism. Exceptions include those patients with a contraindication to warfarin and those younger than 65 years with no structural heart disease (lone AF). Aspirin therapy may be useful for patients with a contraindication to warfarin. Control of ventricular rate by slowing impulse conduction through the AV node has been achieved for longer than a century with digitalis preparations. Although effective at rest, digitalis is unable to control ventricular rate adequately during exercise or other clinical states with elevated levels of catecholamines. In many patients, better control may be achieved by using β-blocking agents or calcium channel blockers such as verapamil or diltiazem. Intravenous agents such as esmolol or diltiazem can be used to rapidly achieve rate control; longer-acting drugs can then be used for chronic therapy. Other antiarrhythmics, such as class Ic drugs and amiodarone, also slow the ventricular rate. Patients with excessive tachycardia due to inadequate rate control (average heart rate over the day faster than 80 beats/min and the maximum heart rate greater than 110% of the maximum predicted heart rate for that patient) may develop cardiomyopathy with progression to congestive heart failure.

Patients whose heart rates are uncontrollable when using combinations of agents (i.e., digoxin and verapamil or propranolol) should be considered for catheter ablative techniques and permanent pacemaker implantation. Antiarrhythmic drugs are useful to restore sinus rhythm and lessen the duration between episodes of AF. Agents used for these purposes include class Ia drugs (quinidine, procainamide, and disopyramide); class Ic drugs (propafenone and flecainide); class II agents; and class III agents (sotalol, amiodarone, and dofetilide). In general, antiarrhythmic drugs do not eliminate recurrent episodes of AF but can increase the duration of sinus rhythm between recurrences. β-blocking drugs are especially useful for this purpose in patients immediately after cardiac surgery. Class III agents (amiodarone, sotalol, and dofetilide) are being used more frequently for control of AF. Ibutilide, a class III agent, is used in bolus fashion to chemically cardiovert patients to sinus rhythm. It has been effective in approximately 40% to 70% of patients. Nonpharmacologic techniques for control of AF are rapidly being developed and include radiofrequency catheter ablation/isolation of pulmonary vein foci, catheter-based or surgical MAZE procedure, and tachy-brady device-based therapies. A large multicenter study has been conducted by the National Institutes of Health to determine whether optimized antiarrhythmic drug therapy administered to maintain sinus rhythm in patients having episodes of AF or atrial flutter (AFL) has an impact on total mortality and disabling stroke when compared with optimized therapy that merely controls heart rate in patients with AF or AFL [Atrial Fibrillation Follow-up Investigation of Rhythm Management (AFFIRM)]. The results indicated that in these selected patients who tolerated AF sufficiently well that they were candidates for rate control, a strategy of rhythm control with the currently available antiarrhythmic drugs, did not have better outcomes. Effective anticoagulation was important for reduction of stroke risk with both approaches. Among available treatments, amiodarone was the most effective in maintaining sinus rhythm.

Atrial Flutter

In many ways, management of AFL is similar to that of AF. Acute control of ventricular rate is usually achieved through intravenous therapy using a β-blocking agent, such as esmolol or propranolol, or a calcium channel blocking drug, such as verapamil or diltiazem. Infusions of esmolol or diltiazem may be preferred due to the short half-life, which permits finer control of ventricular rate with a faster offset in case hypotension or excessive bradycardia develops. Chronic control of ventricular rate with AFL is difficult, but similar types of agents, given orally, are commonly used. Digoxin alone is rarely sufficient except in patients with intrinsic AV nodal dysfunction. Direct current (DC) cardioversion and atrial overdrive pacing are the most rapid methods used to restore sinus rhythm, although pharmacologic conversion may become more frequent in the future. Ibutilide appears uniquely able to rapidly terminate established AFL in most patients. The risks of embolization and stroke after conversion from AFL appear to be less than with AF, although most clinicians also anticoagulate patients with AFL. Oral antiarrhythmic drugs—such as quinidine, procainamide, disopyramide, sotalol, amiodarone, dofetilide, flecainide, moricizine, and propafenone—may be used to restore and maintain sinus rhythm. Particular care must be used when administering class Ia or Ic agents to patients with AFL. These drugs may slow the atrial rate, whereas the anticholinergic effects of some of these agents may facilitate AV nodal conduction, resulting in an acceleration of ventricular rate. Occasionally, 1:1 conduction of the AFL impulse may occur, resulting in a ventricular rate between 220 and 250 beats/min, which may cause hemodynamic compromise. This complication may be averted by ensuring adequate AV nodal blockade before instituting therapy with these agents. Amiodarone slows AV conduction in addition to other antiarrhythmic properties and may be used as a single agent. Administration of adenosine to patients with AFL will increase AV block, thereby allowing visualization of flutter waves. AV conduction may paradoxically improve after adenosine administration and has caused 1:1 AV conduction. Nonpharmacologic therapy for AFL is increasingly being used. Radiofrequency catheter ablation of the isthmus of atrial tissue between the tricuspid valve and inferior vena cava annulus is effective in preventing recurrences of AFL. Alternatively, for intractable cases, ablation of the AV junction to create complete heart block with insertion of a permanent pacemaker may be performed.

AV Nodal Reentrant Tachycardia

After AF and AFL, AV nodal reentrant tachycardia is the most common form of supraventricular tachycardia. This arrhythmia is caused by a reentrant circuit within the AV node and perinodal tissues. Therefore pharmacologic therapies are directed toward the AV node. Acute management includes vagal maneuvers such as carotid sinus massage or Valsalva. Administration of adenosine or verapamil intravenously will universally terminate this arrhythmia. Similarly, intravenous β blockers, diltiazem, or verapamil can be effective. Agents useful for long-term pharmacologic management include digoxin, β-adrenergic-receptor antagonists, and calcium channel antagonists such as verapamil or diltiazem. In unusual cases propafenone, flecainide, or amiodarone may be useful. Patients with this arrhythmia are also effectively being treated with radiofrequency catheter modification of the AV nodal slow pathway.

AV Reentrant Tachycardia (Wolff-Parkinson-White Syndrome)

Patients with Wolff-Parkinson-White (WPW) syndrome have an anatomic fiber of myocardium that directly connects the atria and ventricles. This fiber may conduct cardiac impulses unidirectionally from atria to ventricles or from the ventricles to atria, but bidirectional impulse conduction is also common. Because of the presence of dual pathways (the normal AV conduction system being the antegrade or retrograde limb) for impulse conduction from atria to ventricles, reentrant arrhythmias are possible. The most common tachycardia, orthodromic reciprocating tachycardia, uses the bypass tract in a retrograde (ventriculoatrial) direction and generally results in a narrow QRS tachycardia. AF or AFL commonly occurs in conjunction with the WPW syndrome; if the accessory pathway is capable of antegrade (AV) conduction, an irregular rhythm with wide and narrow QRS complexes, often at rapid rates (if the antegrade effective refractory period of the accessory pathway is short), will occur. Rarely, such patients will develop ventricular fibrillation (VF) from exceedingly rapid ventricular rates. The least common arrhythmia, antidromic reciprocating tachycardia, uses the bypass tract in an antegrade direction and results in a regular wide complex arrhythmia resembling ventricular tachycardia (VT). Any of these arrhythmias should be terminated by using synchronized DC cardioversion if hemodynamic collapse is present. Patients with a narrow QRS tachycardia are best treated with vagal maneuvers followed, if necessary, by intravenous adenosine, esmolol, diltiazem, or verapamil. Caution should be used with adenosine in patients with known WPW syndrome because adenosine may produce AF. If rapid antegrade conduction over the bypass tract is possible, hemodynamic collapse may occur. A DC defibrillator should always be immediately available whenever adenosine is used. Patients with wide complex tachycardias and WPW syndrome should be treated as if they had VT. Intravenous procainamide or ibutilide is the therapy of choice if cardioversion is not required. Digoxin should not be used to treat patients with a bypass tract capable of antegrade conduction because it may accelerate impulse conduction over the tract.

The need for chronic pharmacologic therapy for patients with WPW syndrome has almost been completely eliminated by the success of radiofrequency catheter ablation. When necessary, patients without antegrade bypass tract conduction often may be treated with a β blocker or calcium channel blocking drug. Patients with antegrade bypass tract conduction or those with arrhythmia recurrences during therapy with β blockers or calcium channel blocking drugs should be treated with a class Ia, Ic, or III drug. Flecainide, propafenone, quinidine, procainamide, disopyramide, or moricizine may be used, often in conjunction with a β-blocking agent. Sotalol, with β-blocking and class III activities, may also be used. Amiodarone, although effective, is rarely necessary.

Atrial Tachycardia

Atrial tachycardia is an uncommon supraventricular tachycardia caused by abnormal automaticity or reentry within the atria. Patients with structural heart disease, especially after surgical correction of congenital heart disease, have reentrant atrial tachycardias due to atrial suture lines. Automatic atrial tachycardias are often self-limited and may disappear after several months to years. Patients with atrial tachycardias are often symptomatic, and pharmacologic treatment is justified. Long-standing tachycardias, with heart rates in excess of 130 beats/min, may produce a dilated cardiomyopathy and congestive heart failure.

Inappropriate sinus tachycardia is an uncommon disorder and is poorly understood. Abnormal autonomic influence on the sinus node, either excessive sympathetic tone or reduced vagal tone, is one possible explanation. The first-line therapy should be pharmacologic, including β blockers, calcium channel blockers, and class Ia or Ic agents.

Automatic tachycardias are sometimes amenable to treatment with β-blocking or calcium channel blocking drugs such as propranolol or verapamil. In more resistant cases, class Ic drugs such as flecainide or propafenone may be helpful. Some cases of atrial tachycardia are refractory to pharmacologic therapy and require catheter ablation for control. Reentrant atrial tachycardias often require therapy with class Ia, Ic, or III antiarrhythmic drugs. Sotalol, flecainide, and amiodarone are often used. Unlike automatic arrhythmias, reentrant arrhythmias rarely are self-limited, requiring therapy for life. Patients with these arrhythmias often undergo catheter ablation to avoid lifelong antiarrhythmic drug therapy. Multifocal atrial tachycardia appears to result from a diffuse increase in atrial automaticity. It is commonly seen in patients with severe lung disease and may be facilitated by theophylline, inhaled or oral β-adrenergic stimulants, and possibly digoxin. Therapy with verapamil or metoprolol has been shown to be helpful, although any long-term therapy should include improving underlying lung function.

Ventricular Tachycardia

VT is a heterogeneous collection of ventricular tachyarrhythmias caused by several different arrhythmia mechanisms that occur in patients with different degrees of structural heart disease. Most commonly, VT is a reentrant arrhythmia occurring in a patient with coronary artery disease, prior myocardial infarction, and frequently left ventricular (LV) dysfunction. Hemodynamic collapse is a common result of VT that is not self-terminating; sudden cardiac death is often the final result.

Occasionally, VT may be hemodynamically tolerated. In these individuals, intravenous infusion of lidocaine, procainamide, or amiodarone may result in the slowing and often the termination of arrhythmia. Ventricular overdrive pacing is also effective, but synchronized DC cardioversion (with appropriate sedation and anesthesia) is the quickest method to restore a normal rhythm. However, most episodes of VT terminate spontaneously and produce no symptoms. Optimal management of these patients is currently unknown.

Intravenous lidocaine, procainamide, bretylium, and amiodarone are useful acutely for the prevention of VT recurrences. Class III agents sotalol and amiodarone are increasingly being used as chronic therapy for symptomatic VT. Other useful agents include mexiletine, quinidine, procainamide, disopyramide, propafenone, flecainide, and moricizine. All these agents have appreciable cardiac and noncardiac side effects, and, depending on the method used to judge efficacy, each may be effective in only 10% to 30% of patients. It does appear certain that whatever pharmacologic agent is employed must be proved effective by suppression of ambient ectopy, by Holter monitoring, or by means of electrophysiologic testing. VT with a continuously changing QRS morphology occurring in the setting of a prolonged QT interval (torsades de pointes) is a unique form of VT. This arrhythmia is often due to effects of antiarrhythmic drugs that prolong the action potential (classes Ia and III). Although this form of VT often terminates spontaneously, VF and sudden death may occur. Acute therapy consists of normalization of potassium and magnesium levels and acceleration of the heart rate to 110 to 120 beats/min by pacing or infusion of isoproterenol. Chronic therapy consists of elimination of all agents that prolong the duration of action potentials. If it is necessary to treat other arrhythmias, amiodarone appears safe for use in patients with torsades de pointes despite its ability to markedly prolong the QT interval. Torsades de pointes also can occur as a familial form of arrhythmia as a result of mutations to DNA encoding the cardiac sodium or potassium channel proteins.

Unusual forms of VT may occur in apparently structurally normal hearts. VT with left bundle branch morphology and an inferior frontal plane axis often originates from the right ventricular outflow tract. This arrhythmia is often catecholamine sensitive; it is frequently induced by exercise. β-Blocker drugs, calcium channel blockers, or catheter ablation is usually effective. Another unique type of VT, idiopathic LV VT, has a right bundle branch QRS morphology with a superior frontal plane axis. This VT is often responsive to verapamil; catheter ablation is also effective. However, most patients with right bundle superior axis VT will not have the verapamil-sensitive type. It is also worth noting that verapamil should not be administered to patients during VT except when the VT is known by prior electrophysiologic testing to be verapamil-sensitive. Administration of verapamil to patients with VT and coronary artery disease has resulted in hypotension and several deaths. Implantable cardioverter defibrillators (ICDs) are being used increasingly for patients with recurrent hemodynamically destabilizing VT and for primary prophylaxis in patients with history of coronary artery disease (CAD), LV systolic dysfunction, nonsustained VT, and inducible VT during programmed electrical stimulation. In a large randomized trial of patients with CAD, ejection fraction (EF) below 40%, nonsustained VT, and inducible VT, ICD therapy significantly reduced the incidence of arrhythmic death and total mortality. Other therapies such as endocardial resection and catheter ablative techniques may be useful in selected patients.

Ventricular Fibrillation

Immediate DC countershock is the appropriate response to VF. After a hemodynamically stable rhythm has been restored, antiarrhythmic therapy may be useful to prevent recurrences of this lethal arrhythmia. Acceptable intravenous medications include lidocaine, procainamide, bretylium, and amiodarone. Adjunctive therapies such as relief of myocardial ischemia and correction of electrolyte imbalance are often helpful. Small doses of an intravenous β-blocking agent—such as propranolol, metoprolol, or esmolol—also can have a surprisingly beneficial effect. Patients with frequent recurrences of VF whose intrinsic rhythm is relatively bradycardic may be helped by temporary atrial or ventricular pacing at heart rates of approximately 100 to 120 beats/min. Chronic antiarrhythmic drug therapy for the prevention of recurrences of VF ideally should be guided by serial electrophysiologic testing or serial Holter monitoring to ensure drug efficacy. Common choices include sotalol or amiodarone. Empiric therapy with amiodarone has been evaluated as one therapy arm in the multicenter Antiarrhythmic Drug Versus Implantable Defibrillator study (AVID). In this study 1016 patients with CAD, EFs below 40%, and VF or VT with syncope or hemodynamic compromise were randomized to empiric therapy with amiodarone plus Holter electrophysiologically guided sotalol or ICD. ICD therapy proved to be effective in reducing arrhythmic but not total mortality as compared with antiarrhythmic drugs, and this benefit was most prominent in patients with EFs below 35%. Of course, ICDs do not prevent recurrences of ventricular tachyarrhythmias but immediately resuscitate patients when these arrhythmias are detected. Often combined therapy of an ICD with antiarrhythmic drug therapy is necessary in patients with frequent episodes of ventricular tachyarrhythmias. Unfortunately, no currently available primary antiarrhythmic drug therapy has been demonstrated to substantially reduce the incidence of sudden cardiac death, a major cause of mortality. Only β blockers, when used as adjunctive therapy in patients with heart failure or recent myocardial infarction, have been shown to provide a significant benefit.

CLASS Ia AGENTS

Class Ia drugs block the sodium channel and fast response, predominantly in atrial, ventricular, and Purkinje tissues. The maximum rate of rise of phase 0 of the action potential is depressed, slowing conduction velocity. The potency of channel blockade is moderate, and repolarization (action potential duration) is prolonged. In addition, the drugs kinetics of channel association and dissociation may be on the order of several seconds, and as a consequence, drug effects are typically more profound at more rapid heart rates. Class Ia antiarrhythmic drugs are effective for many atrial and ventricular tachyarrhythmias.

Quinidine

Pharmacologic Description

Quinidine, an optical isomer of quinine, is an alkaloid derived from cinchona bark. First described by van Heynigen in 1848, quinidine was given its present name by Louis Pasteur in 1853. Use of cinchona in patients with AF was described by Jean Baptiste de Senac of Paris in 1749.

Electrophysiologic Action

Quinidine is a prototypic class Ia antiarrhythmic agent. It decreases the slope of phase 0 of the action potential, decreases the amplitude of the action potential, and slows conduction velocity in atrial, ventricular, and Purkinje tissues. In addition, quinidine delays repolarization, thereby increasing the duration of action potentials. Electrocardiographic (ECG) effects include prolongation of the QT and corrected QT (QTc) and QRS intervals. QRS prolongation greater than 35% to 50% of baseline is usually associated with toxicity.

Pharmacokinetics and Metabolism

Quinidine is currently available as quinidine sulfate, quinidine gluconate, and quinidine polygalacturonate. The bioavailability of quinidine ranges from 47% to 96%, with an average of 75%. The milligrams of quinidine base in different preparations differ and thus should be considered in dosing, particularly when switching formulations. The bioavailability of the gluconate preparation is 10% less than that of the quinidine sulfate. After oral ingestion of quinidine sulfate, peak plasma concentrations occur within 60 to 90 min. The gluconate preparation is absorbed more slowly, with peak levels occurring 4 h after dosing. The elimination half-life ranges between 6 and 8 h. The clearance of quinidine is decreased in patients with significant hepatic insufficiency and with advancing age. Smaller maintenance doses are required in these patients. Advanced renal disease has only minimal effects on quinidine clearance. Approximately 90% of quinidine is bound to plasma proteins. Several cardioactive metabolites have been identified including (3S)-3-hydroxyquinidine, (3OH)-quinidine, and quinidine-N-oxide. Although these metabolites are less active than the parent compound (approximately 25% and 4% for [3OH]-quinidine and quinidine-N-oxide, respectively), in approximately one-fourth of patients their concentrations may approach or even exceed that of quinidine and contribute significantly to the overall electrophysiologic effects of the drug. Because these metabolites are not measured in all assays, quinidine levels may underestimate the potential activity of the drug under steady-state conditions.

Hemodynamic Effects

Quinidine is an α-adrenergic receptor antagonist that lowers peripheral vascular resistance. Although large oral doses can produce hypotension through this mechanism, the problem is most common with intravenous dosing. Although quinidine directly depresses myocardial contractility, clinically significant myocardial depression usually does not occur except with large intravenous doses.

Antiarrhythmic Effects

Quinidine can suppress a wide variety of supraventricular and ventricular arrhythmias. In life-threatening ventricular tachyarrhythmias, quinidine has shown long-term efficacy in 15% to 30% of patients with VT or cardiac arrest when guided by electrophysiologic testing. Quinidine can also terminate AFL or fibrillation in many patients, especially when these conditions are of recent onset and if the atria are not enlarged. Quinidine also has vagolytic effects that can enhance AV nodal conduction. In some patients, this can result in an increased ventricular rate with some atrial tachyarrhythmias, such as AFL, unless an AV nodal blocking agent is also given. Typically, therapeutic levels range from 3 to 6 μg/mL.

Side Effects

Gastrointestinal side effects are common, with diarrhea and nausea being the most bothersome. Quinidine may cause tinnitus, blurred vision, dizziness, lightheadedness, and tremor, a syndrome known as *cinchonism*. Rarely, severe antibody-mediated thrombocytopenia, pancytopenia, or hemolytic anemia may occur. Side effects may require cessation of therapy in as many as 30% of patients. Up to 3% to 4% of patients receiving quinidine may develop quinidine syncope, a form of proarrhythmia usually caused by rapid polymorphic VT associated with prolongation of the QT interval (torsades de pointes). Other cases have been attributed to sinus pauses or first-dose hypotension related in part to α-adrenergic receptor blockade. The risk of serious proarrhythmia is greatest during the first few days of dosing, during bradycardia or hypokalemia. Many advocate the initiation of quinidine therapy in the hospital with ECG monitoring, particularly in patients with cardiac dysfunction.

Interactions

Drugs that alter the kinetics of hepatic enzyme systems—such as phenobarbital, phenytoin, and rifampin—can increase hepatic metabolism of quinidine and reduce its concentration. Cimetidine, in contrast, decreases hepatic metabolism of quinidine, thereby increasing the plasma concentration. In addition, the concomitant administration of amiodarone increases the concentration of many antiarrhythmic drugs, including quinidine. Quinidine increases serum levels of digoxin by decreasing digoxin clearance, volume of distribution, and affinity of tissue receptors for digoxin and thus may contribute to digoxin toxicity. Digitoxin levels are also increased. Recently, quinidine has been shown to be a potent inhibitor of cytochrome P450db1, a genetically determined polymorphic enzyme responsible for the oxidative metabolism of many drugs by the liver. Because of inhibition of this enzyme system, quinidine substantially decreases the metabolism of some drugs, such as encainide and propafenone, thus decreasing the concentration of their metabolites and increasing the concentrations of the parent compounds.

Indications and Dosage

Quinidine is indicated for the treatment of incapacitating atrial, AV nodal, and ventricular tachyarrhythmias. The usual adult dose of quinidine sulfate is 200 to 400 mg four times daily, or less frequently with longer-acting preparations. Intravenous quinidine gluconate is occasionally used in special situations such as the electrophysiology laboratory and may be given using a dose of 6 to 10 mg/kg at a rate of 0.3 to 0.5 mg/kg per minute with frequent checks of blood pressure and ECG parameters. In some patients, efficacy can be enhanced by the concomitant use of class Ib or class II antiarrhythmic drugs, such as mexiletine, propafenone, and propranolol.

Procainamide

Pharmacologic Description

Procainamide hydrochloride is an amide analogue of procaine hydrochloride, a local anesthetic agent. It was introduced in 1951 for the treatment of supraventricular and ventricular arrhythmias.

Electrophysiologic Action

Procainamide is a class Ia antiarrhythmic agent. It decreases phase 0 of the action potential, decreases the amplitude of the action potential, and slows conduction velocity in atrial, ventricular, and Purkinje tissues. In addition, procainamide increases the effective refractory periods of atrial and ventricular cells. Its major electrophysiologic effects on myocardial tissues are similar to those of quinidine. Normal sinus node automaticity is not affected. Procainamide is less vagolytic than quinidine and does not induce an adrenergic blockade. The major metabolite of procainamide, NAPA, has different electrophysiologic effects, predominantly prolonging the duration of the action potential, a class III effect. ECG effects of procainamide include prolongation of the QT, QTc, and QRS intervals.

Pharmacokinetics and Metabolism

Procainamide is currently available in parenteral (intravenous or intramuscular), regular, and sustained-release tablet and capsule formulations. The bioavailability of procainamide is approximately 83%. After ingestion of regular release tablets, peak plasma levels are obtained within 60 to 90 min. Approximately 15% of procainamide is bound to plasma proteins. In adults, the elimination half-life varies between 2.5 and 4 h. Elimination is more rapid in children, averaging 1.7 h. Approximately 50% of procainamide is excreted unchanged by the kidney. Of the remainder, a variable portion undergoes hepatic acetylation to NAPA, a cardioactive metabolite. Depending on a patient's genetically determined acetylator phenotype, 16% to 22% (slow acetylators) or 24% to 33% (fast acetylators) of procainamide is metabolized to NAPA. Elimination of NAPA is approximately 85% dependent on the kidney, with an elimination half-life of 7 to 8 h. Small amounts of NAPA may be deacetylated to procainamide.

Hemodynamic Effects

Procainamide can depress myocardial contractility but is usually well tolerated hemodynamically, even by patients with moderately severe cardiac dysfunction. When given intravenously, hypotension may result from vasodilatation due to a mild ganglionic blocking action.

Antiarrhythmic Effects

Procainamide can effectively suppress a variety of atrial, AV nodal, and ventricular tachyarrhythmias, including 20% to 30% of patients with sustained ventricular tachyarrhythmias. It is the drug of choice in the acute medical treatment of wide complex tachycardias including AF with ventricular pre-excitation (WPW syndrome). A mild vagolytic effect may result in an increased ventricular rate due to enhanced AV nodal conduction when given for supraventricular tachyarrhythmias such as AFL. Suppression of ventricular arrhythmias has been shown to occur at plasma levels between 4 and 10 µg/mL of procainamide, but higher levels may be required for suppression of sustained ventricular tachyarrhythmias. In addition, the contribution of NAPA to efficacy cannot always be ascertained. Procainamide has been used extensively with electrophysiologic testing for life-threatening ventricular arrhythmias and cardiac arrest. Failure to respond to procainamide during electrophysiologic testing in these cases often predicts failure with other individual antiarrhythmic agents.

Side Effects

Major side effects of procainamide are gastrointestinal, with nausea, vomiting, anorexia, or diarrhea occurring in up to 30% of patients. A bitter taste, dizziness, mental depression, and psychosis have also been reported. Drug-induced fever, rash, and hepatitis may occur. Agranulocytosis, sometimes fatal, has been described. Most patients will develop a positive antinuclear antibody titer if exposed to the drug for prolonged intervals. Of these, up to 30% can develop a drug-induced systemic lupus-like syndrome. Slow acetylators may be at increased risk of procainamide-induced lupus due to increased production of a hydroxylamine metabolite, which appears to be important in the pathogenesis of this syndrome. Recently, procainamide-induced lupus anticoagulants have been described, which may increase the risk of thrombosis in some patients. As in the case of quinidine, new-onset polymorphic VT in the setting of QT prolongation has been reported. Procainamide usually causes only minimal depression of cardiac function with chronic dosing, but hypotension is not uncommon with rapid intravenous infusions.

Interactions

Unlike quinidine, procainamide does not significantly alter the pharmacokinetics of digoxin. Trimethoprim and cimetidine decrease renal clearance of procainamide and NAPA, resulting in increased plasma levels of both. Concomitant administration of amiodarone also increases procainamide levels.

Indications and Dosage

Procainamide is indicated for the treatment of incapacitating atrial, AV nodal, and ventricular tachyarrhythmias. An average oral daily dose for patients younger than 50 years is 30 to 60 mg/kg, divided into equal doses given every 3, 4, or 6 h. Various sustained-release formulations facilitate dosing on a two-, three-, or four-times-per-day basis with lower peak and higher trough levels. In addition, efficacy may be enhanced in some patients with concomitant use of other agents, including β blockers. Older patients or patients with renal insufficiency require smaller doses. Intravenous therapy can be initiated with a loading infusion of up to 20 mg/kg given at a rate not to exceed 50 mg/min. Frequent blood pressure and ECG checks are required. A maintenance intravenous dose is approximately 30 to 60 mg/kg per minute in a patient with normal renal function.

Disopyramide

Pharmacologic Description

Disopyramide phosphate was first noted to have antiarrhythmic properties in 1962. It was subsequently released for clinical use in the United States in 1978. As currently available, disopyramide exists as a racemic combination of D- and L-enantiomers.

Electrophysiologic Action

The electrophysiologic effects of disopyramide are similar to those of other class Ia agents, such as quinidine and procainamide. It produces a rate-dependent decrease in the rate of rise of phase 0 of the action potential, slows conduction velocity, and prolongs the effective refractory period more than it prolongs the action potential duration. Disopyramide may prolong the action potential duration to a greater extent in normal cells than in cells from infarcted regions of the heart. The different enantiomers of disopyramide have different electrophysiologic effects: the D-enantiomer prolongs action potential duration, whereas the L-enantiomer shortens it. The D-enantiomer has approximately one-third the vagolytic properties as the L-enantiomer. Disopyramide exerts strong anticholinergic effects that tend to counteract some of its direct electrophysiologic effects, particularly in the sinus and AV nodes. In humans, AV nodal conduction is minimally affected by disopyramide. However, in the denervated (transplanted) heart, AV nodal conduction is markedly depressed. Disopyramide can increase or decrease the sinus rate, depending on prevailing cholinergic tone. ECG effects of disopyramide include prolongation of the QRS, QT, and QTc intervals.

Pharmacokinetics and Metabolism

Disopyramide is available in regular and sustained-release capsule formulations. An intravenous preparation is undergoing clinical investigation. After an oral dose, disopyramide is almost completely absorbed, with peak plasma concentrations occurring within 2 h. Peak levels occur from 4 to 6 h after ingestion of sustained-release disopyramide capsules. The elimination half-life is 6 to 9 h, with 40% to 60% excreted unchanged by the kidney; an additional 20% is excreted as the mono-n-dealkylated metabolite, with another 10% excreted as other metabolites. Protein binding is highly variable, ranging from 40% to 90%, depending on plasma concentration. At higher doses, a greater concentration of drug is unbound, resulting in a greater pharmacologic effect than would be predicted based on the total plasma level. The clinical significance of this effect is unknown. α_1-Acid glycoprotein accounts for the majority of protein binding, with albumin accounting for only 5% to 10% of the total.

Hemodynamic Effects

Disopyramide causes significant depression of myocardial contractility, with reductions in systemic blood pressure, stroke index, and cardiac index. Systemic vascular resistance and right atrial pressure increase. Patients with LV dysfunction tolerate disopyramide poorly. In a retrospective study among patients with preexisting congestive heart failure, 55% of patients given disopyramide had clinically significant worsening of their heart failure. In contrast, only 3% of patients without a history of congestive heart failure developed this complication during disopyramide therapy. The drug has been used as a treatment for hypertrophic cardiomyopathy as a monotherapy and in combination with β blockers.

Antiarrhythmic Effects

Like other class Ia antiarrhythmic drugs, disopyramide is effective in a variety of supraventricular and ventricular tachyarrhythmias. Disopyramide can suppress premature ventricular contractions, with plasma concentrations in the range of 3 to 8 μg/mL, but is less effective with sustained VT as assessed by electrophysiologic testing. Disopyramide has been combined with other antiarrhythmic agents, such as mexiletine, for increased efficacy in treating ventricular arrhythmias, with fewer side effects. Disopyramide has been used successfully for the treatment of AFL and AF, including patients with the WPW syndrome. Disopyramide also may be effective for preventing inducible and spontaneous neurally mediated syncope due to its negative inotropic and anticholinergic properties.

Side Effects

Disopyramide significantly depresses myocardial contractility and must be used with caution, if at all, in patients with LV dysfunction. Anticholinergic side effects are frequent, and up to 10% of patients may necessitate discontinuation of the drug. These symptoms include dry mouth, blurred vision, and, particularly in older men, urine retention. Disopyramide can also precipitate acute angle closure glaucoma. Gastrointestinal symptoms are uncommon. As with other drugs that prolong ventricular repolarization and the QT interval, disopyramide can induce polymorphic VT (torsades de pointes). Rare side effects include rash, cholestatic jaundice, psychosis, and agranulocytosis. Hypoglycemia occurs infrequently, apparently owing to increased pancreatic secretion of insulin.

Interactions

Drugs that induce hepatic enzymes, such as phenytoin and phenobarbital, increase hepatic metabolism of disopyramide and result in lower serum levels. Disopyramide does not induce hepatic enzymes, however. Disopyramide does not alter serum digoxin levels. Erythromycin has been reported to increase disopyramide levels, with development of potentially fatal ventricular arrhythmias. The potent negative inotropic effects of disopyramide warrant additional caution in patients with possible cardiac dysfunction requiring therapy with β blockers or calcium channel blockers for indications such as ischemic heart disease.

Indications and Dosage

Disopyramide is indicated for the prevention or suppression of premature ventricular contractions and VT. It has also been used to treat atrial arrhythmias. The usual adult oral dose is 300 to 1600 mg daily, divided into three or four equal doses. Dosage must be reduced in elderly patients and in patients with renal insufficiency. The controlled-release capsules may be given every 12 h.

CLASS Ib AGENTS

Class Ib drugs also block sodium channels, but to a lesser degree than class Ia drugs. The association and disassociation kinetics are more rapid than in class Ia drugs, typically less than 1 s. In addition, repolarization tends to be mildly shortened. Class Ib drugs often suppress premature ventricular contractions but are only occasionally effective as monotherapy for life-threatening ventricular tachyarrhythmias. Class Ib drugs, as a class, are generally ineffective for atrial arrhythmias.

Lidocaine

Pharmacologic Description

Initially synthesized in 1943, lidocaine is widely used as a local anesthetic agent. Its antiarrhythmic properties were noted in the 1950s, but its use did not become common until the advent of coronary care units in the 1960s.

Electrophysiologic Action

Lidocaine is classified as a class Ib antiarrhythmic drug. The action potential duration and effective refractory period of Purkinje and ventricular tissues are shortened. At high concentrations, it depresses the rate of rise of phase 0 of the action potential and decreases conduction velocity in Purkinje fibers. Lidocaine has minimal effects on AV and intraventricular conductions except at high concentrations (>30 μg/mL). In patients with severe His-Purkinje system disease, lidocaine may precipitate complete AV block. Lidocaine decreases phase 4 diastolic depolarizations in Purkinje tissue and decreases automaticity. Consequently, lidocaine may depress the sinus node and potential subsidiary escape pacemakers, rarely causing asystolic pauses. Lidocaine increases the VF threshold. In abnormal myocardium, the effects of lidocaine in depressing conduction may be more pronounced.

Pharmacokinetics and Metabolism

Lidocaine is almost completely absorbed after oral administration, but approximately 70% is rapidly metabolized by hepatic first-pass biotransformation. Less than 10% of an administered dose is recovered unchanged in the urine. For this reason, the drug is almost always given parenterally; however, rectal administration is feasible, as is intramuscular administration, particularly in the prehospital phase of the management of acute myocardial infarction. Lidocaine is approximately 60% to 80% protein bound, depending on the concentration of α_1-acid glycoprotein in the serum. During acute myocardial infarction, serum levels of α_1-acid glycoprotein are increased, resulting in more drug bound to α_1-acid glycoprotein and less free (active) drug. Thus, higher total lidocaine levels may be required during acute myocardial infarction. Lidocaine is almost completely cleared by the liver, with clearance proportional to hepatic blood flow. The mean elimination half-life of lidocaine in humans is 1.5 to 2 h, which is increased in the elderly, patients with reduced cardiac output, and patients with hepatic disease. Elimination is also delayed during prolonged infusions in patients with acute myocardial infarction, the mechanism of which is not understood. The two principal metabolites are glycinexylidide and monoethylglycinexylidide, both of which have weaker antiarrhythmic effects in humans than does lidocaine but can contribute measurably to the central nervous system toxicity of lidocaine. Both metabolites are renally excreted, and glycinexylidide may accumulate in patients with renal failure.

Hemodynamic Effects

At usual doses, lidocaine causes minimal hemodynamic effects. Minimal decreases in cardiac output, arterial blood pressure, heart rate, and ventricular contractility have been reported.

Antiarrhythmic Effects

Lidocaine can be effective for the suppression of ventricular tachyarrhythmias, particularly in patients with myocardial ischemia. Prophylactic use of lidocaine after myocardial infarction, once a common practice, has been abandoned because prophylactic use of any class Ia agents after myocardial infarction has been associated with increased mortality. It also appears to reduce the incidence of VF. Therapeutic plasma concentrations range from 2 to 5 μg/mL.

Side Effects

Adverse effects of lidocaine almost always involve the central nervous system. Early, transient effects include paresthesias, dizziness, and drowsiness, which can be managed by interrupting the drug temporarily. Subsequent, more persistent effects include hallucinations, confusion, somnolence, and muscle tremor, which presage impending seizures, respiratory, or cardiac arrest. Rarely, lidocaine can depress sinus node function or precipitate heart block in patients with severe His-Purkinje system disease; it can also inhibit escape rhythms from His-Purkinje tissue. Adverse effects of lidocaine are common when the plasma concentration exceeds 6 μg/mL.

Interactions

Lidocaine is highly dependent on hepatic metabolism for elimination. Drugs that alter hepatic metabolism cause marked changes in lidocaine pharmacokinetics. Propranolol, metoprolol, cimetidine, and halothane decrease lidocaine clearance.

Indications and Dosage

Lidocaine is indicated for the acute management of ventricular arrhythmias, such as those associated with acute myocardial infarction or cardiac surgery. It may be administered intravenously as a bolus of 0.7 to 1.4 mg/kg at a rate of 25 to 50 mg/min. If necessary, this dose may be repeated in 5 min, followed by a continuous infusion of 0.014 to 0.057 mg/kg (1 to 4 mg/min). Alternative loading and maintenance infusion regimens have been advocated, typically entailing a total of 2 to 4 mg/kg in divided doses over 30 min. Lidocaine may be given by intramuscular injection of 300 to 400 mg (4.3 mg/kg) for use during acute myocardial infarction. The deltoid muscle is the preferred injection site. Lidocaine also has been used in combination with other agents including procainamide, bretylium, and β blockers.

Tocainide

Pharmacologic Description

Tocainide hydrochloride is a primary amine analogue of lidocaine. Minor side-chain differences from lidocaine enable it to avoid substantial first-pass metabolism in the liver, thus allowing oral administration. Its antiarrhythmic effects were described in 1976 and it was approved for oral use in the United States in 1984. As currently available, tocainide is supplied as a racemic mixture of enantiomers D-tocainide and L-tocainide.

Electrophysiologic Action

Tocainide produces dose-dependent decreases in sodium and potassium conductance, thus depressing myocardial excitability. It suppresses the amplitude and rate of depolarization of the action potential and may shorten the action, potential duration, and, to a lesser extent, the effective refractory period of Purkinje tissue. Tocainide increases the fibrillation threshold in normal and ischemic tissues. AV conduction and sinus node automaticity are usually unaffected by tocainide. Tocainide usually produces no significant ECG changes. However, the QT interval may decrease. The individual enantiomers of tocainide may be more effective than the racemic combination for ventricular arrhythmias induced by programmed electrical stimulation.

Pharmacokinetics and Metabolism

After oral administration, the bioavailability of tocainide approaches 100%. Peak plasma concentrations appear between 0.5 and 2 h. Between 10% and 50% of tocainide is bound to plasma proteins. Approximately 40% is excreted unchanged in the urine. The elimination half-life averages 13 to 15 h in healthy subjects but can vary between 9 and 37 h. Elimination is delayed in the presence of renal insufficiency but only minimally changed in the presence of hepatic disease.

Hemodynamic Effects

Intravenous tocainide produces small degrees of left ventricular (LV) depression with no apparent change in cardiac output. Small increases in aortic and pulmonary artery pressures have been observed, probably secondary to increases in vascular resistance. In patients with moderate to severe LV dysfunction, including those receiving β-blocking drugs, hemodynamic changes are often minimal, although more marked and additive effects may occur. In one study, congestive heart failure was precipitated by tocainide in approximately 1.5% of patients.

Antiarrhythmic Effects

Tocainide is a modestly effective agent for suppressing premature ventricular contractions in a number of patients, with approximately 90% suppression in some patients at plasma concentrations of 8.5 mg/mL. Typically, 30% to 75% of patients will have significant suppression of premature ventricular contraction. Tocainide is at times effective in suppressing premature ventricular contractions in patients who are unresponsive to class Ia agents, and the response to lidocaine may predict the response to tocainide. Thus, lidocaine failure is often predictive of tocainide inefficacy, whereas lidocaine efficacy does not necessarily predict tocainide success. Only a small percentage of patients with life-threatening ventricular arrhythmias will respond to tocainide when assessed by electrophysiologic testing. However, the drug may be synergistically effective when combined with class Ia drugs. Dosing tocainide at 600 mg orally twice daily produces levels effective in suppressing premature ventricular contractions in many patients (4 to 10 μg/mL).

Side Effects

Side effects are common with tocainide, having been reported in 20% to 40% of patients. Typically gastrointestinal and central nervous system side effects occur, including nausea, dizziness, tremor, vomiting, paresthesia, tremor, ataxia, and confusion. These effects usually occur with high plasma concentrations and may be minimized by dividing doses and taking the medication with meals to delay absorption. Skin rash occurs frequently. Rarely, more serious adverse effects occur, such as pulmonary fibrosis, a lupus-like syndrome, or hematologic abnormalities, chiefly agranulocytosis.

Interactions

Tocainide has no significant effects on warfarin or digoxin. Concomitant use with β-blocking drugs is safe in most patients. Rifampin has been reported to increase elimination, resulting in reduced plasma levels of tocainide. Cimetidine, but not ranitidine, results in decreased bioavailability of tocainide.

Indications and Dosage

Tocainide is specifically indicated for the treatment of life-threatening ventricular tachyarrhythmias, although it is only infrequently effective for this purpose. It has the same efficacy profile as mexiletine, but its potentially serious systemic side effects have restricted its use. It should not be used as first-line therapy, but only for symptomatic VT resistant to other therapies. Tocainide is available as tablets of 400 and 600 mg. Total daily doses of 800 to 2400 mg are usually administered as divided doses two to four times daily. The dosage should be reduced in the presence of renal insufficiency. Plasma levels above 3 μg/mL are associated with efficacy, whereas levels above 10 μg/mL are associated with increased side effects.

Mexiletine

Pharmacologic Description

Mexiletine hydrochloride is a drug closely related in structure to lidocaine. Initially developed as an anticonvulsant, mexiletine has been recognized to have antiarrhythmic properties since 1972. Used in Europe to treat ventricular arrhythmias since 1976, it became available in the United States in 1986.

Electrophysiologic Action

Mexiletine decreases the rate of rise of phase 0 of the action potential and shortens the action potential's duration. The effective refractory period is decreased in Purkinje tissue but not in ventricular muscle. The slope of phase 4 diastolic depolarization is decreased. The electrophysiologic effects of mexiletine are similar to those of other class Ib agents. Usually no significant changes occur in the PR, QRS, QT, or QTc intervals with intravenous or oral mexiletine. In patients with normal His-Purkinje function, no significant changes are observed after mexiletine. Patients with His-Purkinje system disease may develop prolongation of conduction but rarely block. In addition, prolongation of QRS duration has been reported with mexiletine toxicity.

Pharmacokinetics and Metabolism

Mexiletine is highly bioavailable, with approximately 90% absorption. Absorption occurs in the alkaline environment of the proximal small bowel. Peak plasma levels occur in 2 to 3 h but may be delayed in clinical situations, such as acute myocardial infarction or diabetes mellitus, in which gastric emptying is delayed. Some 50% to 60% of mexiletine is protein bound. Mexiletine is extensively metabolized in the liver; only 10% is excreted unchanged by the kidney. Several metabolites have minor electrophysiologic activity, with the most potent (*N*-methyl mexiletine) having less than 20% of the effect of the parent compound. In healthy subjects, the average elimination half-life is 10 h, with a range of 8 to 12 h. Renal insufficiency has minimal effect on elimination half-life, whereas hepatic insufficiency or reduced hepatic blood flow reduces mexiletine clearance.

Hemodynamic Effects

Mexiletine generally has minimal negative inotropic effects at therapeutic levels. Small decreases in blood pressure and LV contractility with increased LV end diastolic pressure have been observed in some studies. When administered orally, mexiletine produces no changes in LV EF, blood pressure, heart rate, or exercise capacity.

Antiarrhythmic Effects

Mexiletine may be used to suppress frequent and high-grade ventricular arrhythmias, including those that have failed to respond to class Ia antiarrhythmic drugs. Used alone, mexiletine is only infrequently effective in suppressing life-threatening ventricular arrhythmias. Combination therapy with class Ia antiarrhythmic agents can be more effective than with either agent alone, with potentially less toxicity. Mexiletine is effective in suppressing warning ventricular arrhythmias in a number of patients with acute myocardial infarction. The antiarrhythmic response to lidocaine may be used as a sensitive but nonspecific predictor of mexiletine efficacy. Thus, failure to respond to intravenous lidocaine is a strong predictor of mexiletine inefficacy, whereas lidocaine efficacy only weakly predicts mexiletine efficacy. Similarly, the response to tocainide or mexiletine is not necessarily predictive of the response to the other. Plasma concentrations of 0.5 to 2.0 μg/mL are associated with efficacy in many patients.

Side Effects

Side effects are common with mexiletine, occurring in up to 40% to 60% of patients in some series. The most frequent side effects are related to the central nervous system or the gastrointestinal tract and include nausea, vomiting, dizziness, tremor, ataxia, slurred speech, blurred vision, memory impairment, and personality changes. Skin rash and hepatitis occur infrequently. Rarely, seizures have been reported. Gastrointestinal side effects may be reduced by administering the drug with food or by reducing the dosage. Adverse cardiac effects are rare, but worsening of congestive heart failure and proarrhythmic effects have been reported.

Interactions

No specific adverse effects have been reported to date from combining mexiletine with other cardiotonic agents such as β-blocking drugs or other antiarrhythmics. Significant alkalinization of the urine by drugs may decrease renal clearance and result in elevated blood levels. Drugs such as phenobarbital or phenytoin, which induce hepatic enzymes, enhance mexiletine metabolism; cimetidine reduces metabolism and results in increased mexiletine levels.

Indications and Dosage

Mexiletine is indicated for the suppression of incapacitating ventricular arrhythmias, including VT. Effective oral regimens usually require 200 to 400 mg every 8 h. Doses should be given with food to minimize side effects. Dosages may be increased or decreased by 50 to 100 mg at intervals of at least 2 to 3 days. An intravenous preparation is not available in the United States and is associated with a relatively high incidence of side effects. Intravenous therapy has been given as a loading dose of 400 mg over 40 min with 600 to 900 mg/day for maintenance therapy.

CLASS Ic AGENTS

Class Ic drugs are potent sodium channel blocking agents. They have little effect on repolarization and have long half-time kinetics of channel association and dissociation, usually longer than 20 to 30 s. Thus, drug effects are potentiated at moderate to rapid heart rates. They are effective for a variety of atrial and ventricular tachyarrhythmias. As a class, the Ic drugs are highly effective in suppressing chronic ventricular ectopy. Unfortunately, the marked slowing of conduction induced by these agents is an efficient mechanism to induce ventricular proarrhythmia. This effect is most marked in patients with significant structural heart disease but may occur in normal individuals, especially in the setting of rapid heart rates, such as those produced by exercise.

Moricizine

Pharmacologic Description

Moricizine is a phenothiazine derivative first synthesized in the Soviet Union.

Electrophysiologic Action

Intravenous moricizine (3 mg/kg) produces a reduction in the upstroke velocity of phase 0 and a reduction in the action potential duration, effects similar to those of other class Ib antiarrhythmic agents. In contrast to class Ib agents, moricizine has prolonged sodium channel recovery kinetics, similar to class Ic agents. Moricizine does not decrease the slope of phase 4 depolarization in automatic Purkinje fibers unless the fibers are ischemic. Voltage clamp experiments have shown that moricizine reduces the fast sodium current by decreasing maximal conduction of sodium ions. In humans, intravenous moricizine (1.5 to 2 mg/kg) lengthens the P wave to low right atrial, atrial to His bundle (AH), and PR intervals. The sinus rate, QT, and His bundle to ventricular (HV) intervals, and the effective refractory periods of the atrium, AV node, and ventricle were not affected in early studies. However, the refractoriness of an accessory pathway or of the retrograde fast pathway of dual AV nodal pathways was increased by moricizine. When using an oral dose of 10 mg/kg, slight prolongation of the HV interval was noted, whereas at a higher dose of 15 mg/kg, the PR and QRS intervals were prolonged. In patients with sinus node dysfunction, moricizine given intravenously (2 mg/kg) has caused prolongation of the sinus node recovery time and second-degree sinus exit block. Although some properties are similar to those of other class Ib agents, in aggregate moricizine behaves more like a class Ic drug.

Pharmacokinetics and Metabolism

Moricizine is well absorbed when given orally, with peak plasma concentrations occurring 1 to 1.5 h after dosing. The drug undergoes extensive metabolism, with less than 1% of the drug recovered in the urine and feces. Active metabolites have not been identified thus far. After a single oral dose, the elimination half-life is approximately 2 to 5 h. In patients with cardiac disease, the steady-state elimination half-life averages 10 h, but it may be prolonged to 47 h in patients with renal insufficiency. Antiarrhythmic effects of the drug may not be noted for up to 24 h after dosing, an effect that is not completely understood. Therefore, plasma levels may provide little guidance for antiarrhythmic efficacy, and several studies have reported little correlation between plasma concentration and drug toxicity in the form of proarrhythmia.

Hemodynamic Effects

Hemodynamic data in humans are incomplete; however, moricizine appears to have minimal effect on most hemodynamic parameters. Moricizine does not appear to depress myocardial contractility in dogs. However, in patients with preexisting LV dysfunction, moricizine may cause decompensation. In one study, the failure to increase cardiac index by 1.0 L/(min • m^2) or to increase stroke work during bicycle exercise predicted not only patients likely to decompensate but also those patients unlikely to have an antiarrhythmic response.

Antiarrhythmic Effects

Moricizine may be effective for the treatment of supraventricular and ventricular arrhythmias. With doses ranging from 2.4 to 15 mg/kg per day, moricizine was effective in reducing premature ventricular contractions in 50% to 60% of patients and compared favorably with disopyramide in one study. Moricizine appears less effective in the treatment of life-threatening ventricular tachyarrhythmias and has demonstrated an excessive cardiac mortality rate during the first 2 weeks of exposure in patients with ischemic cardiomyopathy and recent myocardial infarction. Unlike other class Ib antiarrhythmic agents, when given intravenously, moricizine has shown efficacy in terminating and preventing initiation of AV nodal supraventricular tachycardias and reciprocating bypass tract tachycardias by slowing retrograde fast pathway conduction. Recently, it has been shown to be safe, well tolerated, and effective in maintaining sinus rhythm in patients with chronic AF and systolic dysfunction.

Side Effects

Moricizine appears to be a generally well-tolerated antiarrhythmic agent. Nausea, vomiting, diarrhea, dizziness, and mild anxiety reactions have been reported. Nervousness, perioral numbness, vertigo, confusion, dry mouth, blurred vision, headache, and insomnia have occurred. Worsening of sinus node dysfunction may occur, and the drug may cause hypotension or worsening of congestive heart failure. Some patients have had transient elevation of hepatic transaminase enzyme levels. Rarely, diaphoresis and memory loss have been reported with long-term therapy. Proarrhythmia reportedly occurred in approximately 3.2% of patients in one review and was reportedly relatively unrelated to dose. Sinusoidal VT, occasionally induced with exercise, has been reported.

Interactions

Serum digoxin levels may increase 10% to 15% during acute but not during chronic dosing in cardiac patients with normal renal function. Other drug interactions have not been reported, but this has not been completely investigated.

Indications and Dosage

At doses of 150 to 250 mg every 8 h, moricizine appears effective for the treatment of atrial and ventricular ectopies. Doses may be given every 8 to 12 h. Therapeutic drug levels appear to be 0.2 to 1.5 µg/mL. The role of moricizine in the treatment of life-threatening ventricular arrhythmias remains undefined.

Flecainide

Pharmacologic Description

Flecainide acetate, a fluorobenzamide, is a derivative of procainamide first synthesized in 1972. Its antiarrhythmic effects were first reported in 1975, and it was released for the treatment of ventricular arrhythmias in the United States in 1985. Subsequently it was approved for the treatment of supraventricular tachyarrhythmias including AFL and AF in patients with structurally normal hearts.

Electrophysiologic Action

Flecainide exhibits potent sodium channel blocking action by depressing phase 0 of the action potential and slowing conduction in a frequency- and dose-dependent manner throughout the heart. His-Purkinje tissue and ventricular muscle are affected the most, followed by atrial muscle, accessory AV pathways, and AV nodal tissue. In most studies, the action potential duration is not significantly affected. Sinus rate, sinoatrial conduction, and sinus node recovery times are usually not affected by flecainide. However, patients with sinus node dysfunction may have significant increases in the corrected sinus node recovery time. Flecainide produces a concentration-dependent increase in PR, QRS, and intraatrial conduction intervals and prolongation of the ventricular effective refractory period. In one study, an intravenous dose of 2 mg/kg (mean level, 335 mg/L) produced a mean QRS increase of 23%. The QT interval increases, reflecting QRS prolongation, with minimal to no change in the JT interval.

Pharmacokinetics and Metabolism

Flecainide is well absorbed (95%), with peak plasma concentrations occurring 2 to 4 h after dosing. Flecainide is 30% to 40% bound to plasma proteins, independent of drug level, over a range of 0.015 to 3.4 µg/mL. Clinically important drug interactions based on protein-binding effects therefore would not be expected. In healthy subjects, 30% (range, 10% to 50%) of flecainide is excreted unchanged in the urine. Approximately 70% of flecainide is metabolized in the liver. The major metabolite (meta-*O*-dealkylated flecainide) is approximately 20% as potent as the parent compound, whereas the minor metabolite (meta-*O*-dealkylated lactam of flecainide) is electrophysiologically inactive. The average elimination half-life is 20 h after repeated doses, but is highly variable and ranges between 12 and 27 h. Steady-state levels are not obtained for 3 to 5 days. Because flecainide is extensively metabolized, the relation between flecainide elimination and creatinine clearance is complex. Reduced doses must be used in patients with renal insufficiency or hepatic insufficiency.

Hemodynamic Effects

Flecainide produces dose-dependent depression of cardiac contractility and cardiac output. Oral treatment is generally well tolerated, but patients with LV dysfunction may develop new or worsening congestive heart failure. Flecainide should not be used in patients with LV dysfunction.

Antiarrhythmic Effects

Flecainide is effective in suppressing supraventricular and ventricular tachyarrhythmias and premature contractions. Flecainide can suppress chronic premature ventricular contractions by more than 75% and repetitive forms by more than 90% in most patients, including patients resistant to other antiarrhythmic drugs. Among patients with life-threatening ventricular tachyarrhythmias, flecainide is reported to prevent induction of VT in 15% to 25%. Flecainide has shown efficacy in the prevention and treatment of AF and arrhythmias in patients with ventricular preexcitation or accessory pathways. Flecainide is most effective in suppressing chronic ectopy in patients with preserved LV function without VT. Patients with LV dysfunction or clinically documented VT are at increased risk for proarrhythmic side effects. Flecainide has been shown to increase cardiac mortality among patients with ventricular ectopy after acute myocardial infarction. Therapeutic levels of flecainide are 0.2 to 1.0 µg/mL; higher levels are associated with an increasing incidence of toxicity.

Side Effects

Most side effects of flecainide are neurologic and cardiac. Neurologic effects include blurred vision, headache, dizziness, paresthesias, and tremor. Skin rash, abdominal pain, diarrhea, and impotence have been reported. Cardiac effects are not uncommon and include worsening of arrhythmia, slowed conduction or heart block, and aggravation of congestive heart failure. Worsening of ventricular arrhythmias occurs in up to 10% or more of patients, more commonly in patients with LV dysfunction and clinical VT. Some episodes of VT induced by flecainide have been resistant to electrical cardioversion. Acute and chronic elevations of the pacing threshold have been reported by some investigators.

Interaction

Small increases in serum digoxin concentrations have been noted with flecainide administration. Flecainide and propranolol concentrations increase mildly with coadministration of both agents. No clinically important interactions have been reported. The concomitant administration of flecainide and a β blocker or calcium channel antagonist can be expected to have additive cardiac depressant effects.

Indications and Dosage

Flecainide is indicated for the treatment of life-threatening ventricular arrhythmias, such as sustained VT, and resistant supraventricular arrhythmias in patients with normal ventricular function. In patients with normal renal and hepatic function, treatment may be begun with 100 mg every 12 h. Dose adjustments should be no larger than 50 mg per dose every 4 days to minimize toxicity. Total daily doses of 200 to 300 mg are associated with efficacy in most patients. Patients with LV dysfunction or a history of VT should have therapy initiated with smaller dosages and continuous ECG monitoring in a hospital environment.

Propafenone

Pharmacologic Description

Propafenone hydrochloride, an antiarrhythmic agent structurally similar to β-blocking drugs, was first synthesized in 1970. Commercially available since 1977 in Europe, propafenone is approved in the United States for the treatment of life-threatening ventricular arrhythmias and supraventricular arrhythmias in patients with structurally normal hearts. Propafenone exists as a racemic mixture of D-propafenone and L-propafenone.

Electrophysiologic Action

Propafenone blocks the fast inward sodium current in atrial, ventricular, and His-Purkinje tissues, thus decreasing the rate of rise of phase 0 of the action potential. The blocking effect is concentration dependent, with ischemic tissue being more susceptible. In patients with ventricular preexcitation or bypass tracts, propafenone decreases conduction velocity and increases refractoriness of the accessory pathway. Sinus node automaticity may be depressed, especially in the presence of preexisting sinus node dysfunction. Propafenone possesses weak β-adrenergic and calcium channel antagonist activities. Both stereoisomers appear to have equal sodium channel blocking ability, and D-propafenone is responsible for the clinically observed β blockade. Propafenone suppresses delayed afterdepolarizations in ischemic Purkinje fibers. Endocardial pacing thresholds are increased. ECG effects include prolongation of the PR and QRS intervals without significant change of the QT interval.

Pharmacokinetics and Metabolism

Absorption of propafenone is almost complete after oral dosing, with peak plasma levels obtained in 2 to 3 h, but extensive first-pass metabolism reduces systemic bioavailability to approximately 12%. The availability appears to vary with the dose, so that higher doses have increased bioavailability, probably due to saturation of hepatic microsomal enzymes with larger doses. About 77% to 79% of propafenone is protein bound, with α_1-acid glycoprotein being the major binding protein. The metabolism of propafenone is polymorphic and segregates with the debrisoquin metabolic phenotype. Extensive metabolizers form two major metabolites: 5-hydroxypropafenone and N-depropyl-propafenone. Poor metabolizers have high levels of propafenone and, hence, greater β-blocking effect and minimal levels of active metabolites. Overall, however, electrophysiologic effects appear similar in both groups given comparable doses. Elimination of propafenone is mostly hepatic; less than 1% is recovered intact in the urine. The average elimination half-life ranges from 3.6 to 7.2 h. In patients with hepatic disease, the elimination half-life is prolonged, with an average of 14 h. Doses must be decreased in these patients.

Hemodynamic Effects

Propafenone has negative inotropic effects. In several studies, occasional patients with depressed cardiac function have had hemodynamic deterioration. Most patients experience no change in resting LV EF, although EF may decrease with exercise. One study using intravenous propafenone (2 mg/kg) reported a slight depression of cardiac index with increased pulmonary vascular resistance but no change in systemic arterial pressure. Thus, caution is necessary if propafenone is used in patients with LV dysfunction.

Antiarrhythmic Effects

Propafenone appears effective in treating supraventricular and ventricular arrhythmias. Like other class Ic antiarrhythmic agents, propafenone is effective in suppressing frequent premature ventricular contractions, including complex forms. It is less effective in treating life-threatening ventricular arrhythmias, but even in this difficult population, up to 25% of patients may respond. Propafenone also has been shown to be effective in treating supraventricular tachyarrhythmias, such as AF or AFL, including patients with the WPW syndrome. Propafenone should be used cautiously in patients with recent myocardial infarction in view of the recent CAST findings showing increased mortality in this population when treated with other class Ic drugs (flecainide or encainide).

Side Effects

Approximately 21% to 32% of patients experience adverse reactions to propafenone, and 3% to 7% require discontinuation of the medication. Worsening of ventricular arrhythmias was reported to occur in 6.1% of 1579 patients in early clinical trials of propafenone. Patients at highest risk include those with LV dysfunction and those with preexisting sustained VT. Noncardiac side effects are predominantly gastrointestinal or related to the central nervous system. Dizziness, lightheadedness, nausea, vomiting, or a metallic taste occurs most frequently. Central nervous system effects and effects related to β-adrenergic blockade may be more frequent in individuals with a poor metabolizer phenotype.

Interactions

Propafenone in a dose of 300 mg every 8 h orally increases digoxin levels an average of 83%; the magnitude of increase seems related to the dose of propafenone. Significant increases in plasma warfarin concentrations and prothrombin times have been reported. Propafenone concentrations may increase with concomitant cimetidine therapy. Propafenone also decreases metoprolol elimination, resulting in increased β-adrenergic blockade. Quinidine in low doses effectively stops hepatic metabolism of propafenone by converting rapid metabolizers to poor metabolizers. The clinical significance of this interaction is unknown.

Indications and Dosage

Propafenone is approved for the treatment of ventricular arrhythmias. Therapy for supraventricular and ventricular arrhythmias may be initiated with a dosage of 150 mg three times a day; doses up to 900 mg (occasionally 1200 mg) daily have been used. High dose oral propafenone (600 mg) also has been shown to be very safe and effective in restoring sinus rhythm in patients with recent onset AF, with conversion rates of up to 76% at 8 h after treatment. Intravenous propafenone has been evaluated for supraventricular and ventricular arrhythmias at doses such as 2 mg/kg followed by a maintenance infusion, but this formulation remains investigational in the United States. A new sustained-release formulation has been proven safe and effective and soon will be available for clinical use.

CLASS II AGENTS

Class II drugs are β-adrenergic blocking agents. Different β blockers will vary with respect to lipid solubility, membrane-stabilizing effect, relative specificity for the β_1 receptor, cardioselectivity, and partial agonist activity (intrinsic sympathomimetic activity). As a class, β blockers are useful for the treatment of many atrial and AV nodal arrhythmias (see Chapter 2). In addition, some β blockers may reduce ventricular ectopy. Several β-blocking agents have been shown to reduce mortality when administered after acute myocardial infarction and may be useful as primary or adjunctive agents in some patients with or at risk for life-threatening ventricular tachyarrhythmias.

Propranolol

Pharmacologic Description

Propranolol hydrochloride is a nonselective β-adrenergic-receptor blocking agent. It is indicated in the United States for the treatment of supraventricular and ventricular arrhythmias. It is also indicated for the treatment of hypertrophic cardiomyopathy, acute myocardial infarction, angina pectoris, hypertension, and numerous noncardiac conditions such as migraine headache and essential tremor.

Electrophysiologic Action

The electrophysiologic effects of propranolol relate primarily to its β-blocking activity, an effect almost entirely mediated by its L-stereoisomer. Propranolol is a competitive nonselective β blocker. β_1 Receptors predominate in cardiac tissue, blockade of which produces an increase in the sinus node cycle length and slowing of AV nodal conduction. At high concentrations, propranolol depresses the inward sodium current in Purkinje fibers, the so-called membrane-stabilizing or quinidine-like effect. This effect generally occurs only at concentrations several times that required for β blockade and thus is probably insignificant clinically. Propranolol can shorten the duration of action potentials acutely in Purkinje fibers and to a lesser extent in atrial and ventricular muscle. With chronic administration, the action potential may lengthen. ECG effects include a slowing of sinus rate and an increase in the PR interval, with minimal or no change in QRS and QTc intervals. The effective refractory period is minimally increased.

Pharmacokinetics and Metabolism

Propranolol is almost completely absorbed after oral administration but undergoes extensive first-pass metabolism in the liver, resulting in a bioavailability of approximately 30%. Peak clinical effects occur between 60 and 90 min after oral dosing. The average biologic half-life is 4 h. A long-acting formulation is also available for once-daily use. Elimination is hepatic and is proportional to hepatic blood flow. With oral dosing, a total of 160 to 240 mg daily is considered necessary for achieving effective β blockade, although smaller doses are often used in antiarrhythmic regimens. With intravenous dosing, a total dose of 0.2 mg/kg achieves effective β blockade, with activity evident almost immediately.

Hemodynamic Effects

Propranolol is a negative inotropic agent by virtue of its β-blocking action. It may precipitate or worsen congestive heart failure. By blocking β_2 receptors in the peripheral circulation, propranolol may increase vascular resistance.

Antiarrhythmic Effects

Propranolol is an effective agent for the treatment of supraventricular arrhythmias such as atrial tachycardia. It will slow the ventricular response to AF or AFL and may terminate arrhythmias requiring participation of the AV node, such as AV nodal reciprocating tachycardias and those associated with the WPW syndrome and accessory pathways. Propranolol has a variable effect on the rapid ventricular response to AF due to accessory pathway conduction. Propranolol can be effective in treating arrhythmias due to digitalis toxicity, thyrotoxicosis, and anesthesia and as adjunctive therapy for pheochromocytoma. Ventricular premature contractions may be suppressed by propranolol, but it is infrequently effective as a single agent in the treatment of life-threatening ventricular tachyarrhythmias. Propranolol may be more effective in preventing rapid polymorphic VTs or VF than in preventing monomorphic VT when assessed by electrophysiologic testing. Propranolol can be an effective adjunctive agent in combination with other agents, with caution to avoid additive depressant effects on conduction and contractility. β Blockers also have been used successfully in some patients with congenital QT prolongation and associated ventricular tachyarrhythmias, including torsades de pointes. Therapeutic plasma levels for propranolol are highly variable but often range from 50 to 100 ng/mL.

Side Effects

Common side effects include bradycardia, hypotension, claudication, Raynaud's phenomenon, and AV block. Worsening of heart failure or asthma may occur. Propranolol is lipophilic and easily penetrates the blood–brain barrier, thereby contributing to central nervous system adverse effects such as vivid dreams, insomnia, mental depression, and possibly fatigue and impotence. Insulin-dependent diabetics may be at increased risk for hypoglycemia. Sudden discontinuation of β blockade may worsen angina pectoris and may even precipitate acute myocardial infarction.

Interactions

Negative inotropic drugs such as verapamil or disopyramide should be used cautiously with propranolol in patients with LV dysfunction. Propranolol and verapamil in combination occasionally may precipitate AV block. Antacids containing aluminum hydroxide significantly reduce absorption of propranolol. Phenytoin, phenobarbital, and rifampin accelerate hepatic metabolism of propranolol, resulting in reduced serum concentrations; cimetidine increases serum concentrations of propranolol. Propranolol, by decreasing cardiac output, can reduce the systemic clearance of lidocaine, theophylline, and antipyrine.

Indications and Dosage

Arrhythmic indications for propranolol include supraventricular arrhythmias and arrhythmias associated with thyrotoxicosis or digitalis toxicity in addition to arrhythmias associated with increased catecholamine states. Propranolol may be effective for ventricular ectopy and some ventricular tachyarrhythmias. Propranolol, in addition to other β-blocking agents, has been shown to reduce cardiovascular mortality for at least 2 to 3 years after acute myocardial infarction. As a class, these drugs are the only antiarrhythmic agents shown to reduce mortality in patients after acute myocardial infarction. Intravenous doses should be given under ECG monitoring beginning with 0.25 to 1.0 mg, with a total dose no greater than 0.2 mg/kg. Oral dosages are highly variable, ranging from 20 to 240 mg or more daily, divided into three or four intervals for antiarrhythmic therapy. Longer-acting preparations may allow once- or twice-daily dosing. Doses of 180 to 240 mg daily in two or three divided doses are recommended to reduce mortality after myocardial infarction.

Acebutolol

Pharmacologic Description

Acebutolol hydrochloride is a relatively cardioselective β_1-adrenergic receptor antagonist with mild intrinsic sympathomimetic activity. It is available in the United States for the treatment of hypertension and ventricular arrhythmias.

Electrophysiologic Action

The electrophysiologic effects of acebutolol are predominantly are related to its β_1-receptor blocking activity. At rest, the sinus cycle length increases minimally owing to intrinsic sympathomimetic activity. The sinus response to exercise is markedly blunted. Although acebutolol possesses membrane-stabilizing activity (sodium channel blocking ability) in high concentrations, this effect does not appear to be important clinically. ECG effects consist of prolongation of the PR interval (AH interval), with minimal, if any, change in the QTc interval. The QRS duration is unchanged.

Pharmacokinetics and Metabolism

After oral administration, acebutolol is well absorbed from the gastrointestinal tract but undergoes extensive first-pass metabolism, resulting in an absolute bioavailability of 40% (range, 20% to 60%). The major metabolite, an *N*-acetyl derivative (diacetolol), is approximately equally active but is more cardioselective than the parent compound. Acebutolol is 26% bound to plasma proteins. Peak plasma concentrations of acebutolol are reached 2.5 h after oral ingestion, whereas peak levels of diacetolol occur at 3.5 h. The elimination half-life of acebutolol is 3 to 4 h, whereas the half-life for diacetolol is 8 to 13 h. Forty percent of acebutolol is eliminated by the kidneys; diacetolol is almost entirely renally excreted. In the presence of renal impairment, plasma concentrations of acebutolol are not significantly changed, but concentrations of diacetolol increase two- to threefold. Therefore, dose reduction is necessary with renal insufficiency.

Acebutolol and diacetolol are hydrophilic; therefore, only minimal concentrations of these compounds are found within the central nervous system.

Hemodynamic Effects

Like propranolol, acebutolol decreases heart rate and cardiac contractility. The potential for heart rate slowing is somewhat less with acebutolol owing to its partial agonist activity. Blood pressure reduction typically is proportional to baseline pressure, but hypotension may occur in previously normotensive individuals.

Antiarrhythmic Effects

The β-blocking activity of acebutolol is approximately 25% that of propranolol on a milligram-to-milligram basis. Acebutolol can suppress premature ventricular contractions, including complex forms, in many patients. Patients with exercise-induced arrhythmias may respond favorably to acebutolol. Acebutolol is also effective for various supraventricular arrhythmias, especially those related to excess catecholamine states or those that require participation of the AV node, such as AV nodal and AV reciprocating tachycardias. A randomized, double-blind, placebo-controlled trial including 600 patients after myocardial infarction (APSI trial) reported that a rather low dose of acebutolol, 200 mg twice daily, decreases cardiovascular mortality by 58%.

Side Effects

Side effects related to acebutolol are similar to those of other β-blocking agents. Patients with congestive heart failure, hypotension, severe peripheral vascular disease, brittle diabetes mellitus, or bronchospastic lung disease should not be treated with acebutolol, despite its partial agonist activity. Similarly, acebutolol may depress sinus node and AV nodal function. Fatigue, headache, reversible mental depression, skin rash, agranulocytosis, development of antinuclear antibodies, alopecia, and Peyronie's disease have been reported.

Interactions

Although specific interactions have not been reported with acebutolol, caution should be used if it is given with other drugs known to depress automaticity, conduction, or cardiac contractility or other drugs known to interact with β blockers.

Indications and Dosage

Acebutolol is indicated for treatment of ventricular premature contractions. It is also effective for some supraventricular arrhythmias. The initial antiarrhythmic dosage usually is 200 mg twice daily, with total daily doses up to 600 to 1200 mg necessary in some patients.

Esmolol

Pharmacologic Description

Esmolol hydrochloride, a phenoxypropanolamine, is a β_1-selective adrenergic-receptor blocking agent. Esmolol is similar in chemical structure to the β-blocker metoprolol but contains an ester linkage on the para position of the phenyl ring. Because of this ester linkage, esmolol has an ultrashort plasma half-life of 9 min. It has no appreciable intrinsic sympathomimetic or membrane-stabilizing activity. On a milligram-to-milligram basis, esmolol is approximately 2% as potent as propranolol.

Electrophysiologic Action

Electrophysiologic effects of esmolol are those typical of β blockade. Esmolol increases the sinus node's cycle length and slows AV nodal conduction. AV nodal refractoriness is increased as a result of decreased sympathetic tone. Thus esmolol may be effective when used to slow the ventricular response to AF or AFL or in treating arrhythmias requiring participation of the AV node, such as reciprocating tachycardias. ECG effects consist of prolongation of the PR interval, with no significant changes in QRS or QTc duration.

Pharmacokinetics and Metabolism

Esmolol is rapidly metabolized by hydrolysis of the ester linkage, chiefly by esterases in the cytosol of red blood cells. The distribution half-life of esmolol is 2 min; the elimination half-life is 9 min, necessitating continuous infusion or repeated boluses for sustained effects. Metabolism of esmolol results in a negligible amount of methanol and an acid metabolite. Less than 2% of esmolol is recovered in the urine. The metabolite has about 0.07% the β-blocking activity of esmolol and is eliminated with a half-life of 3.7 h in individuals with normal renal function. Unlike that of many other agents with ester groups, the metabolism of esmolol is unaffected by plasma cholinesterase. With continuous high-dose infusion of esmolol, levels of methanol approximate endogenous methanol levels, with concentrations reaching only 2% of those associated with methanol toxicity. Esmolol is about 55% bound to plasma proteins, whereas the acid metabolite is only 10% bound.

Hemodynamic Effects

Esmolol produces a dose-dependent decrease in heart rate, cardiac contractility, cardiac output, and blood pressure. Recovery of these effects is nearly complete within 15 to 30 min after discontinuation of the infusion. In clinical trials, approximately 10% to 30% of patients (particularly those with borderline-low or low to normal pretreatment blood pressures) treated with esmolol developed transient hypotension, defined as a systolic pressure less than 90 mm Hg or a diastolic pressure less than 50 mm Hg. Twelve percent of patients were symptomatic.

Antiarrhythmic Effects

Esmolol has been used mainly in acute settings to control the ventricular response to supraventricular arrhythmias. In a multicenter double-blind, randomized study, esmolol was as effective as propranolol, resulting in at least a 20% reduction in ventricular rate in 72% of patients. Conversion to sinus rhythm occurred in 14%. In other studies, esmolol compared favorably with verapamil, with a significantly greater percentage of conversion to sinus rhythm.

Side Effects

The principal side effect of esmolol is hypotension. Other side effects are typical of β blockers and include increased heart failure, dyspnea, bradycardia, decreased peripheral perfusion, nausea, vomiting, irritation at the infusion site, and headache. To avoid phlebitis, esmolol should not be infused at concentrations in excess of 10 mg/mL. For a typical patient requiring 50 to 150 mg/kg per minute, 20 to 60 mL/h of fluid administration is required, necessitating attention to volume status.

Interactions

Esmolol can be very effective when used in combination with digoxin, and the effects on the AV node are additive. Concomitant administration of esmolol and morphine results in a 46% increase in steady-state levels of esmolol. Esmolol prolongs the metabolism of succinylcholine-induced neuromuscular blockade by 5 to 8 min. Esmolol should be administered with caution in patients prone to bradycardia, AV block, or hypotension or in patients on other medications likely to potentiate these effects.

Indications and Dosage

Esmolol is indicated for the acute management and rapid control of ventricular rate in patients with AF or AFL and in some patients with noncompensatory sinus tachycardia. Therapy is usually initiated with a loading dose of 500 µg/kg over 1 min, followed by a maintenance infusion of 25 to 50 µg/kg per minute. Dose titration can be performed after 5 min and consists of additional boluses of 500 µg/kg over 1 min, followed by an increase in the maintenance infusion by 25 to 50 µg/kg per minute. Most patients are controlled with a maintenance infusion of 50 to 200 µg/kg per minute. Esmolol also may be useful in the management of acute myocardial ischemia or infarction, although this has not been studied extensively. The effects of prolonged infusions of esmolol (longer than 48 h) also have not been fully evaluated.

CLASS III AGENTS

Class III drugs prolong the duration of action potential and increase refractoriness. The effect is often mediated by blockade of potassium channels during phase 2 or 3 of the action potential. Some newer agents prolong the duration of the action potential by activating sodium channels during the plateau phase.

Amiodarone

Pharmacologic Description

Amiodarone hydrochloride, an iodinated benzofuran derivative, was initially developed as a vasodilating agent for the treatment of angina pectoris. Thirty-seven percent of its molecular weight is iodine. It was subsequently found to have potent antiarrhythmic properties in 1970. Oral and intravenous preparations are available in the United States for the treatment of life-threatening ventricular arrhythmias.

Electrophysiologic Action

Amiodarone has been shown to have class I, II, III, and IV effects. It is a weak, noncompetitive inhibitor of α- and β-adrenergic receptors. The drug has been shown experimentally to block electrical remodeling induced by atrial tachycardia. Its predominant action on cardiac tissue consists of prolongation of the duration of the action potential and increases in refractoriness. Amiodarone has only slight effects on the rate of rise of phase 0 of the action potential. Conduction velocity is decreased, however, apparently owing to effects on resistance to passive current flow rather than to effects on the inward sodium current. In automatic cells, amiodarone decreases the slope of phase 4 of the action potential, thereby decreasing the depolarization rate of these cells. Amiodarone has differential effects on the two components of cardiac rectifier K^+ current, depending on the length of treatment. ECG effects consist of a slowing of the sinus rate and prolongation of the PR, QRS, and QT intervals. Amiodarone also prolongs the refractory period of accessory AV pathways in patients with bypass tracts or the WPW syndrome. The time course of onset of antiarrhythmic action varies, with effects on the sinus and AV nodes occurring within 2 weeks of therapy, whereas prolongation of the ventricular functional refractory period, QT prolongation, and ventricular antiarrhythmic effects are not maximal for up to 10 weeks.

Pharmacokinetics and Metabolism

When the drug is administered orally, absorption of amiodarone is slow and erratic. Bioavailability ranges from 22% to 65% in most patients. Peak plasma concentrations occur between 3 and 7 h after one oral dose. Even with loading doses, maximal antiarrhythmic effects may not appear for several days to months. Amiodarone is 95% protein bound and has a large but variable volume of distribution of approximately 60 L/kg. Amiodarone and its major metabolite, desethylamiodarone, are highly lipophilic and accumulate throughout the body, including liver, adipose tissue, lung, myocardium, kidney, thyroid, skin, eye, and skeletal muscle. Elimination is principally hepatic via biliary excretion. Enterohepatic recirculation may occur. The elimination of amiodarone is biphasic, with an initial half-life of 2.5 to 10 days; the terminal elimination half-life is 26 to 107 days, with most patients in the 40- to 55-day range. Desethylamiodarone has an elimination half-life averaging 61 days.

Hemodynamic Effects

With intravenous administration, amiodarone decreases heart rate, myocardial contractility, and systemic vascular resistance. Coronary vasodilatation may also occur. Rapid intravenous administration may produce profound hypotension, partly related to systemic vasodilation caused by the vehicle Tween-80. Oral amiodarone usually does not worsen congestive heart failure, even in patients with severe LV dysfunction, although caution is warranted, especially with high doses used during drug loading, because some patients may show hemodynamic deterioration.

Antiarrhythmic Effects

A large number of studies have documented the efficacy of amiodarone in suppressing supraventricular and ventricular arrhythmias even when other agents were ineffective. Amiodarone is very effective in chronic maintenance of sinus rhythm in patients with AF, although it is not approved for this indication in the United States. Daily doses of 200 to 400 mg have shown an efficacy of 53% to 79% for sinus rhythm maintenance. It was more effective than sotalol or propafenone in the maintenance of sinus rhythm in patients with chronic paroxysmal or persistent AF. The drug is often used in patients with life-threatening ventricular tachyarrhythmias who are unresponsive to other antiarrhythmic agents. In a composite of 10 reports from the literature, amiodarone prevented recurrent sustained VT or VF in 66% of 567 patients during a mean follow-up of 13 months. The prognostic utility of electrophysiologic testing with amiodarone remains controversial. The ability to induce VT by using programmed ventricular stimulation during therapy with amiodarone does not preclude a good outcome. Patients rendered not inducible by amiodarone have a good outcome. Induction of a hemodynamically well-tolerated ventricular tachyarrhythmia apparently suggests a relatively favorable prognosis. Suppression of ventricular ectopy on ambulatory monitoring by amiodarone is an unreliable indicator of success, whereas failure to suppress ventricular ectopy appears to indicate a worse prognosis. Therapeutic plasma concentrations are usually between 1.0 and 2.0 µg/mL with chronic dosing. Several trials have shown that amiodarone may improve mortality rates, or at least not worsen mortality rates, when used to treat patients after myocardial infarction or with LV dysfunction. Whether amiodarone is superior in this regard to conventional β-blocking drugs is unknown. Intravenous amiodarone is at least as effective as bretylium for VT or VF and is associated with fewer hemodynamic side effects.

Side Effects

Almost every organ system is affected by amiodarone. Corneal microdeposits of brownish crystals are expected. They may result in blurred vision, halos, or a smoky hue, but such effects reportedly disappear after cessation of therapy. Abnormal thyroid function tests are not uncommon, and in some cases clinical hypothyroidism or hyperthyroidism becomes evident. A bluish-gray skin discoloration and photosensitivity may occur. Liver function abnormalities, neuropathy, and myositis have been reported. Occasionally severe hepatitis has occurred; two cases of fatal hepatic necrosis have been reported after rapid infusion of large intravenous doses. As many as 5% to 15% of patients treated with 400 mg/day will develop pulmonary toxicity. This usually resolves with discontinuation of therapy but may be fatal. Therapy with corticosteroids may be beneficial. Cardiac side effects include bradycardia, AV block, worsening of congestive heart failure, and rarely proarrhythmia. Torsades de pointes occurs only rarely, and many patients having this arrhythmia while on other drugs have not had this recur while on amiodarone. Intravenous amiodarone in concentrations of greater than 2.0 mg/mL should be infused only via a central venous catheter owing to a high incidence of peripheral vein phlebitis. Lower concentrations may be infused using a peripheral vein.

Interaction

Amiodarone interacts with many drugs and increases the plasma concentrations of warfarin (100%), digoxin (70%), quinidine (33%), procainamide (55%), and NAPA (33%). Concentrations of phenytoin and flecainide also have been reported to increase. Appropriate caution should be exercised when using any of these agents with amiodarone.

Indications and Dosage

The oral formulation of amiodarone is indicated in the United States for the treatment of recurrent life-threatening ventricular arrhythmias that have not responded adequately to other agents. Because of the large volume of distribution, large loading doses are required initially. Typically, 1000 to 1600 mg is administered daily for 7 to 14 days, followed by 600 to 800 mg daily for the next 7 to 30 days. Long-term maintenance therapy usually requires 200 to 400 mg daily. Doses should be slowly reduced to the lowest level consistent with adequate arrhythmia control, because higher chronic doses are associated with an increased incidence of toxicity. Given the favorable mortality rate results with amiodarone and its efficacy in treating almost any cardiac arrhythmia, clinical use of amiodarone has increased.

Intravenous Amiodarone

Intravenous amiodarone is indicated for treatment and prophylaxis of frequently recurring VF and hemodynamically unstable VT. Peak serum concentration after one 5-mg/kg 15-min infusion in healthy subjects range between 5 and 41 mg/L. Due to rapid distribution, serum concentrations decline to 10% of peak values within 30 to 45 min after the end of the infusion. It has been reported to produce negative inotropic and vasodilatory effects in animals and humans, with drug-related hypotension occurring in 16% of treated patients. Additional adverse effects were: bradycardia and AV block, VF (<2%), adult respiratory distress syndrome (2%), and torsades de pointes. The recommended starting dose of intravenous amiodarone is about 1000 mg over the first 24 h of therapy, delivered by the following infusion regimen: rapid infusion, i.e., 150 mg over the first 10 min, followed by a slow infusion of 360 mg over the next 6 h, and a maintenance infusion of 540 mg over the remaining 18 h. Concomitant oral therapy may be started simultaneously. Intravenous amiodarone is effective in suppressing refractory VT/VF and provides control of 60% to 80% of recurrent VT/VF when conventional drugs as continuous oral therapy have failed.

Intravenous amiodarone has increased survival to hospital admission in patients with out-of-hospital cardiac arrest due to refractory VT/VF and has been shown to be significantly more effective than lidocaine in improving survival to hospital for out-of-hospital cardiac arrest patients. The most recent Advanced Cardiac Life Support guidelines suggest the use intravenous amiodarone (class IIb) at a dose of 300 mg intravenously as an initial bolus, followed by a second dose of 150 mg intravenously if VF or pulseless VT recurs.

Sotalol

Pharmacologic Description

Sotalol is a nonselective β-adrenergic antagonist introduced in 1965 for the treatment of hypertension. It is without significant intrinsic sympathomimetic activity or membrane-stabilizing activity. Sotalol does prolong the action potential duration, accounting for its class III designation. The antiarrhythmic effects in humans were reported in 1970.

The electrophysiologic effects of sotalol are those of β blockade and class III activity. Sotalol exists as a racemic mixture of D-sotalol and L-sotalol. The D-sotalol form has about 2% the β-blocking activity of L-sotalol, but both are equally responsible for class III effects. Sotalol causes an increase in the duration of the action potential and the refractory period of human atria, ventricles, AV node, Purkinje fibers, and accessory pathways. Conduction velocity is reportedly not decreased by sotalol except for the β-blocking effects on nodal tissues. ECG effects consist of increases in the PR, QT, and QTc intervals. QRS duration and the HV interval are unchanged.

Pharmacokinetics and Metabolism

Sotalol is rapidly absorbed after oral administration, with bioavailability varying from 60% to nearly 100%. Sotalol is not bound to plasma proteins, and greater than 75% of an administered dose is recovered unchanged in the urine. No metabolites have been detected. The elimination half-life averages 10 to 15 h, permitting twice-daily dosing. Sotalol will accumulate in patients with renal but not with hepatic insufficiency.

Hemodynamic Effects

Prolongation of the duration of the action potential allows more time for calcium ions to enter a cell, potentially increasing the inotropic state of the cell. Sotalol appears unique among β-blocking agents in this regard. Studies in isolated muscle preparations, animals, and humans suggest that sotalol may cause less depression of contractility than other β-blocking drugs. Nevertheless, sotalol can reduce blood pressure and precipitate or worsen congestive heart failure in some patients.

Antiarrhythmic Effects

Sotalol has been used effectively for the treatment of supraventricular and ventricular tachyarrhythmias, including WPW syndrome. Sotalol has been effective in terminating many supraventricular arrhythmias or slowing the ventricular response to AF or AFL. In one study, oral sotalol produced a beneficial response in 31 of 33 patients with atrial arrhythmias. Other studies have found sotalol effective in the treatment of life-threatening ventricular arrhythmias when assessed by electrophysiologic testing, including those refractory to class I antiarrhythmic agents. Polymorphic VT (torsades de pointes) in the setting of a prolonged QT interval has occurred with sotalol, often in association with hypokalemia or renal insufficiency (high sotalol levels). Sotalol has also been shown to reduce defibrillation thresholds and the frequency of ICD shocks for VT and VF.

Side Effects

Rates of bronchospasm, fatigue, impotence, depression, and headache are similar to those of other β-blocking drugs. Sinus node slowing, AV block, hypotension, and worsening of congestive heart failure may occur. Rare cases of retroperitoneal fibrosis have been reported. Polymorphic VT is a potentially life-threatening adverse reaction to sotalol. Its incidence may be minimized by careful attention to electrolyte status and avoiding high serum concentrations or excessive bradycardia. Chronic oral therapy with sotalol can increase the serum level of cholesterol as in the case of other β blockers without partial agonist activity. The clinical significance of this effect is unknown.

Interactions

Significant drug interactions have not been reported. However, sotalol should be administered with caution with agents that produce hypokalemia or prolong the QT interval. In addition, sotalol should be used cautiously with drugs that depress cardiac contractility, especially in patients with LV dysfunction and those with contraindications to β blockers.

Indications and Dosage

Sotalol is effective for the treatment of supraventricular and ventricular tachyarrhythmias. Oral therapy is usually begun with 80 mg administered twice daily. Total daily doses greater than 480 mg should be used rarely. Dosage reduction is necessary in patients with mild to moderate renal insufficiency. Sotalol probably should not be used in patients with severe renal insufficiency. Intravenous doses of 0.2 to 1.0 mg/kg have been used in the acute treatment of arrhythmias. The D-stereoisomer of sotalol (D-sotalol) was withdrawn from further clinical testing after it was shown to be associated with increased cardiac and all-cause mortality as compared with placebo in patients with histories of myocardial infarction and reduced LV function.

Ibutilide

Pharmacologic Description

Ibutilide fumarate, a class III antiarrhythmic agent that prolongs repolarization, was approved by the U.S. Food and Drug Administration (FDA) for intravenous use in the United States. Ibutilide is structurally similar to sotalol but is devoid of any clinically significant β-adrenergic blocking activity.

Electrophysiologic Action

Ibutilide affects the duration of action potentials of atrial, ventricular, and His-Purkinje cells in a unique dose-dependent manner. At low concentrations, ibutilide prolongs the duration of action potentials, whereas at higher concentrations the duration decreases. Unlike other class III agents, such as sotalol or *N*-acetylprocainamide, ibutilide prolongs the duration of action potentials by activating an inward sodium current during the plateau phase of the action potential in addition to blocking an outward potassium current.

Pharmacokinetics and Metabolism

Ibutilide is well absorbed after oral administration but, like lidocaine, is rapidly metabolized in the liver, such that oral bioavailability is small. Thus, oral administration does not appear practical. Ibutilide has a large volume of distribution (10 to 15 L/kg), with a terminal elimination half-life of between 6 and 9 h. Rapid distribution after intravenous administration accounts for the disappearance of QT prolongation several minutes after dosing.

Hemodynamic Effects

No significant effects on cardiac contractility have been seen in animal models. In addition, a study of hemodynamic function in patients with EFs above and below 35% showed no clinically significant effects on cardiac output, mean pulmonary artery pressure, or pulmonary capillary wedge pressure at doses of up to 0.03 mg/kg.

Antiarrhythmic Effects

In animal studies and in phase 2 clinical trials, ibutilide has shown efficacy in prevention of induction of VT during programmed electrical stimulation.

Ibutilide appears to decrease the defibrillation threshold in dogs. In human studies, ibutilide has been investigated most extensively for its ability to terminate established AFL or AF. Up to 60% of patients with AFL and approximately 40% of those with AF will revert to sinus rhythm with 0.025 mg/kg of ibutilide given intravenously. Patients with more a recent onset of arrhythmia had a higher rate of conversion. Ibutilide pretreatment also can facilitate electrocardioversion of AF.

Side Effects

To date, the most significant side effect observed in clinical trials of ibutilide is the development of polymorphic VT (torsades de pointes), which has occasionally become sustained and required cardioversion. It occurs in about 1.7% of patients treated and is dose related. The risk of polymorphic VT is higher in patients with systolic dysfunction. Rare episodes of advanced-degree AV block and infra-His conduction block have been reported.

Interactions

Class Ia and III antiarrhythmic drugs should not be given concomitantly with ibutilide infusion or within 4 h after infusion because of their potential to prolong refractoriness. The potential for proarrhythmia may increase with the administration of ibutilide to patients who are being treated with drugs that prolong the QT interval, such as phenothiazines, tricyclic antidepressants, and certain antihistamine drugs.

Indications and Dosage

Ibutilide is indicated for the acute treatment (cardioversion) of recent onset AFL or AF. Patients whose atrial arrhythmias were sustained longer than 90 days were not evaluated in clinical trials. A dose of 1 mg is administered over 10 min intravenously. After an additional 10 min, the dose may be repeated, if needed. Patients weighing less than 60 kg should have the dose reduced.

Dofetilide

Pharmacologic Description

Dofetilide has Vaughn Williams class III antiarrhythmic activity. The mechanism of action is the blockade of the cardiac ion channel carrying the rapid component of the delayed rectifier potassium current I_{Kr}. At all studied concentrations, dofetilide blocks only I_{Kr}, with no relevant block of the other repolarizing potassium currents. It has no effect on sodium channels, α receptors, or β receptors.

Electrophysiologic Action

Dofetilide increases the duration of action potentials in a predictable, concentration-dependent manner, primarily due to delayed repolarization. It increases the effective refractory period of atria and ventricles. It does not have an effect on PR interval or QRS width. Dofetilide does not increase the electrical energy required to convert electrically induced VF, and it significantly reduces the defibrillation threshold in patients with VT and VF undergoing insertion of an ICD.

Pharmacokinetics and Metabolism

The oral bioavailability of dofetilide is greater than 90%, with maximum plasma concentration occurring at about 2 to 3 h. Oral bioavailability is not affected by food intake or antacid use. Steady-state concentration is reached within 2 to 3 days, and the half-life is about 10 h. Plasma protein binding is 60% to 70%, and the volume of distribution is 3 L/kg. Eighty percent of the drug is excreted in urine unchanged, and the remaining 20% comprises five minimally active metabolites. The half-life is longer and the clearance of dofetilide is decreased in patients with renal impairment.

Hemodynamic Effects

In hemodynamic studies, dofetilide had no effect on cardiac output, cardiac index, stroke volume index, and systemic vascular resistance in patients with VT, mild to moderate congestive heart failure or angina, and normal or low LV EF. There was no evidence of a negative inotropic effect related to dofetilide therapy in patients with AF. There was no increase in heart failure in patients with significant LV dysfunction or any significant change in blood pressure. Heart rate was decreased by 4 to 6 beats/min in studies in patients.

Dofetilide use is usually safe in patients with structural heart disease, including patients with impaired LV function (EF $\leq$ 35%; Diamond CHF) or recent myocardial infarction (Diamond MI).

Antiarrhythmic Effects

Dofetilide, like most other class III antiarrhythmic agents, has antifibrillatory activity in the atria; this property is of importance for the conversion and maintenance of sinus rhythm in patients with AF or AFL. In a placebo-controlled blinded study, the conversion rates were 31% in AF patients, 54% in AFL patients, and 0% in those on placebo.

Side Effects

Dofetilide can cause ventricular arrhythmia, primarily torsades de pointes associated with QT prolongation. Prolongation of the QT interval is directly related to the plasma concentration of dofetilide. Factors such as reduced creatinine clearance or dofetilide drug interactions will increase the plasma concentration of dofetilide. The risk of torsades de pointes can be reduced by controlling the plasma concentration through adjustment of the initial dofetilide dose according to creatinine clearance and by monitoring the ECG for excessive increases in the QT interval.

In patients with supraventricular arrhythmias, the overall incidences of torsades were 0.8% to 3.3% in patients with congestive heart failure and 0.9% in patients on dofetilide with recent myocardial infarction. Most episodes of torsades de pointes occurred within the first 3 days of treatment. The rate of torsades de pointes was reduced when patients were dosed according to their renal function. Other adverse reactions reported were headache, chest pain, dizziness, and respiratory tract infection.

Interactions

The use of dofetilide in conjunction with other drugs which prolong the QT interval is not recommended. Such drugs include phenothiazines, cisapride, bepridil, tricyclic antidepressants, and certain oral macrolides. Class I or III antiarrhythmic should be withheld for at least three half-lives before dosing with dofetilide. In clinical trials, dofetilide was administered to patients previously treated with oral amiodarone only if serum amiodarone levels were below 0.3 mg/L or amiodarone had been withdrawn for at least 3 months.

Dofetilide is metabolized to a small degree by the CYP3A4 isoenzyme of the cytochrome P450 system and an inhibitor of this system could increase systemic dofetilide exposure. Concomitant use of the following drugs is contraindicated: cimetidine, verapamil, ketonazole, and trimethoprim alone or in combination with sulfamethoxazole.

Indication and Dosage

The use of dofetilide is indicated for the maintenance of normal sinus rhythm (delay in time to recurrence of AF or AFL) in patients with AF or AFL of longer than 1 week's duration who have been converted to normal sinus rhythm. Because dofetilide can cause life-threatening ventricular arrhythmias, it should be reserved for patients in whom AF or AFL is highly symptomatic. Dofetilide is also indicated for the conversion of AF or AFL to normal sinus rhythm. Dofetilide has not been shown to be effective in patients with paroxysmal AF.

Therapy with dofetilide must be initiated (and, if necessary, reinitiated) in a setting that provides continuous ECG monitoring. Patients should continue to be monitored in this way for a minimum of 3 days. In addition, patients should not be discharged within 12 h of electrical or pharmacologic conversion to normal sinus rhythm.

Because prolongation of QT interval and the risk of torsades de pointes are directly related to plasma concentrations of dofetilide, dose adjustment must be individualized according to calculated creatinine clearance and QTc. The QT interval should be used if the heart rate is slower than 60 beats/min. If the QTc is longer than 440 ms (500 ms in bundle branch block) or creatinine clearance lower than 20 mL/min, dofetilide is contraindicated. During loading, a 12-lead ECG should be done 2 to 3 h after the dose and the QT should be checked.

If patients do not convert to normal sinus rhythm within 72 h of initiation of dofetilide therapy, electrical conversion should be considered, with subsequent monitoring for 12 h postcardioversion.

CLASS IV AGENTS

Class IV antiarrhythmic drugs are the nondihydropyridine calcium channel blocking agents (see Chapter 4).

Verapamil

Pharmacologic Description

Verapamil hydrochloride, a synthetic papaverine derivative, was the first calcium channel blocking agent to be used clinically. It is indicated for the treatment of supraventricular arrhythmias, control of ventricular rate at rest and during exercise in patients with AF or AFL, and certain forms of ventricular tachyarrhythmias that occur in patients with structurally normal hearts.

Electrophysiologic Action

The principal electrophysiologic effect of verapamil is inhibition of the slow inward calcium current. Verapamil prolongs the time-dependent recovery of excitability and the effective refractory period of AV nodal fibers. It has little effect on fibers in the lower AV node (NH region) and no effect on atrial or Purkinje action potentials, which are activated by a rapid sodium current. However, verapamil may be effective in suppressing triggered arrhythmias arising from ventricular or Purkinje tissue. Expected ECG changes consist of prolongation of the PR interval and no significant change in QRS or QT duration. Verapamil also may depress sinus node function (automaticity and conduction), particularly when it is abnormal.

Pharmacokinetics and Metabolism

Verapamil is almost completely (>90%) absorbed after oral administration but undergoes extensive first-pass metabolism. Absolute bioavailability ranges from 20% to 35%, with peak plasma levels occurring 1 to 2 h after dosing. Verapamil is 90% bound to plasma proteins. The L-isomer of verapamil undergoes more rapid metabolism than the D-isomer, and the L-verapamil isomer is more active electrophysiologically. Twelve metabolites of verapamil have been identified; the major one, norverapamil, can reach concentrations equal to those of the parent compound with chronic dosing. The cardiovascular activity of norverapamil is approximately 20% that of verapamil. After single oral doses, the elimination half-life of verapamil varies from 3 to 7 h; with multiple doses, the half-life ranges from 3 to 12 h. Elimination half-life is usually prolonged with advancing age. In one study, the elimination half-life was 7.4 h in patients older than 61 years versus 3.8 h in individuals younger than 36 years. The elimination of verapamil also may be prolonged in patients with AF or with hepatic dysfunction.

Hemodynamic Effects

Verapamil produces negative inotropic, dromotropic (AV and sinoatrial nodes), and chronotropic (sinoatrial node) effects. However, it is well tolerated in most individuals, even in those with LV dysfunction. Hypotension, bradycardia, AV block, and asystole have occurred on occasion. Simultaneous use of verapamil with a β blocker may result in significant hypotension and depression of cardiac function. This risk is more pronounced with intravenous administration of verapamil.

Antiarrhythmic Effects

Verapamil will slow the ventricular response to AF and AFL even in patients with normal AV conduction. Patients with AF and accessory AV pathways may experience increases in ventricular rate after verapamil administration, related to a reflex increase in sympathetic tone after vasodilation or decreased AV nodal conduction with less retrograde penetration of the bypass tract. Verapamil can slow and terminate most arrhythmias by using the AV node as part of the reentrant circuit, such as AV nodal reentry, or AV reciprocating tachycardia by using an accessory pathway. Oral verapamil is consistently less effective than intravenous verapamil in terminating these arrhythmias, a difference that may be explained in part by the differences in bioavailability and metabolism of the more active L-isomer when the racemic mixture of D- and L-verapamil is given by these two routes. Verapamil can be effective monotherapy for long-term control of ventricular rate in patients with AF or as adjunctive therapy in combination with digoxin. Verapamil is generally ineffective in treating reentrant VT but may be effective in certain ventricular tachyarrhythmias, usually seen in younger patients, presumably due to triggered activity. Verapamil also may be used to suppress or reduce the ventricular rate in patients with multifocal atrial tachycardia.

Side Effects

Intravenous verapamil may produce hypotension, bradycardia, AV block, and occasionally asystole. The risk of hypotension may be lessened by the prior administration of 1000 mg of intravenous calcium chloride without interfering with the acute depressant effects of intravenous verapamil on AV nodal conduction. It should be avoided in patients with severe LV dysfunction and in those with wide QRS tachycardias in which VT or AF with preexcitation are considerations. Oral therapy is most commonly associated with constipation, but some patients complain of dizziness, fatigue, or ankle edema. Rarely, increases in liver aminotransferases have been observed.

Interactions

Verapamil reduces the clearance of digoxin by 35%, with an increase in serum digoxin concentrations of 50% to 75% within the first week of verapamil therapy. Concomitant administration of verapamil and quinidine may result in significant hypotension, because both drugs antagonize the effects of catecholamines on α-adrenergic receptors. Other drugs with negative inotropic properties, such as disopyramide or flecainide, should be used cautiously with verapamil. Simultaneous administration of β blockers and verapamil may result in hypotension, bradycardia, or AV block. Verapamil appears to variably increase the bioavailability of metoprolol from 0% to 28%.

Indications and Dosage

Verapamil is indicated for the termination of supraventricular tachycardias involving the AV node. It is also indicated to control the ventricular rate in patients with AF or AFL and normal AV conduction. Intravenous doses of 5 to 10 mg given over no fewer than 2 min are often effective. The dose may be repeated, if necessary, in 30 min. Alternatively, smaller doses (e.g., 2.5 mg) repeated as indicated at more frequent intervals also may be effective. In contrast to certain class I and III antiarrhythmic agents, verapamil is rarely effective in converting AF or AFL to sinus rhythm. Oral therapy using doses of 160 to 480 mg/day, in three or four divided doses, can be effective for chronic control of ventricular response with AF or prophylaxis of paroxysmal supraventricular tachycardia. Sustained-release preparations may allow once- or twice-daily dosing in many patients.

Diltiazem

Pharmacologic Description

Diltiazem hydrochloride is a benzodiazepine derivative that blocks influx of calcium ions during cell depolarization in cardiac and vascular smooth muscles. It is indicated for therapy of supraventricular arrhythmias and for control of ventricular rate in AF and AFL.

Electrophysiologic Action

The principal electrophysiologic effect of diltiazem is inhibition of the slow inward calcium current. It prolongs the time-dependent recovery of excitability and the effective refractory period of AV nodal fibers. Expected ECG changes consist of prolongation of the PR (AH) interval and no significant change in QRS or QT duration. Diltiazem also may depress sinus node function (automaticity and conduction), particularly when it is abnormal.

Pharmacokinetics and Metabolism

Diltiazem binds to α_1-acid glycoprotein (40%) and serum albumin (30%). Diltiazem is extensively metabolized in the liver by the cytochrome P450 system. Little diltiazem is renally eliminated. As such, diltiazem doses do not need to be adjusted in the presence of renal insufficiency or failure. The elimination half-life of intravenous diltiazem is approximately 3.4 h.

Hemodynamic Effects

Intravenous diltiazem produces negative inotropic, dromotropic, and chronotropic effects. When administered acutely, diltiazem lowers systolic and diastolic blood pressures and systemic vascular resistance. Coronary artery vascular resistance also decreases, thus increasing coronary blood flow.

Antiarrhythmic Effects

Diltiazem increases AV nodal conduction time and increases AV nodal refractoriness. The effects of diltiazem on the AV node demonstrate use dependence, being more pronounced at faster heart rates. In addition, diltiazem slows the rate of depolarization of the sinus node. AV nodal reentry and reciprocating tachycardia may be terminated by direct effects on the AV node. Increased AV nodal refractoriness also slows the ventricular response to AF and AFL.

Side Effects

Hypotension is the most common side effect of diltiazem, occurring in approximately 4.3% of patients in clinical trials. Although the sinus rate decreases with intravenous diltiazem, sinus bradycardia or high-grade AV block occurs rarely. Elevations of serum aminotransferase enzyme levels occur rarely.

Interactions

Drugs that produce hypotension or interfere with sinus and AV nodal function would be expected to produce synergistic effects with diltiazem. Agents that interfere or induce the hepatic microsomal enzyme system would be expected to alter diltiazem levels. Diltiazem increases propranolol levels by 50%.

Indications and Dosage

Intravenous diltiazem is indicated for temporary control of the rapid ventricular rate associated with supraventricular tachyarrhythmias such as AF and AFL, AV nodal reentrant tachycardia, or reciprocating tachycardia using an AV bypass tract. Diltiazem should not be used to treat patients with AF or AFL and AV bypass tracts. Initial therapy with intravenous diltiazem is usually administered as a bolus dose of 15 to 25 mg (0.25 mg/kg, followed by an infusion of 5 to 15 mg/h. If ventricular rate control is not achieved after the first bolus, the bolus dose may be repeated in 15 min. An 11-mg/h infusion approximates the steady-state levels achieved with a 360-mg sustained-release preparation of diltiazem. Oral preparations are available in immediate-release tablets of 30 to 120 mg used every 6 to 8 h and a sustained-release form of 180 to 300 mg requiring only once-daily dosing. Although effective, oral forms of diltiazem are not approved for treatment of arrhythmias.

UNCLASSIFIED ANTIARRHYTHMIC AGENTS

Adenosine

Pharmacologic Description

Adenosine is an endogenous compound found within every cell of the human body. It is approved by the FDA for use in the United States. Adenosine has a short half-life, enabling multiple doses without danger of cumulative or long-lasting effects.

Electrophysiologic Action

Adenosine exerts negative chronotropic and dromotropic effects on the sinus and AV nodes. It decreases the duration of action potentials and hyperpolarizes atrial myocardial cells. No direct effect on ventricular tissue has been demonstrated; however, catecholamine-enhanced ventricular automaticity may be suppressed by adenosine. The electrophysiologic effects of adenosine may be mediated in part by a vagal reflex. ECG effects consist of slowing of the sinus rate and prolongation of the PR interval.

Pharmacokinetics and Metabolism

Adenosine has a half-life shorter than 10 seconds. Adenosine is degraded by extracellular deaminases and by intracellular deaminases after it is rapidly transported into cells, forming inosine.

Hemodynamic Effects

Adenosine is a potent vasodilator that tends to reduce systolic blood pressure. Hemodynamic effects are transient after a single bolus dose, which is usually well tolerated. Adenosine is also a potent coronary artery vasodilator.

Antiarrhythmic Effects

Adenosine is effective in terminating supraventricular tachyarrhythmias requiring participation of the AV node, such as AV nodal reentry or AV reciprocating tachycardia in patients with accessory pathways. Compared with verapamil, adenosine may be more likely to unmask latent ventricular preexcitation after termination of AV reentrant tachycardia in patients with WPW syndrome. It also may cause fewer hemodynamically significant arrhythmias after termination of AV reentrant tachycardia. Overall, adenosine has been effective in 60% to more than 90% of patients in different small series, in part reflecting dosing regimens, patient selection, and arrhythmia mechanism. Occasionally, transient AF has been reported after administration of adenosine; therefore, caution is warranted in administering these agents to patients with preexcitation. In patients with various atrial tachyarrhythmias, including AF, adenosine will depress AV nodal conduction, which can be useful diagnostically. Adenosine also can be effective for certain types of VT in animal models and humans, including catecholamine-sensitive tachyarrhythmias in young adults. Further studies are required, however, to determine the efficacy and utility of adenosine in the treatment of ventricular tachyarrhythmias.

Side Effects

Adenosine produces transient flushing and dyspnea after intravenous administration. Additional side effects include bronchospasm, dyspnea, vomiting, retching, cramps, headache, and rarely cardiac arrest. Side effects are transient, and the potential for long-lasting adverse effects is minimal. Nevertheless, the possibility of profound bradycardia, AV block, or AF, especially in WPW patients with accelerated accessory AV conduction, justifies appropriate caution. Selective adenosine agonists are currently being developed to avoid these problems.

Interactions

Numerous drugs affect adenosine transport or degradation, often potentiating the effect of adenosine in experimental models. Examples include dipyridamole, digitalis, verapamil, and benzodiazepines. Aminophylline and other methylxanthines antagonize the effects of adenosine in humans. In one documented case, a patient receiving sustained-release theophylline failed to respond to high-dose adenosine.

Indications and Dosage

Adenosine is an effective agent in the acute management of paroxysmal supraventricular and AV reciprocating tachycardias involving the AV node. Adenosine is usually administered in doses of 3 to 12 mg (3 mg/mL) by rapid intravenous bolus. To be maximally effective, this agent must be given as rapid intravenous bolus injections administered directly in a free-flowing intravenous line; effects are more marked with injection into a central line. Injection into a circuitous line of peripheral tubing may be ineffective.

Digitalis

Pharmacologic Description

Digitalis glycosides are among the oldest antiarrhythmic agents still used today (see Chapter 8). Medicinal use of foxglove (digitalis) was mentioned by Welsh physicians as early as 1250. It was used to treat heart failure and arrhythmias in patients in 1775, and William Withering described his experiences with digitalis 10 years later in the classic monograph, *An Account of the Foxglove and Some of Its Medical Uses*. Digitalis preparations are steroid glycosides mostly derived from the leaves of the common flowering plants *Digitalis purpurea* (digitoxin) and *Digitalis lanata* (digoxin, lanatoside C, and deslanoside). Ouabain, a rapidly acting digitalis preparation, is derived from seeds of *Strophanthus gratus*. Digoxin and, to a much lesser extent, digitoxin are the most commonly used digitalis preparations.

Electrophysiologic Action

Digitalis glycosides produce electrophysiologic effects by a direct effect on myocardial cells and by indirect effects mediated by the autonomic nervous system. Digitalis preparations are specific inhibitors of a magnesium- and adenosine triphosphate (ATP)-dependent sodium-potassium ATPase enzyme. Inhibition of this enzyme indirectly promotes an increased concentration of intracellular calcium ions. Increased intracellular calcium results in an increased force of myocardial contraction and appears to be responsible for many of the arrhythmic effects seen with digitalis toxicity. Indirect effects result from a vagomimetic action and include negative chronotropic and dromotropic (AV node) effects. At toxic levels, digitalis results in increased sympathetic activity. Effective refractory periods of atrial and ventricular muscles generally decrease, whereas those of the AV node and Purkinje fibers increase. Refractory periods of accessory AV pathways may decrease in some patients, which can increase the rate of AV conduction in these patients with AF. In most individuals, digitalis does not appreciably alter the sinus rate. Sinus rate may slow markedly in patients with heart failure treated with digitalis, however, owing in part to vagal effects and to withdrawal of sympathetic tone. ECG effects include prolongation of the PR (AH) interval with various changes in the ST segment and T wave, characteristically with concave caving of downward-sloping ST segments.

Pharmacokinetics and Metabolism

Digoxin is 60% to 80% bioavailable when administered orally in tablets. A capsule preparation of digoxin in solution is 90% to 100% bioavailable. In as many as 10% of patients, intestinal bacteria may degrade up to 40% of digoxin to cardio-inactive products such as dihydrodigoxin, resulting in reduced digoxin serum levels. Digoxin is 20% to 25% protein bound. Elimination is mostly renal, with a half-life averaging 36 to 48 h in normal individuals. Severe renal insufficiency can prolong the elimination half-life up to 4.4 days. Digitoxin is a less polar glycoside that constitutes the principal active ingredient of the digitalis leaf. Digitoxin is nearly completely bioavailable after oral administration and is approximately 95% bound to serum proteins. Elimination is predominantly hepatic, with an elimination half-life averaging 7 to 9 days.

Hemodynamic Effects

Digitalis produces positive inotropic effects in normal and failing hearts. Cardiac output does not increase in normal individuals, however, owing to counteracting changes in preload and afterload. Digitalis increases arterial and venous tone, thus increasing systemic vascular resistance. Vascular resistance may increase before positive inotropic effects. Thus caution is required when digitalis is administered acutely in patients in whom an increase in vascular resistance would be deleterious. Rapid administration increases coronary vascular resistance, an effect that may be avoided by slow administration. In addition, increased mesenteric vascular tone on occasion may result in ischemic bowel necrosis.

Antiarrhythmic Effects

Antiarrhythmic effects result predominantly from conduction slowing within the AV node. Thus digitalis is most useful in controlling the ventricular rate in patients with AF. It is somewhat less effective in adequately slowing AV conduction in patients with AFL or atrial tachycardia or in cases where sympathetic tone is high. Addition of a β blocker or calcium channel antagonist such as verapamil or diltiazem typically results in additive electrophysiologic effects. Whether digitalis can reduce the frequency of these arrhythmias or facilitate their conversion to sinus rhythm has not been clearly established. Digitalis also may be effective in the chronic prophylactic or acute management of patients with AV nodal reentrant tachycardia. Therapeutic plasma levels range from 0.8 to 2.0 ng/mL for digoxin and from 14 to 26 ng/mL for digitoxin.

Side Effects

Adverse reactions most commonly involve the heart, central nervous system, and gastrointestinal tract. Hypersensitivity reactions are rare, and gynecomastia occurs infrequently. Patients with abnormal AV nodal function may experience heart block in the absence of toxicity. Digitalis toxicity results in many cardiac and noncardiac manifestations. Noncardiac effects include nausea, vomiting, abdominal pain, headache, and visual disturbances, especially a yellow-green color distortion. Ventricular premature contractions are perhaps the most common manifestation of cardiac toxicity; however, VT or fibrillation may occur. In addition, advanced-degree AV block, atrial tachycardia, and accelerated junctional rhythms are commonly seen. Combinations of enhanced automaticity (or triggered activity) with AV block (e.g., paroxysmal atrial tachycardia with AV block) are suggestive of digitalis toxicity. Toxicity may be treated with potassium if serum concentrations of potassium are low or normal, with monitoring to avoid high-grade AV block. Magnesium, lidocaine, propranolol, and temporary cardiac pacing may be helpful in selected cases, when withdrawal of digoxin is not sufficient to resolve toxicity. In some patients with WPW syndrome and accelerated AV conduction, digoxin may shorten the refractory period of the bypass tract, making rapid anomalous conduction more likely if atrial fibrillation occurs. In cases of severe digoxin or digitoxin toxicity associated with life-threatening ventricular arrhythmias, hyperkalemia, and/or heart block, rapid reversal of toxicity is possible with the administration of bovine digoxin immune antigen-binding fragments (Fabs). Free levels of digoxin drop to undetectable levels within 1 min of administration, with favorable cardiac effects usually occurring within 30 min. Each vial of antigen fragments (40 mg) will bind approximately 0.6 mg of digoxin or digitoxin. The average dose of Fab used during clinical trials was 10 vials; however, up to 20 vials or more may be necessary in suicidal overdose situations. The Fabs are excreted mainly by the kidneys, with an elimination half-life averaging 15 to 20 h in patients with normal renal function. Patients with significant renal insufficiency must be observed closely for the reemergence of digitalis toxicity. The Fabs may not be excreted from the body in these patients; rather, the fragments are degraded by other processes, with subsequent liberation of previously bound digitalis.

Interactions

Concomitant administration of quinidine, verapamil, amiodarone, flecainide, or propafenone increases digoxin levels and may precipitate digitalis toxicity. Potassium-depleting diuretics and corticosteroids also may precipitate digitalis toxicity. Antibiotics may increase digoxin absorption by reducing metabolism of digoxin by intestinal bacteria. Antacids and resins such as cholestyramine may reduce digoxin absorption. Concomitant administration of calcium channel antagonists or β blockers may produce heart block when administered with digitalis preparations. Digitoxin metabolism may be enhanced by agents such as phenobarbital and phenytoin that enhance hepatic microsomal enzyme activity.

Indications and Dosage

Digitalis preparations are indicated as antiarrhythmic agents to control the ventricular rate in patients with paroxysmal or chronic AF and in those with AV nodal reentrant or AV reciprocating tachycardias. Complete digitalization of an adult typically requires 0.6 to 1.2 mg of digoxin administered in divided doses intravenously or orally; however, differences in bioavailability between preparations must be considered. Maintenance doses of digoxin usually range from 0.125 to 0.25 mg daily but must be substantially reduced in patients with renal insufficiency. When rapid digitalization is not required, therapy may be begun with maintenance doses, with steady-state levels achieved in approximately 7 days in patients with normal renal function. Digitoxin may be useful in patients with renal insufficiency because its metabolism is not dependent on renal excretion. Digitalization may be accomplished by giving 0.2 mg of digitoxin orally twice daily for 4 days. Maintenance therapy ranges from 0.1 to 0.3 mg daily.

Electrolytes

Although not traditionally considered antiarrhythmic agents, serum electrolytes can have a profound effect on many cardiac arrhythmias. Alterations in the concentration of sodium, potassium, magnesium, or calcium may exacerbate many cardiac arrhythmias. In some cases, arrhythmias may be due entirely to electrolyte imbalance, and correction of electrolyte imbalance may be all that is required to treat these patients. Electrolyte abnormalities may be particularly arrhythmogenic in the setting of hypoxemia, ischemia, high-catecholamine states, cardiac hypertrophy or dilatation, altered pH, and in the presence of digitalis. During myocardial infarction, hypokalemia increases the risk of VT and fibrillation. In addition, hypokalemia diminishes the effectiveness of class I antiarrhythmic agents; it may also increase the risk of toxicity or proarrhythmia, especially with class Ia antiarrhythmic agents (torsades de pointes). Arrhythmias due to digitalis toxicity often may be treated successfully with potassium supplementation provided that the serum potassium concentration is not elevated and with monitoring to avoid high-degree AV block. Hypokalemia, hypoxia, and high-catecholamine states also may cause or exacerbate abnormal atrial tachyarrhythmias, especially multifocal atrial tachycardia. In some patients, hypokalemia may be refractory to oral repletion unless concomitant magnesium replacement is undertaken.

Magnesium

Pharmacologic description Magnesium is the second most abundant intracellular cation (after potassium). It is involved as a cofactor in many diverse intracellular biochemical processes (see Chapter 7), including cellular energy production, protein synthesis, DNA synthesis, and maintenance of cellular electrolyte composition (potassium and calcium). All enzymatic reactions involving ATP have an absolute requirement for magnesium. Use of magnesium to treat cardiac arrhythmias was first documented by Zwillinger in 1935. Until recently, its use in the treatment of arrhythmias has been largely ignored, with only occasional case reports being published. Magnesium deficiency has become more common with the widespread use of thiazide and loop diuretics.

Electrophysiologic action Magnesium's effects on the heart may be direct or indirect via effects on potassium and calcium homeostasis. Magnesium increases the length of the sinus cycle, slows AV nodal conduction, and slows intraatrial and intraventricular conductions. It also increases the effective refractory periods of the atria, AV node, and ventricles. Hypomagnesemia often produces opposite effects, such as sinus tachycardia and shortening of effective refractory intervals. Magnesium is essential for the proper functioning of sodium-potassium ATPase; thus, magnesium deficiency reduces the ability of a cell to maintain a normal intracellular potassium concentration, thereby producing intracellular hypokalemia. These alterations increase automaticity and excitability and reduce conduction velocity, thus predisposing to arrhythmogenesis. In addition, magnesium is a physiologic calcium channel antagonist. ECG effects of magnesium administration include prolongation of the PR and QRS intervals and a shortening of the QT interval. Magnesium deficiency may produce ST-segment and T-wave abnormalities; occasionally a prolonged QT interval and U wave are seen. In general, however, hypomagnesemia cannot be recognized with certainty on the ECG, and many of these changes may reflect hypokalemia, which is a commonly associated abnormality.

Pharmacokinetics and metabolism Magnesium is contained mostly within bones and soft tissues. Only 1% of total body magnesium is found in the serum. Thus, serum concentrations may not accurately reflect total body magnesium content. Absorption of magnesium occurs in the small bowel, typically beginning within 1 h of ingestion and continuing at a steady rate for 2 to 8 h. The kidney is the principal organ responsible for the maintenance of magnesium homeostasis. In the presence of hypomagnesemia, urinary excretion decreases to less than 1 mEq/day. Parathyroid hormone and vitamin D also may be important in magnesium regulation. In the case of hypomagnesemia, both parathyroid release and bone action are diminished. This effect on parathyroid hormone is the major determinant of the hypocalcemia that accompanies hypomagnesemia. In the presence of normal renal function, hypermagnesemia is difficult to maintain.

Hemodynamic effects Administration of magnesium may cause an increase in stroke volume and coronary blood flow related to arterial dilatation, which also may result in mild blood pressure reduction. Conversely, cardiac output may decrease owing in part to a decrease in heart rate.

Antiarrhythmic effects Antiarrhythmic effects of magnesium have been demonstrated for the treatment of digitalis toxicity and polymorphic VT associated with a prolonged QT interval (torsades de pointes). Accumulating evidence also suggests that magnesium may be beneficial in the treatment of VF and VT. Correction of magnesium deficiency has been shown to reduce the frequency of ventricular ectopy. Administration of magnesium sulfate in doses sufficient to double the serum magnesium concentration (65 mmol/day) significantly reduced the number of deaths and serious ventricular arrhythmias in patients with acute myocardial infarction in one study.

Side effects Progressive increases in magnesium concentration produces hypotension, PR and QRS interval prolongation, and peaked T waves. At concentrations greater than 5.0 mmol/L, areflexia, respiratory paralysis, and cardiac arrest may occur. Hypermagnesemia most commonly occurs in patients with renal insufficiency.

Indications and dosing Magnesium may be beneficial in the treatment of many arrhythmias; however, arrhythmias secondary to magnesium deficiency, digitalis toxicity, and torsades de pointes appear especially responsive. Acute treatment of arrhythmias may be accomplished by the administration of 2 g of magnesium sulfate intravenously. If necessary, an additional 2 g may be administered in 5 to 15 min. Doses should be administered over 1 to 2 min. Maintenance infusions may be used, with doses ranging from 3 to 20 mg/min. Continuous ECG monitoring is required, and serum magnesium levels should be checked frequently, especially in patients with renal insufficiency. Oral therapy with magnesium chloride (e.g., two to six 500-mg tablets daily) or magnesium oxide (e.g., 400 to 800 mg daily) may be used to prevent or treat diuretic-induced magnesium depletion. Substitution or addition of potassium- and magnesium-sparing diuretics (e.g., spironolactone, amiloride, or triamterene) also may be beneficial.

ADDITIONAL READINGS

ACC/AHA/ESC Guidelines for the Management of Patients with Atrial Fibrillation: Executive summary. *Circulation* 104:2118, 2001.

Antiarrhythmics Versus Implantable Defibrillators (AVID) Investigators: A comparison of antiarrhythmic-drug therapy with implantable defibrillators in patients resuscitated from near-fatal ventricular arrhythmias. *N Engl J Med* 337:1576, 1997.

Atrial Fibrillation Follow-up Investigation of Rhythm Management (AFFIRM) Investigators: A comparison of rate control and rhythm control in patients with atrial fibrillation. *N Engl J Med* 347:1825, 2002.

Brendorp B, Elming H, Jun L, et al, for the DIAMOND Study Group: QTc interval as a guide to select those patients with congestive heart failure and reduced left ventricular systolic function who will benefit from antiarrhythmic treatment with dofetilide. *Circulation* 103:1422, 2001.

Buxton AE, Lee K, Fisher JD, et al: A randomized study of the prevention of sudden death in patients with coronary artery disease. *N Engl J Med* 341:1882, 1999.

Canadian Trial of Atrial Fibrillation Investigators: Amiodarone to prevent recurrence of atrial fibrillation. *N Engl J Med* 342:913, 2000.

Cannom DS, Prystowsky EN: Management of ventricular arrhythmias. Detection, drugs and devices. *JAMA* 281:172, 1999.

Connolly SJ: Evidence-based analysis of amiodarone efficacy and safety. *Circulation* 100:2025, 1999.

Dorian P, Cass D, Schwartz B, et al: Amiodarone as compared with lidocaine for shock-resistant ventricular fibrillation. *N Engl J Med* 346:884, 2002.

Frishman WH, Murthy VS, Strom JA, Hershman DL: Ultrashort-acting β-adrenoreceptor blocking drug: Esmolol, in Messerli FH (ed): *Cardiovascular Drug Therapy*, 2nd ed. Philadelphia, Saunders, 1996

Giri S, White CM, Dunn AB, et al: Oral amiodarone for prevention of atrial fibrillation after open heart surgery, the Atrial Fibrillation Suppression Trial (AFIST): A randomised, placebo-controlled trial. *Lancet* 357:830, 2001.

Glatter KA, Dorostkar PC, Yang Y, et al: Electrophysiological effects of ibutilide in patients with accessory pathways. *Circulation* 104:1933, 2001.

Glatter K, Yang Y, Chatterjee K, et al: Chemical cardioversion of atrial fibrillation or flutter with ibutilide in patients receiving amiodarone therapy. *Circulation* 103:253, 2001.

Kuck K-H, Cappato R, Siebels J: Randomized comparison of antiarrhythmic drug therapy with implantable defibrillators in patients resuscitated from cardiac arrest. The Cardiac Arrest Study Hamburg (CASH). *Circulation* 102:748, 2000.

Lau C-P, Chow MSS, Tse H-F, et al: Control of paroxysmal atrial fibrillation recurrence using combined administration of propafenone and quinidine. *Am J Cardiol* 86:1327, 2000.

Lau W, Newman D, Dorian P: Can antiarrhythmic agents be selected based on mechanism of action? *Drugs* 60:1315, 2000.

Members of the Sicilian Gambit: New approaches to antiarrhythmic therapy, part I. Emerging therapeutic applications of the cell biology of cardiac arrhythmias. *Circulation* 104:2865, 2001.

Members of the Sicilian Gambit: New approaches to antiarrhythmic therapy, part II. Emerging therapeutic applications of the cell biology of cardiac arrhythmias. *Circulation* 104:2990, 2001.

Moss AJ, Zareba W, Hall WJ, et al, for the Multicenter Automatic Defibrillator Implantation Trial II Investigators: Prophylactic implantation of a defibrillator in patients with myocardial infarction and reduced ejection fraction. *N Engl J Med* 346:877, 2002.

Mounsey JP, DiMarco JP: Dofetilide. *Circulation* 102:2665, 2000.

Natale A, Newby KH, Pisano E, et al: Prospective randomized comparison of antiarrhythmic therapy versus first-line radiofrequency ablation in patients with atrial flutter. *J Am Coll Cardiol* 35:1898, 2000.

Pacifico A, Hohnloser SH, Williams JH, et al: Prevention of implantable-defibrillator shocks by treatment with sotalol. D, L-Sotalol Implantable Cardioverter-Defibrillator Study Group. *N Engl J Med* 340:1885, 1999.

Roden DM: Antiarrhythmic drugs, in Hardman JG, Limbird LE (eds): *Goodman & Gilman's the Pharmacological Basis of Therapeutics*, 10th ed. New York, McGraw-Hill, 2001, p 933.

Roy D, Talajic M, Dorian P, et al, for the Canadian Trial of Atrial Fibrillation Investigators: Amiodarone to prevent recurrence of atrial fibrillation. *N Engl J Med* 342: 913, 2000.

Shinagawa K, Shiroshita-Takeshita A, Schram G, Nattel S: Effects of antiarrhythmic drugs on fibrillation in the remodeled atrium. Insights into the mechanism of the superior efficacy of amiodarone. *Circulation* 107:1440, 2003.

Sica DA, Frishman WH, Cavusoglu E: Magnesium, potassium, and calcium as potential cardiovascular disease therapies, in Frishman WH, Sonnenblick EH, Sica DA (eds): *Cardiovascular Pharmacotherapeutics*, 2nd ed. New York, McGraw-Hill, 2003, p 177.

Singh SN, Fletcher RD, Fisher S, et al: Veterans Affairs congestive heart failure antiarrhythmic trial: CHF STAT investigators. *Am J Cardiol* 72:99F, 1993.

Singh S, Zoble RG, Yellen L, et al: Efficacy and safety of oral dofetilide in converting to and maintaining sinus rhythm in patients with chronic atrial fibrillation and atrial flutter. The Symptomatic Atrial Fibrilation Investigative Research on Dofetilide (SAFIRE-D) Study. *Circulation* 102:2385, 2000.

Sljapic TN, Kowey PR, Michelson EL: Antiarrhythmic drugs, in Frishman WH, Sonnenblick EH, Sica DA (eds): *Cardiovascular Pharmacotherapeutics*, 2nd ed. New York, McGraw-Hill, 2003, p 225.

Stanton MS: Antiarrhythmic drugs: Quinidine, procainamide, disopyramide, lidocaine, mexiletine, tocainide, phenytoin, moricizine, flecanide, propafenone, in Zipes DP, Jalife J (eds): *Cardiac Electrophysiology: From Cell to Bedside*. Philadelphia, WB Saunders, 2000, p 890.

Torp-Pedersen C, Moller M, Bloch-Thomsen PE, et al, for the Danish Investigations of Arrhythmia and Mortality on Dofetilide Study Group: Dofetilide in patients with congestive heart failure and left ventricular dysfunction. *N Engl J Med* 341:857, 1999.

Van Gelder IC, Hagens VE, Bosker HA, et al, for the Rate Control vs Electrical Cardioversion for Persistent Atrial Fibrillation Study Group: A comparison of rate control and rhythm control in patients with recurrent persistent atrial fibrillation. *N Engl J Med* 347:1834, 2002.

13 | Antiplatelet and Antithrombotic Drugs

William H. Frishman   Robert G. Lerner

Remarkable advances have occurred in the management of ischemic heart disease, with innovative antiplatelet, antithrombotic, and thrombolytic therapies leading the list of breakthrough drugs. In this chapter, antiplatelet drugs and antithrombotic drugs are reviewed, with a focus on the management of cardiovascular diseases.

ANTIPLATELET DRUGS

The chief function of blood platelets is to interact with the vascular endothelium and soluble plasma factors in the hemostatic process. Under normal physiologic conditions, platelets are mostly inert; an intact vascular wall prevents their adhesion to the subendothelial matrix. In response to vessel trauma, platelets will spontaneously adhere to newly exposed adhesive proteins, forming a protective monolayer of cells. Within seconds, these platelets will be activated by agonists such as thrombin, collagen, and adenosine 5'-diphosphate (ADP), causing them to change shape and to release stored vesicles. The constituents of the vesicles are mostly involved in the further activation of platelets and the propagation of the hemostatic process. Ultimately, these activated platelets will aggregate to form a hemostatic plug closing the vent in the endothelium and preventing further loss of blood from the site. Under certain pathologic conditions (i.e., rupture of an atherosclerotic plaque), these platelet aggregates can form thrombi and be associated with multiple cardiovascular ischemic events, including unstable angina and myocardial infarction (MI).

CONVENTIONAL ANTIPLATELET THERAPY

The efficacy of acetylsalicylic acid (ASA), or aspirin, as an antiplatelet agent has been thoroughly investigated, and it remains the most widely used and cost-efficient drug in the prevention of platelet aggregation. Ticlopidine, an alternative drug with demonstrated antithrombotic properties in the prevention of strokes, is approved for use in aspirin-sensitive patients; however, its higher cost, its additional adverse side effects (in particular thrombotic thrombocytopenic purpura and agranulocytosis), and the essentially similar results obtained with aspirin preclude its general use. Clopidogrel, a similar drug, is now commonly used instead of ticlopidine because it has a lower incidence of side effects. Until recently, dipyridamole was regarded as an antiplatelet agent, but a significant antithrombotic benefit of the drug when used alone has not been demonstrated.

Aspirin

By virtue of aspirin's antiplatelet properties, it has become an essential part of the treatment of ischemic cardiac syndromes. Aspirin diminishes the production of thromboxane A_2 through its ability to irreversibly inhibit the cyclooxygenase (COX) activity of prostaglandin H synthases 1 and 2, known also as COX-1 and COX-2. As a result, platelets exposed to aspirin exhibit diminished aggregation in response to thrombogenic stimuli. Aspirin's ability to inhibit cyclooxygenase is impressive, as only 30 mg/day is required to eliminate the production of thromboxane A_2 completely. The cyclooxygenase is irreversibly inhibited and cannot be replaced by new protein synthesis because the platelet has no nucleus. As a result, because the body's reservoir of platelets is renewed only every 10 days, one dose of aspirin exhibits detectable inhibition of platelet aggregation for longer than 1 week, although a clinical antithrombotic effect may be of shorter duration. In addition, there is evidence that aspirin may reduce clotting ability by inhibiting the synthesis of vitamin K–dependent factors and by stimulating fibrinolysis. These non-prostaglandin mechanisms are dose dependent and less clearly defined.

In addition to inhibiting platelet cyclooxygenase, aspirin inhibits the production of prostacyclin by the vascular endothelium. Prostacyclin is a substance that promotes vasodilation and inhibits platelet aggregation. Because its inhibition theoretically promotes thrombosis, it has been postulated that the beneficial effects of aspirin are reduced because of reduced prostacyclin levels. Unlike platelets, however, prostacyclin production recovers within hours after aspirin administration. Various formulations of aspirin have been studied in an attempt to selectively inhibit thromboxane A_2 without inhibiting prostacyclin. However, even low doses of conventionally formulated aspirin will inhibit both. Selective inhibition of thromboxane A_2 has been achieved with a low-dose (75 mg), sustained-release aspirin preparation. Platelets in the prehepatic circulation have their cyclooxygenase irreversibly inhibited. Because extensive first-pass metabolism occurs, the endothelium in the systemic circulation is exposed to insufficient drug to inhibit prostacyclin production. Whether this is related to the now well-established clinical benefit is unknown. It has been suggested that using the lowest effective dose is the most sensible strategy to maximize efficacy and minimize toxicity. The ASA and Carotid Endarterectomy Trial reported a lower risk of stroke, MI, or death in patients taking 81 or 325 mg of aspirin than in those patients taking 650 or 1300 mg.

Aspirin in Chronic Stable Angina

One arm of the Physician's Health Study examined 383 male physicians with chronic stable angina. The subjects were randomized to 325 mg of aspirin every other day or to placebo. Treatment was over a 5-year period. Although no change in symptom frequency or severity was noted between groups, the occurrence of a first MI was reduced by 87% in those subjects treated with aspirin. Although there was no change in disease progression (as noted by unchanged symptomatology), the addition of aspirin likely reduced the risk of thrombosis in the event of plaque instability. This conclusion has been supported by data from Chesebro and colleagues who noted that the use of aspirin and dipyridamole decreases the incidence of MI and new atherosclerotic lesions without affecting the progression of old atherosclerotic plaques. The Swedish Angina Pectoris Aspirin Trial found that the addition of low-dose aspirin to sotalol treatment provides additional benefit in terms of cardiovascular events, including a significant reduction in the incidence of first MI in patients with angina pectoris.

Unstable Angina

Unstable angina represents the midpoint of the spectrum of ischemic cardiac syndromes, which spans chronic stable angina and MI. Its pathogenesis lies in the rupture of an intracoronary plaque, which promotes platelet aggregation, thrombus formation, and luminal compromise. Theoretically, because aspirin has potent antiplatelet properties, it should be beneficial in the treatment of unstable angina.

Numerous studies have examined the use of aspirin in patients with unstable angina, all of which have reported marked clinical benefit. The Veterans Administration study examined 1384 patients with unstable angina within 48 h of hospital admission. These patients were randomized to receive 325 mg of aspirin per day or placebo for 12 weeks. Death or nonfatal MI occurred in 11% of those treated with placebo versus only 6.3% of those treated with aspirin ($P < 0.004$). Although treatment was limited to 12 weeks, 1-year mortality was reduced from 9.6% in the placebo group to 5.5% in those treated with aspirin ($P < 0.01$). Cairns and associates randomized 555 patients with unstable angina within 8 days of admission to 325 mg of aspirin four times a day or to placebo. Treatment was for 48 h and nonfatal MI or cardiac death was reduced from 14.7% in those treated with placebo to 10.5% in those treated with aspirin ($P < 0.07$). Similarly, total mortality was reduced from 10% in the placebo group to 5.8% in the aspirin group ($P < 0.04$). Theroux and coworkers randomized 479 patients with unstable angina to 325 mg of aspirin two times per day or to placebo. The patients were enrolled at presentation to the hospital and were treated for 3 to 9 days. Nonfatal MI was reduced from 6.4% in the placebo group to 2.5% in the aspirin group ($P < 0.04$). The Research Group on Instability in Coronary Artery Disease in Southeast Sweden (RISC) study investigated the effects of a reduced dose of aspirin in un-stable angina. In the aspirin versus placebo arm, it enrolled 388 patients to receive 75 mg of aspirin or placebo for 3 months. This study demonstrated a reduction in the rate of nonfatal MI or noncardiac death from 17% in the placebo group to 7.4% in the aspirin group ($P = 0.0042$).

It is clear from these studies that aspirin is effective in reducing the morbidity and mortality of unstable angina with and without heparin. Specifically, nonfatal MI and cardiac death were reduced by 50% to 70%. This benefit seemed to occur across a broad spectrum of daily doses, from 1300 mg/day in the study by Cairns and associates to only 75 mg/day in the RISC trial. Because platelets are exquisitely sensitive to aspirin, this finding is not unexpected. A study of the effect of aspirin on C-reactive protein (CRP), a marker of risk in unstable angina, assessed whether the beneficial effects of aspirin are related to aspirin's ability to influence CRP release. The investigators concluded that the association between CRP and cardiac events in patients with unstable angina is influenced by pretreatment with aspirin, and that modification of the acute-phase inflammatory responses to myocardial injury is the major mechanism of this interaction.

Primary Prevention of Myocardial Infarction

The rupture of an intracoronary atheromatous plaque causes most MIs. This rupture exposes subendothelial collagen to local blood products, which results in the attraction and activation of platelets. These activated platelets release growth factors and vasoactive compounds that produce vasoconstriction, additional platelet aggregation, and, ultimately, the formation of an occlusive mural thrombus.

Although aspirin was shown to improve outcomes in patients with unstable angina, its benefit in primary prevention of MI was largely unknown until the results of the U.S. Physicians' Health Study were reported. In this study, 22,071 male U.S. physicians were randomized to 325 mg of aspirin every other day or to placebo. Ninety-eight percent of those involved were free of cardiac-related symptoms and treatment took place over a 5-year period. Whereas the frequency of angina, coronary revascularization, or death was unchanged between groups, the incidence of MI was impressively reduced in the aspirin-treated group. Specifically, the risk of fatal or nonfatal MI was reduced by 44%.

The observations made in the U.S. Physicians' Health Study were challenged by a similar study from Europe. The British Physicians' Health Study was an uncontrolled trial that involved 5139 British male physicians, two-thirds of whom were treated with 500 mg of aspirin per day. In contrast to the U.S. study, there was no significant reduction in MI or total mortality. Criticisms of this trial were many and included its uncontrolled design, its smaller sample size, the higher dose of aspirin, its older subjects with poorer compliance, and its high confidence intervals. Its results, however, were sufficient to cast some doubt on aspirin's utility in the primary prevention of MI.

Any doubts as to aspirin's role in the primary prevention of MI were largely put to rest by a large, observational study of U.S. nurses and their aspirin usage. In this study, aspirin usage by 87,000 U.S. nurses was analyzed over a 6-year period. All the nurses involved were free of cardiac-related symptoms. In women older than 50 years, the study associated ingestion of one to six 325-mg tablets of aspirin per week with a 32% reduction in first MI. This benefit was most striking in women with risk factors for coronary artery disease including tobacco use, hypercholesterolemia, and hypertension. In women who took more than seven tablets per week, there was no reduction in the rate of MI. In addition, women who took more than 15 tablets per week were at a significantly increased risk of hemorrhagic stroke.

It appears from these studies that 325 mg of aspirin every other day is effective in preventing a first MI in asymptomatic individuals. An aspirin dose as low as 75 mg/day is the minimum dose that effectively reduces the risk of a first MI. The benefit of aspirin is most pronounced in patients who are at high risk for coronary artery disease, specifically older individuals with multiple cardiac risk factors. The corollary of this is that the risk-to-benefit ratio for aspirin use is lowest in healthy individuals and highest in high-risk individuals. Higher doses of aspirin do not appear to confer any additional benefit and most likely impart additional risk of developing hemorrhagic stroke. Despite its proven benefit, aspirin is being underutilized in clinical practice.

Secondary Prevention of Myocardial Infarction

Seven prospective, randomized, placebo-controlled trials have examined the use of aspirin in the secondary prevention of MI. As a cumulative total, these studies enrolled more than 15,000 survivors of MI whose treatment consisted of various aspirin regimens, with doses ranging from 325 to 1500 mg/day. Patients were enrolled from 4 weeks to 5 years post-MI. When each of these trials was examined individually, no statistically significant decrease in mortality was observed. Because the numbers of patients in each study may have been too small to provide adequate statistical power, a meta-analysis of six of the trials was performed. This meta-analysis contained 10,703 patients and showed that, when aspirin was compared with placebo, cardiovascular morbidity was reduced by 21%. In another meta-analysis from the Antiplatelet Trialists Collaboration, the risk of developing a nonfatal reinfarction was shown to be reduced by 31% and death from vascular causes was reduced by 13% in those patients treated with aspirin during the 1- to 4-year follow-up period. In a 23-month follow-up of 931 patients with acute infarction or unstable angina, 80% of subjects were found to use aspirin on a regular basis. Their cardiac death rate was markedly reduced compared with non-aspirin users and was not explicable by imbalances in predictors of postinfarction risk, by concurrent drug therapy, or by preinfarction thrombolysis or angioplasty.

In addition to the cardiac benefits demonstrated by these studies, aspirin seems to reduce the risk of stroke in post-MI patients. In a subset of the Antiplatelet Trialists Collaboration, the risk of stroke in those patients treated with aspirin was examined. A 42% reduction in nonfatal strokes in the aspirin group was demonstrated, as compared with placebo treatment. With these results in mind, treatment of post-MI patients with low-dose aspirin (perhaps 75 mg/day) seems reasonable. Although many of these trials relied on pooled data and meta-analysis to demonstrate aspirin's benefit in the post-MI population, the data are compelling to that effect. Aspirin does not appear to increase the risk of nonfatal cerebrovascular accident (CVA) and most likely will reduce the risk of future cardiac events. The optimal dose of aspirin for long-term postinfarction prophylaxis is unclear at this time and needs to be determined in future studies.

A recent meta-analysis of five randomized trials of primary prevention included 52,251 participants randomized to aspirin doses ranging from 75 to 650 mg/day; the mean overall stroke rate was 0.3% per year during an average follow-up of 4.6 years. Meta-analysis showed no significant effect on stroke (relative risk = 1.08; 95% confidence interval, 0.95 to 1.24) in contrast to a decrease in MI (relative risk = 0.74; 95% confidence interval, 0.68 to 0.82). The investigators concluded that the effect of aspirin therapy on stroke differs between individuals based on the presence or absence of overt vascular disease, in contrast with the consistent reduction in MI by aspirin therapy observed in all populations.

Acute Myocardial Infarction

Localized coronary thrombosis due to the rupture of an unstable, intracoronary, atheromatous plaque is thought to be responsible for more than 90% of Q-wave MIs. Although thrombolytic agents break down the primary clot responsible for the acute event, substances liberated during this process can themselves promote platelet aggregation and reocclusion. Although spontaneous recanalization may occur, thrombus reformation is common and may perpetuate the ischemic process. By virtue of aspirin's potent antiplatelet properties, it is an effective agent, when used alone or with thrombolytic agents, at reducing the mortality from acute MIs (AMIs).

The Second International Study of Infarct Survival (ISIS-2) was a double-blind, placebo-controlled trial that defined aspirin's role in the treatment of AMI. ISIS-2 enrolled 17,187 patients with suspected AMI and randomized them to intravenous streptokinase (1.5 million U over 60 min), aspirin (162 mg/day for 1 month), both, or neither. Five weeks after randomization, aspirin reduced the risks of nonfatal reinfarction by 51% and vascular mortality by 23% when compared with placebo. The addition of intravenous streptokinase further reduced mortality in conjunction with aspirin. These results indicated that aspirin reduces mortality to a similar degree as streptokinase alone and that, there is a cumulative benefit when the two are combined. Aspirin's reduction in mortality also extended to groups treated with various heparin dosages, ranging from no heparin (288 vs. 347 deaths), to subcutaneous heparin (338 vs. 431 deaths), and to intravenous heparin (178 vs. 238 deaths; $P < 0.001$). Mortality benefits were similar in men and women and remained present after 24 months of follow-up. Importantly, treatment with aspirin did not result in any increased incidence of major bleeds (31 vs. 33 bleeds) and seemed to decrease the risk of nonfatal CVA by 46% ($P = 0.003$). It seems clear that aspirin, with or without thrombolytic therapy, is effective in reducing the mortality and morbidity of an evolving MI.

Non–Q-wave MI results when an intracoronary occlusion is incomplete or occurs for only a short time. The pathophysiology of a non–Q-wave MI is similar to unstable angina and to Q-wave MI in that a ruptured atheromatous plaque results in acute intracoronary thrombus formation. Although it seems likely that aspirin would confer a benefit in evolving non–Q-wave MIs, no adequate trials have been performed in this subgroup of patients.

Current recommendations of the American College of Chest Physicians Sixth Consensus Conference are that all patients with AMI who receive fibrinolytic therapy also receive adjunctive treatment with aspirin (165 to 325 mg) on arrival to the hospital and daily thereafter. They also recommend that patients receive heparin or hirudin as an adjunct, depending on patients' risk factors for systemic or venous thromboembolism and the fibrinolytic agent with which they are treated.

Percutaneous Transluminal Coronary Angioplasty and Arterial Stenting

When percutaneous transluminal coronary angioplasty is performed, the intracoronary atheromatous plaque that is acted upon is "cracked" or "fissured" by the destructive action of balloon inflation. This fissure results in the exposure of underlying subendothelial collagen to circulating blood products, which activates platelets and promotes thrombogenesis. It has been shown that the magnitude of platelet deposition after angioplasty is related to the depth of arterial injury and that in animals pretreatment with aspirin reduces the degree of thrombus formation.

There have been two randomized, prospective trials that have evaluated the role of aspirin in preventing abrupt closure after angioplasty. In these studies, aspirin (650 to 990 mg/day) and dipyridamole (225 mg/day) were started 24 h preangioplasty and continued indefinitely. These studies demonstrated that the incidence of abrupt closure is significantly reduced when compared with placebo. In another trial, Barnathan and colleagues retrospectively analyzed the coronary angiograms of patients undergoing angioplasty and found that the incidence of coronary thrombosis decreases significantly in patients treated with aspirin or aspirin plus dipyridamole. Although aspirin does appear to lower the risk of acute thrombosis after angioplasty, it has not been shown to affect the rate of late restenosis. With regard to coronary artery stenting, aspirin remains an important prophylactic treatment in preventing acute thrombosis, especially in combination with ticlopidine or clopidogrel. In a randomized trial of 700 patients with 899 lesions, after the placement of coronary artery stents, antiplatelet therapy with aspirin and clopidogrel was as safe and effective as aspirin and ticlopidine, and noncardiac events were significantly reduced with aspirin plus clopidogrel.

Coronary Artery Bypass Surgery

In coronary artery bypass grafting (CABG) surgery, native coronary arteries whose blood flow is compromised by atherosclerotic blockages are "bypassed" by using venous or arterial conduits. The arterial conduit usually consists of the left or right internal mammary arteries, and the venous conduit is usually a reversed, saphenous vein from the leg. Although this surgery is one of the mainstays of treatment for coronary artery disease, occlusion of the bypass vessels acutely or over time is not uncommon. For example, 40% to 50% of saphenous vein grafts have been found to occlude within 10 years of their implantation. Reasons for graft occlusion depend on the age of the conduit. "Acute" closure (less than 1 month after placement) is usually due to thrombosis, whereas "intermediate" closure (1 month to 1 year) is caused by accelerated intimal hyperplasia. "Late" occlusion (more than 1 year) results from atherosclerosis within the bypass graft.

Multiple studies have demonstrated a decreased incidence of early thrombosis when aspirin is used in the perioperative period. Goldman and coworkers randomized 50 groups of CABG patients to receive (a) aspirin 325 mg/day, (b) aspirin 325 mg twice daily, (c) aspirin 325 mg twice daily and dipyridamole 75 mg twice, (d) sulfinpyrazone 267 mg twice daily, or (e) placebo. This study demonstrated a significantly decreased risk of early thrombosis in all groups treated with aspirin (73% graft patency with placebo at 2 months vs. 93% with aspirin, $P < 0.05$). The addition of dipyridamole resulted in no additional benefit, and sulfinpyrazone was ineffective in reducing the risk of thrombosis. Although those patients treated with aspirin had increased blood loss and need for reoperation, perioperative mortality was unchanged. The benefits noted in this study remained after 1 year of follow-up. In a follow-up to this study, predictors of patency 3 years after CABG were analyzed. For a patient with patent vein grafts 7 to 10 days after the operation, predictors of 3-year graft patency were more closely related to operative techniques and underlying disease and not to aspirin treatment.

Despite the lack of effect on patency at 3 years, it is recommended that aspirin should be given to all patients undergoing bypass surgery unless a clear contraindication exists. A dose of 325 mg/day is reasonable because higher doses do not add any clinical benefit. The medication may be started preoperatively or within 48 h postoperatively if preoperative administration is not possible.

Transient Ischemia Attack and Stroke

The capacity of aspirin in doses of 50 to 1500 mg/day, alone or in combination with other antiplatelet agents (dipyridamole or sulfinpyrazone), to reduce the risk of recurrent cerebrovascular events was studied in 10 trials involving approximately 8000 patients with stroke (CVA) or transient ischemic attacks (TIAs). Based on these studies, treatment of 1000 patients with aspirin for 3 years will reduce fatal and nonfatal cardiovascular events including recurrent CVA by about 25%. Optimal daily dose of aspirin for secondary prophylaxis in cerebrovascular disease remains somewhat controversial, but doses between 300 and 1200 mg/day are within the recommended dose range. The U.S. Food and Drug Administration (FDA) published its rules for labeling aspirin products for over-the-counter human use and recommended aspirin doses from 50 to 325 mg/day for prevention of ischemic stroke. The ASA and

Carotid Endarterectomy Trial suggested that low-dose aspirin is at least as effective as high-dose aspirin.

The Clopidogrel Versus Aspirin in Patients at Risk of Ischemic Events (CAPRIE) study included 19,185 patients, 6431 of whom entered the trial with stroke. There was a statistically nonsignificant relative risk reduction of 8% for stroke favoring clopidogrel. The European Stroke Prevention Study 2 demonstrated that aspirin combined with sustained-release dipyridamole is more effective than either alone in reducing the risk of stroke. The results were independent of age. Based on this study, a combination formulation of aspirin and dipyridamole has been approved for clinical use.

Systemic Lupus Erythematosus

Prophylactic aspirin should be given to all patients with systemic lupus erythematosus to prevent arterial and venous thrombotic manifestations, especially in patients with antiphospholipid antibodies.

Venous Thromboembolism

Aspirin use has also been shown to reduce the risk of thromboembolism after major orthopedic surgery. It has not been compared with low-molecular-weight heparin (LMWH) or evaluated in combination with LMWH.

Atrial Fibrillation

Aspirin has been used to reduce the hazard of thromboembolic stroke in non-valvular atrial fibrillation (NVAF) and compared with the efficacy of warfarin. Data from randomized trials supported aspirin use for thromboembolism prophylaxis in younger NVAF patients (<60 years), especially in the absence of associated risk factors of hypertension, recent congestive heart failure, or remote thromboembolism. A slightly greater hazard for intracranial bleeding with warfarin might make aspirin a suitable alternative to warfarin in selected other patients. An ongoing clinical trial (SPAF III) was designed to evaluate the relative efficacy and safety of aspirin as an adjunct to low-intensity, fixed-dose warfarin in preventing thromboembolism in high-risk NVAF patients. The trial is ongoing in low-risk patients. The trial was stopped prematurely in high-risk patients due to an excess of strokes in patients receiving aspirin plus low-dose warfarin. The published results thus far support the use of conventional dose warfarin in most patients with atrial fibrillation.

Adverse Effects and Drug–Drug Interactions

The most common side effect of aspirin treatment is gastrointestinal (GI) intolerance. In the Aspirin Myocardial Infarction Study, in which patients with known peptic ulcer disease were excluded, 24% of those treated with aspirin (1000 mg/day) reported GI intolerance as compared with 15% in the placebo group. In the United Kingdom TIA Trial, GI symptoms were reduced by 30% when the dose of aspirin was decreased from 1200 mg/day to 300 mg/day. In the Physicians' Health Study (patients with known peptic ulcer disease were excluded), 325 mg of aspirin every other day resulted in only a 0.5% increase in GI symptoms when compared with placebo. Therefore, GI intolerance due to aspirin appears to occur in a dose-dependent manner and treatment with 325 mg/day appears to be well tolerated. Two forms of cyclooxygenase enzymes have been identified, one which produces the "good" prostaglandins that act in the stomach and other tissues (COX-1) and another (COX-2) that is involved in thromboxane formation.

Agents are now available to inhibit COX-2 and spare COX-1, which could provide a stomach-sparing aspirin. The relative risk of GI bleeding with such drugs as compared with other nonsteroidal anti-inflammatory drugs is reduced. However, a recent study suggested that COX-2 inhibitors have a prothrombotic effect in patients at risk for coronary artery disease. Therefore, until this issue is resolved, the COX-2 inhibitors cannot be used as aspirin substitutes for cardiovascular prophylaxis.

Bleeding complications are a common side effect of aspirin therapy. Specifically, the risk of developing a hemorrhagic event such as bruising, melena, or epistaxis is increased with aspirin use. The Physicians' Health Study confirmed this observation by reporting that 27% of those treated with aspirin (325 mg every other day) experience bleeding complications, as compared with only 20% in the placebo group. In the United Kingdom TIA Trial, there was a significant increase in the risk of GI bleeding when the dose of aspirin was increased to 1200 mg/day. For these reasons, the risks and benefits of aspirin therapy need to be weighed against one another in patients who are at increased risk of bleeding. Further, the dose of aspirin used should be as low as possible because higher doses do not appear to confer additional benefits but do increase bleeding risk substantially.

Aspirin also may interfere with the clinical benefit of angiotensin-converting enzyme inhibitors (see Chapter 5) and with furosemide in patients with heart failure.

Aspirin Resistance

Aspirin does not block thromboxane A_2 in some patients, making them resistant to the protective effects of the drug. Patients taking aspirin who had high levels of thromboxane in their urine were found to have a three to five times higher risk of cardiovascular death than patients who had lower levels. High levels of 11-dehydrothromboxane B_2 in urine can identify patients who are resistant to aspirin. Those patients may benefit from alternative antiplatelet therapies or treatments that more effectively block thromboxane production.

Conclusion

Aspirin is effective at reducing the morbidity and mortality associated with ischemic cardiac syndromes. In particular, it is effective as primary prevention against MI in asymptomatic patients and in those with chronic stable and unstable angina. It also reduces the risk of reinfarction in the peri- and post-MI periods. Aspirin decreases the incidence of acute thrombosis after percutaneous transluminal coronary angioplasty (PTCA) and stenting and reduces the risk of bypass graft thrombosis after CABG surgery. These benefits must be weighed against the increased risk of bleeding associated with aspirin therapy. In those patients who are at a low risk for bleeding complications and who fall into one of the above categories, 325 mg of aspirin, daily or every other day, is recommended. In patients with a greater likelihood of bleeding, these risks and benefits need to be taken into account, and therapy must be individualized.

Dipyridamole

Dipyridamole is a pyramidopyrimidine compound that can act as a vasodilator and an antithrombotic. The drug inhibits platelet action in vitro only at doses that are higher than those commonly used in patients, but it has been clinically effective in reducing platelet adherence to prosthetic surfaces in vivo at lower doses when combined with other agents. A number of mechanisms for its antiplatelet activity has been proposed, including the inhibition of phosphodiesterase or the indirect activation of adenylate cyclase through its effects on prostacyclin and/or the inhibition of adenosine uptake by the vascular endothelium. The exact mechanism of action requires further definition, although the common pathway involves elevated levels of intraplatelet cyclic adenosine monophosphate, a platelet inhibitory substance. The usual dose of dipyridamole is 400 mg/day in three to four divided doses. It is also used as a provocative agent in patients undergoing diagnostic testing for coronary artery disease.

Clinical Studies

Its primary use in humans has been as an adjunct to anticoagulant therapy in the prevention of thromboembolic events in patients with prosthetic heart valves. Although current American College of Chest Physicians' guidelines do not include dipyridamole as a first-line therapy in a patient with prosthetic heart valves, it is a useful adjunct to anticoagulant therapy. It is recommended as part of the therapy in a patient with a prosthesis-related thromboembolic event, especially in those patients with peptic ulcer disease in whom aspirin may need to be avoided. Dipyridamole is not associated with an excess of hemorrhage when combined with anticoagulant therapy. Dipyridamole also has been used as part of the therapy for patients with prosthetic grafts. Experimental and clinical evidence suggests a superiority of an aspirin/and dipyridamole combination to either drug used alone in terms of platelet survival and graft patency.

A controlled trial comparing aspirin and dipyridamole alone and in combination against placebo for secondary prevention of ischemic stroke in 6602 patients found an 18% reduction with aspirin alone, a 16% reduction with dipyridamole alone, and a 37% reduction with combination therapy. Although there was no effect on the death rate, there was a significant reduction in TIAs. Bleeding was significantly more common in patients receiving aspirin. A combination formulation of aspirin and dipyridamole is currently available for stroke prevention.

Controlled trials comparing aspirin with dipyridamole in patients with stable angina are few. The limited data suggest no statistically significant difference between aspirin and dipyridamole used together as compared with aspirin alone. No trial has shown a definitive superiority of combination therapy over aspirin alone in stable coronary disease, graft survival after CABG, or in the need for emergency revascularization after angioplasty.

Adverse Effects

The primary side effects of dipyridamole are gastrointestinal and consist of nausea and vomiting. In rare cases, angina has been provoked through what is believed to be a coronary steal phenomenon.

Ticlopidine

Ticlopidine is a thienopyridine compound that acts by blocking ADP receptors within the platelet membrane and acts independently of arachidonic acid pathways. Ticlopidine produces a thrombasthenia-like state, with a resultant reduction in platelet aggregation, a prolongation of the bleeding time, a decrease in platelet granule release, and a reduction in platelet and fibrin deposition on artificial surfaces.

Cerebrovascular and Peripheral Vascular Diseases

Ticlopidine has been tested thoroughly in the prevention of cerebrovascular disease. When compared with placebo in 1000 patients as part of a study in secondary prevention after stroke, the administration of ticlopidine resulted in a 30% reduction in the relative risk of stroke, MI, or vascular death. When compared with aspirin in the Ticlopidine Aspirin Stroke Study (TASS), ticlopidine was superior in terms of all-cause mortality and nonfatal stroke. This benefit persisted throughout the 5-year duration of the trial.

In patients with peripheral vascular disease and claudication, treatment with ticlopidine was associated with reductions in mortality, MI, and cerebrovascular events. Patients with cerebrovascular and peripheral vascular diseases appear to benefit from ticlopidine therapy in terms of stroke, MI, and vascular events.

Cardiovascular Disease

Ticlopidine has been used in the therapy of patients after CABG. In a randomized trial involving 173 patients, ticlopidine therapy resulted in a reduction in vein graft closure at 1 year as compared with placebo. The graft closure rate, as assessed by digital angiography on days 10, 180, and 360, was decreased in the ticlopidine group as compared with the placebo group. When used in the therapy of patients with electrocardiographic (ECG) evidence of unstable coronary syndromes, the addition of ticlopidine to standard therapy was associated with a reduction in vascular death and nonfatal MI and the composite end point of fatal and nonfatal MIs. In those patients who undergo coronary stent implantation, ticlopidine and aspirin have demonstrated a superiority over anticoagulant therapy with heparin and phenprocoumon. In patients undergoing stenting, ticlopidine should be administered at a 500-mg loading dose and then given 250 mg twice daily for 10 to 14 days.

In patients with AMI, the drug appears to be similar to aspirin with regard to subsequent mortality, recurrent AMI, stroke, and angina. The drug in combination with aspirin reduces the plasma levels of procoagulant tissue factor in patients with unstable angina.

Adverse Events

Neutropenia can occur in up to 4% of patients receiving ticlopidine. It is generally reversible, although cases of agranulocytosis have been reported. It is recommended that, during the first 2 months of therapy, white blood cell counts should be checked. The most common side effects of the medication are gastrointestinal, occurring in about 12% of patients, and include nausea, vomiting, diarrhea, and dyspepsia. A rash has been reported within the first 3 months of ticlopidine treatment. Ticlopidine is associated with a risk of thrombotic thrombocytopenic purpura estimated at 0.02%. Although this complication also has been reported with clopidogrel, ticlopidine has been supplanted by clopidogrel because of an overall better safety profile.

Clopidogrel

Clopidogrel is a thienopyridine antiplatelet drug in the same class as ticlopidine. Similar to ticlopidine, clopidogrel is a prodrug that is not active in vitro but is active in vivo. It functions as an ADP-selective agent whose anti-aggregating properties are several times higher than those of ticlopidine and are apparently due to the same mechanism of action (i.e., inhibition of ADP binding to its platelet receptor and triggering the release of thrombogenic factor-containing α granules). In various experimental animal models, one oral or intravenous administration of clopidogrel inhibited ADP-induced platelet aggregation for several days and potently reduced thrombus formation.

Clinical Trials

Clopidogrel has been evaluated in a large phase III clinical trial (CAPRIE), a randomized, blinded, clinical study comparing clopidogrel 75 mg/day with aspirin 325 mg/day in 19,185 patients who had a recent ischemic stroke or MI or who had symptomatic atherosclerotic peripheral vascular disease. The study showed a more favorable effect on clinical outcomes with clopidogrel as compared with aspirin, and based on this study, clopidogrel was approved by the FDA. Clopidogrel is also of benefit when started with aspirin at the time patients present with acute coronary syndrome and may be a useful alternative in patients having aspirin resistance.

In addition to aspirin and glycoprotein (GP) IIb/IIIa integrin receptor blockers, clopidogrel has become an important drug for use in patients undergoing angioplasty and stenting to reduce thrombotic complications. In patients undergoing coronary stenting, it should be given as a 300-mg oral loading dose followed by a maintenance dose of 75 mg for 1 year. The drug is also as effective as aspirin and ticlopidine as an antiplatelet agent after MI and can be combined with aspirin to achieve a greater antiplatelet effect. In patients who had had prior cardiac surgery, clopidogrel was shown to be better than aspirin in reducing events with less bleeding.

THE GLYCOPROTEIN IIB/IIIA INTEGRIN RECEPTOR ANTAGONISTS

Platelet aggregation is mediated by the GP IIb/IIIa receptor, a member of the integrin superfamily of membrane-bound adhesion molecules. Integrins are defined as subunit receptors composed of an α subunit (i.e., GP IIb) and a β subunit (i.e., GP IIIa) capable of mediating adhesive interactions between cells or matrix. Although integrins are distributed widely throughout the vasculature, where they are expressed on endothelial, smooth muscle cells, and leukocytes, expression of the GP IIb/IIIa integrin is restricted to platelets. It is the chief receptor responsible for platelet aggregation because of its ability to bind soluble fibrinogen, thus forming bridges between platelets and leading, ultimately, to thrombus formation. GP IIb/IIIa is widely distributed on platelet surfaces (approximately 50,000 per cell) but cannot bind fibrinogen unless the platelet is first stimulated by agonists (such as ADP, thrombin, arachidonic acid, etc.) and undergoes a conformational change. It is believed that the adhesive binding pocket is somehow hidden until platelet activation, although this process is unclear. Although fibrinogen is the peptide that mediates aggregation, mostly because of the large concentration of fibrinogen in plasma, GP IIb/IIIa can bind von Willebrand factor, fibronectin, and vitronectin. It has been demonstrated that aggregation can be supported by von Willebrand factor in the absence of fibrinogen. Therefore, these molecules also may play a role in aggregation at high shear rates, such as is found in the coronary arteries.

GP IIb/IIIa, a heterodimer of two subunits, was the first integrin to be identified and has served as a model for characterization of other integrins. It has been demonstrated by electron microscopy that the receptor is composed of a globular head and two flexible tails that are imbedded in the platelet membrane. The GP IIb subunit has calcium-binding sites that have homology with calmodulin. In the presence of the calcium chelating agent ethylenediamine tetraacetic acid, the receptor function is lost and the integrin dissociates into its two individual subunits. Each subunit contains a portion of the head and one tail (Fig. 13-1).

The GP IIb/IIIa domains responsible for binding adhesive proteins have been identified and in general are characterized by their ability to recognize the peptide sequence RGD. The RGD recognition sequence originally was described for fibronectin, but is now known to be present in fibrinogen, von Willebrand factor, vitronectin, and thrombospondin. Fibrinogen is a symmetrical protein composed of two α chains, two β chains, and two γ chains. Both of its RGD sequences are located on the α chain at residues 95 to 97 and 572 to 574. Fibrinogen also contains a 12–amino acid residue that possesses the ability to bind to the GP IIb/IIIa receptor. This dodecapeptide (HHLGGAKQAGDV) is located at residues 400 to 411 on the fibrinogen γ chain. It has been proposed that the RGD residues and the dodecapeptide competitively bind to GP IIb/IIIa. By initiating a conformational change in

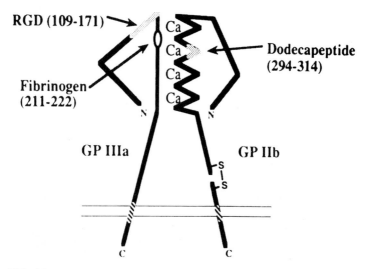

FIG. 13-1 Structure of glycoprotein (GP) IIb/IIIa complex. Transmembrane domains are near carboxyl termini of GP IIb and GP IIIa. RGD peptides have been cross-linked to domain within amino acids 109 to 171 of GP IIIa, whereas dodecapeptide from the γ chain of fibrinogen cross-links to domain within residues 294 to 314 of GP IIb. The third region in GP IIIa involved in fibrinogen binding corresponds to residues 211 to 222. (*Adapted with permission from Charo et al., in Colman RW, et al (eds): Hemostasis and Thrombosis: Basic Principles and Clinical Practice, 3rd ed. Philadelphia, JB Lippincott, 1994, p 489–507.*)

the receptor after binding, one recognition sequence on fibrinogen renders the other sequence inaccessible for binding. This alteration in receptor shape may be a self-regulatory mechanism of the GP IIb/IIIa receptor.

If two activated platelets with functional GP IIb/IIIa receptors each bind to the same fibrinogen molecule, a fibrinogen bridge is created between the two platelets (Fig. 13-2). When this process of aggregation is repeated thousands of times, a thrombus will form. Experiments have indicated that the RGD peptides bind to the GP IIIa subunit at residues 109 to 171. In contrast, the dodecapeptide binds to the GP IIb subunit at residues 294 to 314. Genetic defects in either of these two subunits can lead to the rare hemostatic disorder of Glanzmann's thrombasthenia. Patients with Glanzmann's thrombasthenia usually have a bleeding disorder during childhood. Although they have a normal platelet count, the GP IIb/IIIa receptor is nonfunctional or absent. Platelet aggregation in response to agonists such as thrombin, ADP, or arachidonic acid is therefore completely absent.

GP IIb/IIIa Antagonists as Antiplatelet Agents

As discussed earlier in this chapter, aspirin is the most common antiplatelet drug in use today. However, it is a relatively weak drug that is effective against only one of the many platelet activators, thromboxane A_2. Other drugs similar to clopidogrel, ticlopidine, and hirudin, which are effective against ADP and thrombin, respectively, also are limited in their activity because of the platelet's ability to be activated by multiple agonists. Many patients with vascular disease take the current antiplatelet drugs and still sustain thromboembolic complications that often develop into ischemic conditions. Of importance, therefore, is the development of more effective antiplatelet agents. A drug able to inhibit platelet activation in response to all endogenous agonists would constitute a more effective therapy.

The binding of fibrinogen to activated platelets is the final step in platelet aggregation, and this binding is completely mediated by GP IIb/IIIa. Therefore, expression of the GP IIb/IIIa integrin is the final common pathway for platelet aggregation by *all* agonists. GP IIb/IIIa also is unique to platelets and is the most abundant platelet surface glycoprotein. These factors make GP IIb/IIIa an extremely favorable target for therapeutic pharmacologic blockade. A drug that could block the binding of fibrinogen to GP IIb/IIIa theoretically could abolish thrombosis resulting from vessel damage or atherosclerotic plaque rupture, regardless of the platelet's degree of activation. Discussed below are three classes of GP IIb/IIIa antagonists: disintegrins (naturally occurring GP IIb/IIIa blocking agents), monoclonal antibodies to the GP IIb/IIIa receptor, and synthetic peptide- and non–peptide-receptor antagonists capable of blocking fibrinogen binding to platelets.

Murine Monoclonal Antibodies (7E3)

Abciximab is a highly effective antithrombotic agent, specifically in preventing arterial thrombi in canines and primates, including humans. To eliminate the binding of fibrinogen to activated platelets, large doses of abciximab must be given to block GP IIb/IIIa receptor function effectively on all circulating platelets. However, by blocking all GP IIb/IIIa receptors and, consequently, inhibiting platelet aggregation, the risk of concurrent hemorrhage is increased. This bleeding risk is increased when combining

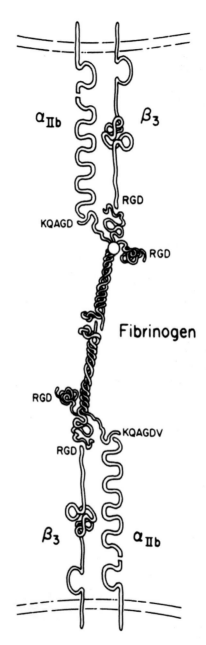

FIG. 13-2 Glycoprotein IIb/IIIa structure and interactions of binding platelets by divalent fibrinogen. *(Reproduced with permission from Harker et al, in Colman RW, et al (eds): Hemostasis and Thrombosis: Basic Principles and Clinical Practice, 3rd ed. Philadelphia, JB Lippincott, 1994, p 1638–1660.)*

antiplatelet therapy with invasive treatments such as coronary angioplasty or bypass surgery.

The results of a larger study demonstrated the effectiveness of 7E3 in the prevention of postangioplasty restenosis. The Evaluation of 7E3 for the Prevention of Ischemic Complications (EPIC) study highlighted the importance of the GP IIb/IIIa receptor in abrupt vessel closure after high-risk coronary angioplasty and atherectomy. A random population (2099 patients) scheduled to undergo these procedures received a bolus and infusion of placebo, a bolus of 0.25 mg/kg 7E3 and a 12-h infusion of placebo, or a bolus and infusion of 7E3. Results were measured as the risk of experiencing a composite primary end point (which included death, nonfatal MI, or unplanned invasive revascularization procedures) by 30 days. Data indicated that, as compared with those patients given placebo, patients who received administration of the bolus and infusion of 7E3 had a 35% risk reduction in the composite event rate. Patients who received only a 0.25 mg/kg bolus of 7E3 (and placebo infusion) showed a 10% reduction in the risk of experiencing a primary end point (Fig. 13-3). On the basis of the results of the EPIC trial and other pharmacologic studies, the 7E3 antibody, abciximab, was approved for use in patients undergoing high-risk angioplasty. The drug is now also approved for unstable angina. The FDA-approved dose is a 0.25-mg/kg bolus and a 10-μg/min infusion for 18 to 24 h before percutaneous coronary intervention (PCI) and continued for 1 h after PCI. This may not be the optimal dose, and a 12-h infusion after PCI is recommended. In addition, during a 6-month follow-up period, the number of ischemic events was reduced by 26% in patients who received the 7E3 antibody, suggesting a long-term benefit against clinical coronary artery stenosis.

Although these results demonstrate the importance of pharmacologic blockade of GP IIb/IIIa as therapy for ischemic events, the use of abciximab results in several negative complications. In 14% of the patients in the EPIC

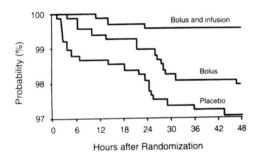

FIG. 13-3 Probability of no urgent repeated percutaneous revascularization procedures in three treatment groups (Kaplan-Meier plots). Events began to occur shortly after the index procedure in placebo group, between 6 and 12 h after the procedure in the group given bolus of c7E3 antibody fragments, and even later in the group given bolus and infusion; the y axis is truncated at 97% to demonstrate differences in this end point, which occurred with low frequency. *(Reprinted with permission from EPIC Investigators: Use of a monoclonal antibody directed against the platelet glycoprotein IIb/IIIa receptor in high-risk coronary angioplasty. N Engl J Med 330: 956, 1994).*

trial who received the 7E3 bolus and infusion, a significant amount of bleeding, twice the number of major bleeding episodes in the placebo group, occurred and often required transfusion. The bleeding usually occurred at the site of vascular puncture in the groin. The increased bleeding time is compounded because the antibodies are inherently long-lived and do not dissociate from platelets during the platelets' survival time in the plasma. Thus, the inhibitory effect on systemic platelet aggregation is nonreversible and may last several days. This situation may prove to be deleterious for patients with unstable conditions that may require unplanned invasive procedures. Thrombocytopenia and pseudothrombocytopenia have been described with the use of abciximab, and altered leukocyte adhesion has been observed when with the combination of abciximab and ticlopidine. Further, the use of large doses of monoclonal antibodies could stimulate the proliferation of neutralizing antibodies and therefore may restrict 7E3 therapy to a single use. Despite these complications, the positive results obtained by monoclonal antibody blockade of GP IIb/IIIa receptors have advanced the development of high-affinity, synthetic peptide antagonists.

The Evaluation of PTCA to Improve Long term Outcomes by 7E3 GPIIb/IIIa Receptor Blockade Trial (EPILOG) evaluated the use of high- and low-risk PTCA with 7E3. The original study design called for the enrollment of 4800 patients randomized to receive placebo and high-dose heparin [activated clotting time (ACT) > 300], 7E3 and high-dose heparin, or 7E3 and low-dose heparin. The trial was double blind and placebo controlled, with an interim analysis to be done after 1500 patients. After the interim analysis, the study was terminated prematurely for the following reasons. In those patients treated with 7E3, a three-time decrease in creatine kinase levels was noted, as was a 68% reduction in the combined end point of MI and death. In addition, in contrast to the results from the EPIC trial, bleeding complications in the group receiving 7E3 and low-dose heparin were not significantly different than with placebo (<2% with treatment, 3.1% with placebo). These reductions in the rate of bleeding complications may have been due to the use of early sheath removal in the EPILOG trial.

The use of abciximab (7E3) in patients who developed unstable angina with ECG changes before scheduled PTCA was evaluated in the Chimeric c7E3 Antiplatelet Therapy in Unstable Angina Refractory to Standard Therapy Trial. In this trial, patients who were scheduled for PTCA the following day and who developed unstable angina and ECG changes the night before were randomized to standard therapy with or without 7E3. The medication was continued into the PTCA the next day. Although 1200 patients were to be enrolled, the trial was stopped prematurely after 1050 patients because of strongly favorable results in those treated with abciximab. Specifically, the primary end points of MI—death and recurrent PTCA— were reduced from 16.4% to 10.8% in the treatment group. In addition, the incidence of MI was reduced from 9.4% to 4.9%, and the secondary end points of emergent CABG/repeat PTCA/emergent stent placement were significantly reduced in those patients who received abciximab. No increased risk of intracranial bleeding was noted, although the incidence of major bleeding was increased from 1.7% to 2.8%.

When abciximab was used as an adjunct to standard therapy for unstable angina, there was no additional benefit on outcomes in patients not undergoing invasive procedures. In contrast, patients receiving abciximab plus stenting had better outcomes than did MI patients receiving thrombolysis.

Abciximab also has been combined with thrombolytic agents in AMI, with no additional benefit observed when compared with thrombolytics used alone. The drug has been used as an alternative to thrombolysis after unsuccessful thrombolytic therapy.

A recent placebo-controlled trial showed that the early administration of abciximab in patients with AMI improves coronary patency before stenting, the success rate of the stenting procedure, the rate of coronary patency at 6 months, left ventricular function, and clinical outcomes. It is now well accepted that abciximab improves outcome when used in conjunction with PCI in high-risk patients with acute coronary syndromes, and that the early use of GP IIb/IIIa inhibitors before percutaneous coronary revascularization may qualify the discrepancies noted in earlier trials.

Synthetic Peptide and Nonpeptide Antagonists

As an alternative to monoclonal antibodies, researchers have attempted to develop small synthetic peptides with the ability to block fibrinogen from binding to the GP IIb/IIIa platelet receptor. The goal of this effort has been to create a peptide with the same affinity and specificity exhibited by monoclonal antibodies, but without the negative side effects of prolonged bleeding time, immunogenicity, and irreversibility. In many cases, the synthetic peptides were modeled on the "disintegrin" or natural antiplatelet antagonists, but were smaller and therefore less immunogenic. By using the RGD binding sequence found in circulating adhesive proteins, researchers have developed a series of modified RGD analogues capable of binding to GP IIb/IIIa. One modification includes the addition of disulfide bonds for the creation of cyclic peptides. The cyclic conformation has not only rendered the peptides more stable in plasma but also imparted a higher affinity for the integrin receptor. Another modification has been to substitute lysine (K) in the RGD sequence for arginine (R). This substitution creates a peptide similar to the disintegrin barbourin (discussed earlier in this chapter), which has absolute specificity for GP IIb/IIIa integrin.

The cyclic heptapeptide eptifibatide (Integrelin) is now approved for use in acute coronary syndromes on the basis of the Platelet Glycoprotein IIb/IIIa in Unstable Angina: Receptor Suppression using Integrelin Therapy (PURSUIT) trial. The recommended dose for acute coronary syndromes is a 180-μg/kg bolus followed by an infusion of 2.0 μg/min for 72 to 96 h. The approved dose for PCI on the basis of the IMPACT-II trial is a bolus of 135 μg/kg followed by an infusion of 0.5 μg/kg per minute for 20 to 24 h. However, a dose based on the Enhanced Suppression of the Platelet IIb/IIIa Receptor with Integrelin Therapy (ESPRIT) trial is now recommended, which is two 180-μg/kg boluses 10 min apart and a 2.0-μg/kg per minute infusion for 18 to 24 h.

The nonpeptide tirofiban (Aggrastat) is approved for use in acute coronary syndromes at a dose of 0.4 μg/kg per minute for 30 min and then 0.1 μg/kg per minute for 48 to 108 h. When tirofiban was used in patients with coronary syndromes and undergoing invasive therapy, a more favorable outcome was observed when compared with conservative therapy. A comparison trial of two platelet glycoprotein IIb/IIIa inhibitors, tirofiban and abciximab, for the prevention of ischemic events with percutaneous coronary revascularization demonstrated that tirofiban offers less protection than abciximab against major ischemic events.

Although the peptide antagonists to the GP IIb/IIIa integrin appear to compensate for the shortcomings of the monoclonal antibodies (i.e., decreased bleeding time, reversibility, and non-immunogenicity), they have one major limitation: none is orally bioavailable in human beings. Currently, all antagonists, peptide or monoclonal antibody, must be administered intravenously. Therefore, their therapeutic use is limited to acute thrombotic situations, such as maintenance of coronary flow after angioplasty or thrombolysis [with tissue plasminogen activator (t-PA) or streptokinase]. To be effective as preventative therapy (i.e., for unstable angina and MI), an orally active form must become available.

However, a meta-analysis of oral GP IIb/IIIa inhibitor trials found a highly significant excess in mortality that was consistent across four trials with three different oral GP IIb/IIIa inhibitor agents and was associated with a reduction in the need for urgent revascularization and no increase in MI. The investigators believed that these findings suggest a direct toxic effect with these agents that is not related to a prothrombotic mechanism.

Conclusion

Antiplatelet therapy is an effective treatment for patients with coronary and cerebral vascular diseases. Aspirin is effective in reducing mortality risk in survivors of AMI, and aspirin, ticlopidine, and clopidogrel are useful in preventing strokes in persons at high risk. The development of monoclonal antibodies and intravenous peptide and nonpeptide compounds that bind to the GP IIb/IIIa receptor in activated platelets show great potential for treating patients undergoing coronary angioplasty to prevent short- and long-term complications and for treating patients with unstable angina and MI. The clinical development of oral GP IIb/IIIa inhibitor agents suitable for long-term use has been disappointing and is an area for future research.

OTHER ANTICOAGULANTS AND DIRECT ANTITHROMBINS

In this section, the anticoagulant drugs heparin, heparin derivatives, and warfarin are reviewed, and the new direct thrombin inhibitors hirudin, hirulog, argatroban, melagatran, and ximelagatran are discussed.

Heparin

Mechanisms of Action

Heparin, a glycosaminoglycan, is composed of alternating residues of D-glucosamine and iduronic acid. Its principal anticoagulant effect depends on a critical pentasaccharide with high-affinity binding to antithrombin III (ATIII). When bound to the critical pentasaccharide, ATIII changes its configuration so that it can directly inhibit activated factor X (Xa). If the polysaccharide chain is long enough (>18 saccharides), the heparin/ATIII complex can also bind thrombin and inactivate its active site. Heparin catalyzes the inactivation of thrombin by ATIII (Fig. 13-4) by providing a template to which thrombin (factor IIa) and the naturally occurring serine protease inhibitor, ATIII, can bind. In addition, heparin catalyzes thrombin inactivation via a specific pathway involving heparin cofactor II, a mechanism requiring higher heparin doses but not involving the ATIII-binding pentasaccharide. In contradistinction to direct thrombin inhibitors that impede thrombin activity, heparin indirectly inhibits thrombin activity and thrombin generation; the heparin/ATIII complex also inhibits other anticoagulation proteases, including factors IXa, Xa, XIa, and XIIa.

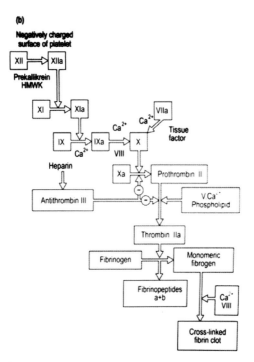

FIG. 13-4 Antithrombin III inactivates factor Xa and thrombin (factor IIa). This effect is enhanced by heparin.

The molecular weight of heparin ranges from 5000 to 30,000 kDa, with a mean value of 15,000 kDa containing an average of approximately 50 saccharide chains. Heparin's pharmacokinetic properties in anticoagulant activity are heterogeneous for two reasons. First, its plasma clearance is influenced by molecular size, with larger molecules being cleared more rapidly than smaller molecules, resulting in an increased antifactor Xa to antifactor IIa (thrombin) activity ratio. Second, the anticoagulant activity of heparin is also influenced by molecular chain length; only about 33% of standard unfractionated heparin molecules in clinical usage are sufficiently long (containing more than 18 saccharides) to possess the ability to inhibit thrombin via ATIII-mediated anticoagulant action.

Pharmacokinetics

Because it is not absorbed orally, heparin is given subcutaneously or intravenously. When given in sufficient doses, the safety and efficacy of both routes are comparable for treating venous thrombosis if the reduced bioavailability of subcutaneous heparin is taken into account. At clinically therapeutic doses, a substantial proportion of heparin is cleared via the dose-dependent rapid pathway. Hence, the anticoagulant response to heparin is not linear but increases disproportionately in intensity and duration with larger heparin doses. The apparently biologic half-life of heparin increases from 30 to 60 to 150 min after bolus intravenous doses of 25, 100, and 400 U/kg, respectively.

Pharmacodynamics

The intensity of heparin's anticoagulant effect is monitored by the activated partial thromboplastin time (aPTT) test, which is sensitive to antithrombin (antifactor IIa) and antifactor IXa and Xa effects. Experimental data have suggested than an aPTT of 1.5 times control could prevent venous thrombus extension. When heparin is used clinically, consideration must be given to (1) interpatient variability in plasma and tissue binding that alters heparin pharmacokinetics; (2) potential increases in factor VIII (occurring as part of an acute phase reaction in seriously ill patients) that can blunt the aPTT response to a given heparin level; and (3) the variable potency of commercially employed aPTT reagents. It has been recommended that the therapeutic range for each aPTT reagent be calibrated to be the equivalent to a heparin level of 0.2 to 0.4 U/mL by protamine titration or to an antifactor Xa level of about 0.3 to 0.7 U/mL.

Clinical Use: Venous Thrombosis

Randomized clinical trials have established the efficacy of heparin usage in venous thrombosis. Heparin may be given in an initial intravenous bolus of 5000 U, or a weight-adjusted bolus, followed by at least 30,000 U/24 h by continuous infusion with additional heparin dose adjustments to maintain a therapeutic aPTT range. Heparin's effectiveness depends on using an adequate starting dose and a maintenance infusion that produce an adequate anticoagulant effect as measured by aPTT or by heparin levels, provided that the heparin level is above 0.3 U/mL of antifactor Xa activity.

Orthopedic and General Surgery

Heparin has been recommended for routine usage in the prevention of venous thromboembolism, especially in surgical patients undergoing elective hip or knee repair or replacement who are at high risk for perioperative venous thrombosis and pulmonary embolism. The prevalence of venous thromboembolism after total knee or hip replacement surgery has been summarized as between 45% and 84% and that after hip fracture surgery as being between 36% and 60%, with corresponding pulmonary embolism rates of 2% to 30% and 4% to 24%, respectively. A meta-analysis comparing the efficacy of LMWH to low-dose unfractionated heparin (LDUH) indicated that LMWH was more effective in suppressing venous thromboembolism. Elective neurosurgery and acute spinal cord injury patients also have a high risk for venous thromboembolism that averages 24%. Although there has been concern regarding intracranial or intraspinal bleeding, a recent study has demonstrated the efficacy and safety of LDUH and LMWH prophylaxes.

Acute Myocardial Infarction and Unstable Angina

Heparin has been used in AMI patients to prevent venous thromboembolism, mural thrombosis, and systemic embolism. Among AMI patients not treated with antithrombotic agents, the incidence of deep vein thrombosis (DVT) is about 24%. Subcutaneous LDUH in doses of 5000 to 7500 U twice daily and high-dose intravenous heparin, 40,000 U/day, reduce DVT without adverse bleeding events. In the contemporary AMI patient, heparin anticoagulation coupled with aspirin and other antiplatelet therapy has become a mainstay of treatment. However, no benefit was seen on early coronary patency in MI patients receiving heparin before primary angioplasty. In acute coronary syndromes, it has been used to reduce the frequency of unstable angina. It also has become a standard adjunct to thrombolytic drugs despite definitive proof of its efficacy, where it is used concurrently with t-PA, tenecteplase, reteplase, or anisoylated plasminogen streptokinase activator complex (APSAC), or subsequent to streptokinase, thereby minimizing thrombolytic drug activation of the coagulation system during fibrinolysis. The increased plasmin generated during fibrinolytic drug therapy mediates platelet activation and plasmin-mediated prothrombinase activity, thus requiring ancillary antithrombotic drug treatment.

Studies examining the efficacy of heparin therapy for the treatment of MI in the thrombolytic era are reviewed next. The Studio sulla Calciparina nell' Angina e nella Trombosi Ventricolare nell' Infarto (SCATI) study examined 711 patients randomized to receive subcutaneous heparin or no heparin as part of therapy for MI. Approximately 50% of patients received thrombolytic therapy with streptokinase. In the heparin plus thrombolytic group and the heparin-alone group, a reduction in mortality associated with heparin was noted. In addition, a trend toward a reduction in the number of postinfarction ischemic episodes was noted in those patients who received thrombolytic therapy plus heparin. Heparin therapy was clearly effective alone or as an adjunct to thrombolytic therapy in the treatment of AMI. In a larger trial, the Gruppo Italiano per lo Studio della Streptochinase nell' Infarto Miocardico (GISSI-2) study, subcutaneous heparin therapy was not associated with a statistically significant difference in mortality, reinfarction, or unstable angina. However, it did highlight an excess of bleeding. The International Study Group, which incorporated some of the GISSI-2 data, examined 20,891 patients who underwent thrombolytic therapy with APSAC or streptokinase. The group that received subcutaneous heparin experienced an excess of bleeding episodes without the benefit of a reduction in reinfarction or stroke. In addition, ISIS-3 examined 41,300 patients treated with thrombolytic therapy. The addition of heparin to aspirin resulted in an excess of transfused or major bleeding, with a trend toward a reduction in reinfarction and no differences in mortality or stroke. However, a meta-analysis of the data from the ISIS-3 and GISSI trials supported a decrease in mortality during the treatment period. This mortality benefit came at the expense of increased bleeding. Taken together with a review of prior data on the use of heparin as adjuvant therapy for MI published in 1985, heparin did not appear to significantly influence the rates of reinfarction or death.

A few trials using heparin have demonstrated an improved patency rate of the infarct-related artery up to 3 days after thrombolysis for AMI. The HART study, in which 205 patients received t-PA plus heparin or aspirin, associated the improved 18-h patency of the infarct-related artery with heparin therapy. There were no significant differences between groups in terms of patency at 7 days or in terms of hemorrhagic events. Examination of the data from the TAMI and the Global Use of Strategies to Open Occluded Coronary Arteries (GUSTO) trials did not demonstrate an effect of heparin on mortality, reinfarction, major hemorrhage, infarct-related artery patency, or reocclusion. These angiographic trials highlighted the fact that heparin may improve coronary patency in some patients, with improvement being greatest in those patients not treated or under-treated with aspirin.

In all, the data available with heparin as adjunctive therapy for MI do not support its routine use with streptokinase. Anticoagulant therapy should be reserved for use in those patients who are at higher risk for additional events—specifically, those patients with atrial fibrillation, heart failure, or who have suffered a large MI. The data regarding the use of heparin with t-PA are even more limited. However, its short duration of activity, its more specific fibrinolytic effect, and the angiographic data lend some support to its use with t-PA.

Randomized clinical trials have compared the effectiveness of intravenous heparin (an indirect thrombin inhibitor) with intravenous hirudin (a direct thrombin antagonist). In the Thrombolysis in Myocardial Infarction (TIMI) 9B study, heparin (5000 U bolus and 1000 U/h) and hirudin (0.1 mg/kg bolus and 0.1 mg/kg per hour) were found to be equally effective and to have similar major hemorrhagic side effects (4% to 5%) when used as adjuncts to t-PA or streptokinase to prevent unsatisfactory thrombotic outcomes in AMI patients.

Dosing

There are several methods for optimizing intravenous heparin dose adjustments. These nomograms have been used for the treatment of venous thromboembolism and AMI patients. A weight-based heparin nomogram also has been recommended in the current treatment guidelines for unstable angina. Such algorithms are convenient to use, are successful in achieving therapeutic aPTT levels in an expeditious manner, and reduce thromboembolism.

Side Effects

Bleeding is the major side effect associated with heparin use and is partly a function of the drug's complex pharmacokinetics, its use in severely ill patients who are often on other antithrombotic or fibrinolytic agents, and the numerous other actions of heparin on a variety of processes besides anticoagulation.

Of special concern is heparin-induced thrombocytopenia (HIT). Two mechanisms for HIT have been elucidated: an early reversible nonimmune thrombocytopenia, possibly related to weak platelet activation by the drug, and a late, serious immune thrombocytopenia with immunoglobulin G–mediated platelet activation and thrombotic complications. Immune-related HIT was seen in 1% and 3% of patients receiving LDUH for 7 and 14 days, respectively, but was not observed with LMWH. When present, HIT becomes manifest 5 to 15 days after initiating heparin therapy but may arise within hours in patients exposed to heparin within the previous 3 to 6 months. In vitro studies have suggested that LMWH can cross-react to activate platelets in serum from HIT patients.

Low-Molecular-Weight Heparins

LMWHs are fragments of commercial-grade standard heparin produced by enzymatic or chemical depolymerization, with a resultant molecular weight of 4000 to 6500 kDa (Table 13-1). Because smaller heparin molecules (molecular weight < 4000) are not able to bind to thrombin (factor II) and ATIII simultaneously, LMWHs have a diminished ability to accelerate the inactivation of thrombin by ATIII. However, LMWH retains its ability to catalyze the inhibition of factor Xa by ATIII. Therefore, in contrast to standard heparin (average molecular weight, 12,000 to 15,000) with an anti-Xa/anti-IIa inhibitory ratio of 1:1, commercial LMWH has anti-Xa/anti-IIa ratios from 2:1 to 4:1 when tested in vitro. The persistence of anti-IIa activity by LMWH emanates from the larger oligosaccharide chains in its polydispersed spectrum.

Other properties that distinguish LMWH from standard heparin include lack of inhibition of activity by platelet factor IV, a potent inhibitor of stan-

TABLE 13-1 Low-Molecular-Weight Heparins

Generic name	Brand name	Mean (range) molecular weight	Anti-Xa/ anti-IIa ratio	Plasma half-life (min)
Ardeparin	Normiflow	5000		
Certroparin	Sandoparin	6000 (5000–9000)	2.0/1.0	270
Dalteparin*	Fragmin	5000 (2000–9000)	2.7/1.0	119–139
Enoxaparin*	Lovenox	4500 (3000–8000)	3.8/1.0	129–180
Naroparin	Fraxiparine	4500 (2000–8000)	3.2/1.0	132–162
Parnaparin	Flaxum	—	—	—
Reviparin	Clivarine	3900 (2000–4500)	5.0/1.0	—
Tinzaparin*	Innohep	4500 (3000–6000)	2.8/1.0	111

*FDA approved.
Key: IIa, activated factor II; Xa, activated factor x.

dard heparin release during coagulation; persistence of inactivation of Xa bound to platelet membranes in the prothrombinase complex, a feature lacking in standard heparin; and lack of LMWH binding by plasma proteins, histidine-rich glycoprotein, fibronectin, vitronectin, and von Willebrand factor, as opposed to the plasma binding of standard heparin, which partly neutralizes its anti-Xa inhibition. In addition, unfractionated heparin (UH) binds to endothelium, monocytes, and osteoclasts. The diminished binding of LMWH to osteoclasts may account for the decreased incidence of osteoporosis as compared with that seen with the prolonged use of UH.

These features of LMWH that distinguish it from standard heparin can result in certain clinical advantages: (1) a more predictable dose response with patient variability to a fixed dose, (2) a long half-life and reduced bleeding for equivalent antithrombotic effects, and (3) enhanced safety and efficacy in the treatment of patients with venous thrombosis. Table 13-1 lists several LMWHs.

Clinical Trials

A meta-analysis of the relevant randomized clinical trials comparing UH with LMWH examined total mortality, pulmonary embolism mortality, rates of recurrent venous thromboembolism, change in venography scores, and incidence of bleeding. LMWH significantly reduced short-term and pulmonary embolism mortalities and caused less major bleeding as compared with UH. Longer-term mortality and serious bleeding rates were influenced by case mix and efficacy of subsequent oral anticoagulation but favorably influenced by LMWH as compared with UH, with relative risks of 0.30 (95% confidence interval, 0.3 to 0.4; $P = 0.0006$) for mortality and 0.42 (95% confidence interval, 0.2 to 0.9; $P < 0.01$) for major bleeding. Additional data favoring the safety of LMWH versus UH were provided from a study of 3809 patients undergoing major abdominal surgery with heparin prophylaxis for at least 5 days perioperatively. The 4-week incidence of major bleeding was reduced from 4.8% to 3.6% ($P < 0.058$), and that of major hematoma was reduced from 2.7% to 1.4% when LMWH was compared with UH. Individual trials and a meta-analysis have associated LMWH as opposed to UH use in venous thromboembolism with a decreased mortality. This decreased mortality incidence appears to be seen only in cancer patients and is the subject of new trials.

Acute Ischemic Stroke

Thrombolytics have a place in the treatment of acute stroke, but full-dose anticoagulation with UH or LMWH is generally not recommended, except possibly for prevention of recurrent cardioembolic stroke. The International Stroke Trial compared aspirin, subcutaneous heparin, both, and neither and found no significant advantage from heparin but did find a higher rate of bleeding with higher doses of the drug.

Kay and associates, in a randomized double-blind, placebo-controlled trial, compared the effect of two dosages of LMWH with placebo. Three hundred twelve patients with acute ischemic stroke were randomized within 48 h of symptom onset to high-dose nadroparin (4100 IU of antifactor Xa, subcutaneously, twice daily), low-dose nadroparin (4100 IU subcutaneously once daily), or placebo subcutaneously for 10 days. The primary end point of death and dependency regarding daily living were analyzed for 306 patients at a 6-month time point. A significant, favorable dose-dependent effect of LMWH on outcomes was noted as follows: high-dose group, 45%; low-dose group, 52%; and placebo, 65% ($P = 0.005$). No statistically significant differences in hemorrhagic transformation of the infarct were noted across groups. LMWH improved the 6-month outcome of acute ischemic stroke. However, these findings could not be duplicated in a very similar trial that used the same agent.

Myocardial Infarction

LMWH can be used as an alternative to weight-adjusted UH in patients with AMI undergoing thrombolysis. In a recent trial, tenecteplase plus enoxaparin reduced the frequency of ischemic complications of an AMI as compared with UH. The tenecteplase–enoxaparin combination also was shown to be as effective as tenecteplase plus abciximab but was easier to administer to patients.

Unstable Angina

The use of antithrombotic agents for unstable angina, a process that results from platelet aggregation and thrombus formation, has been well studied. Gurfinkel and colleagues, in a prospective, single-blind, randomized trial of patients with unstable angina, compared the effects of nadroparin calcium, an LMWH (214 IU/kg anti-Xa, subcutaneously, twice daily), and ASA with those of UH and ASA (200 mg/day) and those of ASA (200 mg/day) alone in 211 patients. Primary outcomes were recurrent angina, AMI, urgent revascularization, major bleeding, and death. There was a significant benefit with the use of LMWH and ASA versus UH and ASA in the rate of recurrent angina: 21% versus 44%, respectively.

Fragmin During Instability with Coronary Artery Disease was a multicenter study that randomized 1506 patients with unstable angina to LMWH (120 IU/kg subcutaneously every 12 h up to day 6 and then 7500 U every day at home until day 40) or placebo. At day 6, there were differences between the LMWH and placebo groups in the occurrence of new MI and death (1.8% and 4.7%, respectively) and severe angina (7.8% and 13.9%, respectively). The benefit continued through day 40. By day 150 no differences were noted between the two groups. FRIC, another multicenter, randomized study, enrolled 1482 patients with unstable angina. Patients were randomized to UH (5000 U intravenous bolus, 1000 U/infusion, and then 1250 U subcutaneously twice daily) versus LMWH (120 IU/kg every 12 h). Therapy continued for

6 weeks. The initial data at 7 days indicated no differences between groups in death, MI, urgent revascularization, non–Q-wave MI, or unstable angina.

In a study of thrombolytic therapy with enoxaparin plus aspirin versus UH plus aspirin, enoxaparin plus aspirin was more effective in reducing the incidence of ischemic events in patients with unstable angina or non–Q-wave MIs in the early stage. This greater efficacy was sustained at a 1-year follow-up. A recent meta-analysis found no difference in efficacy or safety between UH and LMWH in aspirin-treated patients with acute coronary syndromes. Both therapies halved the risk of MI and death. There is no evidence to support the use of LMWH after 7 days. The American College of Chest Physicians Consensus Conference currently recommends that unstable angina be treated with aspirin or an alternative antiplatelet agent combined with intravenous heparin (about 75 U/kg as an intravenous bolus; initial maintenance, 1250 U/h intravenously; aPTT, 1.5 to 2 times control) or LMWH (dose regimen from trial), dalteparin (120 IU/kg subcutaneously every 12 h), enoxaparin (1 mg/kg subcutaneously twice daily), nadroparin (86 IU anti-Xa/kg twice daily for 4 to 8 days or the same dose given intravenously and then subcutaneously twice daily for 24 days) for at least 48 h, or until the unstable pain pattern resolves. The newest American College of Cardiology/American Heart Association guidelines for managing acute coronary syndromes also recommend LMWH as an alternative to UH.

Prevention of Venous Thromboembolism After Knee Arthroplasty

In patients undergoing major knee surgery, 60% to 70% develop DVT. Proximal DVT occurs in 20% of these patients. Initially, pneumatic compression cuffs and warfarin were used as prophylaxis. In a double-blind, randomized trial, Levine and associates compared the use of ardeparin (Normiflo), an LMWH, and compression stockings with stockings alone for the prevention of thromboembolism postoperatively. The study group received ardeparin 0.005 mL/kg (50 anti-Xa U/kg) subcutaneously every 12 h. At day 14, venography was performed. Of the patients receiving LMWH, 29 of 97 (29.9%) were found to have DVT or pulmonary embolism and 2 (2%) had proximal DVT, whereas 61 of the 104 patients (58.7%) with compression stockings alone developed DVT or pulmonary embolism with 16 (15%) being proximal DVT. One patient in each group developed pulmonary embolism. There was no difference in the rate of major bleeding between groups. LMWH was found to be safe and effective.

Leclerc and coworkers compared the use of the LMWH enoxaparin with placebo in patients undergoing knee replacement. The incidences of distal and proximal DVTs in the placebo group were 45% and 20%, respectively. The LMWH group had only a 19% incidence of distal DVT and no proximal DVT. In a recent randomized, double-blind trial, Leclerc compared enoxaparin with warfarin. Patients undergoing knee replacement were randomized to enoxaparin (30 mg subcutaneously every 12 h) or warfarin [dose adjusted to keep the international normalized ratio (INR) between 2.0 and 3.0]. The primary end point was the incidence of DVT as per bilateral venography. The secondary end point was the incidence of hemorrhage. The incidences of DVT were 36.9% for the enoxaparin group and 51.7% for the warfarin group. There was no difference in the incidence of major bleeding, 1.8% versus 2.1%, respectively, or proximal DVT.

Other studies have compared LMWH with warfarin in patients undergoing knee arthroplasty (Table 13-2). All but one of the studies showed that fixed-

TABLE 13-2 Comparative Studies of Warfarin and Low-Molecular-Weight Heparin After Knee Arthroplasty

Study	Intensity	Warfarin*				Regimen	Low-molecular-weight-heparin*			
		DVT	Proximal DVT	Wound hematoma	Major bleeding		DVT	Proximal DVT	Wound hematoma	Major bleeding
Hull et al	INR 2.0–3.0	152/277 (55)	34/277 (12)	19/324 (6)	3/321 (1)	Tinzaparin 75 U/(kg per d)	116/258 (45)	20/258 (8)	28/317 (9)	9/317 (3)
RD Heparin	Prothrombin time ratio 1.2–1.5	60/147 (41)	15/147 (10)	NA	NA	Ardeparin 90 U/(kg per d)	41/149 (28)	7/149 (5)	NA	NA
				NA	NA	Ardeparin 50 U/kg twice daily	37/150 (25)	9/150 (6)	NA	NA
Spiro et al	INR 2.0–3.0	72/122 (59)	16/122 (13)	6/176 (3)	4/176 (2)	Exoxaparin 30 mg twice daily	41/108 (38)	3/108 (3)	12/173 (7)	9/173 (5)
Heit et al	INR 2.0–3.0	81/222 (36)	15/222 (7)	NA	NA	Ardeparin 50 U twice daily	58/230 (25)	14/230 (6)	NA	NA
Leclerc	INR 2.0–3.0	109/211 (52)	22/211 (10)	18/334 (5)	6/334 (2)	Enoxaparin 30 mg	76/206 (37)	24/206 (12)	18/336 (5)	7/336 (2)

*Values are the number of patients with events/number of patients studied (%).

Key: DVT, deep venous thrombosis; INR, international normalized ratio; NA, not available.

Source: Leclerc JR, Goerts WH, Desjardins L, et al: Prevention of venous thromboembolism after knee arthroplasty. A randomized, double-blind trial comparing enoxaparin with warfarin. Ann Intern Med 124:619, 1996.

dose LMWH is more effective than adjusted-dose warfarin in preventing DVT postoperatively. Hull and colleagues compared Logiparin (tinzaparin) subcutaneously every day with warfarin. The incidences of DVT were 45% and 55%, respectively. The high incidence of DVT in the LMWH group was believed to be secondary to the daily dosing required instead of the usual twice-a-day dosing regimen. The American College of Chest Physicians Consensus Conference reviewed six randomized trials that directly compared oral anticoagulants with LMWH in total knee replacement and found total DVT rates of 46.2% and 31.5%, respectively, with some increase in bleeding. However, because one high-quality study found a 3-month cumulative incidence of only 0.8%, it was concluded that adjusted-dose warfarin was also effective after total knee replacement.

Acute Proximal Deep Vein Thrombosis and Superficial Vein Thrombosis

Acute proximal DVT is associated with the risk of pulmonary embolism and recurrent thromboembolism. Management of this condition has traditionally required a hospitalization of 5 to 7 days for treatment with UH and initiation of oral anticoagulation with warfarin. Recent studies compared the hospital use of LMWH with UH for the treatment of proximal DVT. Hull and coworkers randomized 418 patients to receive UH or LMWH (Logiparin, now called tinzaparin; 175 U/kg subcutaneously once daily) and found a significantly lower recurrence and bleeding rate with LMWH and a decreased mortality rate. Subsequent studies took this type of treatment to the outpatient setting. Levine and associates randomized 253 patients to receive UH intravenously and 247 patients to receive LMWH (enoxaparin 1 mg/kg, subcutaneously twice daily) for the management of acute proximal DVT. They found no statistically significant difference in recurrent thromboembolism or major bleeding between the two groups. There was a major difference in the average length of hospitalization, 1.1 days for the LMWH group and 6.5 days for the UH group. Similarly, Koopman and colleagues randomized 198 patients to receive UH intravenously and 202 patients to receive weight-dosed nadroparin-Ca (Fraxiparine) subcutaneously twice a day. Rates of recurrent thromboembolism and major bleeding were low and similar between groups. There was a significant reduction in the length of hospitalization for the LMWH group. The outpatient treatment of proximal DVT with LMWH is safe and effective. Gould and associates conducted a meta-analysis of 11 randomized, controlled studies comparing LMWH with UH for the acute treatment of DVT and confirmed the finding of Hull and colleagues, that there is a significant decrease in mortality with LMWH and similar rates of recurrence and bleeding. Subset analysis suggested that this decrease in mortality is seen only in cancer patients with DVT, and new trials are addressing this issue.

Treatment with LMWH or with an oral nonsteroidal anti-inflammatory agent has been suggested to prevent thromboembolic complications in patients with superficial vein thrombosis.

Management of Intermittent Claudication

Several small studies have demonstrated clinical improvement when using LMWH in patients with intermittent claudication and Raynaud's phenomenon. Mannarino and colleagues randomized 44 patients into a double-blinded controlled study evaluating LMWH versus placebo. Patients were treated for 6 months with daily subcutaneous injections of LMWH or placebo. After 6 months of treatment, the LMWH group had a 25% improvement in pain-free walking time ($P < 0.05$) with no adverse bleeding effects. Although patients were clinically improved, no angiographic changes were found. Calabro and associates randomized 36 patients in a double-blinded study to receive LMWH or placebo for 6 months. Patients receiving LMWH had statistically significant increases in claudication time, absolute claudication distance, and interval free of pain. These small studies showing clinical improvement with LMWH as opposed to placebo suggest that LMWH may have a role in the management of intermittent claudication (see Chapter 22), but larger and more definitive studies are needed.

Another small study tested the hypothesis that LMWH would be more effective than aspirin and dipyridamole in maintaining graft patency in patients undergoing femoropopliteal bypass grafting. Patients were randomized to receive a daily injection of 2500 IU LMWH or 300 mg aspirin with 100 mg dipyridamole for 3 months. Ninety-four patients were randomized to LMWH and 106 were randomized to aspirin and dipyridamole. Patients were stratified according to indication for surgery and were followed for 1 year. Benefit was confined to those having salvage surgery. For those having surgery for claudication, there was no significant benefit. No major bleeding events occurred in either group. The investigators concluded that LMWH is better than aspirin and dipyridamole in maintaining femoropopliteal graft patency in patients with critical limb ischemia undergoing salvage surgery. This study also used small numbers of patients, and LMWH has not yet gained a standard role in the management of intermittent claudication.

Thromboembolic Prophylaxis in Patients With Atrial Fibrillation

The increased risk of arterial embolism associated with chronic atrial fibrillation is well known. Aspirin and oral anticoagulation with warfarin reduce the incidence of embolic events in patients with chronic nonrheumatic atrial fibrillation. Harenberg and coworkers randomized 75 patients with nonrheumatic atrial fibrillation to receive the LMWH CY 216 or no specific treatment. Patients with a history of cerebral or peripheral embolism were included in the study. Overall mortality in the control group was 43%; it was 7.5% in the treatment group. The number of embolic events was reduced in the treatment group from 20% to 8.6%. The most striking difference was seen in the group of patients with a history of prior cerebral embolism. In the 15 patients from this subset who were treated with LMWH, one extracerebral nonfatal embolism occurred, and three of the seven patients with prior stroke who received no treatment experienced fatal re-embolism. No major bleeding complications were reported in either group. Further studies to evaluate the efficacy and safety of LMWH versus oral anticoagulation are necessary, particularly in patients with prior embolic events. There is no evidence that LMWH is superior to aspirin for the treatment of acute ischemic stroke in patients with atrial fibrillation. The use of LMWH as bridging therapy to warfarin with cardioversion or other procedures is attractive from an economic point of view. This approach has been carried out in small trials, but it requires further study.

Thromboprophylaxis for Hemodialysis

Standard UH is used to prevent clotting in the membrane filter during hemodialysis. Because many azotemic patients have increased risk for bleeding complications due to abnormal platelet function, an alternative to UH is being sought in LMWHs in the hope of reducing bleeding complications in hemodialysis patients. Several preliminary studies have demonstrated adequate antithrombosis with fewer hemorrhagic effects. An additional benefit of LMWH prophylaxis is a decrease in lipid blood levels. Schmitt and Schneider switched 22 patients on chronic hemodialysis from UH to the LMWH dalteparin. They found significant decreases in total cholesterol, low-density lipoprotein cholesterol, apolipoprotein B, and a minor decrease in high-density lipoprotein cholesterol levels. Triglycerides increased during the first 2 months of LMWH therapy but then normalized to previous levels. Hyperlipidemia presents a high risk for developing cardiovascular disease, and LMWH may become the antithrombotic of choice in hemodialysis patients if further trials indicate its safety, efficacy, and significant lipid-lowering effects. Recent small studies have found no difference in lipid profiles over 24 weeks of LMWH or UH for hemodialysis and small or no differences in anticoagulant efficacy, so that the increased cost of LMWH has resulted in UH remaining the standard product used for standard and venovenous hemodialyses.

Angina

Preliminary studies have suggested that LMWHs may play a role in the control of stable angina, but no definitive recommendation can be made at present. Melandri and colleagues conducted a randomized, double-blind, placebo-controlled trial of 29 patients with stable exercise-induced angina pectoris and angiographically proven coronary artery disease. Patients aged 40 to 79 years received 6400 U of the LMWH parnaparin or placebo subcutaneously. All patients were treated with β blockers and calcium channel blockers, nitrates, and aspirin. Treadmill exercise testing was conducted at the beginning of the study and repeated at the end of the 3-month treatment period, with myocardial ischemia being defined as ST depression greater than 1 mm. Exercise time to ischemia (ST depression) in the treatment group increased from 285 to 345 s. There was no significant increase in the placebo group. The time to onset of symptoms increased insignificantly in the treatment group, although there was a significant improvement ($P = 0.016$) in terms of the Canadian Cardiovascular Society classification for angina reflecting subjective improvement in symptoms.

Cost Effectiveness

Cost minimization analyses have addressed the issue of the higher cost of LMWH versus UH. These analyses showed that the higher medication cost of LMWH was outweighed by the reduction in cost attributable to reduced incidences of DVT, pulmonary embolism, and major and minor bleeding associated with LMWH for general and orthopedic surgical patients undergoing perioperative heparin thromboembolic prophylaxis.

Danaparoid

The heparin analogue danaparoid sodium is a mixture of sulfated glycosaminoglycans of porcine origin. Danaparoid consists of heparan sulfate ($\approx 84\%$), dermatan sulfate ($\approx 12\%$), and a small amount of chondroitin sulfate ($\approx 4\%$). The drug is FDA approved for prophylaxis of postoperative DVT in patients undergoing elective hip replacement surgery. In contrast to LMWHs, which have an 80% to 90% incidence of cross-reactivity in HIT, danaparoid has a cross-reactivity rate of approximately 10%. Although danaparoid is effective for total DVT prophylaxis, it does not offer a significant advantage over comparators for prophylaxis of the more clinically important proximal DVT. For this reason, its high cost prohibits routine use for this indication. It has been used as an option in patients who have documented HIT and require anticoagulation. However, new agents (see below) have been approved that have no cross-reactivity with the antibodies found in HIT.

Hirudin (Direct Thrombin Inhibition)

The rationale for developing direct thrombin inhibitors came from the realization that: (1) the acute coronary syndromes, MI, and unstable angina are the result of plaque rupture and in situ thrombosis; and (2) thrombin plays a central role in the activation of clotting factors V and VIII, platelet activation and aggregations, cross-linking of fibrin, and stabilization of the hemostatic plug. Therefore, investigators have looked to thrombin and thrombin inhibitors as prime targets for anticoagulant drug therapy.

Brief Review of Thrombin's Action

Thrombin is a key regulator of the hemostatic process responsible for the conversion of fibrinogen to fibrin. Thrombin is generated from prothrombin through the action of activated factors V and X, calcium, and phospholipid. Thrombin not only acts to catalyze the conversion of fibrinogen to fibrin, it also acts with factor XIII to cross-link and stabilize the clot. It amplifies the clotting cascade by activating other clotting factors and acts as a potent agonist for platelet activity and recruitment. In terms of its interaction with the endothelial surface, it can act as a vasodilator in areas where the endothelial surface has not been damaged, but it can be a potent vasoconstrictor when it comes into contact with injured or denuded endothelial surfaces. This action is dependent on endothelin release. In addition, it stimulates the release of platelet-derived growth factor and interleukin 1, and therefore may be an important mediator of smooth muscle growth and proliferation; thus, it may play an important role in subacute coronary artery closure and in postangioplasty restenosis.

Shortfalls of Heparin

The search for more potent and more direct antagonists to the clotting cascade was brought about by the realization that heparin actions are incomplete, unpredictable, and dependent on cofactors not consistently found from patient to patient. Heparin's shortfalls have included a dependence on ATIII and cofactor II for its anticoagulant effect; varied activity from preparation to preparation; binding to plasma proteins, leukocytes, and osteoclasts; and an inability to inactivate clot-bound thrombin.

Meticulous monitoring of the anticoagulant effect is necessary to retain heparin in a therapeutic range for several reasons. First, heparin is a heterogeneous mixture of molecules, each with variable biologic effects. Second, the concentrations of cofactors ATIII and II vary from individual to individual. Third, heparin can be bound by a number of plasma proteins with variable concentrations from individual to individual, with a resultant difference in the amount of heparin available to exert an anticoagulant effect. In addition, activated platelets release platelet factor IV and heparinase, both of which can act to counter the anticoagulant activity of heparin. Fourth, much of the active thrombin is clot bound, which protects it from inactivation by heparin. Thus, the nidus for clot formation and propagation cannot be activated.

In contrast, the direct thrombin inhibitors are ATIII independent, provide a stable, anticoagulant effect, and can inhibit clot-bound thrombin.

Properties and Mechanism of Action

Hirudin is a 65–amino acid polypeptide that originally was isolated from leech salivary glands and is now available as a recombinant product derived from yeast.

Hirudin is a specific inhibitor of thrombin that binds to the active and substrate recognition sites of thrombin. The attachment of hirudin to thrombin is not limited to these two sites, and other areas of contact have been described. Hirudin is specific for thrombin and does not inhibit other serine proteases. Although binding is not covalent, the process of deattachment is slow and for most purposes is irreversible. This is in contrast to many of the other direct thrombin inhibitors, in which binding to thrombin is not as extensive. Lepirudin is one of several recombinant hirudins. It is FDA approved for use in patients with HIT on the basis of two clinical trials.

Argatroban and melagatran are other potent thrombin inhibitors. Argatroban is safe and effective for patients requiring anticoagulation who have HIT or a prior episode of HIT and was approved recently for clinical use in patients with HIT. Before administering argatroban, heparin should be discontinued. The recommended dose of argatroban is 2 μg/kg per minute administered as a continuous infusion. Therapy with argatroban is monitored with the aPTT, and the dose of the drug should not exceed 10 μg/kg per minute.

Although melagatran has complete subcutaneous bioavailability and low interindividual variability with parental administration, its oral bioavailability is low. To improve the oral bioavailability of melagatran, it has been converted into an orally absorbable prodrug, H376/95 (ximelagatran). Subcutaneous melagatran combined with oral H376/95 has shown promise as a therapeutic modality in patients with DVT; additional studies are in progress.

Thrombin aptamers bind to the substrate recognition site and demonstrate potent thrombin inhibition with a short half-life. Alternate antithrombin strategies include the development of factor Xa inhibitors that can block thrombin formation (e.g., fondaparinux).

Myocardial Infarction

Trials in MI have demonstrated the efficacy and safety of hirudin. In the TIMI 5 trial, which involved 246 patients, hirudin was associated with a significant reduction in the composite end point of death, reinfarction, congestive heart failure, or shock. Hirudin use was associated with improved patency of the infarct related artery at 18 to 36 h. Major hemorrhage occurred in 23% of heparin-treated patients and in 17% of hirudin-treated patients. The HIT trial also showed a low incidence of spontaneous hemorrhage and low incidence of reocclusion with low doses of hirudin. HIT also associated higher doses of hirudin with cerebral bleeds. The TIMI 6 data confirmed the results of TIMI 5, with favorable trends in the incidence of death, reinfarction, and shock without increases in major hemorrhage. In the phase III clinical trials, TIMI 9A and GUSTO 2A, an excess of cerebral hemorrhage associated with hirudin was found, without a clear mortality benefit. TIMI 9B also did not demonstrate a superiority to heparin in terms of efficacy or safety. More recently, the GUSTO 2B data did not show an advantage of hirudin over heparin in the composite end point of death or reinfarction at 30 days. However, treatment with hirudin resulted in fewer adjustments of anticoagulant doses and a significant reduction in the combined end point at 48 h. In patients with unstable angina, hirudin improved the minimal luminal diameter of the culprit artery to a greater extent than did heparin and slightly reduced the incidence of MI.

Percutaneous Transluminal Coronary Angioplasty

There have been a number of trials comparing heparin with hirudin and hirulog in patients undergoing angioplasty. In a pilot trial involving 113 patients, coronary flows 24 h postprocedure were 100% for hirudin and 91% for heparin. The end point of ischemia on 24-h Holter monitor and MI, and the composite end point of death, MI, and coronary artery bypass were reduced in the hirudin group. The HELVETICA trial involved more than 1000 patients and compared angiographic evidence of restenosis at 6 months postangioplasty. This trial reported no significant differences in restenosis. However, the incidences of death, MI, and repeat intervention within the first 24 h were lower with hirudin. The rates of major bleeds were similar. Hirulog reduces bleeding complications after angioplasty but is ineffective in reducing important clinical events.

Monitoring Therapy and Dose

There are a number of issues that should be considered in the dosing and monitoring of hirudin activity. Hirudin levels can be monitored with the aPTT and the thrombin time. The thrombin time is the most accurate indicator of hirudin activity. However, the assay system may be too cumbersome for routine clinical use. The aPTT system is the most widely used system despite the fact that the aPTT values may not be completely reliable. Many studies have found the aPTT is insensitive at high and low doses of hirudin. In addition, the dose range of heparin that has been effective in the treatment of cardiovascular disease was determined empirically, which may not be true for hirudin. Antithrombotic doses of hirudin that appear to be equipotent with heparin prolong the aPTT to a lesser degree in animal and human models. However, clinical studies in humans have demonstrated efficacy for hirudin and hirulog. Weight-adjusted dosing with a target aPTT of 65 to 90 s was effective and safe in the TIMI 6 trial. In TIMI 9A, a hirudin dose of 0.6-mg/kg bolus with an infusion rate of 0.2 mg/kg per hour was excessive. GUSTO 2B evaluated a bolus dose of hirudin of 0.1-mg/kg bolus followed by an infusion of 0.1 mg/kg per minute and found that it was safe and effective, but not superior to heparin. The dosage regimen approved for clinical use in the United States for patients with HIT and associated thromboembolic disease is 0.4 mg/kg as a bolus dose followed by a 0.15 mg/kg per hour infusion for 2 to 10 days.

Adverse Effects

The major reported complication with hirudin has been bleeding. Initial trials have demonstrated efficacy and safety of its use as compared with heparin. Unlike heparin, hirudin does not have a commercially available antagonist. If significant bleeding occurs, the clinician should be familiar with the therapies available to neutralize the effects of hirudin. Some studies have suggested that activated prothrombin complex concentrates may be useful. The mechanism of this reversal has not been elucidated; presumably the production of thrombin generated by the activated complexes overcomes the effects of hirudin. Recombinant factor VIIa also restores platelet function and reverses the bleeding effect of hirudin. Monoclonal antibodies or plasma infusions have been used to neutralize the effects of hirudin. In addition, physical methods of removing hirudin from the circulation are available; these include hemofiltration and hemodialysis.

OTHER DIRECT THROMBIN INHIBITORS

Other direct thrombin inhibitors have been developed. Hirulog, also known as bivalirudin, binds at the active and substrate recognition sites of thrombin and does not exhibit other multiple areas of contact. In addition, there is evidence that it is degraded at the active site, making it a less-potent thrombin inhibitor. Bivalirudin has been used as an adjunct to thrombolytic therapy, with initial results indicating favorable trends in terms of vessel patency, clinical events, and bleeding complications. The drug is FDA approved for use as an anticoagulant in patients with unstable angina undergoing PTCA on the basis of trials showing that it is as effective as heparin and causes less bleeding. The recommended dose of bivalirudin is 1 mg/kg as an intravenous bolus followed by a 4-h infusion at a rate of 2.5 mg/kg per hour. After the completion of the initial 4-h infusion, an additional infusion may be initiated at a rate of 0.2 mg/kg per hour for up to 20 h. The drug has also been combined with GP IIb/IIIa inhibitors in patients undergoing PTCA, showing comparable efficacy to heparin combined with GP IIb/IIIa inhibitors, and less bleeding.

Factor Xa Inhibitors

The direct thrombin inhibitors do not affect thrombin generation and may not inhibit all available thrombin. The inhibition of factor Xa can prevent thrombin from being generated and disrupt the thrombin feedback loop, which amplifies additional thrombin production.

A novel approach to factor Xa inhibition has been taken by synthesizing the critical pentasaccharide of heparin that is the binding site of heparin to ATIII. This agent, previously known as SR90107A/ORG 31540, is now called fondaparinux. It has been used successfully as a prophylactic anticoagulant for the prevention of DVT during hip surgery and as a treatment for DVT. It is now approved by the FDA for prophylaxis to prevent venous thromboembolic disease in total hip replacement, total knee replacement, and hip fracture surgery at a dose of 2.5 mg daily by subcutaneous injection. In clinical trials in orthopedic surgery, fondaparinux was started 6 h postoperatively and shown to be more effective than LMWH. When used in patients undergoing coronary angioplasty, administration of the pentasaccharide led to the inhibition of thrombin generation without modification of the aPTT and activated clotting time. Vessel closure rate was similar to rates seen in prior trials. Additional clinical trials are underway.

Although the results with fondaparinux were better than those with LMWH, the improved results may have been due to the timing of dosing in close proximity to surgery instead of the next day, and not to an inherent superiority of fondaparinux to LMWH. Others believe that the difference is due to the longer duration of action of fondaparinux. It should be noted that the aPTT is not affected by this dose of fondaparinux, and clinical monitoring is not recommended. Additional clinical data have supported its potential benefits in arterial thrombotic disorders.

Warfarin

Mechanism of Action

Warfarin is a vitamin K antagonist that blocks the cyclic interconversion of vitamin K_{H2} and its 2,3 epoxide by inhibiting two regulatory enzymes, vitamin K epoxide reductase and vitamin K reductase. Vitamin K_{H2} is an essential cofactor for the carboxylation of glutamate residues on N-terminal portions of inactive coagulant proenzymes (factors II, VII, IX, and X) in a reaction that is catalyzed by a vitamin K–dependent carboxylase. Because γ-carboxylation of vitamin K–dependent coagulation enzymes is a requisite step in the ability of the enzymes to bind metals, undergo conformational changes, bind to cofactors, and become activated, warfarin impedes the activity of these essential reactions in the coagulation pathway.

Pharmacokinetics

Warfarin, a racemic mixture of R and S isoforms, undergoes rapid and extensive gastrointestinal absorption, reaching maximal plasma concentrations in 90 min. In the blood, it has a half-life of 36 to 42 h and is extensively bound to plasma proteins, principally albumin. Only 1% to 3% of warfarin circulates in the free state, but it rapidly accumulates in the liver, where it is metabolized microsomally to inactive catabolites, the R isomers are metabolized to warfarin alcohols and excreted in the urine, and the S isomers are oxidized and eliminated via the bile. Numerous drugs and disease entities that alter warfarin absorption, plasma protein binding, liver microsomal activity, or basal vitamin K levels can increase or decrease warfarin anticoagulant intensity (see Chapter 21). Because many of these agents may be prescribed concurrently with warfarin, adjustment in the daily anticoagulant dose is necessary to avoid inadequate or excessive anticoagulation. A dietary inventory, including all drug and vitamin supplementation, is equally important: massive amounts of dietary vitamin K can increase warfarin resistance; dietary vitamin K deficiency, malabsorption problems, liquid paraffin laxatives, and hypocholesterolemic bile-binding resins can reduce warfarin absorption or increase warfarin excretion; and large doses of vitamin E used as an antioxidant can antagonize vitamin K action. Moreover, variations in dose response to warfarin can occur during extended periods of anticoagulation, variations that may have one or several patient, medication, or laboratory causes.

Laboratory Monitoring of Warfarin

Historically, the most commonly used test to monitor warfarin anticoagulation has been the prothrombin time (PT). This test is sensitive to reduced activity of factors II, VII, and X but not to reduced activity of factor IX. Interpretation of the PT results, although satisfactory for individual patient measurement, has been complicated, because thromboplastin reagents in standard usage vary in their sensitivity to the reduction of vitamin K–dependent clotting factors. Hence, the PT result can reflect very different degrees of anticoagulation when different thromboplastins are used as reagents.

Efforts to resolve the problem of variability in thromboplastin sensitivity have led to the adoption of the INR system based on a World Health Organization (WHO) International Reference Thromboplastin Reagent. The INR is the PT ratio (PTR) obtained by testing a given anticoagulated patient plasma sample against the WHO reference thromboplastin. The INR for any PTR measured with any thromboplastin reagent can be calculated if the international sensitivity index (ISI) of the reagent is known, where INR equals the measured PTR^{ISI}. Figure 13-5 shows the relation between PTR and INR for thromboplastins reagents of different ISIs. The INR value is the preferred method for expressing the degree of anticoagulation with warfarin, for com-

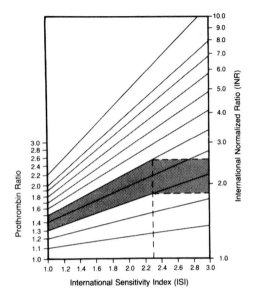

FIG. 13-5   Relation between the prothrombin time ratio (PTR) and the international normalized ratio (INR) for thromboplastin reagents over a range of international sensitivity index (ISI) values. The example shown is for a PTR of 1.3 to 1.5 for a thromboplastin preparation with an ISI of 2.3. From the formula INR = PT^{ISI}, the INR is calculated as $1.3^{2.3}$ to $1.5^{2.3}$, or 1.83 to 2.54. *[Modified with permission from Hirsh J, Polker L, Deykin D, et al: Optimal therapeutic range for anticoagulants. Chest 95(suppl 2):5s, 1989.]*

paring various results of clinical trials using warfarin, and for setting standard ranges of anticoagulation for specific clinical entities.

Certain caveats regarding the use of an INR measurement system should be kept in mind. First, during induction of warfarin anticoagulation, the PT may more accurately define the warfarin effect because the INR standard is based on ISI values derived from patients anticoagulated for at least 6 weeks, when factors II, VII, and X are decreased in activity. During the initial 2 to 3 days of warfarin therapy, the PT increase is attributable mainly to decreased functional factor VII and, to a lesser extent, factor X. Second, the naturally occurring anticoagulant protein C is decreased by warfarin anticoagulation. During the early stages of warfarin anticoagulation, protein C falls rapidly, just as factor VII does. Thus, there is a period when the full impact of anticoagulation is not manifest, but a natural protective mechanism has been diminished. This is particularly important when considering switching from argatroban or lepirudin to warfarin anticoagulation in the treatment of HIT. Third, individual thromboplastin reagents differ in their sensitivity to differing proportionate reductions in the activity of the three of four vitamin K–dependent procoagulant factors impeded by warfarin. Fourth, the calculated INR value is less accurate when the PT is measured with insensitive thromboplastin having high ISI values. Despite these limitations, expert panels continue to recommend the INR as a grading system for warfarin dosing during induction and maintenance anticoagulation, especially when sensitive thromboplastin (INR ≤ 1.5) reagents are used, careful calibration of laboratory automated clot detectors are employed, and mean normal PT is calculated according to recommended guidelines.

Warfarin Dosing: Initiation of Treatment

Upon inception of warfarin, a measurable anticoagulation effect is delayed until circulating factors II, VII, and X are cleared and replaced by dysfunctional vitamin K–dependent factors with fewer carboxy-glutamate residues. An initial anticoagulant effect will occur within 24 h as factor VII (half-life, 6 to 7 h) is cleared. Peak anticoagulation action of warfarin is delayed for 72 to 96 h because of the longer half-lives of factors II (50 h), IX (24 h), and X (36 h). Warfarin suppression of the anticoagulant activity of proteins C (half-life, 8 h) and S (30 h) also may contribute to the initial delay in anticoagulant effect.

Selection of an initial warfarin dose will depend on an appraisal of the age and nutrition status of the patient and concomitant medical conditions and drugs that could alter the impact of warfarin on anticoagulation. Expeditious but safe anticoagulation is also an economic concern for hospitalized patients with decreased inpatient length of stay. For rapid effect, a dose of 10 mg warfarin can be given on day 1. If the INR is lower than 1.5 on day 2, an additional 10 mg can be given. If the INR is higher than 1.5 on day 2, then a smaller warfarin dose may be given (5.0 to 7.5 mg). By day 3, an INR lower than 1.5 suggests a higher-than-average maintenance dose (≥5 mg), an INR of 1.5 to 2.0 suggests an average maintenance dose (4 to 6 mg), and an INR of at least 2.0 suggests that a lower-than-average maintenance dose is needed. When urgent anticoagulation is required, intravenous heparin should be used concurrently for 3 to 4 days.

When less urgent outpatient anticoagulation is desired, warfarin can be initiated at 5 mg/day. In many patients, an INR of 2.0 can be attained in about 4 to 5 days. Daily maintenance doses will depend on the clinical condition being treated and the targeted INR range.

Warfarin Dosing: Maintenance Therapy

Chronic warfarin therapy is used in the prevention of venous and arterial thromboembolisms. Specific clinical indications, generally recommended INR ranges, and duration of therapy are outlined in Fig. 13-6, and are summarized in greater detail in a consensus report on antithrombotic therapy and a detailed report of anticoagulation in patients with artificial cardiac valves. Recently it was shown that long-term, low-intensity warfarin therapy (target INR 1.5 to 2.0) was highly effective in preventing recurrent venous thromboembolism. However, another study emphasized the importance of maintaining the INR between 2.0 and 3.0 to maximize the long-term benefit. The use of specialized anticoagulation clinics can enhance the quality of care in patients receiving warfarin treatment by ensuring that the INR remains within the desired range. Thromboembolic strokes arising from inadequate anticoagulation and serious bleeding adverse events stemming from excessive anticoagulation are thereby kept to a minimum.

Persistent questions regarding the optimal benefit-to-risk ratio of specific or combined drug therapy with warfarin and aspirin in the treatment of arterial thromboembolism have been addressed recently. Three hundred seventy cardiac surgical patients receiving a mechanical or tissue valve replacement

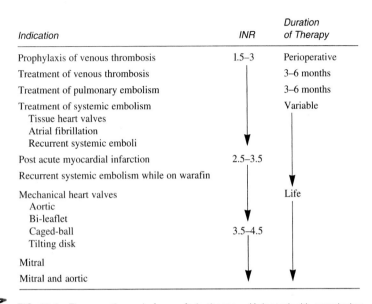

Indication	INR	Duration of Therapy
Prophylaxis of venous thrombosis	1.5–3	Perioperative
Treatment of venous thrombosis		3–6 months
Treatment of pulmonary embolism		3–6 months

Treatment of systemic embolism
  Tissue heart valves
  Atrial fibrillation
  Recurrent systemic emboli
		Variable

Post acute myocardial infarction	2.5–3.5	
Recurrent systemic embolism while on warafin		

Mechanical heart valves
  Aortic
  Bi-leaflet
  Caged-ball
  Tilting disk
	3.5–4.5	Life

Mitral		
Mitral and aortic		

FIG. 13-6 Therapeutic goals for warfarin therapy. *(Adapted with permission from Chest 108:231s, 1995.)*

were randomized to 100-mg delayed-release enteric aspirin or placebo, in addition to warfarin adjusted to an INR of 3.0 to 4.5. Combined aspirin and warfarin therapy reduced total and cardiovascular mortality and major systemic and cerebral emboli, with an additional overall risk reduction of 61% (9.9% per year for placebo plus warfarin, 3.9% per year for aspirin plus warfarin), albeit with increased minor bleeding events. The average INR value in these patients was 3.0 to 3.1, and the average warfarin dose was 5.5 to 5.8 mg/day. Low-dose aspirin and low-dose warfarin studies have tested the efficacy and safety of such combinations, with no apparent benefit seen. Clinical experience with well-controlled adequate warfarin anticoagulation continues to be the mainstay of treatment for prosthetic valve patients and for patients with rheumatic mitral valve disease who have a history of systemic embolism or who have paroxysmal or chronic atrial fibrillation. Warfarin is also recommended as a prophylaxis in patients with nonrheumatic atrial fibrillation. Recent recommendations have stratified such patients according to the presence of risk factors for embolization, including left ventricular systolic dysfunction, history of prior embolism, hypertension, or age older than 75 years. Warfarin is recommended for patients with any of these high-risk factors, and aspirin or warfarin is recommended for lower-risk patients.

Further studies using a case control methodology have indicated that, among patients with nonrheumatic atrial fibrillation, warfarin anticoagulation prophylaxis is highly effective against ischemic stroke at an INR of at least 2.0. Adjusted odds ratio for ischemic stroke rose to 1.5 at an INR of 1.8 and more precipitously at lower INRs. Secondary stroke prevention in non-valvular atrial fibrillation patients was also found to be effective at an INR of at least 2.0, and hemorrhagic risk increased at INRs above 4.5. In older patients, low-intensity warfarin (INR = 1.5 to 2.1) appears to be safer than conventional-intensity treatment. Although higher INRs are required for mechanical heart valves, adverse bleeding events also increase at INR levels of at least 4.5.

Clinical Recommendation for Myocardial Infarction

Data from the prethrombolytic era showed significant reductions in pulmonary embolism, stroke, and, in one case, reductions in mortality associated with anticoagulant use after MI. A meta-analysis of several trials from this era found reductions in the combined end point of mortality and nonfatal reinfarction. Recently, the ASPECT trial demonstrated a 50% reduction in reinfarction and a 40% reduction in stroke associated with the use of warfarin after MI. Many studies from the thrombolytic era support the use of warfarin after MI, particularly in the prevention of embolic events in those patients who are at high risk (anterior wall MI, atrial fibrillation, significant left ventricular dysfunction). The Warfarin Aspirin Reinfarction Study examined the effect of low-dose warfarin in combination with aspirin in the long-term treatment of postinfarction patients. Warfarin doses of up to 3 mg/day in combination with aspirin doses of 80 mg/day did not improve mortality when compared with aspirin doses of 160 mg/day. In fact, the combination group showed a stroke rate that was higher than that in the aspirin-alone group. At this juncture, we recommend the use of oral anticoagulants in those patients with an anterior MI, significant left ventricular dysfunction, atrial fibrillation, or history of a thromboembolic event.

Unstable Angina

The Antithrombotic Therapy in Acute Coronary Syndromes Trial showed that the long-term combination of aspirin plus warfarin is superior to aspirin alone in preventing ischemic events.

Prosthetic Valves

There are clear indications for anticoagulation after the placement of prosthetic heart valves. For those patients with bioprosthetic heart valves in the aortic position, we do not recommend routine anticoagulation. However, evidence exists for a high rate of embolic events in the first 3 months, and some recommend anticoagulants for the first 3 months postoperatively. For those patients with bioprosthetic valves in the mitral position, the rate of embolic events ranges from 0.4% to 1.9% per year in those patients without atrial fibrillation, without prior history of emboli, and without enlarged atria. However, given a thromboembolic rate of up to 80% within the first 3 months of replacement, all patients after mitral valve replacement should be anticoagulated for the first 3 months. However, it remains unclear whether these patients should be anticoagulated long term. If atrial fibrillation has become evident, left atrial thrombus is present, or there is a history of embolic events, then these patients probably should be anticoagulated.

Those patients with mechanical heart valves should be anticoagulated regardless of location. Those patients with a prosthetic valve in the mitral position are more likely to have a thromboembolic event than those patients with a prosthetic valve in the aortic position. Other risk factors for high rates of thromboembolic events include patients with prior thromboembolic events, atrial fibrillation, enlarged left atria, ball-and-cage type valves, and dual-valve replacement. Given the data for the different types of valves, each with its own optimal regimen, our recommendations are bound to be over-simplified. For those patients without a prior embolic event, we recommend a PTR of 2.5 to 3.5, with a slightly higher INR for those patients with a ball-and-cage valve. For those patients with a prior embolic event, aspirin at an initial dose of 80 mg or dipyridamole at a dose of 400 mg/day should be added. Although the risk of bleeding will be greater if significant bleeding occurs in patients with prosthetic valves, anticoagulation can be stopped for up to 2 weeks with a low risk of thromboembolism.

Atrial Fibrillation

There have been several randomized, placebo-controlled trials of anticoagulant therapy in atrial fibrillation. The current recommendations for anticoagulant therapy can be divided into several major groups. Those patients with valvular disease and atrial fibrillation should be anticoagulated. Those patients younger than 75 years with non-valvular atrial fibrillation without structural heart disease and without risk factors for heart disease can be managed without anticoagulant therapy and, in many cases, without aspirin. Those patients older than 75 years should be anticoagulated. However, the decision to treat should be balanced with the risk of an age-related increase in bleeds. For those patients older than 65 years and younger than 75 years, the presence of risk factors plays a major role in the decision to anticoagulate. Those patients with a prior thromboembolic event, hypertension, diabetes, existing coronary disease, or reduced left ventricular function are at increased risk of a thrombotic event. Those patients with none of these risk factors are at a risk of thromboembolic events of 2% to 4% per year, and the benefit of therapy with oral anticoagulants as compared with aspirin is much reduced. In the Stroke Prevention in Atrial Fibrillation Trial II, there was no significant difference between aspirin therapy and warfarin therapy for some patients. Patients with atrial fibrillation complicating thyrotoxicosis are at increased risk of thromboembolism and should be anticoagulated.

Angioplasty and Thrombolysis

In a clinical trial of warfarin started before PCI and continued for 1 year, there was also a reduction in early and long-term ischemic events.

Adverse Effects

The main complication associated with warfarin therapy is bleeding. The risk of bleeding is directly related to the intensity of therapy, with higher anticoagulant levels being associated with the greatest risk of hemorrhage. The risk of bleeding is also reported to be associated with advancing age, prior history of gastrointestinal bleeding, prior stroke, and concomitant use of aspirin and other nonsteroidal anti-inflammatory agents. If bleeding does occur, anticoagulation can be stopped.

Additional adverse events with warfarin have been described, the most important of which is warfarin-induced skin necrosis. The mechanism is unclear, but an association with protein C and protein S deficiencies have been described. In addition, a similarity between these lesions and those seen in neonatal purpura fulminans (complicating homozygous protein C deficiency) has been noted. The lesion is caused by thrombosis of venules and capillaries in subcutaneous fatty tissue. In this group of patients, anticoagulation with warfarin must be overlapped with heparin, and warfarin therapy is begun at very low doses (0.03 mg/kg). Warfarin therapy should be avoided in pregnancy because it is associated with birth defects, central nervous system abnormalities, and fetal bleeding.

ADDITIONAL READINGS

ACC/AHA Guidelines for the Management of Patients with Acute Myocardial Infarction: Executive Summary and Recommendations. A Report of the American College of Cardiology/American Heart Association Task Force on Practice Guidelines (Committee on Management of Acute Myocardial Infarction). *Circulation* 100:1016, 1999.

Armstrong PW: Heparin in acute coronary disease-requiem for a heavyweight? (editorial). *N Engl J Med* 337:492, 1997.

Ault KA, Cannon CP, Mitchell J, et al: Platelet activation in patients after an acute coronary syndrome: results from the TIMI-12 trial. *J Am Coll Cardiol* 33:634, 1999.

Awtry EH, Loscalzo J: Aspirin. *Circulation* 101:1206, 2000.

Berge E, Abdelnoor M, Nakstad PH, et al: Low-molecular-weight heparin versus aspirin in patients with acute ischaemic stroke and atrial fibrillation: A double-blind randomised study. *Lancet* 355:1205, 2000.

Boden WE, McKay RG: Optimal treatment of acute coronary syndromes—an evolving strategy. *N Engl J Med* 344:1939, 2001.

Bonnefoy E, Lapostolle F, Leizorovicz A, et al: Comparison of angioplasty and prehospital thrombolysis in acute myocardial infarction study group. Primary angioplasty versus prehospital fibrinolysis in acute myocardial infarction: A randomized study. *Lancet* 360:825, 2002.

Braunwald E, Antman EM, Beasley JW, et al: ACC/AHA guideline update for the management of patients with unstable angina and non–ST-segment elevation myocardial infarction: 2002: Summary article. A report of the American College of Cardiology/American Heart Association Task Force on Practice Guidelines (Committee on the Management of Patients with Unstable Angina). *Circulation* 106:1893, 2002.

Cannegeiter SC, Rosendaal FR: Optimal oral anticoagulation for patients with mechanical heart valves. *N Engl J Med* 333:11, 1995.

Cannon CP, Weintraub WS, Demopoulos LA, et al, for the TACTICS—Thrombolysis in Myocardial Infarction 18 Investigators: Comparison of early invasive and conservative strategies in patients with unstable coronary syndromes treated with the glycoprotein IIb/IIIa inhibitor tirofiban. *N Engl J Med* 344:1879, 2001.

CAPRIE Steering Committee: A randomised, blinded, trial of clopidogrel versus aspirin in patients at risk of ischaemic events (CAPRIE). *Lancet* 348:1329, 1996.

Clopidogrel in Unstable Angina to Prevent Recurrent Events Trial Investigators: Effects of clopidogrel in addition to aspirin in patients with acute coronary syndromes without ST-segment elevation. *N Engl J Med* 345:494, 2001.

Cohen M, Demers C, Gurfinkel EP, et al: A comparison of low-molecular-weight heparin with unfractionated heparin for unstable coronary artery disease. Efficacy and Safety of Subcutaneous Enoxaparin in Non–Q-Wave Coronary Events Study Group. *N Engl J Med* 337:447, 1997.

Coller BS: Platelets and thrombolytic therapy. *N Engl J Med* 322:33, 1990.

de Gaetano G for the Collaborative Group of the Primary Prevention Project (PPP): Low-dose aspirin and vitamin E in people at cardiovascular risk: A randomised trial in general practice. *Lancet* 357:89, 2001.

Elkelboom JW, Anand SS, Malmberg K, et al: Unfractionated heparin and low-molecular-weight heparin in acute coronary syndrome without ST elevation: A meta-analysis. *Lancet* 355:1936, 2000.

EPIC Investigators: Use of a monoclonal antibody directed against the platelet glycoprotein IIb/IIIa receptor in high-risk coronary angioplasty. *N Engl J Med* 330:956, 1994.

Eriksson BI, Bauer KA, Lassen MR, et al, for the Steering Committee of the Pentasaccharide in Hip-Fracture Surgery Study: Fondaparinux compared with enoxaparin for the prevention of venous thromboembolism after hip-fracture surgery. *N Engl J Med* 345:1298, 2001.

Frishman WH, Cheng-Lai A, Chen J (eds): *Current Cardiovascular Drugs,* 3rd ed. Philadelphia, Current Medicine, 2000, p 85.

Frishman WH, Lerner RG, Klein MD, Roganovic M: Antiplatelet and antithrombotic drugs, in Frishman WH, Sonnenblick EH, Sica DA (eds): *Cardiovascular Pharmacotherapeutics,* 2nd ed. New York, McGraw-Hill, 2003, p 259.

Gaspoz J-M, Coxson PG, Goldman PA, et al: Cost effectiveness of aspirin, clopidogrel, or both for secondary prevention of coronary heart disease. *N Engl J Med* 346: 1800, 2002.

Goodman SG, Fitchett D, Armstrong PW, et al for the INTERACT Trial Investigators: Randomized evaluation of the safety and efficacy of enoxaparin versus unfractionated heparin in high-risk patients with non-ST-segment elevation acute coronary syndromes receiving the glycoprotein IIb/IIIa inhibitor eptifibatide. *Circulation* 107:238, 2003.

Gould MK, Dembitzer AD, Doyle RL, et al: Low-molecular-weight heparins compared with unfractionated heparin for treatment of acute deep venous thrombosis. A meta-analysis of randomized, controlled trials. *Ann Intern Med* 130:800, 1999.

GUSTO IV-ACS Investigators: Effect of glycoprotein IIb/IIIa receptor blocker abciximab on outcome in patients with acute coronary syndromes without early coronary revascularisation. *Lancet* 357:1915, 2001.

GUSTO V Investigators: Reperfusion therapy for acute myocardial infarction with fibrinolytic therapy or combination reduced fibrinolytic therapy and platelet glycoprotein IIb/IIIa inhibition: The GUSTO V randomised trial. *Lancet* 357:1905, 2001.

Greinacher A, Lubenow N: Recombinant hirudin in clinical practice. *Circulation* 103:1479, 2001.

Hart RG, Halperin JL, Pearce LA, et al, for the Stroke Prevention in Atrial Fibrillation Investigators: Lessons from the Stroke Prevention in Atrial Fibrillation trials. *Ann Intern Med* 138:831, 2003.

Hirsh J: New anticoagulants. *Am Heart J* 142:S3, 2001.

Hirsh J, Fuster V, Ansell J, Halperin JL: American Heart Association/American College of Cardiology Foundation guide to warfarin therapy. *Circulation* 107:1692, 2003.

Hull RD, Raskob GE, Pineo GF, et al: Subcutaneous low-molecular-weight heparin compared with continuous intravenous heparin in the treatment of proximal-vein thrombosis. *N Engl J Med* 326:975, 1992.

Jackson EA, Sivasubramian R, Spencer FA, et al: Changes over time in the use of aspirin in patients hospitalized with acute myocardial infarction (1975–1977): a population-based prospective. *Am Heart J* 144:259, 2002.

Janz TG: Using thrombolytic therapy for life-threatening pulmonary embolism. *J Crit Illness* 18:102, 2003.

Juul-Moller S, Edvardsson N, Jahnmatz B, et al: Double-blind trial of aspirin in primary prevention of myocardial infarction in patients with stable chronic angina pectoris. The Swedish Angina Pectoris Aspirin Trial (SAPAT) Group. *Lancet* 340:1421, 1992.

Keam SJ, Goa KL: Fondaparinux sodium. *Drugs* 62:1673, 2002.

Kearon C, Ginsberg JS, Kovacs MJ, et al for the Extended Low-Intensity Anticoagulation for Thrombo-Embolism Investigators: Comparison of low-intensity warfarin therapy with conventional-intensity warfarin therapy for long-term prevention of recurrent venous thromboembolism. *N Engl J Med* 349:631, 2003.

Kennon S, Price CP, Mills PG, et al: The effect of aspirin on C-reactive protein as a marker of risk in unstable angina. *J Am Coll Cardiol* 37:1266, 2001.

Lee AYY, Levine MN, Baker RI, et al for the CLOT Investigators: Low-molecular-weight heparin versus a coumarin for the prevention of recurrent venous thromboembolism in patients with cancer. *N Engl J Med* 349:146, 2003.

Lerner RG, Frishman WH, Mohan KT: Clopidogrel. A new antiplatelet drug. *Heart Dis* 2:168, 2000.

Lincoff AM, Bittl JA, Harrington RA, et al for the REPLACE-2 Investigators: Bivalirudin and provisional glycoprotein IIb/IIIa blockade compared with heparin and planned glycoprotein IIb/IIIa blockade during percutaneous coronary intervention. REPLACE-2 randomized trial. *JAMA* 289:853, 2003.

Majerus PW, Tollefsen DM: Anticoagulant, thrombolytic and antiplatelet drugs, in Hardman JG, Limbird LE (eds): *Goodman & Gilman's the Pharmacological Basis of Therapeutics,* 10th ed. New York, McGraw-Hill, 2001, p 1519.

Massel D, Little SH: Risks and benefits of adding anti-platelet therapy to warfarin among patients with prosthetic heart valves: A meta-analysis. *J Am Col Cardiol* 37:569, 2001.

McKeage K, Plosker GL: Argatroban. *Drugs* 61:515, 2001.

Mehta SR, Yusuf S, Peters RJG, et al, for the Clopidogrel in Unstable Angina to Prevent Recurrent Events trial (CURE) Investigators. Effects of pretreatment with clopidogrel and aspirin followed by long-term therapy in patients undergoing percutaneous coronary intervention: The PCI-CURE study. *Lancet* 358:527, 2001.

Muller C, Buttner HJ, Petersen J, Roskamm H: A randomized comparison of clopidogrel and aspirin versus ticlopidine and aspirin after the placement of coronary-artery stents. *Circulation* 101(6):590, 2000

Nawarskas JJ, Anderson JR: Bivalirudin: A new approach to anticoagulation. *Heart Dis* 3:131, 2001.

Patrono C, Coller B, Dalen JE, et al: Platelet-active drugs: The relationships among dose, effectiveness, and side effects. *Chest* 119(suppl 1):39S, 2001.

Pulmonary Embolism Prevention (PEP) Trial Collaborative Group: Prevention of pulmonary embolism and deep venous thrombosis with low-dose aspirin: Pulmonary Embolism Prevention (PEP) Trial. *Lancet* 355:1295, 2000.

Prandoni P, Bilora F, Marchiori A, et al: An association between atherosclerosis and venous thrombosis. *N Engl J Med* 348:1435, 2003.

Ridker PM, Goldhaber SZ, Danielson E, et al for the PREVENT Investigators: Long-term low-intensity warfarin therapy for the prevention of recurrent venous thromboembolism. *N Engl J Med* 348:1425, 2003.

Schulman S: Care of patients receiving long-term anticoagulant therapy. *N Engl J Med* 349:675, 2003.

Stein PD, Alpert JS, Bussey HI, et al: Antithrombotic therapy in patients with mechanical and biological prosthetic heart valves. *Chest* 119(suppl 1):220S, 2001.

Steinhubl SR, Berger PB, Tift Mann J III, et al for the CREDO Investigators: Early and sustained dual oral antiplatelet therapy following percutaneous coronary intervention. A randomized controlled trial. *JAMA* 288:2411, 2002.

Stone GW, Grines CL, Cox DA, et al: Comparison of angioplasty with stenting, with or without abciximab in acute myocardial infarction. *N Engl J Med* 346:957, 2002.

The Superficial Thrombophlebitis Treated by Enoxaparin Study Group: A pilot randomized double-blind comparison of a low-molecular-weight heparin, a nonsteroidal anti-inflammatory agent, and placebo in the treatment of superficial vein thrombosis. *Arch Intern Med* 163:1657, 2003.

Taylor DW, Barnett HJ, Haynes RB, et al: Low-dose and high-dose acetylsalicylic acid for patients undergoing carotid endarterectomy: A randomised controlled trial. ASA and Carotid Endarterectomy (ACE) Trial Collaborators. *Lancet* 353:2179, 1999.

Turpie AG, Gallus AS, Hoek JA: Pentasaccharide Investigators. A synthetic pentasaccharide for the prevention of deep-vein thrombosis after total hip replacement. *N Engl J Med* 344:619, 2001.

Wallentin L, Goldstein P, Armstrong PW, et al: Efficacy and safety of tenecteplase in combination with the low-molecular-weight heparin enoxaparin or unfractionated heparin in the prehospital setting. The ASSENT-3 Plus randomized trial in acute myocardial infarction. *Circulation* 108:135, 2003.

Wilde MI, Markham A: Danaparoid: A review of its pharmacology and clinical use in the management of heparin induced thrombocytopenia. *Drugs* 54:903, 1997.

Yusuf S, Mehta SR, Zhao F, et al for the CURE Trial Investigators. Early and late effects of clopidogrel in patients with acute coronary syndromes. *Circulation* 107:966, 2003.

14 | Thrombolytic Agents

Robert Forman   William H. Frishman

Thrombolytic agents are drugs administered to patients for dissolution by fibrinolysis of established blood clot by activating endogenous plasminogen. Although some of these agents have been available for longer than 50 years, it was not until the 1980s that they came into wide use for the treatment of patients with acute myocardial infarction and other thrombotic states.

Thrombolytic agents act by converting the proenzyme plasminogen into the active enzyme plasmin (Fig. 14-1) by cleavage of the arginine–valine peptide bond. Plasmin lyses fibrin clot and is a nonspecific serum protease that is capable of breaking down plasminogen factors V and VIII. The action of plasmin is neutralized by circulating plasma inhibitors, primarily α-antiplasmin. Endogenous thrombolysis is also inhibited by plasminogen activator inhibitor type 1. Thrombolytics also affect platelet function in response to pathologic shear stress by inhibiting platelet aggregation in stenotic arteries.

SPECIFIC THROMBOLYTIC AGENTS

Streptokinase

Streptokinase is a single-chain polypeptide derived from β-hemolytic streptococci. It is not an enzyme and thus has no enzymatic action on plasminogen. It binds with plasminogen in a 1:1 ratio, resulting in a conformational change in the plasminogen, which thus becomes an active enzyme. This

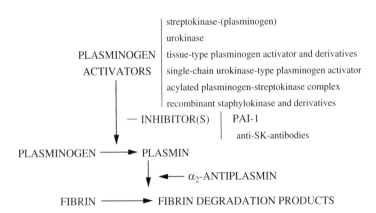

FIG. 14-1   Schematic representation of fibrinolytic system. Plasminogen is a proenzyme and is activated by plasminogen into the active enzyme plasmin. Plasmin degrades fibrin into fibrin degradation products. Fibrinolysis may be inhibited at the level of plasminogen activators by plasminogen activator inhibitor type 1 and anti-streptokinase antibodies or the level of plasmin by α_2-antiplasmin. *(Reproduced with permission from Collen D: Fibrin-selective thrombolytic therapy for acute MI. Circulation 93:857, 1996.)*

active plasminogen–streptokinase complex catalyzes the conversion of another plasminogen molecule to active plasmin. This activation of plasminogen is enhanced in the presence of not only fibrinogen but also other coagulation proteins, resulting in a systemic fibrinolytic state. In contrast to plasmin, the plasminogen–streptokinase complex is not rapidly neutralized by α_2-antiplasmin.

Anistreplase

Anisoylated plasminogen–streptokinase activator complex (APSAC) is a second-generation agent consisting of streptokinase bound in vitro to plasminogen by the insertion of an anisoyl group. This results in a much more stable enzyme complex, thereby protecting it from plasmin inhibitors and resulting in a prolonged half-life, thus permitting the agent to be administered as a single bolus. APSAC is currently unavailable in the United States.

Urokinase

Urokinase is available in single- and double-chain forms. The double-chain form originally was isolated from urine and more recently from human kidney cells in culture. Urokinase activates plasminogen directly and has no specific affinity for fibrin; hence, urokinase activates fibrin-bound and circulating plasminogens. Because urokinase is a naturally occurring product, it is not antigenic and is not neutralized by antibodies.

Tissue Plasminogen Activator

Single-chain tissue plasminogen activator (tPA), known as alteplase, occurs naturally but is synthesized for commercial use by using a recombinant DNA technique. A double-chain form of tPA, duteplase, also was synthesized and appeared to have similar activity when tested in vitro, but this form is not commercially available. The tPA molecule has a binding site enabling it to bind specifically to fibrin in thrombus. Thus it theoretically should be clot specific and not result in activation of generally circulating plasminogen. Plasminogen activator inhibitor type 1 is important and under natural conditions neutralizes endogenous tPA but not with administration of therapeutic doses of tPA.

The currently available thrombolytic agents are listed in Table 14-1. The doses listed are for patients with acute myocardial infarction.

Reteplase

Recombinant plasmin activator, or reteplase, is a deletion mutant of naturally occurring tPA that has a kringle-2 domain that lacks the finger, epidermal growth factor, and a kringle-1 domain. Its slower clearance permits reteplase to be given as a double bolus injection.

Tenecteplase

Tenecteplase tPA (TNK-tPA) is a genetically engineered variant of tPA with amino acid substitutions at three sites. These substitutions lead to a longer

TABLE 14-1 Thrombolytic Agents Currently Available in the United States

Characteristic	Streptokinase	tPA	Reteplase	Tenecteplase
Molecular weight (daltons)	47,000	70,000	40,000	70,000
Plasma clearance time (min)	15–25	4–8	13–16	20–24
Fibrin specificity	Minimal	Moderate	Mild-moderate	High
Plasminogen binding	Indirect	Direct	Direct	Direct
Potential allergic reaction	Yes	No	No	No
Typical dose	1.5 million units	100 mg	20 million units	40 mg
Administration	1-h IV infusion	15 mg IV bolus, 0.75 mg/kg over 30 min (max 50 mg) then 0.5 mg/kg over 60 min (max 35 mg)	Double bolus: 10 million U then 10 million U 30 min later	Single bolus: according to weight <60 kg:30 mg 60–69 kg: 35 mg 70–79 kg: 40 mg 80–89 kg: 45 mg ≥90 kg: 50 mg
Approximate cost ($)	340	2000	2000	2000

Key: IV, intravenously; tPA, tissue plasminogen activator.

half-life, increased fibrin specificity, and an increased resistance to plasminogen activator inhibitor. The longer half-life of TNK-tPA makes it the only thrombolytic agent currently available that can be given as a single bolus injection.

FIBRIN SPECIFICITY

An agent that is fibrin specific is activated in the presence of fibrin clot and will not indiscriminately activate circulating plasminogen. Agents that are non–fibrin specific will activate circulating plasminogen, which is not indiscriminately clot bound. This may result in depletion of circulating plasminogen and lead to "plasminogen steal," i.e., leaching fibrin-bound plasminogen from the clot and reducing the intensity of the thrombolysis.

USE IN ACUTE MYOCARDIAL INFARCTION

Enthusiasm for the use of thrombolytic agents with the ensuing trials only became popular after the pathophysiology of acute myocardial infarction was understood. Davies and Thomas observed in pathologic specimens that most cases with acute myocardial infarction are due to sudden occlusion of a coronary artery by a thrombus at the site of a ruptured atherosclerotic plaque. DeWood and colleagues confirmed this observation by demonstrating an occlusive thrombus in more than 85% of coronary angiograms performed in patients within the first 3 h of presentation with a transmural myocardial infarction. A decade previously, established that a "wavefront" of myocardial infarction progresses from the subendocardium to the subepicardium, with a longer duration of temporary occlusion of a circumflex coronary artery in dogs.

Rentrop and colleagues demonstrated the successful dissolution of the offending coronary thrombus with the use of intracoronary streptokinase. Subsequent trials using intracoronary administration of streptokinase found significant improvement in survival, particularly in those patients in whom the thrombus was successfully lysed. However, it was not until intravenous thrombolytic agents were administered that large multicenter trials could be undertaken successfully.

Effect on Mortality

Intravenous administration of thrombolytic agents has been shown to significantly reduce the mortality rate of acute myocardial infarction by approximately 25%. The results of the larger multicenter randomized trials in which different intravenous thrombolytic agents were used are shown in Table 14-2.

The first large-scale trial conducted in 1986 by the Gruppo Italiano per lo Studio della Streptochinasi nell' Infarto Miocardico (GISSI) convincingly showed that intravenous streptokinase administered within 6 h of acute myocardial infarction significantly reduces 21-day mortality by 18%. A similar 25% reduction in vascular mortality with the use of intravenous streptokinase was shown in the Second International Study of Infarct Survival (ISIS-2) trial. In this trial, patients were admitted with symptoms suggestive of acute myocardial infarction, and only 55% had significant ST-segment elevation. One smaller trial of Intravenous Streptokinase in Acute Myocardial Infarction (ISAM) showed no significant survival benefit

TABLE 14-2 Early Mortality After Thrombolysis

| Thrombolytic agent | Trial | *n* | Mortality (%) | | Survival benefit (%) |
			Control	Agent	
Streptokinase	ISAM	1,741	7.10	6.30	11 (NS)
	GISSI-1	11,806	13.0	10.70	18
	ISIS-2	17,187	12.0	9.20	25
APSAC	AIMS	1,004	12.2	6.40	47
tPA	ASSET	5,011	9.80	7.20	27

Key: AIMS, APSAC Interventional Mortality Study; APSAC, anisoylated plasminogen streptokinase activator complex; ASSET, Anglo-Saxon Scandinavian Study of Early Thrombolysis; GISSI, Gruppo Italiano per lo Studio della Streptochinasi nell' Infarto Miocardico; ISAM, Intravenous Streptokinase in Acute Myocardial Infarction; ISIS, International Study of Infarct Survival; *n*, number of patients randomized in trial; NS, not significant; tPA, tissue plasminogen activator.

despite improved ventricular function and smaller infarct size in the thrombolysed group.

In the APSAC Interventional Mortality Study (AIMS), patients with acute myocardial infarction and ST-segment elevation were randomized within 6 h of onset of symptoms. The trial was terminated prematurely because of the significant 47.5% reduction in mortality in the actively treated group.

The effect of tPA on mortality was studied in the Anglo-Saxon Scandinavian Study of Early Thrombolysis (ASSET) by using the then standard 3-h dosing regimen and randomizing the patients within 5 h of the onset of symptoms. As with the ISIS-2 trial, no electrocardiographic criteria were required for enrollment; as a consequence, only 72% of these patients were considered to have an acute myocardial infarction, but there was a significant 26% reduction in mortality in patients receiving tPA.

Because of the proven efficacy of thrombolytic agents, it would be unethical to test new agents against placebo. Thus, thrombolytic agents are now tested for equivalency or superiority to standard thrombolytic agents.

Comparison of Thrombolytic Agents

The early mortality rates comparing thrombolytic agents used in the treatment of acute myocardial infarction are shown in Table 14-3.

Streptokinase Versus tPA

In the GISSI-2 and ISIS-3 trials, the mortality rates were similar in the patients who received streptokinase and tPA. In the ISIS-3 trial, the mortality rate in 33% of patients who also received APSAC was similar. However, in these two trials, conducted predominately in Europe, heparin was administered subcutaneously and not intravenously, as is customary in the United States. In the Global Utilization of Streptokinase and Tissue Plasminogen Activator for Occluded Coronary Arteries (GUSTO) trial, there were 14% relative and 1% absolute reductions in mortality rate in patients assigned to receive tPA as opposed to those receiving streptokinase. In this trial, tPA was administered as per an accelerated protocol in which a thrombolytic agent was administered over 1 h 30 min, with two-thirds of the dose being given in the first 30 min rather

TABLE 14-3 Early Mortality Comparing Different Thrombolytic Agents

Trial	n	Mortality (%)				P
		Streptokinase	tPA	Reteplase	Tenecteplase	
ISIS-3		41,299	10.6	10.3		NS
GISSI-2	12,490	8.6	9.0			NS
GUSTO-1	41,021	7.3	6.3			0.001
INJECT	6,010	9.53		9.02		NS
GUSTO-3	15,059		7.24	7.47		NS
ASSENT-2	16,949		6.18		6.15	NS

Key: ASSENT, Assessment of the Safety and Efficacy of a New Thrombolytic; GISSI, Gruppo Italiano per lo Studio della Streptochinasi nell' Infarto Miocardico; GUSTO, Global Utilization of Streptokinase and Tissue Plasminogen Activator for Occluded Coronary Arteries; INJECT, International Joint Efficacy Comparison of Thrombolytic; ISIS, International Study of Infarct Survival; n, number of patients in trial; NS, not significant; tPA, tissue plasminogen activator.

than the conventional 3 h. The tPA used in the ISIS-3 trial was duteplase rather than the standard alteplase, but the 90-min patency rate was regarded as similar.

Double Bolus Versus Continuous Infusion of tPA

In the Continuous Infusion Versus Double Administration of Alteplase trial, more than 7000 patients were randomized to receive tPA in the form of double boluses separated by 30 min or a 90-min continuous infusion. The 30-day mortality was 7.98% for the patients receiving double boluses versus 7.44% for those receiving continuous infusion. Thus, the double bolus of alteplase failed to show equivalency to the 90-min front-loaded infusion despite its superiority in achieving 90-min patency.

Reteplase Versus Streptokinase and tPA

In the International Joint Efficacy Comparison of Thrombolytic trial (INJECT), reteplase was shown to be at least equivalent to streptokinase. The size of the trial was not large enough to determine whether the 0.5% lower mortality in patients treated with reteplase was significant. The early mortality rate in patients treated with reteplase and front-loaded tPA was shown to be similar in the GUSTO-3 trial, despite the apparent superiority of 90-min patency rates when these two agents were specifically tested.

TNK-tPA Versus tPA

Single-bolus TNK-tPA was compared with front-loaded tPA in the Second Assessment of the Safety and Efficacy of a New Thrombolytic (ASSENT-2) trial. The rate of intercerebral hemorrhage was 0.9% and similar for both agents, whereas there were significantly less noncerebral bleeding complications in patients receiving TNK-tPA. The ease of administration of TNK-tPA has made its use more convenient than that of conventional tPA, with the sole advantage of tPA being that it can be discontinued should major hemorrhage occur within the first 90 min of its infusion.

TABLE 14-4 Patency Rates (Timi Grades 2 and 3) at 90 Min After Thrombolysis with Different Agents

| Agent | n | TIMI grade (%) | |
		2 and 3	3
Streptokinase	283	60	32
tPA: 3-h infusion	1,648	70	52
tPA: front loaded	629	83	65
tPA: double bolus	84	93	88
Reteplase	157	83	60
Tenecteplase	148	79	63

Key: *n,* number of patients randomized; TIMI, thrombolysis in myocardial Infarction; tPA, tissue plasminogen activator.

Effect of Time on Efficacy

In the GISSI-1 trial, there was a nearly 50% reduction in mortality when streptokinase was administered within 1 h of the onset of symptoms, a 23% reduction in mortality when thrombolytic agent was administered within 3 h, and a 17% reduction in mortality when the agent was administered between 3 and 6 h. There was no significant reduction in mortality when streptokinase was administered 6 to 12 h after the onset of symptoms. However, in the AIMS trial, there was a similar reduction in mortality when the APSAC was administered within 4 h or between 4 and 6 h after the onset of symptoms, but the relatively small number of patients randomized in the trial makes these results less generalizable. In the ASSET trial, in which tPA was administered, there was a similar reduction in mortality in patients who received thrombolysis within 3 h or between 3 and 5 h. In the ISIS-2 trial, the greatest reduction in vascular mortality (35%) occurred when streptokinase was administered within 4 h of the onset of chest pain, although there was still a significant reduction in mortality in those patients who were randomized between 5 and 24 h. In the South American EMERAS (Estudio Multicentrico Estreptoquinasa Republicas de America del Sur) trial, there was no improvement in survival when streptokinase was administered between 7 and 12 h or up to 24 h after chest pain.

The Late Assessment of Thrombolytic Efficacy (LATE) study prospectively randomized patients to receive tPA between 6 and 24 h after the onset of chest pain. However, only 55% of the patients had significant ST-segment elevation. There was a significant relative reduction (25.6%) in the 35-day mortality rate in patients randomized to receive tPA between 6 and 12 h compared with placebo (8.9 vs. 12.0%, respectively). There was no significant difference in mortality when these patients were randomized between 12 and 24 h after the onset of symptoms. However, if patients whose thrombolysis was delayed longer than 3 h after being initially assessed in the hospital were excluded from the study, patients who received their thrombolytic agents 12 to 24 h after the onset of symptoms had a 22.4% reduction in mortality.

Thus, it has become standard practice to administer thrombolytic agents up to 12 h after the onset of chest pain in patients with acute myocardial infarction. Whether patients should receive thrombolytic agents if they present 12 to 24 h after the onset of chest pain is controversial. However, patients who have continued chest pain beyond 12 h, have staggered onset of pain, or are at higher risk with, e.g., anterior wall or complicated inferior wall myocardial infarction, can be considered for late administration of these agents.

It is not clear why patients benefit from late thrombolysis, as it is assumed that myocardial necrosis would have been completed within 6 h. Thus, its benefits may be attributed to a reduction in post–myocardial infarction remodeling and ventricular arrhythmias. In addition, infarction may not be completed if significant collateral blood flow is present to maintain viability beyond 6 h or if the occluded coronary vessel is intermittently or partly spontaneously reperfused.

A prehospital treatment strategy for ST elevation MI has been shown to reduce time to treatment by 0.5 to 1.0 h and to reduce mortality, and compares favorably with the results of primary angioplasty. In the ASSENT-3 PLUS study, it was shown that half of the MI patients could be treated with the combination of TNK-tPA and the low-molecular weight heparin, enoxaparin, with a greater benefit over TNK-tPA plus unfractionated heparin. However, there was a greater risk of intracerebral bleeding in patients over 75 years of age.

Patency

The mechanism whereby thrombolysis improves survival is by achieving and maintaining patency of the infarct related artery. Early or 90-min patency has been shown to be an important determinant of survival after thrombolysis. The thrombolysis in myocardial infarction (TIMI) grade classification is generally used to evaluate patency: grade 0, no perfusion; grade 1, penetration without perfusion; grade 2, partial perfusion with a rate of entry or clearance of contrast material beyond the occlusion that is impaired; and grade 3, complete reperfusion.

The patency rates (TIMI grades 2 and 3) at 90 min, from grouped studies, are shown in Table 14-4. Treatment with the front-loaded or accelerated tPA regimen is associated with high patency rates, whereas streptokinase is associated with the lowest patency rates. Administration of double bolus tPA, reteplase, and TNK-tPA resulted in similar patency rates. By 2 to 3 h, there was no significant difference in the patency rates between the different agents, and by 24 h, there was no further increase in the patency rates.

Reocclusion and Reinfarction

Reocclusion and reinfarction after successful thrombolysis carries a significant increase in morbidity and mortality.

For a diagnosis of reocclusion to be made, angiograms must be performed immediately after thrombolysis and at a later date, generally before hospital discharge. The diagnosis of reinfarction is often difficult, because it may immediately follow successful thrombolysis. In a meta-analysis combining the results of randomized trials, Granger and colleagues reported a reocclusion rate of 13.5% when patients received tPA and intravenous heparin compared with 8.0% when non–fibrin-specific thrombolytic agents (streptokinase, APSAC, and urokinase) were used. Thus, it was somewhat surprising to observe the lower reported rates of reinfarction in those patients who received tPA with subcutaneous heparin as opposed to streptokinase in the GISSI-2 and ISSI-3 trials. Because more than 50% of the reocclusions occur within 24 h, these events may have been undetected in clinical trials. However, there was no difference in the reocclusion rates reported with streptokinase versus tPA in the GUSTO and angiographic substudy.

Reocclusion after successful thrombolysis was recorded in 9.2% of patients in the Thrombolysis and Angioplasty in Myocardial Infarction (TAMI) I, II, and III trials but was 16.9% in those patients who required emergency angioplasty after thrombolysis. The reocclusion was clinically recognized in 58% of the patients and was associated with deleterious effects, whether silent or clinically evident. The mortality rate was 4.5% if the infarct-related artery remained patent and 11.0% if the artery reoccluded.

Patients who reinfarct while in the hospital are generally managed by performing immediate angioplasty without repeat administration of a thrombolytic agent. However, should performing an angioplasty not be feasible or appropriate, the patient can receive a second dose of a thrombolytic agent. Streptokinase resistance titers increase by the fifth day after administration of streptokinase or APSAC and remain raised for at least 1 year. Therefore, if a patient has received either of these two agents in the previous year (and probably longer ago), it is advisable that tPA or reteplase be used. Recurrence of reinfarction after thrombolysis with tPA or streptokinase was successfully treated with tPA in 85% of patients (67% within 1 h of completion of thrombolysis) without an increase in bleeding complications, but reocclusion occurred in more than 50% of these patients.

A nonrandomized study of 2301 patients who reinfarcted in the GUSTO-I and ASSENT-2 trials reported that the 30-day mortality was similar in those who received repeat thrombolysis or revascularization (11% vs. 11%), whereas the mortality in patients who were treated conservatively was higher (28%).

Completeness of Reperfusion

In the Western Washington Trial, in which intracoronary streptokinase was administered, the 30-day survival was significantly improved in those patients receiving thrombolysis compared with controls (3.7% vs. 11.2%, respectively), but by 1 year there was no difference in survival. However, when survival was analyzed for completeness of reperfusion, there was a significant improvement in survival in those patients who had complete reperfusion (and presumably TIMI grade 3 flow) compared with patients with partial (presumably TIMI grade 2 flow) or no reperfusion (98% vs. 77% vs. 85%, respectively), suggesting that partial reperfusion might be harmful.

The Third Thrombolysis Trial of Anistreplase in Acute Myocardial Infarction, in which APSAC or tPA was administered and the patients were studied 30 h after administration of their thrombolytic agents, patients with TIMI grade 3 perfusion had better left ventricular systolic function and a trend toward lower mortality than did patients with TIMI grade 2 and TIMI grade 0 or 1.

The angiographic substudy of the GUSTO trial reported that the 24-h mortality was 2.93% and highest in patients who had TIMI grade 2 at 90 min after thrombolysis. The mortality rates were 0.89% and lowest in patients with TIMI grade 3 flow and 2.35% in patients with TIMI grade 0 or 1 flow. In this angiographic substudy, in which 1210 patients were randomized to have a 90-min coronary angiogram, 54% of the patients who received tPA had TIMI grade 3 flow compared with 31% of patients who received streptokinase. However, irrespective of the treatment regimen the patient received, the 30-day mortality rates were 4% in patients with TIMI grade 3 flow and 8.4%, 9.2%, and 7.8% in patients with TIMI grades 0, 1, and 2, respectively. When the 90-min patency data and the corresponding 30-day mortality rates from the angiographic substudy were extrapolated to the 41,021 patients in the main GUSTO trial, the investigators accurately predicted the mortality in the different subgroups of the thrombolytic regimen.

Thus, it appears that the 90-min patency rate after thrombolysis and, in particular, the TIMI grade 3 flow can predict an improved survival when compared with patients with TIMI grade 2 flow who may have no difference in survival compared to patients who have TIMI grade 0 or 1 flow.

Thrombolysis in Clinical Subgroups

Anterior Wall Myocardial Infarction

The mortality rate of patients with anterior wall myocardial infarction has been reduced significantly by thrombolysis, with a 37% reduction in mortality in the ISSI-2 trial and a 21% reduction in mortality in the GISSI-1 trial. These rate reductions were significantly greater with anterior than with inferior wall myocardial infarctions. The GUSTO-1 trial found a significant 18% reduction, or a 1.9% absolute reduction, in mortality in patients with anterior wall myocardial infarction who received tPA compared with those receiving streptokinase, whereas the 11% reduction in mortality in patients with inferior wall myocardial infarction who received tPA as opposed to streptokinase was of borderline significance.

Inferior Wall Myocardial Infarction

Inferior wall myocardial infarction is generally associated with a lower mortality rate because of the smaller mass of myocardium supplied by the right coronary artery. Thus, it is not surprising that there was no statistical difference with regard to mortality in the individual trials among patients treated with thrombolysis as opposed to placebo. However, when the data were pooled, there was a significant 22% relative reduction in mortality, from 8.7% to 6.8%, with the use of thrombolytic agents. In a more recent overview that included patients in the ISIS-3, EMERAS, and LATE trials, the reduction in mortality was only 11% in patients randomized to receive thrombolysis.

Patients with inferior wall myocardial infarcts with the highest mortality rates are most likely to derive the greatest benefit from thrombolysis; these include patients with right ventricular infarction, accompanying anterior ST-segment depression, and heart block. Thus, the use of thrombolytic agents should be considered in all patients with an inferior wall myocardial infarction, particularly those who are considered to be at highest risk.

Non–Q-Wave Myocardial Infarction

Approximately 50% of patients presenting with acute myocardial infarction do not have ST-segment elevation or left bundle branch block. Administration of thrombolytic agents to patients in the GISSI-1 and ISIS-2 trials who presented with ST-segment depression did not result in improvement in survival despite a significant mortality in these groups (16% to 20%). This question was specifically addressed in a prospective manner in the TIMI-3B trial, in which patients who presented with non–Q-wave myocardial infarction or unstable angina with ST-segment depression or T-wave inversion were randomized to receive tPA or placebo. The mortality rate did not differ significantly between the tPA group and those receiving placebo (10.9% vs. 8.9%, respectively). Thrombolytic agents actually may be harmful in patients with non–Q-wave myocardial infarction, because thrombolytic therapy has a prothrombotic action, activating platelets and exposing thrombin, thus resulting in progression of the partly occluded coronary artery to complete occlusion. A post hoc analysis of the LATE study found that thrombolysis is beneficial to patients presenting 6 h after the onset of chest pain with non–Q-wave myocardial infarction. However, the investigators cautioned against accepting these results without further prospective testing in a larger number of patients.

Left Bundle Branch Block

The diagnosis of acute myocardial infarction in the presence of left bundle branch block may be masked; even when using the criteria developed from the GUSTO-1 study, in which the sensitivity of diagnosis was as low as 36%. Unfortunately, relatively few patients with left bundle branch block have been randomized in the mega-trials. In an overview of all the fibrinolysis trials, only 2032 patients with bundle branch blocks were enrolled. There was a significant reduction in 35-day mortality in patients having thrombolysis compared with those receiving placebo (18.7% vs. 23.6%, respectively). However, it has become standard practice to administer thrombolytic agents to all patients with presumed new left bundle branch block and typical symptoms of acute myocardial infarction.

Cardiogenic Shock

Patients with cardiogenic shock generally have been excluded from most of the thrombolysis trials. Thus, there are limited data concerning the efficacy of these agents. In the GISSI-1 trial, there was no significant difference in the survival of patients who presented in cardiogenic shock, whether they received thrombolysis or placebo. In the ISIS-2 trial, patients who were hypotensive with a systolic blood pressure below 100 mm Hg had a 24% significant relative reduction in 5-week mortality of 28.5% in the streptokinase group compared with 37.5% in the control group. In an overview of the mega-trials of patients presenting with blood pressures below 100 mm Hg, the 35-day mortality was 28.9% in patients receiving thrombolysis compared with 31.5% in the control subjects.

A problem in treating patients in cardiogenic shock with streptokinase is that the patients are already hypotensive before administration of a drug, which itself may cause a decrease in blood pressure. However, in the GUSTO-1 trial, patients treated with tPA were much less likely to develop cardiogenic shock, whereas those who were in cardiogenic shock at the time of randomization and who received streptokinase with intravenous heparin had a better 30-day mortality of 54%, compared with 59% in those patients receiving tPA. The poor results with administration of thrombolytic agents in patients with cardiogenic shock likely are related to the low patency rates achieved even with the use of intracoronary streptokinase. The low patency rate has been attributed to the poor delivery of thrombolytic agents to the occluded coronary vessel in the presence of cardiogenic shock, but this does not explain the poor results with administration of intracoronary thrombolysis. Because of the high mortality associated with thrombolysis and administration of thrombolytic agents, it has become standard practice not to use thrombolytic agents and to transfer these patients directly to the cardiac catheterization laboratory for immediate angiography and coronary revascularization.

Elderly Patients

There is a general reluctance to use thrombolytic agents in the elderly because it is widely believed that the complication rate from their use is higher among these patients and that their effectiveness is inferior in the elderly. In addition, a higher percentage of elderly patients will have contraindications to thrombolytic therapy, including severe hypertension, recent cerebrovascular accident and bleeding disorders, or too late an arrival in an emergency room.

Streptokinase is the only thrombolytic agent that was administered to patients older than 70 years in these early trials. In the GISSI-1 trial, there was a significant reduction in mortality compared with controls among patients younger than 65 years who were treated with streptokinase. Although the mortality rate was lower among patients older than 65 or 75 years who were thrombolysed, the reduction in mortality was not significantly different. However, the number of lives saved was larger than 4 in 100 patients among the elderly who were treated and only 2 in the younger group. The ISAM trial was the only study in which a greater mortality in the elderly was reported, but the total number of patients in this age group was small and results were not statistically significant. By far the largest number of elderly patients was randomized in the ISIS-2 trial; the mortality rate was significantly reduced among the elderly, but particularly when aspirin was combined with streptokinase. In the ASSET trial, in which patients received tPA or placebo, all patients were younger than 75 years. In this trial, a reduction in mortality for patients younger than 66 years was not significant, but it was highly significant for those older than 65 years. The results of the AIMS trial were similar to those of the ASSET trial in that the mortality rate was reduced in patients randomized to receive APSAC, but it was significant only in the older and not in the younger patients. In this trial, all patients were younger than 70 years and the numbers were relatively small.

Three large trials directly compared the outcome of streptokinase with tPA. In the GISSI-2 trial, 22.5% of the 12,490 patients were older than 70 years, but the results were not analyzed separately according to age. In the ISSI-3 trial, 26.1% of the 41,299 patients were 70 years or older, and those results were not analyzed separately according to age.

In the GUSTO-1 trial, in which 12% of the 31,021 patients were older than 75 years, there was no significant difference in the mortality rate of 19.3% in patients receiving tPA compared with 20.6% receiving streptokinase. In the angiographic substudy, regional left ventricular dysfunction was greater in patients older than 75 years; in contrast to the younger patients, this dysfunction was maintained at follow-up despite patency of the infarct-related artery. This finding led the investigators to speculate that a more rapid progression or impaired recovery of ischemic injury occurs in the elderly.

A recent observational study of 7864 Medicare patients who had received thrombolytic treatment found that patients older than 75 years have a higher 30-day mortality than those who do not receive thrombolysis (18.0% vs. 13.6%). This study has been criticized because there were significant imbalances between the groups, which were adjusted for prognostic factors. Selection for treatment was based on physician preferences, and only 33% of the electrocardiographically eligible patients were included in the study. The Fibrinolytic Therapy Trialist reviewed 58,600 patients who were randomized to thrombolytic trials and found, among the 5788 patients older than 75 years, a nonsignificant difference in mortality benefit in those patients who receive thrombolytic therapy compared with those who do not (24.3% vs. 25.3%).

Thus, elderly patients with acute myocardial infarction can benefit significantly from the administration of thrombolytic agents, but it should be remembered that the incidence, albeit small, of intracerebral hemorrhage increases with age (see Intracranial Hemorrhage, below) and that thrombolytic agents generally should be reserved for those patients who are at high risk, i.e., presenting with large anterior wall myocardial infarction and/or complicated inferior wall infarction.

Combination of Fibrinolytic Agents and Platelet Glycoprotein IIb/IIIa Receptor Inhibitors

The use of a fibrinolytic agent alone or with conventional use of aspirin and heparin has achieved a ceiling of approximately 60% TIMI grade 3 flow at 90 min. This is less than that achieved with primary percutaneous transluminal coronary angioplasty, at 80% to 95%. Because acute myocardial infarction is associated with a thrombus rich in fibrin and platelets, recent trials have added platelet glycoprotein (GP) IIb/IIIa receptor antagonists to a thrombolytic agent to improve the reperfusion rate without significantly increasing bleeding events. These agents may both potentiate fibrinolysis and reduce distal microembolism and platelet-leukocyte clumping.

In the IMPACT trial, integrelin was added to full-dose front-loaded tPA and resulted in a 66% TIMI grade 3 flow at 90 min compared with 39% in patients who received tPA alone. Abciximab was used with a lower dose of reteplase (5 µg + 5 µg) in the Strategies for Patency Enhancement in the Emergency Department trial, resulting in a 61% TIMI grade 3 flow at 60 min compared with 47% in those patients receiving full-dose reteplase. Abciximab also has been used with lower-dose tPA (5-mg bolus plus 35-mg infusion over 60 min) in the TIMI 14 study. This resulted in a 76% TIMI grade 3 flow at 90 min compared with 50% in those patients receiving front-loaded tPA. This combination of thrombolytic and GP IIb/IIIa inhibitor resulted in an even more pronounced difference at 60 min. The combination of streptokinase and abciximab was found to be ineffective and resulted in a significant increase in bleeding complications.

Despite the superior early patency rates in patients receiving the combination of thrombolytic and platelet GP IIb/IIIa inhibitors, when 16,588 patients were randomized to receive reteplase with or without abciximab, in the GUSTO V trial there was no difference in the 30-day mortality rate (5.6% vs. 5.9%). In the ASSENT-3 trial, 6095 patients were randomized into three groups: full dose TNK-tPA with unfractionated heparin or low-molecular-weight heparin or half-dose TNK-tPA with abciximab. The rate of in-hospital refractory ischemia and reinfarction was higher in the group receiving unfractionated heparin and similar in the groups receiving low-molecular-weight heparin or abciximab, but the 30-day mortality rates did not differ across groups. There was no difference in the incidence of intracranial hemorrhage, but major hemorrhage was significantly greater in the patients receiving abciximab (4.3%) than in those receiving unfractionated heparin (2.2%).

OTHER ADJUNCTIVE ANTITHROMBOTIC THERAPIES

Successful thrombolysis paradoxically results in conditions that favor re-thrombosis. In the process of thrombolysis, thrombin bound to fibrin is exposed to reperfused blood on the thrombus surface. This clot-bound thrombus activates fibrinogen and platelets, which are major contributors to re-thrombosis and, hence, reocclusion of successfully thrombolysed coronary arteries.

The objective of adjunctive treatment is to improve patency and reduce the high incidence of reocclusion after successful thrombolysis by inhibiting thrombin activity and platelet function. It is not clear whether adjunctive therapy can enhance thrombolysis.

Aspirin and Other Antiplatelet Drugs

Aspirin inhibits platelet aggregation by irreversibly inhibiting cyclooxygenase and the consequent production of thromboxane A_2. Aspirin has been convincingly shown to reduce mortality and presumably prevent reocclusion after successful thrombolysis. In the ISIS-2 trial, there was a 23% reduction in mortality among patients receiving aspirin alone as opposed to placebo, and this was similar to the 25% reduction in mortality among those who received streptokinase alone. When aspirin was combined with streptokinase, there was an additional 19% reduction in mortality. Because aspirin administration after thrombolysis decreased late but not early mortality, it is postulated that the mechanism whereby it is beneficial is in preventing reocclusion and consequently reinfarction rather than by accelerating thrombolysis.

Thromboxane is one of the many activators of the GP IIb/IIIa receptors on the platelet surface that permit the binding of fibrinogen to platelets and the consequent aggregation. Thus, aspirin is a relatively weak antiplatelet drug in comparison with the recently developed and more powerful GP IIb/IIIa receptor inhibitors.

Ticlopidine is an orally active antiplatelet agent that blocks adenosine diphosphate–induced platelet activation, but it is more expensive and has potential adverse effects on the bone marrow. However, it can be used in patients who cannot tolerate aspirin. Clopidogrel has a similar antiplatelet action without significant adverse bone marrow effect and can be used in similar circumstances. The role of clopidogrel has expanded in these syndromes, although its cost effectiveness has been called into question.

Heparin and Other Antithrombin Drugs

The anticoagulant affect of heparin is primarily related to its antithrombin activity. Thus, heparin has been administered to improve patency, particularly after thrombolysis with tPA, but it is also used with streptokinase. Heparin has been shown to improve patency but not clearly to improve mortality and reduce reinfarction. In the TAMI study, patency at 90 min after thrombolysis with tPA was 79% whether or not the patients received heparin. This led the investigators to conclude that heparin does not facilitate the fibrinolytic effect of tPA. In the Heparin Aspirin Reperfusion Trial, coronary artery patency in 205 patients who had been thrombolysed was assessed at 18 h after patients had received aspirin or heparin. The patency rate was 82% in the heparin group and significantly greater than that in the aspirin group, but a low dose of aspirin (80 mg) was used. In the European Cooperative Study Group 6 trial, patency rate at the mean of 81 h after thrombolysis with tPA was 80% in those patients who received aspirin and heparin and was significantly greater than the 75% in patients who received aspirin alone. The study group concluded that intravenous heparin in a 5000-U bolus followed by 1000/h increases patency during the first few days after thrombolysis with tPA, probably by preventing re-thrombosis.

The effect of heparin on mortality is less convincing. In the GISSI-2 study, patients received aspirin with streptokinase or tPA and were randomized to 12-h delayed administration of subcutaneous heparin or to placebo. It was surprising to observe that the mortality rate improved with addition of heparin to streptokinase rather than to tPA (GISSI International). Similar results were reported in the Studio sulla Calciparina nell'Angina e nella Trombosi Ventricoliare nell'Infarto study. Addition of subcutaneous heparin 4 h after thrombolytic therapy in the ISIS-3 study resulted in a nonsignificant reduction in reinfarction and 35-day mortality. Addition of heparin to aspirin resulted in a small absolute excess of 0.16% cerebral bleeds and 0.2% of serious noncerebral bleeds. The data from these trials did not assess the benefit of intravenously administered heparin. In the GUSTO-1 trial, there was no additional clinical benefit with regard to mortality or patency when intravenous versus subcutaneous heparin was added to streptokinase.

There are insufficient data from randomized trials to assess the efficacy of intravenous versus subcutaneous heparin on mortality after thrombolysis with tPA. In the LATE trial, in which patients were randomized to tPA or placebo, intravenous heparin did not have a beneficial effect on mortality, but the administration of heparin was not random.

The basis for use of heparin in addition to thrombolysis is not clear, although it is current practice. It is advised that heparin be given concomitantly with tPA or delayed 2 to 3 h after streptokinase.

In recent trials, high-dose heparin has been used in conjunction with tPA and resulted in an excess of intracerebral hemorrhage (GUSTO-IIa, TIMI 9A). An increase in intracerebral bleeding also has been recorded with the use of hirudin, an antithrombin agent; it acts directly to inhibit thrombin independently of antithrombin III. Compared with heparin, the antithrombin argatroban enhanced reperfusion when it was coadministered with tPA, with a lower incidence of major bleeding.

With the high incidence of intracerebral bleeding recorded, particularly in elderly patients, the current recommendation is that heparin be given according to weight: 60 U/kg (maximum, 4000 U) as a bolus followed by a maintenance infusion of 12 U/kg per hour.

COMPLICATIONS

Intracranial Hemorrhage

An intracerebral bleed is the most feared complication after administration of thrombolytic agents. Results are generally devastating, with the event usually occurring within 24 h of thrombolysis and carrying a high mortality rate of approximately 50%. However, it should be realized that the incidence of stroke in the prethrombolytic era was 1.7% to 2.4%. A meta-analysis of the major thrombolytic trials has shown that administration of thrombolytic agents is associated with an 0.4% absolute increase in the incidence of stroke (1.2% for patients receiving thrombolysis vs. 0.8% in controls). This increase was attributed mostly to the 0.4% to 0.5% incidence of intracerebral bleeding that occurs on the first day. The 0.3% incidence of stroke is very significantly lower in patients younger than 55 years compared with 0.7% in patients 75 years and older (Table 14-5).

Patients admitted to thrombolytic trials are believed to be at lower risk for intracerebral bleeding; therefore it is important to note the results from two separate surveys that were conducted outside the trials. The incidence of intracerebral hemorrhage in a group of nonrandomized patients admitted to 61 hospitals in Holland over 18 months was 1.0% (95% confidence limits, 0.62 to 1.3%). Analysis of events from a Myocardial Infarction Triage and Intervention Study, where patients in the Seattle area with myocardial infarction were monitored, reported an equal incidence of stroke in patients receiving thrombolysis (1.6%) as in patients not receiving thrombolysis (2.2%). The incidence of hemorrhagic stroke was 1.1% among the patients who received thrombolysis compared with 0.4% among those who did not.

The incidence of intracranial hemorrhage was as high as 1.3% in the TIMI-2 trial, in which patients were treated with 150 mg of tPA. The incidence decreased to 0.4% when the dose of tPA was decreased to 100 mg; thus, the larger dose of tPA is no longer used.

Although hypertension is generally regarded as a significant risk factor in the development of an intracranial bleed after administration of thrombolytic agents, this has not been proven from the trials or general surveys. A multivariant logistic regression analysis found that only prior treatment with other anticoagulants, body weight less than 70 kg, and age older than 65 years were associated with a significantly greater incidence of intracerebral bleeding.

Patients who had a cerebrovascular episode more than 6 months before the myocardial infarction were believed to be at low risk for an intracerebral bleed. When such patients were randomized to receive tPA in the TIMI study, the incidence of cerebral hemorrhage remained very high, at 3.4%, compared with 0.5% in the later part of the trial, when such patients were excluded.

There appears to be a small difference in hemorrhagic stroke according to the thrombolytic agent used. A significant difference in intracerebral bleeding was found in the ISIS-3 trial between patients who received tPA (0.7%) and those who received streptokinase (0.3%). This difference was attributed to a higher dose of duteplase compared with a lower dose of alteplase, which is the current form of tPA. In the GISSI-2 trial, the incidences of hemorrhagic stroke were 0.3% in the tPA group and 0.25% in patients receiving streptokinase. However, in the GUSTO trial, the incidence of hemorrhagic stroke was 0.7% and significantly greater than 0.5% in patients receiving streptokinase. In patients older than 75 years, the incidence of hemorrhagic stroke was 2.08% in those treated with tPA and significantly greater than the 1.23% in the patients receiving streptokinase. Thus, it may be more judicious to use streptokinase in very elderly patients presenting with acute myocardial infarction.

TABLE 14-5 Incidence of Stroke After Thrombolysis

Age (years)	Control (%)	Thrombolytic (%)	Excess /1000 (SD)
<55	0.4	0.3	−1.7 (1.1)
55–64	0.6	1.1	5.1 (1.5)
65–74	1.0	1.4	4.8 (1.9)
>75	1.2	2.0	7.6 (3.7)

Key: SD, standard deviation.

Noncerebral Hemorrhage

Major noncerebral bleeds that require blood transfusion occurred more frequently in patients who received thrombolysis, with an excess of 7.3 per 1000 patients (1.1% in patients receiving thrombolysis and 0.4% in the patients in the control group).

Treatment of Bleeding with Thrombolysis

Massive bleeding accompanied by hemodynamic compromise, particularly if the bleeding site is not compressible, should be treated with coagulation factors and volume replacement. If the patient is receiving heparin, it should be discontinued and protamine administered. In the absence of heparin therapy, a prolonged partial thromboplastin time will identify patients with a persistent fibrinolytic state. Such a patient should immediately receive 10 U of cryoprecipitate. The fibrinogen level should be monitored only after the cryoprecipitate has been given; if that level is less than 100 mg/100 mL, the patient should receive an additional 10 U of cryoprecipitate. If bleeding persists after fibrinogen has been restored, 2 U of fresh frozen plasma should be given. If the bleeding continues to be uncontrolled, it is recommended that bleeding time be monitored. If this bleeding time is longer than 9 min, the patient should receive 10 U of platelets; if the bleeding time is shorter than 9 min, the patient should receive an antifibrinolytic agent such as aminocaproic acid.

Cardiac Rupture

Myocardial rupture is a consequence of transmural myocardial necrosis and occurs in approximately 4% of patients admitted with acute myocardial infarction. It has been reasoned that early administration of thrombolytic therapy will reduce cardiac rupture by preventing transmural necrosis, whereas late thrombolysis, which promotes hemorrhage into a transmural myocardial infarct, will increase the incidence of myocardial rupture. A meta-analysis of placebo-controlled trials in which thrombolysis was administered to 1638 patients found that 58 patients had developed myocardial rupture. Regression-line analysis showed that the incidence of myocardial rupture increases with the interval between the onset of symptoms and the administration of the thrombolytic agent and that the odds ratio of developing cardiac rupture is

---

TABLE 14-6 Criteria for Thrombolysis in Acute Myocardial Infarction

Chest pain consistent with acute myocardial infarction lasting 30 min
Electrocardiographic changes
    ST-segment elevation in at least two contiguous limb leads of 0.1 mV
    V_1–V_3 of 0.2 mV
    V_4–V_6 of 0.1 mV
    ST-segment depression in V_{1-3} with tall R in V_2 with diagnosis of
      posterior infarction
    New or presumed left bundle branch block
Time from onset of symptoms
    <6 h: most beneficial
    6–12 h: intermediate benefit
    >12 h: least benefit; consider if chest pain present or staggered pain
      course in high-risk patients

TABLE 14-7 Contraindications to Thrombolytic Therapy

Absolute contraindications:
    Prior intracranial bleed
    Thromboembolic stroke within 2 months
    Neurosurgery within 1 month
    Active internal bleeding (excluding menstruation)
    Dissecting aortic aneurysm
Relative contraindications:
    Persistent hypertension ≥180/110 mm Hg despite therapy
    Recent puncture of noncompressible vessel
    Gastrointestinal and genitourinary bleeding within 1 month
    Bleeding diathesis
    Anticoagulant therapy
    Significant liver and renal disease
    Pericarditis
    Proliferative diabetic retinopathy
    Pregnancy
    Recent surgery or biopsy of internal organ within 2 weeks

greater than 1.0 when the thrombolytic agents are administered 11 h after the onset of symptoms. However, in the prospectively designed LATE study, the incidence of myocardial rupture was greater with thrombolysis between 6 and 12 h than at 12 and 24 h after the onset of symptoms.

Thus, the time course of rupture may be accelerated by thrombolysis, but the overall incidence may not be increased.

INDICATIONS AND CONTRAINDICATIONS TO THROMBOLYSIS

The indications for thrombolysis in patients with acute myocardial infarction are listed in Table 14-6 and the contraindications are listed in Table 14-7. A more detailed discussion of the following items is provided in the earlier part of the text: time after myocardial infarction, site of myocardial infarction, non–Q-wave myocardial infarction, cardiogenic shock, elderly patients, and hypertension. The distinction between absolute and relative contraindications to thrombolysis becomes less important when a cardiac catheterization laboratory is available for the performance of immediate coronary angioplasty.

THROMBOLYSIS FOR CONDITIONS OTHER THAN ACUTE MYOCARDIAL INFARCTION

Obstructive Mechanical Prosthetic Valve

The incidence of thrombosis of mechanical mitral prostheses is greater than that in the aortic position, with an annual incidence of less than 0.5%. The operative mortality has been reported to be 11% to 12% but was significantly higher, 17.5%, in patients with New York Heart Association class IV symptoms. Roudaut and colleagues described successful thrombolysis in 73% of 75 thrombotic events, with a 92% success rate in patients with functional class I and II and 63% in patients with functional class III and IV symptoms. Embolic events occurred in 12 of the 64 patients, four of which were major. Thrombosis recurred in 11 patients in approximately 1 year. In a meta-analysis, thrombolysis was reported to be effective in 84% of patients, and streptokinase appeared to be more effective than urokinase.

Others have reported a very low rate of embolic events after thrombolysis in the presence of mobile thrombi. However, most believe that a mobile thrombus is a relative contraindication to thrombolysis. Successful thrombolysis is frequently achieved with one to three courses of thrombolytic agent on a daily basis, with streptokinase 60,000 to 100,000 U/h over 16 to 24 h or tPA with a 10-mg bolus followed by 90-mg infusion over 3 h. Patients should continue taking warfarin during thrombolysis and receive heparin until the international normalized ratio is therapeutic. If the patient requires emergent surgery, it is advantageous to use tPA rather than streptokinase, because the latter is associated with a systemic thrombolytic state and depletion of thrombin.

It has been recommended that patients who have obstructed prostheses with minimal clot seen on transesophageal echocardiography receive thrombolysis, which has an expected success rate of 92%. Surgery is also recommend for patients with large substantial clots or those who have class IV symptoms with obstructive prostheses.

Pulmonary Embolism

In the Urokinase Pulmonary Embolism Trial (UPET) conducted in the early 1970s, in which urokinase followed by heparin was compared with heparin alone in 160 patients, there was a trend toward reduction in mortality and recurrent emboli in patients receiving thrombolysis. There was a significantly more rapid and complete dissolution of thrombi but also more bleeding complications in the patients receiving thrombolysis.

Unfortunately, subsequent trials used even fewer patients than the UPET. The PAIMS-2 (Plasminogen Activator Italian Multicenter Study 2) trial in Italy showed that thrombolysis produces a more efficient dissolution of thrombus and more rapid reduction in pulmonary arterial pressure after 2 h of tPA infusion than does heparin. When tPA was compared with urokinase in the European Cooperative Study Group, there was a more significant and rapid reduction in pulmonary vascular resistance at 2 h, but the results were similar at 6 h.

In the series of trials carried out by Goldhaber and coworkers, after tPA infusion, there was significantly greater clot lysis after 2 h when compared with urokinase administered over 24 h; at 24 h, however, there was no difference in clot lysis between these two groups. Similar efficacy resulted when a condensed dose of urokinase was administered. This group also demonstrated a significantly greater improvement in right ventricular systolic function as measured by echocardiography at 24 h when tPA was administered as compared with heparin. In addition, tPA administered via a pulmonary catheter or a peripheral vein resulted in similar rate of thrombolysis; thus, thrombolytic agents do not have to be administered via a pulmonary catheter.

The use of heparin and a thrombolytic agent was compared in a report from a multicenter registry of 719 consecutive patients with major pulmonary embolism and specifically excluded patients who were hemodynamically unstable. The mortality rates were 4.7% for 169 patients receiving thrombolytic treatment and 11.1% for 555 patients receiving heparin. Although the groups were not similar, multivariate logistic regression analysis demonstrated that thrombolytic treatment is an independent predictor of survival. The patients receiving thrombolysis had a significantly higher rate of major hemorrhage than did patients receiving heparin (21.9% vs. 7.8%, respectively). Only 1.2% of the patients receiving thrombolysis developed intracranial hemorrhage.

It has become accepted practice to treat massive pulmonary embolism associated with hemodynamic instability with thrombolysis. The presence of right ventricular dysfunction seen on echocardiography is also considered an indication for thrombolysis.

Regimens approved by the U.S. Food and Drug Administration for the treatment of pulmonary embolism are as follows: streptokinase 250,000 U loading dose over 30 min followed by 100,000 U/h for 24 h; urokinase 4400 U/kg loading dose over 10 min followed by 4400 U/h for 12 to 24 h; and tPA 100 mg over 2 h. It is recommended that heparin not be given simultaneously with a thrombolytic agent.

Ischemic Stroke

The use of thrombolytic agents in the treatment of ischemic stroke remains controversial. Previous studies using streptokinase were prematurely stopped because of excess intracranial hemorrhage or because treatment was of no benefit when tPA was used. These trials treated patients up to 6 h after the onset of stroke. In a subsequent study, patients were randomized to receive tPA or placebo within 3 h after the onset of stroke. After computed tomography had excluded intracranial hemorrhage, patients who received thrombolysis were 30% to 50% more likely to have minimal or no disability at 3 months.

Thrombolysis with intravenous tPA is now accepted treatment when administered within 3 h of the onset of nonhemorrhagic ischemic stroke, with some consideration for its administration in the time window up to 6 h after onset of symptoms. In addition, several strategies combining antiplatelet and thrombolytic therapies for stroke are now being refined. Unfortunately, only 5% of stroke patients receive intravenous thrombolysis in the United States. Pro-urokinase has been given intraarterially in patients with middle cerebral artery occlusion up to 6 h after onset, with significant success.

Deep Venous Thrombosis

Standard treatment of deep venous thrombosis with heparin reduces the extension and embolization of thrombus but does not increase the rate of clot lysis. Thus, permanent damage to the venous valvular system may ensue, with a resultant postthrombotic syndrome of pain, edema, stasis, and dermatitis.

Significantly faster resolution of deep venous thrombosis has been reported with the use of streptokinase, urokinase, and tPA, with approximately 45% complete resolution when using a thrombolytic agent compared with 4% when using heparin. Complete lysis of thrombus may require several days of treatment and is less successful for older thrombi, particularly those beyond 7 days. However, using selective catheter infusion of a thrombolytic agent may improve the rate of thrombolysis. A more recent study reported that systemically administered thrombolytic agents result in higher recanalization and a lower incidence of postthrombotic syndrome. Because of a 6% rate of major bleeding complications, the investigators advised its use only in patients with limb-threatening situations.

Subclavian and axillary venous thromboses have been treated successfully with direct infusion of thrombolytic agents into the distal vein, and thrombectomy generally has been avoided. Those patients with primary thrombosis of the subclavian or axillary veins may require additional surgery to correct thoracic outlet syndrome.

The doses of thrombolytics used are as follows: streptokinase 2500 U bolus, followed by 100,000 U/h for up to 3 days; streptokinase 3 million U over 4 h; and tPA 0.05 mg/kg per hour for 8 to 24 h. For local or regional infusion, the doses are urokinase 100,000 U/day and tPA 20 mg/day.

Thrombotic Arterial Occlusion

Patients with acute arterial occlusion of the lower limbs and pelvis are potential candidates for intraarterial infusion of thrombolytic agents. With acute ischemia that threatens the viability of the limb, surgery should be considered the primary option and thrombolysis used only if surgery is not feasible or the limb is not threatened. Thrombolytic therapy should be infused by a directed catheter into the occluded artery. This has been performed successfully with streptokinase, urokinase, and tPA and has resulted in fewer lower limb amputations and a significant increase clot lysis and recanalization. Thrombolytic arterial occlusion therapy also has been used as a treatment for mesenteric thrombosis.

A recent consensus statement indicated that catheter-directed thrombolysis is more likely to be superior to surgery if the guidewire passes through the thrombus, the occlusion is less than 14 days old, the occlusion is thrombotic rather than embolic, and significant comorbid cardiopulmonary disease is coexistent.

Doses of catheter-directed thrombolytic agents used are: urokinase 4000 U/h over 4 h, and tPA 0.5 to 0.1 mg/kg per hour for up to 12 h.

Arterial emboli are better removed by balloon catheter techniques or surgery, because thrombolysis in such instances has not been as successful.

Hemodialysis Catheters, Grafts and Fistulas, and Central Venous Catheters

Thrombolytic agents can be used to clear occluded central venous catheters. They also have been shown to be efficacious in treating occluded hemodialysis accesses that include native arteries and vascular grafts.

CONCLUSION

Modification of the molecular structure of thrombolytic agents has improved their potency and fibrin specificity and delayed their plasma clearance. Addition of more potent antiplatelet regimens also has enhanced their thrombolytic efficacy. However, these modifications in treatment of patients with acute myocardial infarction have not always translated into improved survival.

ADDITIONAL READINGS

ACC/AHA Task Force on Practice Guidelines: 1999 Update: ACC/AHA guidelines for management of patients with acute myocardial infarction: Executive summary and recommendations *Circulation* 100:1016, 1999.

Albers GW, Bates VE, Clark WM, et al: Intravenous tissue-type plasminogen activator for treatment of acute stroke. The Standard Treatment with Alteplase to Reverse Stroke (STARS) study. *JAMA* 283:1145, 2000.

Assessment of the Safety and Efficacy of a New Thrombolytic (ASSENT-2) Investigators: Single bolus tenecteplase compared with front-loaded alteplase in acute myocardial infarction: the ASSENT-2 double-blind trial. *Lancet* 354:716, 1999.

Assessment of the Safety and Efficacy of a New Thrombolytic regimen (ASSENT-3) Investigators: Efficacy and safety of tenecteplase in combination with enoxaparin, abciximab or unfractionated heparin: The ASSENT-3 randomized trial in acute myocardial infarction. *Lancet* 358:605, 2001.

Berger AK, Radford MJ, Wang Y, Krumholz HM: Thrombolytic therapy in older patients. *J Am Coll Cardiol* 36:366, 2000.

Cannon CP, Fuster V: Thrombogenesis, antithrombotic, and thrombolytic therapy, in Fuster V, Alexander RW, O'Rourke RA (eds): *Hurst's the Heart,* 10th ed. New York, McGraw-Hill, 2001, p 1373.

Clase CM, Crowther MA, Ingram AJ, Cina CS: Thrombolysis for restoration of patency to haemodialysis central venous catheters: A systematic review. *J Thromb Thrombolysis* 11:127, 2001.

Continuous Infusion Versus Double-Bolus Administration of Alteplase (COBOLT) Investigators: A comparison of continuous infusion of alteplase with double-bolus administration for acute myocardial infarction. *N Engl J Med* 337:1124, 1997.

Forman R, Frishman WH: Thrombolytic agents, in Frishman WH, Sonnenblick EH, Sica DA (eds): *Cardiovascular Pharmacotherapeutics,* 2nd ed. New York, McGraw-Hill, 2003, p 301.

Frishman WH, Cheng-Lai A, Chen J: Antithrombotic therapy, in Frishman WH, Cheng-Lai A, Chen J (eds): *Current Cardiovascular Drugs,* 3rd ed. Philadelphia, Current Medicine, 2000, p 85.

Goldhaber SZ: Pulmonary embolism thrombolysis. Broadening the paradigm for its administration. *Circulation* 96:716, 1997.

Goldman LE, Eisenberg MJ: Identification and management of patients with failed thrombolysis after acute myocardial infarction. *Ann Intern Med* 132:556, 2000.

GUSTO V Investigators: Reperfusion therapy for acute myocardial infarction with fibrinolytic therapy or combination reduced fibrinolytic therapy and platelet glycoprotein IIb/IIIa inhibition: The GUSTO V randomized Trial. *Lancet* 357:1905, 2001.

Hochman JS, Sleeper LA, Webb JG, et al: Early revascularization in acute myocardial infarction complicated by cardiogenic shock. *N Eng J Med* 341:625, 1999.

Keller NM, Feit F: Thrombolytic therapy in acute MI, part 2: Update on adjuvants. *J Crit Illness* 13:646, 1998.

Multicenter Acute Stroke Trial—Europe Study Group: Thrombolytic therapy with streptokinase in acute ischemic stroke. *N Engl J Med* 335:145, 1996.

Ozkan M, Kaymaz C, Kirma ,C et al: Intravenous thrombolytic treatment of mechanical prosthetic valve thrombosis: A study using serial transesophageal echocardiography. *J Am Coll Cardiol* 35:1881, 2000.

Patel SC, Mody A: Cerebral hemorrhage complications of thrombolytic therapy. *Prog Cardiovasc Dis* 42:217, 1999.

Schweizer J, Kirch W, Koch R, et al: Short- and long-term results after thrombolytic treatment of deep venous thrombosis. *J Am Coll Cardiol* 36:1336, 2000.

Strategies for Patency Enhancement in the Emergency Department (SPEED): Group trial of abciximab with and without low-dose reteplase for acute myocardial infarction. *Circulation* 101:2788, 2000.

van de Werf F, Cannon CP, Luyten A, et al, for the ASSENT-1 Investigators: Safety assessment of single-bolus administration of TNK tissue-plasminogen activator in acute myocardial infarction: The ASSENT-1 trial. *Am Heart J* 137:786, 1999.

van Domburg RT, Boersma E, Simoons ML: A review of the long term effects of thrombolytic agents. *Drugs* 60:293, 2000.

Verstrate M: Third-generation thrombolytic drugs. *Am J Med* 109:52, 2000.

15 | Lipid-Lowering Drugs
Neil S. Shachter   William H. Frishman

A direct relationship between elevated serum cholesterol levels, especially elevated low-density-lipoprotein (LDL) cholesterol levels, and the incidence of coronary artery disease (CAD) is now well established. The lowering of LDL cholesterol levels by means of diet and/or drug therapy has been shown to reduce the progression of coronary artery lesions and the incidence of clinical coronary artery events. As predicted from the Framingham Study, a 10% decrease in cholesterol levels is associated with a 20% decrease in the incidence of combined morbidity and mortality related to CAD. Elevations in triglycerides and reductions in high-density-lipoprotein (HDL) cholesterol levels also may contribute to an increased CAD risk.

Advances in the understanding of lipid metabolism and the development of new drugs and dietary strategies for the treatment of lipid and lipoprotein disorders have made effective therapy of hyperlipidemia, and thus CAD risk intervention, an understandable and attainable goal.

In the following introductory section, a framework for understanding the treatment of lipid disorders is presented. Recommendations are provided, based on the Third Expert Panel Report of the National Cholesterol Education Program (NCEP), regarding screening and dietary and drug interventions in human populations with hyperlipidemia at risk for premature CAD.

RATIONALE FOR THE TREATMENT OF HYPERLIPIDEMIA IN PREVENTION OF CORONARY ARTERY DISEASE

The basis for the treatment of hyperlipidemia is the theory that abnormalities in lipid and lipoprotein levels are risk factors for CAD and that the lowering of blood lipids can decrease the risk of disease and its complications. Levels of plasma cholesterol and LDL cholesterol consistently have been shown to be directly correlated with the risk of CAD.

The results of the clinical trials with cholesterol and LDL cholesterol–lowering interventions support the premise that cholesterol-lowering therapies aimed at reducing cholesterol by at least 20% to 25% produce clinically significant reductions in cardiovascular events in patients having preexisting vascular disease across a broad range of cholesterol values within 5 years of starting treatment. The greatest impact of cholesterol lowering still occurs in individuals with the highest baseline cholesterol levels. The absolute magnitude of these benefits would be even greater in those individuals having other risk factors for CAD, such as cigarette smoking and hypertension. These risk relationships are the basis for recommending lower cholesterol cutoff points and goals for those who are at high risk for developing clinical CAD.

Thus, taking into consideration the recommendations of the NCEP and data from recently published trials, two general groups of patients that warrant aggressive therapy for hypercholesterolemia can be identified: those without evidence of CAD who are at high risk for developing CAD (primary prevention, target LDL <130 mg/dL) and those with known CAD or other atherosclerotic processes and high cholesterol (secondary prevention, target LDL <100 mg/dL). Patients with lesser degrees of risk are treated to less aggressive

LDL targets (<160 mg/dL). The current guidelines have identified a fourth group whose risk factors mark them as having a "coronary risk equivalent." Such patients are treated in keeping with the aggressive goals recommended for known CAD (now all atherosclerotic diseases). The most important categories are diabetes and chronic renal disease, but due to the important influence of age on coronary risk, many older individuals with other risk factors also meet current criteria for treatment to the target of below 100 mg/dL LDL. Recommendations for the treatment of elevated triglycerides are less definitive.

Several prospective studies have shown a correlation between levels of plasma triglycerides and CAD. Data from the Framingham Study, however, have indicated that when other risk factors—such as obesity, elevated serum cholesterol (or hypercholesterolemia), hypertension, and diabetes—are accounted for, triglycerides are not a potent independent risk factor for CAD. However, there is a select group of patients with isolated hypertriglyceridemia who are at increased risk of CAD and who can be identified by a strong family history of premature CAD. It should be kept in mind that, to some extent, the epidemiologic studies evaluating the independent risk associated with hypertriglyceridemia have been exercises of little relevance to clinical decision-making. Clearly, once one adjusts for some of the risk factors that are causes of hypertriglyceridemia (obesity, diabetes, lack of exercise, low dietary fiber, family history, etc.), risks associated with the correlates of hypertriglyceridemia (other manifestations of the insulin resistance syndrome, such as hypertension) and the risks associated with the consequences of hypertriglyceridemia (low HDL, small dense LDL), then little measurable risk will remain. However, hypertriglyceridemia is a valuable marker of the insulin resistance syndrome, and therapy addressed at the basis of that syndrome will benefit all the causes and correlates of hypertriglyceridemia. In addition, the level of plasma triglycerides is a primary determinant of the level of HDL, the most potent predictor of the risk of atherosclerotic disease; the two measurements exhibit a strong inverse correlation. In general, the direction of causation is clearly that of the level of triglycerides determining the level of HDL, and most therapies that raise the level of HDL are, in fact, directed at modifying triglyceride metabolism. Therefore, whether triglycerides or HDLs are the more important element in the physiologic mediation of atherosclerotic risk cannot be determined from epidemiologic studies or intervention trials. HDL is the more potent statistical predictor, but this is likely due to "ascertainment bias." Triglyceride levels are quite variable, whereas HDL levels are fairly stable, leading to greater predictive value for the HDL measurement. In part, this is likely due only to its being a more accurately ascertained surrogate for the level of plasma triglycerides. There is now evidence that, by lowering triglyceride levels or raising HDL levels (or both), the risk of CAD will be diminished. The Veterans Affairs Low HDL Intervention Trial (VA-HIT), showed a significant reduction in coronary events in otherwise high-risk patients with normal LDL levels associated with the use of an agent (gemfibrozil) that markedly lowered triglycerides and modestly raised HDL but had no effect on the level of LDL. However, similar benefit was not observed in another trial that used a related drug (Bezafibrate Infarction Prevention Study).

Although CAD is the most important clinical manifestation of atherosclerosis, it bears emphasis that lipid-lowering therapy has been shown to decrease the incidence of all atherosclerotic diseases. Comprehensive meta-analyses of the *3-hydroxy-3-methylglutaryl coenzyme A* (HMG-CoA) reductase inhibitor trials have specifically confirmed the value of these agents in preventing stroke in hyperlipidemic subjects.

RISK ASSESSMENT

For many years clinicians depended on total cholesterol and triglyceride measurements for patient management. More sophisticated lipoprotein measurements were available only in research facilities. Methodologic advances have made lipoprotein subclass and apolipoprotein (apo) determinations available from many clinical laboratories. As a result, LDL cholesterol has been shown to be a more accurate predictor of CAD risk than has total cholesterol. Likewise, low levels of HDL cholesterol have been demonstrated to be more powerful predictors of CAD than elevated total cholesterol. Levels of plasma lipoprotein(a), apo A-I and apo B, and the distribution of HDL subfractions (HDL2 and HDL3) are also accurate univariate predictors of CAD risk. However, in most cases, these measurements contribute little to the assessment of coronary risk provided by LDL, HDL, and triglyceride. Mean serum cholesterol and calculated LDL cholesterol values for various population groups have been reported and document a progressive decline in plasma cholesterol in the United States; this is consistent with the decreased mortality from atherosclerotic disease that has been observed simultaneously. A number of nonlipid measurements (homocysteine and a variety of inflammatory markers, including C-reactive protein) can contribute to the assessment of coronary risk. Only C-reactive protein, as measured by the high-sensitivity assay, appears to provide significant prediction independent of the traditional lipid risk factors.

WHO SHOULD BE SCREENED FOR HYPERLIPIDEMIA?

The Third Report of the NCEP Expert Panel on Detection, Evaluation and Treatment of High Blood Cholesterol in Adults continues to suggest that total cholesterol be measured in all adults 20 years and older at least once every 5 years. A controversy was raised when the American College of Physicians recommended only general cholesterol screening for middle-age men—an approach that was vigorously challenged and did not receive acceptance. An NCEP panel recommended that cholesterol screening should not be done routinely in children unless there was a history of familial hyperlipidemia or a family history of premature CAD. Cholesterol values in the general pediatric population may not always predict the future development of hypercholesterolemia in adults.

WHO SHOULD BE TREATED FOR HYPERCHOLESTEROLEMIA?

Ideally, a fasting lipid profile (total cholesterol, HDL cholesterol, total triglycerides, and calculated LDL) should be obtained in all cases. If this is not practical, then screening cholesterol and HDL values should be obtained (Table 15-1). A total cholesterol above 200 mg/dL or an HDL cholesterol below 40 mg/dL mandates obtaining a fasting lipid profile. The presence of high cholesterol should always be confirmed with a second lipid profile to make a more precise estimate of CAD risk. The standard deviations of repeated measurements in an individual over time have been reported as 0.39 mm/L (15 mg/dL) for total cholesterol and 0.39 mm/L (15 mg/dL) for LDL

TABLE 15-1 Adult Treatment Panel III Classification of LDL, Total, and HDL Cholesterol (mg/dL)

LDL cholesterol	
<100	Optimal
100–129	Near or above optimal
103–159	Borderline high
160–189	High
≥190	Very high
Total cholesterol	
<200	Desirable
200–239	Borderline high
≥240	High
HDL cholesterol	
<40	Low
≥60	High

Key: HDL, high-density lipoprotein; LDL, low-density lipoprotein.
Source: Reproduced with permission from Executive Committee of the Third Report of the National Cholesterol Education Program (NCEP) Expert Panel on Detection, Evaluation, and Treatment of High Blood Cholesterol in Adults (Adult Treatment Panel III). *JAMA* 285:2486, 2001.

cholesterol. Patients should be maintained on the same diet during these initial determinations before therapy is instituted. Secondary causes of hypercholesterolemia (hypothyroidism, nephrotic syndrome, or diabetes mellitus) also should be considered.

The NCEP recommends an approach in adults based on LDL cholesterol, which is shown in Tables 15-2 and 15-3. In most cases, management should begin with dietary intervention. When the response to diet is inadequate or when the target LDL is unlikely to be achieved by diet alone, the addition of pharmacologic therapy is recommended. Specific drug therapies are discussed in subsequent sections of this chapter.

TABLE 15-2 LDL Goals, Cutoff Points for Therapeutic Lifestyle Changes, and Drug Therapy in Different Risk Categories

Therapy risk category	LDL goal (mg/dL)	Initiate lifestyle changes	Initiate drug regimen
CHD or CHD risk equivalents (10-y risk >20%)	<100	≥100	≥130 (100–129: drug optional)
2+ Risk factors (10-y risk ≤20%)	<130	≥130	10-y risk 10–20% ≥130 10-y risk <10% ≥160
0–1 Risk factor	<160	≥160	≥190 (160–189: LDL-lowering drug optional)

Key: CHD, coronary heart disease; LDL, low-density lipoprotein.
Source: Reproduced with permission from Executive Committee of the Third Report of the National Cholesterol Education Program (NCEP) Expert Panel on Detection, Evaluation, and Treatment of High Blood Cholesterol in Adults (Adult Treatment Panel III). *JAMA* 285:2486, 2001.

TABLE 15-3 Major Risk Factors (Exclusive of LDL Cholesterol)
That Modify LDL Goals

Cigarette smoking
Hypertension (BP ≥140/90 mm Hg or on antihypertensive medication)
Low HDL cholesterol (<40 mg/dL)*
Family history of premature CAD
     CHD in male first-degree relative <55 y
     CHD in female first-degree relative <65 y
Age (men ≥45 y; women ≥55 y)
Diabetes (fasting glucose ≥127 mg/dL) in and of itself mandates an LDL
   goal of <100 mg/dL

*HDL cholesterol ≥60 mg/dL counts as a "negative" risk factor; its presence removes one risk factor from the total count.
Key: BP, blood pressure; CHD, coronary heart disease; HDL, high-density lipoprotein; LDL, low-density lipoprotein.
Source: Adapted with permission from Executive Committee of the Third Report of the National Cholesterol Education Program (NCEP) Expert Panel on Detection, Evaluation, and Treatment of High Blood Cholesterol in Adults (Adult Treatment Panel III). *JAMA* 285:2486, 2001.

WHO SHOULD BE TREATED FOR HYPERTRIGLYCERIDEMIA?

Interest in the link between serum triglyceride levels and CHD has grown in recent years. Triglyceride levels correlate positively with levels of LDL cholesterol and inversely with HDL. Clinical trials with the triglyceride-lowering drugs, nicotinic acid, and gemfibrozil have shown a benefit on the frequency of coronary artery events as compared with placebo therapy. However, therapy in these trials was not targeted to patients with primary hypertriglyceridemia. The currently recommended approach to the problem of hypertriglyceridemia is presented in the report of the NCEP.

Normal triglycerides are defined as levels below 150 mg/dL, borderline high triglycerides as 150 to 199 mg/dL, high triglycerides as 200 to 499 mg/dL, and very high triglycerides as levels higher than 500 mg/dL. Most hypertriglyceridemias up to 5.65 mm/L (500 mg/dL) are due primarily to insulin resistance related to the "metabolic syndrome." Criteria for the diagnosis of this syndrome are shown in Table 15-4. Common contributors to this syndrome include obesity (body mass index >30 kg/m²), overweight (body mass index > 25 kg/m²), physical inactivity, excess alcohol consumption, and high consumption of low-fiber carbohydrate sources (>60% of total energy). Other contributors to hypertriglyceridemia may include diabetes mellitus, hypothyroidism, marked obesity, chronic renal disease (failure or nephrotic syndrome), and certain drugs (glucocorticoids, estrogens, retinoids, and higher doses of β-adrenergic blocking agents or thiazide diuretics). Weight loss, exercise, dietary change (decreased saturated fat, increased omega-3 unsaturated oils, and increased dietary fiber), reduction or elimination of triglyceride-raising drugs, and/or treatment of the primary disease process (e.g., improved glycemic control of diabetes) may be sufficient to reduce triglycerides.

Patients with familial combined hyperlipoproteinemia often have associated hypertriglyceridemia. Patients with this condition are at risk for premature CAD. These patients should have dietary treatment first and then, if necessary, drugs. Patients with borderline hypertriglyceridemia with clinical

TABLE 15-4 Clinical Identification of the Metabolic Syndrome

Risk factor	Defining level
Abdominal obesity* (waist circumference†)	
Men	>102 cm (>40 in.)
Women	>88 cm (>35 in.)
Triglycerides	>150 mg/dL
HDL cholesterol	
Men	<40 mg/dL
Women	<50 mg/dL
Blood pressure	>130/>85 mm Hg
Fasting glucose	>110 mg/dL

*Overweight and obesity are associated with insulin resistance and the metabolic syndrome. However, the presence of abdominal obesity is more strongly correlated with the metabolic risk factors than is an elevated body mass index. Therefore, the simple measure of waist circumference is recommended to identify the body weight component of the metabolic syndrome.
†Some male patients can develop multiple metabolic risk factors when the waist circumference is only marginally increased, e.g., 94 to 102 cm (37 to 40 in.). Such patients may have a strong genetic contribution to insulin resistance; for example, men with categorical increases in waist circumference should benefit from changes in life habits.
Key: HDL, high-density lipoprotein.
Source: Reproduced with permission from Executive Committee of the Third Report of the National Cholesterol Education Program (NCEP) Expert Panel on Detection, Evaluation, and Treatment of High Blood Cholesterol in Adults (Adult Treatment Panel III). *JAMA* 285:2486, 2001.

manifestations of CAD can be treated as if they had combined hyperlipoproteinemia, with lifestyle, LDL-lowering, and triglyceride-lowering therapies.

APPROACH TO LOW SERUM HDL CHOLESTEROL

A low serum HDL cholesterol level is a strong lipoprotein predictor of CAD. In one prospective study, after adjustment for other risk factors in predicting the risk of myocardial infarction, a change in one unit in the ratio of total to HDL cholesterol was associated with a 53% change in risk. However, it is still unclear how low HDL levels are linked to CAD. A recent trial of combined

TABLE 15-5   Major Causes of Reduced Serum High-Density Lipoprotein Cholesterol

Cigarette smoking
Obesity
Lack of exercise
Androgenic and related steroids
Androgens
Progestational agents
Anabolic steroids
β-Adrenergic blocking agents
Hypertriglyceridemia
Genetic factors
Primary hypoalphalipoproteinemia

LDL-lowering and HDL-raising therapy showed benefit well beyond that anticipated from LDL lowering alone. HDL metabolism is complex, and the utility of interventions to raise HDL will likely depend on the specific HDL-raising pathway that is targeted. The major causes of reduced serum HDL cholesterol are listed in Table 15-5. Clearly, attempts should be made to raise low HDL cholesterol by hygienic means. When a low HDL is associated with an increase in plasma triglycerides, as is typically the case, the latter deserves consideration for therapeutic modification. However, when the HDL is reduced without hypertriglyceridemia or other associated risk factors, the utility of raising low HDL levels by drugs for primary prevention has not been adequately addressed in clinical trials.

SPECIAL PROBLEMS

Myocardial Infarction

The post–myocardial infarction setting is the paradigm of known atherosclerotic disease. Virtually all such patients require aggressive lipid lowering with the maintenance of an LDL cholesterol below 100 mg/dL. All patients with known CAD should have a fasting lipoprotein analysis. If this is not accomplished promptly (within a few hours of presentation), the measured cholesterol levels will be artifactually depressed by the acute-phase response. Under these circumstances, the initial dosage of lipid-lowering therapy may have to be empiric, with the dosage adjusted subsequently based on the levels at least 3 months after the acute event, at which point the effects of the acute-phase response will have substantially resolved. The value of the immediate institution of high-dose LDL-lowering therapy in the setting of acute myocardial infarction is an area of controversy. An observational study adjusted for possible confounders found a significantly lower incidence of short-term (30 days and 6 months) mortality in individuals discharged on lipid-lowering therapy. A randomized trial of high-dose (80 mg) atorvastatin after presentation with acute non–Q-wave myocardial infarction or unstable angina found a significant decrease in re-hospitalizations for ischemia within 16 weeks and a decrease in complicating stroke without any difference in death, recurrent myocardial infarction, or heart failure.

Aggressive lipid-lowering therapy results in a marked reduction of cardiovascular thrombotic events, with only minimal change in the size of the coronary artery plaque; but exactly how this happens is still uncertain. Once a plaque develops, it may remain stable for long periods. What triggers acute ischemic syndromes, such as myocardial infarction or unstable angina, is the development of lesion instability. An unstable lesion has an increased tendency to rupture or crack, leading to exposure of the highly thrombogenic interior, with superimposed thrombosis and, thereafter, acute ischemic syndromes. Several studies have suggested that the lipid content of a plaque correlates with the risk of a subsequent rupture. Most commonly, the crack occurs at the junction of the plaque and the normal intima. Progressive accumulation of lipids appears to promote macrophage accumulation, which destabilizes the plaque, leading to thinning and destruction of the fibrous cap and resulting in rupture at points of high pressure. Thus, limiting the lipid pool of the atherosclerotic plaque may prevent plaque thinning and facilitate the conversion of an unstable, vulnerable plaque to a stable one. Changes in plaque composition that predict vulnerability are not detectable by coronary angiography but have been shown to be detectable by specialized cardiac magnetic resonance imaging techniques.

It is well established that atherosclerosis and hypercholesterolemia are associated with endothelial cell dysfunction, which may play a part in the pathogenesis of acute ischemic syndromes via an increased tendency to vasospasm and decreased secretion of prostaglandins, which suppress platelet aggregation. An important mediator of normal endothelial function is nitric oxide, which is released continuously, thereby maintaining vascular tone and preventing platelet and leukocyte adhesion. Hypercholesterolemia and coronary atherosclerosis have been shown to impair nitric oxide release, whereas aggressive lipid lowering can improve nitric oxide–mediated responses. This likely represents an additional mechanism by which cholesterol reduction reduces the risk of myocardial infarction.

Coronary Artery Bypass Grafts

In an important observational study, investigators at the Montreal Heart Institute performed angiography 1 and 10 years after surgery to determine the patency of vein grafts in 82 patients who had undergone saphenous vein bypass surgery. The 10-year examination confirmed that atherosclerotic changes are common in saphenous vein bypass grafts. Of 132 grafts that were patent at the 1-year examination, only 50 (37.5%) showed no change at the 10-year examination, whereas evidence of atherosclerosis was found in 43 (33%) and complete occlusion was found in 30 (29.5%). Progressive atherosclerosis was identified as the single most important cause of occlusion in these grafts. When the investigators analyzed the relation between cardiovascular risk factors and the development of atherosclerosis, they found no significant difference for smoking, hypertension, or diabetes between the group that developed disease and the group that did not. However, in a multivariate analysis, the investigators found low HDL cholesterol, high LDL cholesterol, and high apo B to be the most significant predictors of atherosclerotic disease in grafts. Almost 80% of those who did not develop disease had normal lipid levels and normal LDL and apo B levels, in contrast to 8% of patients who developed disease.

There is now evidence that aggressive dietary and LDL-lowering drug therapy with niacin/colestipol and with the hydroxymethylglutaryl-coenzyme A reductase inhibitor lovastatin can slow down, arrest, and even reverse atherosclerotic disease in patients with saphenous vein coronary bypass grafts. Detailed lipoprotein analysis of the patients in the study using lovastatin indicated that the beneficial effects were achieved, as expected, by LDL lowering and not via effects on triglyceride-rich lipoproteins and HDL. However, a similar trial that used a triglyceride-lowering agent (gemfibrozil) in patients who had coronary artery bypass grafts and low HDL also showed a beneficial effect on atherosclerosis progression. Of note, internal thoracic artery and other arterial grafts have a significantly lower rate of atherosclerosis than have saphenous vein grafts and are now performed whenever it is feasible.

Coronary Angioplasty

Restenosis after successful isolated coronary angioplasty has been observed in 25% to 40% of patients undergoing this procedure. This incidence has been reduced significantly by the routine use of coronary stenting, but the problem of restenosis has not been eliminated. Attempts have been made to decrease the incidence of restenosis by using a wide array of pharmacologic interventions. Restenosis after angioplasty appears to result from the proliferation of intimal smooth muscle cells. Results of experiments in cholesterol-fed animals after balloon injury of the arterial wall have suggested that restenosis occurs primarily from the migration and proliferation of smooth muscle cells in response to platelet-derived growth factor released from platelets adherent to the site of de-endothelialization. Antiplatelet drugs and calcium channel blocking drugs have had little or no benefit in reducing the rate of postangioplasty restenosis. A recent study with fluvastatin has shown benefit in reducing the risk of recurrent cardiac events, and some positive results have been achieved with probucol and a related antioxidant compound, drugs not currently approved in the United States. Local irradiation and specific drug-containing stents have been the most promising of the currently available modalities.

Heart Transplantation

Elevated plasma lipids and an increased risk of having accelerated CAD are commonly found in recipients of cardiac transplants. Although many of the drugs used to treat and/or prevent rejection (high-dose steroids, cyclosporine) can raise LDL cholesterol, hypercholesterolemia has not been found to be a primary risk factor for developing graft atherosclerosis. Pathologically, the CAD is often different from that seen in nontransplanted patients and is characterized as a diffuse, necrotizing vasculitis or, more commonly, intimal hyperplasia of the entire coronary arterial system. It has been proposed that the development of CAD in transplant recipients may be a manifestation of chronic tissue rejection.

Monitoring of lipids after cardiac transplantation is still worthwhile, and intake of dietary fats and cholesterol should be modified. Use of lipid-lowering drug therapy does carry with it an increased risk of potential complications. However, prospective studies with pravastatin and simvastatin have shown a prominent benefit from lipid-lowering drug therapy in this population, without excessive risk. Early administration of diltiazem is also indicated as part of a regimen to prevent graft vasculopathy.

Cerebrovascular Disease

The results of recent trials have indicated that lipid-lowering treatment can reduce the risk of stroke in patients with existing heart disease. The mechanism for risk reduction includes plaque stabilization and the retardation of plaque progression.

Calcific Aortic Stenosis

Hypercholesterolemia is associated with calcific aortic stenosis and may be implicated in its pathogenesis and progression. A randomized controlled trial of cholesterol-lowering therapy in patients with calcific aortic stenosis is indicated at this time.

Chronic Renal Disease and Nephrotic Syndrome

The nephrotic syndrome is associated with increased levels of cholesterol and triglycerides. The elevated serum concentrations of LDL cholesterol, other lipids, and apo B in patients with uncomplicated nephrotic syndrome are due to reversible increases in lipoprotein production. These lipid disorders are difficult to treat, and they predispose patients to early-onset CAD. It has been suggested that the treatment guidelines adopted by the NCEP be extended to patients with unremitting nephrotic syndrome and chronic renal disease, which is to reduce LDL cholesterol below 100 mg/dL. Statins have been shown to reduce plasma concentrations of very low-density lipoprotein (VLDL) and LDL cholesterol in patients with nephrotic syndrome with kinetic evidence of enhanced LDL receptor activity. In addition, statins may reduce renal protein excretion in hypertensive patients who are already receiving angiotensin-converting enzyme inhibitors or angiotensin receptor blockers.

Diabetes Mellitus

The NCEP recommends that all diabetic patients (fasting glucose at or above 127 mg/dL) have their LDL cholesterol reduced below 100 mg/dL. The dyslipidemia associated with diabetes is typically a combined hyperlipidemia with elevations in LDL cholesterol, an increase in triglycerides, and a decrease in HDL cholesterol. Combination drug therapy is usually necessary to normalize lipid levels and to control diabetes. The combined hyperlipidemia associated with diabetes appears to be more prevalent in women than in men, which may explain a greater susceptibility for atherosclerosis in women.

Metabolic Syndrome

The metabolic syndrome, or insulin resistance syndrome, is associated with an increased risk for cardiovascular disease and related mortality. Dyslipidemia in the syndrome is characterized by hypertriglyceridemia, low HDL cholesterol, and small, dense LDL particles in the context of normal to slightly elevated LDL cholesterol. Outcomes in treatment studies including diabetic patients have suggested that a variety of therapies may be of benefit in reducing cardiovascular risk in patients with metabolic syndrome, including physiologic therapies and pharmacologic treatments such as aspirin, antihypertensive therapy, anti-ischemic therapy, and lipid-modifying therapies. The NCEP guidelines identify the metabolic syndrome as a secondary target of lipid-lowering therapy after LDL cholesterol reduction and recommend the use of weight reduction and increased physical activity to address the underlying risk factors, in addition to therapies to address specific lipid and nonlipid risk factors.

Conclusion

Hyperlipidemia, specifically elevations in plasma cholesterol and LDL cholesterol, is associated with an increased risk of morbidity and mortality from CAD. Elevations in plasma triglycerides and lower HDL cholesterol values may contribute to increased risk. It is now clear that dietary and/or drug therapy of hypercholesterolemia can modify this risk favorably. Guidelines for selecting subjects for drug treatment have been established. In the subsequent sections, pharmacologic interventions designed to treat hyperlipidemia and the associated cardiovascular disease risk are presented and discussed. These guidelines will continue to be refined as more information becomes available from clinical trials in a wide range of patient populations.

BILE ACID SEQUESTRANTS

The bile acid–binding resins cholestyramine and colestipol have long been among the drugs of first choice for hypercholesterolemia in patients without concurrent hypertriglyceridemia. Despite the mounting data on the safety, efficacy, and tolerability of HMG-CoA reductase inhibitors, this remains true for children, adolescents, and women who may become pregnant. Colesevelam, a newer bile acid sequestrant (BAS) with increased bile acid–binding specificity—and consequently a decrease in bulk, in gastrointestinal (GI) side effects, and the potential for vitamin and drug malabsorption—has reawakened interest in this class.

Cholestyramine originally was used for treatment of pruritus caused by elevated concentrations of bile acids secondary to cholestasis. However, attention has focused on the ability of the BASs to lower the concentration of LDL cholesterol in plasma. The resins have been tested extensively in large-scale, long-term follow-up clinical trials to explore their efficacy for such an application. These drugs are not absorbed in the GI tract and therefore have a limited range of systemic side effects. For this reason they are particularly useful for the treatment of pregnant women with hypercholesterolemia and are the drugs generally recommended in children with heterozygous familial hypercholesterolemia. The disadvantage of the early sequestrants cholestyramine and colestipol lie in their mode of administration and the frequency of GI side effects.

Chemistry

Cholestyramine (Questran powder) is the chloride salt of a basic anion-exchange resin. The ion-exchange sites are provided by the presence of trimethyl-benzyl-ammonium groups in a large copolymer of styrene and divinyl benzene. The resin is hydrophilic yet insoluble in water. It is given orally after being suspended in water or juice. It is not absorbed in the GI tract and not altered by digestive enzymes, thus permitting it to remain unchanged while traversing the intestines.

Colestipol (Colestid), supplied as the powder colestipol hydrochloride, is a basic anion-exchange copolymer made up of diethylenetriamine and 1-chloro-2,3-epoxypropane. It has approximately one of its five amine nitrogens protonated (chloride form). Like cholestyramine, colestipol is not altered by digestive enzymes, nor is it absorbed in the digestive tract. It is supplied in powder form and is taken orally after being suspended in liquid.

Colesevelam is poly(allylamine hydrochloride) cross-linked with epichlorohydrin and alkylated with 1-bromodecane and (6-bromohexyl)-trimethyl-ammonium bromide; it has been engineered to bind bile acids specifically. It is a non-absorbed hydrophilic polymer that is unmodified by digestive enzymes. It is supplied in tablet form and taken orally.

Pharmacology

Bile acids are synthesized in the liver from cholesterol, their sole precursor. They are then secreted into the GI tract, where they interact with fat-soluble molecules, thereby aiding in the digestion and subsequent absorption of these substances. Bile acids are absorbed with the fat-soluble molecules and are subsequently recycled by the liver via the portal circulation for re-secretion into the GI tract. The bile acids remain in the enterohepatic circulation and never enter the systemic circulation.

Cholestyramine, colestipol, and colesevelam bind bile acids in the intestine. The complex thus formed is then excreted in the feces. By binding the bile acids, the resins deny the bile acids entry into the bloodstream and thereby remove a large portion of the acids from the enterohepatic circulation. The decrease in hepatic concentrations of bile acids allows a disinhibition of cholesterol 7a-hydroxylase, the rate-limiting enzyme in bile acid synthesis. Also seen is an increase in activity of phosphatidic acid phosphatase, an enzyme responsible for the conversion of α-glycerol phosphate to triglyceride. The increased activity of this enzyme causes a shift away from phospholipid production and ultimately an increase in the triglyceride content and size of VLDL particles. There is also evidence to suggest that the BASs cause an increase in the activity of HMG-CoA reductase, the rate-limiting enzyme in the hepatic cholesterol synthesis pathway. Although cholesterol synthesis is increased when BASs are used, there is no rise in plasma cholesterol, presumably because of the immediate shunting of the newly formed cholesterol into the bile acid–synthesis pathway. The apparent shortage of cholesterol causes the hepatocyte cell surface receptors for LDL particles to be altered quantitatively, by increasing in number, or qualitatively, by increasing their affinity for the LDL particle. By sequestering the cholesterol-rich LDL particles, the liver decreases the plasma concentration of cholesterol.

Pharmacokinetics

Cholestyramine, colestipol, and colesevelam bind bile acids in the intestines, forming a chemical complex that is excreted in the feces. There is no chemical modification of the resins while in the GI tract; however, the chloride ions of the resins may be replaced by other anions with higher affinity for the resin. Colestipol and colesevelam are hydrophilic but virtually insoluble in water (99.75%). The high-molecular-weight polymers of cholestyramine, colestipol, and colesevelam are not absorbed in the GI tract. Less than 0.05% of ^{14}C-labeled colestipol or ^{14}C-labeled colesevelam is excreted in the urine.

Because the resins are not absorbed into the systemic circulation, any interactions that occur between the resins and other molecules occur in the intestines, usually with substances ingested at or near the time of resin ingestion. In the case of cholestyramine and colestipol, interaction between resins and fat-soluble substances, such as the fat-soluble vitamins, causes a decrease in absorption of these substances. Malabsorption of vitamin K, for instance, has been associated with hypoprothrombinemia. It is therefore recommended that vitamins K and D be supplemented in patients on long-term resin therapy. Likewise, medications taken with or near the time of resin ingestion may be bound by the resin and not be absorbed. Drugs at risk include phenylbutazone, warfarin, chlorothiazide (acidic), propranolol (basic), penicillin G, tetracycline, phenobarbital, thyroid and thyroxine preparations, and digitalis preparations. In the case of colesevelam, such interactions essentially do not occur, although modest and variable effects on verapamil absorption have been described.

The dose–response curves for the bile acid resins are nonlinear, with increases in the antihypercholesterolemic effect being minimal for doses higher than 30 g/day. Further, there tend to be compliance problems when large doses of resin are used, making doses higher than 15 g twice daily nonefficacious. In the case of colesevelam, which has a lower dosing range, nonlinearity was evident in the 3.75-g dose, which had about twice (19%) the cholesterol-lowering efficacy of the 3-g dose (9%).

Because the BASs are polymeric cations bound to chloride anions, continued ingestion of the resins imposes a chloride load on the body. This chloride load may cause a decrease in the urine pH and an increase in the urinary excretion of chloride, which can reach 60% of the ingested resin load. Further, there may be an increase in the excretion of calcium ions, which is dependent on the extent of chloride ion excretion. Because of this increase in calcium ion excretion, care should be taken, especially in treating a person at risk for osteoporosis, to limit the extent of calcium excretion by controlling the dietary chloride load.

Clinical Experience

Numerous studies have shown the BASs cholestyramine and colestipol to be efficacious in lowering LDL and total cholesterol levels in the plasma. Studies have further correlated the decreased levels of LDL cholesterol with the slowing of progression of coronary atherosclerosis and a lowered incidence of coronary events. Similarly, the use of BASs retards the progression of femoral atherosclerosis. Further, studies of the lipoprotein content in resin-treated individuals have detected a qualitative effect that may contribute to the anti-atherosclerotic effects of the drug. Sequestrants are limited to use in those patients having hypercholesterolemia that is not associated with severe hypertriglyceridemia. Therefore, unless bile acid resins are combined with other antihyperlipidemic drugs, their use is typically limited to treatment of individuals with isolated hypercholesterolemia.

Clinical Use of Resins

Bile acid resins are indicated as adjunct therapy to diet for reduction of serum cholesterol in patients with primary hypercholesterolemia. Dietary therapy should precede resin usage and should address the patient's specific type of hyperlipoproteinemia and his or her body weight, because obesity has been shown to be a contributing factor in hyperlipoproteinemia. Because resin use can cause a 5% to 20% increase in VLDL levels, it should be restricted to hypercholesterolemic patients with only slightly increased triglyceride levels. The increase in VLDL seen with resin use usually starts during the first few weeks of therapy and disappears 4 weeks after the initial rise. It is thought that excessive increases in the VLDL particles may dampen the LDL-lowering effect of the drug by competitively binding the upwardly regulated LDL receptors on the hepatocyte. The resins therefore should not be used in patients whose triglyceride levels exceed 3.5 mmol/L unless accompanied by a second drug that has antihypertriglyceride effects; some suggest not using resins if the triglyceride level exceeds 2.5 mmol/L. A general rule of thumb is that, if the triglyceride level exceeds 7 mmol/L, the LDL concentration is seldom raised; therefore, treatment with a bile acid resin would not be effective.

Cholestyramine and colestipol are available as powders that must be mixed with water or fruit juice before ingestion; they are taken in two to three divided doses with or just after meals. BASs can decrease absorption of some antihypertensive agents, including thiazide diuretics and propranolol. As a general recommendation, all other drugs should be administered 1 h before or 4 h after the BAS. The cholesterol-lowering effect of 4 g of cholestyramine appears to be equivalent to that of 5 g of colestipol. The response to therapy is variable in each individual, but a 15% to 30% reduction in LDL cholesterol may be seen with colestipol given at 20 to 30 g/day or cholestyramine at 16 to 24 g/day. The fall in LDL concentration becomes detectable 4 to 7 days after the start of treatment and approaches 90% of maximal effect in 2 weeks. Initial dosing should be 4 or 5 g of cholestyramine or colestipol, respectively, two times daily. The drugs are also useful if they are administered once daily. In patients who do not respond adequately to initial therapy, the dosing can be increased to the maximum mentioned above.

Dosing above the maximum dose does not increase the antihypercholesterolemic effect of the drug considerably but does increase side effects and therefore decreases compliance. Because both resins are virtually identical in action, the choice of one over the other is based on patient preference, specifically taste and the ability to tolerate ingestion of bulky material.

To avoid some of the difficulties with use of the powders, colestipol is available in 1-g tablets that are swallowed whole. In addition, colestipol is available in a flavored powdered form. Cholestyramine is also available in a low-calorie, lower-volume formulation that contains 1.4 calories per packet.

If resin treatment is discontinued, cholesterol levels return to pretreatment levels within 1 month. In patients with heterozygous hypercholesterolemia who have not achieved desirable cholesterol levels on resin plus diet, the combination therapy of colestipol hydrochloride and nicotinic acid has been shown to provide further lowering of serum cholesterol, triglycerides, and LDL and cause an increase in serum HDL concentration. Other drug combinations have been studied; of particular promise is the combination therapy of a BAS and HMG-CoA reductase inhibitor.

Oral colesevelam can be administered alone or in combination with an HMG-CoA reductase inhibitor as an adjunctive therapy to diet and exercise for the reduction of elevated LDL cholesterol. The recommended dose is three 625-mg tablets taken twice daily with meals or six tablets once a day with a liquid meal. The dose can be increased to seven tablets a day.

Adverse Effects of Resins

Because cholestyramine and colestipol are not absorbed in the body, the range of adverse effects is limited. A majority of patients' complaints stems from the resins' effect on the GI tract and from subjective complaints concerning the taste, texture, and bulkiness of the resins. The most common side effect is constipation, which is reported in approximately 10% of patients on colestipol and 28% of patients on cholestyramine but is less common with colesevelam. This side effect is seen most commonly in patients taking large doses of the resin and most often in patients older than 65 years. Although most cases of constipation are mild and self-limiting, progression to fecal impaction can occur. A range of 1 in 30 to 1 in 100 patients on colestipol and approximately 12% on cholestyramine experience abdominal distention and/or belching, flatulence, nausea, vomiting, and diarrhea. Peptic ulcer disease, GI irritation and bleeding, cholecystitis, and cholelithiasis have been reported in 1 of 100 patients taking colestipol but have not been shown to be purely drug related.

Fewer than 1 of 1000 patients on colestipol experience hypersensitivity reactions such as urticaria or dermatitis. Asthma and wheezing were not seen with colestipol treatment but were reported with cholestyramine treatment in a small number of patients. In a small percentage of patients, muscle pain, dizziness, vertigo, anxiety, and drowsiness have been reported with both drugs. With cholestyramine treatment, hematuria, dysuria, and uveitis have also been reported. Resin therapy has been associated with transient and modest elevations of serum glutamic oxaloacetic transaminase and alkaline phosphatase. Some patients have shown an increase in iron-binding capacity and serum phosphorus with an increase in chloride ions and a decrease in sodium ions, potassium ions, uric acid, and carotene.

Case reports have described hyperchloremic acidosis in a child taking cholestyramine suffering from ischemic hepatitis and renal insufficiency, in a child with liver agenesis and renal failure, and in a patient with diarrhea due to ileal resection. For these reasons, those patients at risk for hyperchloremia should have serum chloride levels checked during the course of resin treatment.

In the Lipid Research Clinics—Coronary Primary Prevention Trial study, the incidence of malignancy in the cholestyramine-treated group was equal to that in the control group; however, the incidence of GI malignancy in the treated group was higher than that in the untreated group (21 vs. 11, respectively), with more fatal cases in the treated group (eight deaths in the treated group vs. one in the control group). In animal studies, cholestyramine was shown to increase the mammary tumorigenesis capabilities of 7,12-dimethylbenzanthracene in Wistar rats. In the rats treated with cholestyramine plus 7,12-dimethylbenzanthracene, there was a fivefold increase in the incidence of mammary cancer over control. Owing to the resin's ability to disrupt the normal absorption of fat-soluble vitamins in the gut, there have been a number of reports concerning the occurrence of hypoprothrombinemic hemorrhage secondary to vitamin K malabsorption. In both of the cases cited above, the patients responded to adjunctive vitamin K therapy. An early study showed that colestipol can bind thyroxine (T_4) in the gut and in vitro. This binding theoretically can upset the normal reabsorption of T_4 from the gut and thereby disrupt normal T_4 recycling, thus causing hypothyroidism. However, a subsequent study showed that, for euthyroid patients, thyroid function tests can remain normal throughout resin treatment. It is advisable for patients on thyroid replacement therapy to avoid taking the replacement drug at the same time as the resin to avoid any malabsorption problems.

Colesevelam appears to have a better side effect profile than cholestyramine and colestipol and fewer associated drug interactions. Compared with placebo, a significantly greater incidence of dyspepsia, constipation, and myalgia has been reported in clinical trials with cholestyramine and colestipol.

GEMFIBROZIL, FENOFIBRATE, AND OTHER FIBRIC ACID DERIVATIVES

Fibric acid derivatives (FADs) are a class of drugs that have been shown to inhibit the production of VLDL and enhance VLDL clearance, principally owing to decreased hepatic synthesis of the endogenous lipoprotein lipase inhibitor apo C-III and, to some extent, via stimulation of lipoprotein lipase gene expression. The drugs can reduce plasma triglycerides and concurrently raise HDL cholesterol levels, primarily due to the effects of lower plasma triglycerides but, in part, also to a modest direct effect on the production of the principal HDL apolipoproteins, apo A-I and apo A-II. Their effects on LDL cholesterol are less marked and more variable. FADs also modify intracellular lipid metabolism by increasing the transport of fatty acids into mitochondria and improving peroxisomal and mitochondrial fatty acid catabolism. All effects of the currently available FADs are felt to be due to ligation and activation of the ligand-activated transcription factor peroxisome proliferator-activated receptor (PPAR) α. PPARs (there are three: PPAR-α,

PPAR-γ, and PPAR-δ) heterodimerize with the retinoid X receptor and bind to characteristic DNA sequence elements.

This section reviews the clinical pharmacology of gemfibrozil and the other FADs, discusses the therapeutic experiences with these agents, and provides recommendations for their clinical use.

Pharmacokinetics

Gemfibrozil is well absorbed from the GI tract, with peak plasma levels seen 1 to 2 h after administration. The plasma half-lives are 1.5 h after a single dose and 1.3 h after multiple-dose therapy. The plasma drug concentration is proportional to dose and steady state and is reached after 1 to 2 weeks of twice-daily dosing. Gemfibrozil undergoes oxidation of the ring methyl group in the liver to form hydroxymethyl and carboxyl metabolites (in total, there are four major metabolites). No reports as yet have described distribution of the drug into human breast milk or across the placenta. Two-thirds (66%) of the twice-daily dose is eliminated in the urine within 48 h, 6% is eliminated in the feces within 5 days of dosing, and less than 5% of the drug is eliminated unchanged in the urine. Regardless of the dosing schedule, there is no drug accumulation with normal or impaired renal function.

In vitro, gemfibrozil is 98% bound to albumin at therapeutic levels. There have been reports that, when gemfibrozil is combined with warfarin in vitro, a doubling of the unbound warfarin fraction ensues. Similarly, clofibrate has been found to potentiate the anticoagulant activity of warfarin.

The other FADs behave in much the same way as gemfibrozil. Fenofibrate has been studied most extensively. It is well absorbed after oral administration and is hydrolyzed to fenofibric acid, subsequently undergoing carbonyl reduction, which results in reduced fenofibric acid. Fenofibrate and reduced fenofibric acid are active pharmacologically. Sixty-five percent of fenofibrate is excreted into the urine, principally as fenofibryl glucuronide (<20% is excreted through the bile). Drug elimination is completed within 24 to 48 h, and the half-life of the drug is approximately 4.9 h. Steady-state equilibrium is established within 2 to 3 days. Unlike gemfibrozil, the newer FADs—in particular ciprofibrate, fenofibrate, and bezafibrate—can accumulate in patients with renal and hepatic failure; therefore, dose adjustments may be necessary. No pharmacokinetic interaction exists between fenofibrate and BAS.

Mechanism of Action of Gemfibrozil and Other FADs

The PPAR-α transcription factor has a central role in coordinating fatty acid metabolism in the liver, kidney, heart, and muscle. Much of current knowledge of the role of this transcription factor has emerged from studies on the effects of the fibrate drugs on individual lipoprotein components and cholesterol–triglyceride metabolic pathways.

One direct action of FADs appears to be an increase in the level of plasma lipoprotein lipase (LPL). LPL is deficient in patients with type I hyperlipoproteinemia, types I and II diabetes mellitus, hypothyroidism, heart failure, and nephrotic syndrome. LPL is increased by insulin treatment of diabetes mellitus, aerobic exercise, and FADs. LPL is the rate-limiting enzyme governing the removal of triglycerides from lipoproteins in the plasma. It functions at the luminal surface of the vascular endothelium and depends on the presence of apo C-II on chylomicrons, VLDL, and HDL to activate its hydrolytic capacity. The level of LPL has been found to be increased after the addition of gemfibrozil. Enhancement of LPL is also found with fenofibrate therapy. Similarly, bezafibrate has been found to increase LPL activity. When coupled with the decrease in apo C-III, the catabolism of VLDL is dramatically increased. An increase in lipoproteins containing apo B and apo C-III has been shown to be an important discriminator of atherosclerotic risk in a number of clinical trials. A decrease in these lipoproteins may be part of the anti-atherosclerotic benefit of the FAD.

VLDL is produced in the liver and circulates in the plasma, where LPL hydrolyzes it to a VLDL remnant by removing triglyceride. The VLDL remnant is then taken up by an apo E receptor–mediated process in the liver or converted to LDL. FADs have been shown to decrease the production of VLDL and to increase its fractional catabolic rate.

Gemfibrozil has been studied predominantly in subjects with hypertriglyceridemia. The newer FADs have been studied in subjects with hypertriglyceridemia and in those with hypercholesterolemia. Although the FADs have similar triglyceride-lowering abilities, fenofibrate, bezafibrate, and ciprofibrate appear to have a greater cholesterol-lowering effect than do gemfibrozil and clofibrate, which may relate to their having additional HMG-CoA reductase–inhibiting activity.

In the hypertriglyceridemic state, there are alterations in the usual homogeneity of lipoprotein subfractions. For instance, much of the LDL of hypertriglyceridemic patients contains a smaller amount of cholesterol ester and a greater amount of triglyceride than is usual. Presumably, this aberration results from an exchange of triglyceride for cholesterol between VLDL and LDL. The triglyceride-enriched LDL is then hydrolyzed by hepatic triglyceride lipase, leading to a further reduction in size and increase in density of the LDL molecule. Thus, in the hypertriglyceridemic state, there are LDL fragments of normal composition coexisting with triglyceride-enriched and triglyceride-depleted forms. The clinical consequences of this heterogenous LDL population are not yet apparent.

In the hypertriglyceridemic state, the production and fractional clearance of LDL are also increased. Thus, patients with isolated hypertriglyceridemia may have low to normal LDL levels. Correction of the hypertriglyceridemic state with gemfibrozil restores the normal LDL population and reduces the production and catabolism of LDL. The result is often a slight increase in LDL levels. Similarly with fenofibrate or bezafibrate, when there are normal or low LDL levels, treatment increases levels of LDL. An explanation is that during fibrate therapy the increased lipolysis of VLDL and triglyceride promotes increased hepatic uptake of VLDL remnants, leaving fewer receptors for clearance of LDL and thus increased plasma LDL. It has been suggested that the short-term result of FAD therapy is an increased production of LDL-cholesterol secondary to increased VLDL catabolism and a resultant downregulation of hepatic LDL receptors. As the VLDL levels decrease, the LDL cholesterol content increases, thus establishing a more normal LDL particle. Regardless of the mechanism for changes in LDL levels, the importance of inhibiting production of VLDL and enhancing catabolism has been well documented. Studies have shown that, in the primary hypertriglyceridemic state, gemfibrozil increases LDL less than does clofibrate, a drug that enhances VLDL catabolism without altering production. Fenofibrate treatment of hypertriglyceridemic patients improves the conversion of VLDL to LDL and causes LDL levels to increase by 25% as VLDL levels decrease by 77%. However, the drug also increases the clearance rate of apo B and causes a decrease in apo B levels of approximately 35%. Thus these changes would be expected to be, on balance, antiatherogenic. Similar observations have been made with bezafibrate treatment of hypertriglyceridemia.

The composition of HDL is also altered in hypertriglyceridemia. Normally, HDL2a, the cholesterol ester–rich subfraction, predominates in the circulation. HDL2a is transformed to HDL2b when it acquires triglyceride. HDL3 is formed from the removal of triglyceride from HDL2b by hepatic triglyceride lipase and LPL. HDL3 then acquires new cholesterol ester via lecithin cholesterol acetyl transferase and forms HDL2a. Hypertriglyceridemia markedly reduces HDL2a concentration and increases HDL2b concentrations. Essentially, hypertriglyceridemia decreases the cholesterol content of HDL. FAD therapy reverses this process, leading to increased cholesterol content of HDL. Gemfibrozil also has been found to stimulate the synthesis of apo AI, the major apoprotein on HDL, without altering its catabolism. Similarly, fenofibrate and bezafibrate increase apo AI levels during treatment of hypertriglyceridemia. However, the levels of apo AI rarely increase to the extent that HDL rises.

The hypertriglyceridemic state is thought to be associated with an increase in cholesterol synthesis. One explanation for this is that hypertriglyceridemic LDL is altered and may present less cholesterol to the cells, thus leading to less effective downregulation of LDL receptors and less inhibition of HMG-CoA reductase. Consequently, cholesterol synthesis is increased. There is some evidence that FADs inhibit cholesterol synthesis. From comparison studies, it would appear that the newer FADs—fenofibrate, bezafibrate, and ciprofibrate—are more effective than gemfibrozil and clofibrate in reducing cholesterol levels. The results of animal studies appear to confirm that these new agents inhibit HMG-CoA reductase. Although the older agents may have some minimal activity in inhibiting HMG-CoA reductase, the results of animal studies have shown much greater activity with the newer agents, such as bezafibrate, versus clofibrate. In vivo, fenofibrate has been shown to decrease HMG-CoA reductase activity on human mononuclear cells in type IIa and IIb patients. Similarly, bezafibrate has been found to inhibit HMG-CoA reductase activity from mononuclear cells of normal and hypercholesterolemic patients. Other data suggest an increased peripheral mobilization of cholesterol from tissues with FADs and feedback inhibition of hepatic cholesterol synthesis.

FADs increase the secretion of cholesterol into bile and decrease the synthesis of bile acids. This effect is modulated by LDL receptor activity, with FADs increasing hepatic uptake of cholesterol, and the subsequent secretion of cholesterol into the bile. This increased lithogenicity of bile accompanying clofibrate therapy was first noticed in 1972, and since then, other investigators have reported decreased fecal bile acid secretion and increased fecal excretion of neutral steroid with gemfibrozil therapy. The net effect of decreased bile acid concentration and increased cholesterol concentration is a cholesterol supersaturation of bile, providing the potential nidus for gallstone formation. Studies with the newer FADs, especially fenofibrate, have shown variable results in terms of total bile acid synthesis and subsequent possible bile acid saturation. Thus far, European and American studies have shown no increase in gallstone formation in patients on fenofibrate therapy. Thus, the newer FADs may have less potential for gallstone formation.

In addition, fenofibrate has been shown to decrease platelet-derived growth factor in vitro, which inhibits smooth muscle proliferation in rabbit aorta. Thus, the FADs may directly inhibit atherosclerotic plaque formation. An additional property unique to fenofibrate is the ability to decrease uric acid by 10% to 28% in 90% to 95% of all treated patients, with an increase in renal uric acid secretion. The exact mechanism and clinical significance of this observation are unclear.

Clinical Experience

The effects of FADs are largely dependent on the pretreatment lipoprotein classification of the patient. In short, most patients respond to therapy with a decrease in triglyceride levels and an increase in HDL levels. Hypertriglyceridemic patients without hypercholesterolemia often have a slight increase in cholesterol and LDL levels. However, patients with hypercholesterolemia often have a decrease in their cholesterol and LDL levels. The predominant difference between gemfibrozil and the newer FADs is that the FADs appear to lower LDL to a greater degree. One explanation for this is that these new derivatives may also inhibit HMG-CoA reductase to some extent.

The clinical data for FADs are best summarized according to their effect on hypertriglyceridemic patients, subjects with combined hypertriglyceridemia and hypercholesterolemia, and subjects with only hypercholesterolemia. Patients with type I chylomicronemia would benefit little from FADs because these individuals lack LPL, the enzyme responsible for the increased clearance mediated by the FADs.

The Helsinki Heart Study, a 5-year, double-blind, intervention trial, used gemfibrozil on 2051 middle-age men, 8.8% of whom had isolated hypertriglyceridemia (type IV hyperlipidemia). In this subgroup there was a 5% increase in LDL with gemfibrozil compared with a 7% increase with placebo. There was a 10% increase in HDL and a significant decrease in total cholesterol. Type IV patients experienced the greatest drop in triglycerides as compared with type IIa or IIb subjects. There was a 2% incidence in cardiovascular end points in this treated group as compared with 3.3% in the placebo group. A relation between the decreased triglyceride levels and the decreased cardiovascular morbidity was not observed. Instead, it was proposed that the elevated HDL, perhaps resulting from triglyceride lowering, conferred protection.

The Lopid Coronary Angiographic Trial, which used gemfibrozil in 372 men with prior coronary artery bypass graft surgery, showed a significant benefit in decreasing angiographic progression and new lesion development in native vessels and saphenous vein grafts. The VA-HIT study, which used gemfibrozil to detect an effect on clinical end points in more than 2500 men with normal LDL (<140 mg/dL) and low HDL (<40 mg/dL), also showed a significant benefit with this agent, including a favorable effect on stroke incidence.

Clinical Use

It is well established that FADs are first-line therapy to reduce the risk of pancreatitis in patients with very high levels of plasma triglycerides. Results from the Helsinki Heart Study have also suggested that the hypertriglyceridemic patient with low HDL values can derive a cardioprotective effect from gemfibrozil. Isolated low HDL levels are not as responsive to fibrate therapy. Niacin therapy, when tolerated, may be preferable in these patients. Nevertheless, the benefit in decreased coronary end points demonstrated in such patients in the VA-HIT study is supportive of the use of gemfibrozil to reduce coronary risk in patients with isolated low HDL, despite the rather modest increase in HDL that was achieved.

FADs, particularly the newer generation, decrease total cholesterol and LDL levels. However, in the absence of elevated triglycerides, they should not be first-line therapy for hypercholesterolemic patients. Type IIb patients comprise the subset most commonly seen in clinical practice that would benefit from FAD therapy. HMG-CoA reductase inhibitors combined with FADs are excellent therapy for severe type IIb disease; however, the development of symptoms of myositis must be monitored. Bile acid resins plus gemfibrozil also constitute a reasonable combination for type IIb disease; however, HDL levels may drop slightly.

Gemfibrozil is approved for clinical use in the United States for the treatment of patients with very high serum triglycerides who are at risk of developing pancreatitis and for reducing the risk of clinical CAD in patients with type IIB hypercholesterolemia who are not symptomatic and who have low HDL cholesterol and elevated LDL cholesterol and triglyceride levels. The recommended dose for gemfibrozil is 600 mg before the morning meal and 600 mg before the evening meal. Some patients may respond to 800 mg/day, but in most instances the therapeutic benefit is augmented with an increase to 1200 mg daily. Some patients derive benefit from increasing the dosage of gemfibrozil to 1600 mg daily.

Fenofibrate tablets are approved for clinical use as adjunctive therapy to diet for the reductions of LDL cholesterol, total cholesterol, triglycerides, and apo B in adult patients with primary hypercholesterolemia or mixed dyslipidemia (types IIA and IIB). The drug is also indicated as adjunctive therapy to diet for the treatment of patients with hypertriglyceridemia (type IV and V hyperlipidemias). For treatment of primary hypercholesterolemia or mixed hyperlipidemia, the initial dose of fenofibrate is 160 mg once daily. For patients with hypertriglyceridemia, the initial dose is 54 to 160 mg once daily. Dosage should be individualized according to the patient's response and should be adjusted as necessary after repeat lipid determinations at 4- to 8-week intervals. The maximum dose is 160 mg daily.

Adverse Effects

Clofibrate, one of the earliest FADs, became unpopular because of its causative association with cholelithiasis and cholecystitis in the Coronary Drug Project. The World Health Organization trial then reported a 29% increase in overall mortality in clofibrate-treated as compared to placebo-treated subjects. The mortality was principally due to postcholecystectomy complications, pancreatitis, and assorted malignancies. The Helsinki Heart Study reported a decrease in cardiovascular mortality but not in overall mortality in gemfibrozil-treated subjects. The reason for the similarity of overall mortality rates with placebo and gemfibrozil remains a mystery at this time. Obviously, these findings have led to careful scrutiny of currently used and tested FADs. The significant adverse effects noted in the Helsinki Heart Study included atrial fibrillation, acute appendicitis, dyspepsia, abdominal pain, and nonspecific rash. The review of the European clinical trials of fenofibrate with 6.5 million patient-years showed a 2% to 15% adverse reaction rate, the most common adverse reactions being GI disturbances, dizziness and headache, muscle pains, and rash. However, the only side effect significant in frequency was skin rash. In a United States multicenter study of fenofibrate in 227 patients, there was a 6% increase in side effects from the drug, similar to the observations of the European studies.

In the Helsinki Heart Study, there were a 55% excess incidence of gall-stones and a 64% excess incidence of cholecystectomy in the drug-treated as compared with placebo-treated group. Although European studies of fenofibrate may show some increased lithogenicity of the bile, there has been no increase in the incidence of gallstone formation during the trials or during post-marketing surveillance.

The manufacturers of gemfibrozil and fenofibrate have reported mild depressions of hemoglobin, white blood cell count, and hematocrit with the drugs. The Helsinki Heart Study did not find significant alterations in these parameters.

The combination of fibrates and HMG-CoA reductase inhibitors has been shown repeatedly to predispose to rhabdomyolysis and, in some cases, renal failure. The Helsinki Heart Study did not report any cases of myopathy in patients treated with only gemfibrozil.

Fenofibrate therapy is associated with increases in liver function tests, leading to discontinuation of treatment in 1.6% of patients in double-blind trials. Like treatment with other fibrates, fenofibrate treatment may cause myopathy, especially in patients with impaired renal function, which interferes with the drug's excretion. Uric acid is noted to increase 10% to 28% on fenofibrate therapy; the clinical significance of this is unknown.

HMG-CoA REDUCTASE INHIBITORS

In 1987 the U.S. Food and Drug Administration (FDA) approved the marketing of lovastatin, a competitive inhibitor of HMG-CoA reductase, the rate-limiting enzyme step in cholesterol synthesis in the body. The pharmacology and clinical efficacy of this cholesterol-lowering drug and other drugs in this class that were also approved for marketing are reviewed in this section.

Lovastatin

Chemistry

Lovastatin (Mevinolin) is a fermentation product of the fungus, *Aspergillus terreus*. It is similar in structure to an earlier compound, mevastatin, a less potent inhibitor of HMG-CoA reductase, whose clinical development was limited by its possible carcinogenicity in animals.

Pharmacology

Lovastatin, as a competitive inhibitor of HMG-CoA reductase, interferes with the formation of mevalonate, a precursor of cholesterol. Mevalonate also is a precursor of ubiquinone and dolichol, non-sterol substances essential for cell growth. It was initially thought that the HMG-CoA reductase inhibitors might inhibit formation of these substances, but this is not the case. Non-sterol synthesis does not appear to be inhibited by HMG-CoA reductase inhibitors.

Pharmacokinetics

Lovastatin is an inactive lactone (prodrug) that is hydrolyzed in the liver to an active β-hydroxy acid form. The prodrug was developed rather than the active hydroxy acid form because the prodrug undergoes more efficient shunting to the liver on first pass. The potential result of this enhanced liver uptake is lower peripheral drug concentrations and fewer systemic side effects. This principal metabolite is the inhibitor of the enzyme HMG-CoA reductase. The dissociation constant of the enzyme inhibitor complex is approximately 1029 mol/L.

An oral dose of lovastatin is absorbed from the GI tract, with greater absorption at meals. The drug undergoes extensive first-pass metabolism in the liver, its primary site of action, with subsequent excretion of drug equivalents in the bile. It is estimated that only 5% of an oral dose reaches the general circulation as an active enzyme inhibitor. The drug is excreted via the bile (83%) and the urine (10%).

Lovastatin and its β-hydroxy acid metabolite are highly bound to human plasma proteins. Lovastatin crosses the blood–brain and placental barriers. The major active metabolites present in human plasma are the β-hydroxy acid of lovastatin, its 6-hydroxy derivative, and two unidentified metabolites. Peak plasma levels of active and total inhibitors are attained 2 to 4 h after lovastatin ingestion. The half-life of the β-hydroxy acid is approximately 1 to 2 h. This rapid metabolism would seem to necessitate multiple doses per day. Clinical trials, however, have indicated that once- or twice-daily dosing is optimum. With a once-daily dosing regimen, within the therapeutic range of 20 to 80 mg/day, steady-state plasma concentration of total inhibitors after 2 to 3 days was about 1.5 times that of a single dose. Single daily doses administered in the evening are more effective than the same dose given in the morning, perhaps because cholesterol is mainly synthesized at night (between 12 and 6 A.M.). A substantial clinical effect of lovastatin is noted within 2 weeks and a maximal effect is found at 4 to 6 weeks; the effect dissipates completely 4 to 6 weeks after the drug is stopped. A tachyphylaxis effect has been suggested with prolonged use of statins.

Clinical Experience

Several investigators have demonstrated that lovastatin lowers the cholesterol levels of normal and hypercholesterolemic animals. These studies have demonstrated that the increased LDL receptor activity and decreased LDL synthesis are responsible for the hypocholesterolemic effect of the drug. Several studies in humans have confirmed this observation. This increase in LDL receptor activity occurs in response to a decrement in cholesterol synthesis by HMG-CoA reductase inhibition. LDL may be reduced by its increased clearance from the plasma or its decreased production.

Clinical End Points

In a report from the Familial Atherosclerosis Treatment Study, the combination of 40 mg of lovastatin and 30 g of colestipol daily was more effective than colestipol and diet alone in reducing LDL and raising HDL in patients with CAD and elevated apo B levels. There were also fewer cardiovascular events, less progression of coronary lesions, and more regression.

In the Monitored Atherosclerotic Regression Study (MARS), patients whose cholesterol was 190 to 295 mg/dL and who were receiving 80 mg of lovastatin per day and a cholesterol-lowering diet showed a slower rate of progression and an increase in the regression in coronary artery lesions, especially in more severe lesions, as compared with placebo plus diet. These anatomic changes on coronary angiography with lovastatin were associated with a significant reduction in total cholesterol, LDL cholesterol, and apo B levels, with a modest increase in HDL cholesterol. In this study, lovastatin also was shown to reduce the progression of early, pre-intrusive atherosclerosis of the carotid artery as evaluated by B-mode ultrasonography.

In the Canadian Coronary Atherosclerosis Intervention Trial (CCAIT), 331 patients with diffuse but not necessarily severe coronary atherosclerosis on coronary angiography and cholesterol between 220 and 300 mg/dL were randomized to receive diet plus lovastatin (20, 40, and 80 mg), titrated to achieve an LDL cholesterol below 130 mg/dL, or diet plus placebo. Lovastatin treatment slowed the progression of coronary atherosclerosis, especially of the milder lesions, and inhibited the development of new lesions. In a substudy analysis of female participants in the CCAIT, lovastatin was effective in slowing the progression and neogenesis of coronary atherosclerotic lesions.

The effects of lovastatin on atherosclerotic lesions in the carotid arteries was assessed in the Asymptomatic Carotid Artery Progression Study (ACAPS). In this study, 919 asymptomatic men and women with early carotid atherosclerosis as defined by B-mode ultrasonography and LDL-cholesterol levels between 130 and 159 mg/dL were randomized to receive 20 to 40 mg of lovastatin or placebo. In addition, all patients received 80 mg of aspirin daily, and 50% were treated with 1 mg of warfarin daily.

Lovastatin reduced LDL cholesterol levels and, after 3 years of follow-up, slowed the progression of mean intimal–medial thickness of the common carotid arteries and decreased mortality and major cardiovascular events.

As in the findings in ACAPS, Familial Atherosclerosis Treatment Study (FATS), MARS, and CCAIT, reductions in cardiac event rates were observed with lovastatin as opposed to placebo.

The Air Force/Texas Coronary Atherosclerosis Prevention Study (AFCAPS/TexCAPS) was a double-blind, placebo-controlled, primary prevention study using lovastatin that targeted 5608 men and women with average LDL levels (mean 60th percentile) and low HDL level (25th percentile for men, 16th for women). Its primary end point was the development of a first major acute coronary event (myocardial infarction, unstable angina, or sudden cardiac death). The drug was well tolerated, with no clinical differences in liver enzyme abnormalities, myositis, and so forth. After a mean 5.2 years of follow-up, lovastatin reduced the incidence of the primary end point by 37% ($P < 0.001$), with a similar benefit on a variety of other atherosclerotic end points (coronary revascularizations, etc.), presumably via the noted 25% reduction in LDL and 6% increase in HDL. Mortality was limited in this relatively low-risk population, and the apparent benefit of treatment did not reach statistical significance. Most of these individuals would not have met criteria for therapy under the NCEP guidelines then in force. However, post hoc subgroup analysis showed that the benefit is substantially confined to the 66% of subjects with HDL levels below 40 mg/dL. Redefinition of the low-HDL risk factor from below 35 mg/dL to below 40 mg/dL would have led to most of these subjects meeting criteria for therapy under the guidelines. This analysis was a prominent factor in the redefinition of the low-HDL risk factor to below 40 mg/dL in the current (third) edition of the guidelines.

Clinical Use

Lovastatin is approved as an adjunct to diet for the reduction of elevated total and LDL cholesterol in patients with primary hypercholesterolemia (types IIa and IIb) when the response to a diet restricted in saturated fat and cholesterol has not been adequate. In individuals without symptomatic cardiovascular disease, average to moderately elevated total cholesterol and LDL cholesterol levels, and below average HDL cholesterol, lovastatin is indicated to reduce the risk of myocardial infarction, unstable angina, and coronary revascularization procedures. The drug is also indicated for slowing the progression of atherosclerosis in patients with CHD.

Lovastatin doses as low as 5 mg twice daily produce significant reductions in serum cholesterol. Patients should be placed on a standard cholesterol-lowering diet before drug treatment. The recommended starting dose is 20 mg once daily given with the evening meal. The recommended dosing range is 20 to 80 mg daily in single or divided doses. Adjustments should be made at intervals of 4 weeks or longer. A dose of 40 mg daily can be initiated in patients with cholesterol levels above 7.76 mm/L (>300 mg/dL).

Twice-daily dosing appears to be the most effective treatment regimen, with daily evening doses being slightly less effective and daily morning doses least effective. Maximal and stable cholesterol reduction typically is achieved within 4 to 6 weeks of treatment initiation. A new extended-release formulation of lovastatin has been approved for once-daily clinical use in doses of 10, 20, 40, and 60 mg. Unlike immediate-release lovastatin, this formulation is best absorbed in the absence of food.

In patients with high cholesterol, diet and lovastatin may not reduce cholesterol to the desired level. Niacin, BAS, and fibrates, in combination with lovastatin, may provide additional efficacy. A combination formulation of niacin and lovastatin has been approved for clinical use.

Adverse Effects

Several hypercholesterolemic agents are available, each having a significant side effect profile. Lovastatin and other HMG-CoA reductase inhibitors have an acceptable rate of adverse reactions but must to be used with some caution.

In the published trials, approximately 2% of patients were withdrawn from treatment because of adverse reactions. GI side effects (diarrhea, abdominal pain, constipation, and flatulence) are the most commonly reported adverse effects. Marked, persistent, but asymptomatic increases (to greater than three times the upper limit of normal) in serum transaminases have been reported in 2% of patients receiving the drug for 1 year. The increases are predominantly in serum glutamate pyruvate transaminase and serum glutamic-oxaloacetic transaminase rather than in alkaline phosphatase, suggesting a hepatocellular, not cholestatic, effect. These abnormalities rapidly return to normal after the discontinuation of the drug, and no permanent liver damage has been reported with the drug. Symptomatic hepatitis in patients without underlying disease or other known hepatotoxic medications has been observed. It is recommended that liver function tests be performed before the initiation of treatment, at 6 and 12 weeks after initiation of therapy or elevations of dose, and semiannually thereafter.

The side effect of greatest concern with lovastatin is a myopathy, which appears to develop in three clinical patterns. The first, a moderate elevation in plasma creatine kinase levels, is asymptomatic. Second, patients may develop muscle pain, primarily in the proximal muscle groups. Creatine phosphokinase (CPK) elevations may or may not be present. Third, patients may develop a severe myopathy marked by extreme elevations in CPK, muscle pain with weakness, myoglobinuria, and, rarely, acute renal failure. This finding most often occurs in the setting of concurrent immunosuppressive therapy (cyclosporine), particularly when gemfibrozil, erythromycin, or niacin is added. Similarly, the use of itraconazole, an antimycotic drug, has been shown to drastically increase plasma concentrations of lovastatin and lovastatin acid. Inhibition of CYP3A4-mediated hepatic metabolism likely explains the increased toxicity of lovastatin caused not only by itraconazole but also by cyclosporine, erythromycin, and other inhibitors of CYP3A4.

Cases of myopathy have been identified as soon as a few weeks and as late as 2 or more years after the initiation of therapy. CPK elevations appear to correlate little with the severity of the symptoms, but if CPK levels rise or muscle pain develops, it is recommended that lovastatin be reduced. If levels rise drastically (>10 times the upper limits of normal) with muscle pain, therapy should be discontinued.

In a study of 11 cardiac transplant patients, all were treated with lovastatin and cyclosporine, monitored closely for 1 year, and were not treated with other hepatotoxic medications or lipid-lowering agents. None developed any evidence of hepatic, muscle, or renal toxicity, and the investigators concluded that, in the absence of other effective therapy, cardiac transplantation should not be a contraindication to the use of lovastatin. Combinations of lovastatin with hepatotoxic agents, in the absence of cyclosporine, also have been associated with myositis. The FDA has documented multiple cases of myopathy and rhabdomyolysis associated with lovastatin–gemfibrozil combination therapy and has discouraged the use of this regimen. Although the reason that myopathy has been associated with lovastatin is not well understood, drugs that impair hepatic function may alter the first-pass extraction of lovastatin and produce elevated levels, which in turn may be responsible for the myotoxicity. Lovastatin may disrupt the proper assembly of membrane glycoproteins, the oxidation-reduction reactions of the mitochondrial respiratory chain, or the regulation of DNA replication. However, four cases of myositis with lovastatin monotherapy were reported, but three of these patients had biliary stasis leading to decreased clearance of the drug.

Bleeding, increase in prothrombin time, or both have been observed in patients on concomitant warfarin anticoagulation. Although these accounts have not been attributed to lovastatin, it is recommended that prothrombin time be carefully regulated in these patients, as in all patients receiving oral anticoagulation.

In addition to reports of rashes during the clinical trials, there have been several accounts of serious hypersensitivity reactions during prescription use: anaphylaxis, arthralgia (a lupus-like syndrome), angioedema, urticaria, hemolytic anemia, leukopenia, and thrombocytopenia have been reported. Twenty-five cases were considered serious, but all of these patients recovered with discontinuation of lovastatin therapy. Because these adverse effects were never reported during the clinical trials, it is likely that the incidence is significantly less than 1 per 1000. Sleep disturbances, characterized by insomnia or shortening of the sleep period, also have been described.

Lovastatin (40 mg daily) and pravastatin (40 mg daily) were compared in a double-blind study of effects on quality of life and drug tolerability in men 20 to 65 years of age with primary hypercholesterolemia who received treatment for 12 weeks. No significant differences between the two groups were observed in tolerability, health-related quality-of-life measures, or changes in lipid profile.

Simvastatin

Simvastatin (synvinolin) is a prodrug that is enzymatically hydrolyzed in vivo to its active form. In clinical trials since 1985 and approved in 1992, simvastatin is synthesized chemically from lovastatin and differs from lovastatin by one methyl group. Like lovastatin, it has a very high affinity for HMG-CoA reductase; but on a milligram-per-milligram basis, simvastatin is twice as potent. Peak plasma concentrations of active inhibitor occur within 1.3 and

2.4 h. One 12-week, multicenter, double-blind study comparing simvastatin with probucol found that a daily dose of simvastatin, 20 and 40 mg, lowered LDL cholesterol by 34% and 40%, respectively. Simvastatin also reduced total cholesterol, triglycerides, and apo B. HDL was increased. As with lovastatin, interactions with warfarin and digoxin have been noted. Another multicenter study comparison with cholestyramine demonstrated that a low dose of simvastatin (10 mg) is sufficient to reduce total cholesterol by 21% and LDL by 30%; HDL increased by 17%. In comparisons of simvastatin with FADs and BAS, simvastatin produced greater reductions in total and LDL cholesterol, whereas FADs and BASs had a greater effect on the serum triglycerides. A small study of patients with familial hypercholesterolemia showed that 40 mg of simvastatin in combination with 12 g of cholestyramine can reduce total cholesterol by 43% and LDL cholesterol by 53%.

The effects of simvastatin are achieved with a single evening dose. Despite its potency, simvastatin has never been shown to disrupt adrenocortical function. Side effects are predominantly headaches and dyspepsia, but asymptomatic myositis has been noted. It is interesting that some patients who experienced enzyme elevations with lovastatin and lovastatin rechallenge tolerated simvastatin well on rechallenge.

Simvastatin has been shown to be useful in all the hypercholesterolemic conditions in which other HMG-CoA reductase inhibitors are used. On a milligram-per-milligram basis, it is about twice as potent as lovastatin. Simvastatin, 10 mg daily, or 20 mg of pravastatin or lovastatin usually produce about 25% to 30% reductions in LDL cholesterol versus about 20% to 25% reductions with 20 mg of fluvastatin. Lovastatin (80 mg), pravastatin (40 mg), or simvastatin (40 mg) generally decrease LDL cholesterol by about 30% to 40%; maximum doses of fluvastatin (40 mg) decrease LDL cholesterol by about 25%. The maximum approved daily dose of simvastatin is 80 mg.

As a treatment for nephrotic hyperlipidemia, simvastatin was noted to be more effective and better tolerated than cholestyramine. Simvastatin also has been evaluated for its effect on the cholesterol saturation index of gallbladder bile, a potential side effect of several hypocholesterolemic agents. A mean decline of 23% was noted in the 10 hypercholesterolemic patients studied, raising the possibility that an HMG-CoA reductase inhibitor may play a future role in the treatment of gallstones.

Effect on Clinical End Points

Like lovastatin and pravastatin, simvastatin was shown to slow the progression of coronary atherosclerosis as assessed by coronary angiography. In the Multicentre Anti-Atheroma Study, simvastatin, 20 mg daily, was compared with placebo in 381 patients with CAD receiving a similar lipid-lowering diet. Patients on simvastatin had a 23% reduction in total cholesterol, a 31% reduction in LDL cholesterol, and a 9% increase in HDL cholesterol as compared with placebo over 4 years. Patients on simvastatin had less progression and more regression of existing lesions and a lower rate of new lesion development.

In a landmark secondary prevention study, the Scandinavian Simvastatin Survival Study (4S), simvastatin was shown to reduce mortality and morbidity in patients with known CAD and hypercholesterolemia. In this study, 4444 patients with prior angina pectoris or myocardial infarction and elevated total serum cholesterol levels (220 to 320 mg/dL or 5.5 to 8.0 mm/L) were randomized in double-blind fashion to receive simvastatin, 20 to 40 mg, or placebo and were followed for a median of 5.4 years (Fig. 15-1). All patients were on a cho-

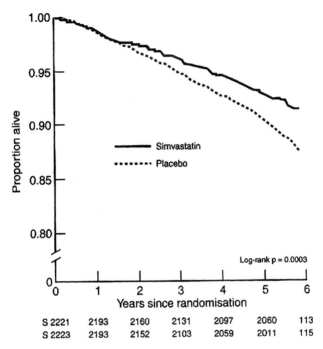

FIG. 15-1 Kaplan-Meier curves for all-cause mortality. The number of patients at risk at the beginning of each year is shown below the horizontal axis. *(Reproduced with permission from the Scandinavian Simvastatin Survival Study Group: Randomized trial of cholesterol lowering in 4444 patients with coronary heart disease: the Scandinavian Simvastatin Survival Study (4S). Lancet 344:1383, 1994.)*

lesterol-lowering diet. Compared with placebo, simvastatin reduced total cholesterol by 25% and LDL cholesterol by 35% and increased HDL cholesterol by 8%. Compared with placebo, there were highly statistically significant reductions of all fatal coronary events by 42% with simvastatin; all fatal cardiovascular events were reduced by 35%, and all-cause mortality was reduced by 30%. Patients older than 60 years had a 27% reduction in mortality, essentially identical to the findings in the younger group. Results on secondary end points (myocardial infarction, revascularization, etc.) paralleled the results on mortality. There was also a 30% reduction in cerebrovascular events with simvastatin. Results in women were essentially the same as the results in men. In comparing placebo with simvastatin treatment, there was no difference in noncardiovascular mortality. Based on this study, subsequent pharmacoeconomic analysis has demonstrated the cost effectiveness of simvastatin in secondary prevention.

The Heart Protection Study enrolled 20,536 patients, ages 40 to 80 years, with CAD, noncoronary arterial disease, diabetes, and treated hypertension. Patients were randomized to simvastatin (40 mg daily), a vitamin cocktail (1600 mg of E, 250 mg of C, and 20 mg of β-carotene), or placebo. Patients were followed for 5 years. There was no effect from the vitamin therapy. Simvastatin caused a one-third reduction in the risk of myocardial infarction, stroke, and coronary and noncoronary revascularization regardless of baseline cholesterol levels.

Based on experimental studies, the suggestion has been made that simvastatin may reduce cardiovascular events beyond the effect on lipid lowering. The possibility of such effects is a continuing area of controversy. Simvastatin and other HMG-CoA reductase inhibitors have been shown to reduce factor VIIc activity and inhibit platelet activation and reduce the propensity of LDL to oxidation. In addition, the drug has been shown to depress blood clotting by inhibiting activation of prothrombin, thrombin factor V, and factor XIII. A beneficial effect to statins has been associated with a lower risk of deep venous thrombosis. Simvastatin also was shown to have a favorable action in causing regression of cardiac hypertrophy in an animal model of hypertrophic cardiomyopathy.

Clinical Use

Similar to other marketed HMG-CoA reductase inhibitors, simvastatin is approved for use in patients with primary hypercholesterolemia and mixed dyslipidemia (Fredrickson types IIa and IIb). In addition, based on the results of the 4S study, the drug has been approved in patients with CHD as long-term treatment for hypercholesterolemia and to reduce the risk of total mortality by reducing coronary death, the risk of nonfatal myocardial infarction, the risk for undergoing myocardial revascularization, and the risk of stroke or transient ischemic attack. In addition, the drug is approved for use in patients with hypertriglyceridemia (Fredrickson type IV) and primary dyslipoproteinemia (Fredrickson type III). Simvastatin is administered orally as a single dose in the evening. The recommended starting dose is 20 mg daily, which is then titrated according to the individual patient's response at 4-week intervals to a maximum 80-mg daily dose. Simvastatin can be combined with FADs, niacin, and BASs—including colesevelam—to achieve maximal cholesterol lowering. A combination formula of simvastatin and ezetimibe, a cholesterol absorption inhibitor, is now in clinical development.

In patients with severe renal insufficiency or those receiving cyclosporine, the recommended starting dose is 5 mg daily, and close monitoring is required. Drug–drug interactions with amiodarone and verapamil require dosing adjustments. The dose of simvastatin should not exceed 20 mg/day. In patients taking fibrates, niacin, or cyclosporin, the simvastatin dose should not exceed 10 mg/day. The low risk of liver enzyme abnormalities and their lack of clinical severity have led to less stringent requirements for liver function testing. Testing is now recommended before initiating or increasing the dose of therapy and twice during the subsequent year, with routine laboratory monitoring ceasing 1 year after the last dosage increment if liver function tests remain normal.

Adverse Effects

The side effects profile of simvastatin is similar to that of lovastatin and other HMG-CoA reductase inhibitors. The rare occurrence of a lupus-like syndrome has recently been reported with lovastatin and simvastatin.

Pravastatin

Pravastatin (Pravachol CS 514, SQ 3100, epstatin) is the 6-α-hydroxy acid form of compactin. It is the first HMG-CoA reductase inhibitor to be administered in the active form and not as a prodrug. In vitro studies demonstrated that pravastatin has a greater specificity than lovastatin for hepatic cells. In vivo animal studies comparing pravastatin with lovastatin and simvastatin, however, found that the concentration of pravastatin in the liver was only half that of the latter two, whereas the concentrations in peripheral tissues were three to six times greater.

Pravastatin also was found to be a specific inhibitor of hepatic HMG-CoA reductase in humans. Other enzymes involved in cholesterol metabolism (α-hydroxylase, which governs bile acid synthesis and acyl-coenzyme A; cholesterol O-acetyltransferase, which regulates cholesterol esterification) were not affected by treatment. Inhibition of hepatic HMG-CoA reductase activity by pravastatin results in an increased expression of hepatic LDL receptors, which explains the lowered plasma levels of LDL cholesterol.

Multiple studies have been conducted on humans to establish efficacy and dosage. Despite its short plasma half-life of approximately 2 h, a single daily dose of pravastatin has been shown to be as effective as twice-daily doses. As with all HMG-CoA reductase inhibitors, the sustained duration of benefit relates to the relatively long half-life of plasma LDL and is independent of the systemic half-life of the drug, most of which is removed in the first pass through the liver in any event. As with other drugs in this class, administration of the drug in the evening rather than in the morning appears to bring about greater cholesterol-lowering activity. Patients with heterozygous familial hypercholes-terolemia (FH), treated with pravastatin 10 and 20 mg, were found to have 26% and 33% decreases in LDL, respectively. HDL was significantly increased. Others also found that 5-, 20-, and 40-mg doses lowered the total serum cho-lesterol by 11.1%, 18.8%, and 25.3%, respectively, in hypercholesterolemic patients. The investigators reported some mild side effects but no myositis.

The efficacy and safety of pravastatin have been evaluated in various patient subgroups. A low dose (10 mg) of pravastatin daily was shown to be a safe and effective method of reducing total and LDL cholesterol in hyper-cholesterolemic, hypertensive elderly patients who were receiving concurrent antihypertensive drug therapy. The safety and efficacy of using lovastatin (20 and 40 mg) in the elderly were confirmed in the Cholesterol Reduction in Seniors Program. The effect of pravastatin on morbidity and mortality in the elderly has been evaluated in the Antihypertensive Lipid Lowering Heart Attack Trial (ALLHAT), which is funded by the National Institutes of Health. Pravastatin (20 mg daily) has been shown to be well tolerated and effective in lowering total cholesterol and LDL cholesterol in patients with type I or II diabetes mellitus and hypercholesterolemia. Moreover, pravastatin (20 mg daily) has been found to be an effective and safe lipid-lowering agent, as have other drugs in this class, in African Americans with primary hypercholes-terolemia and in the elderly.

Lovastatin, simvastatin, and pravastatin have been directly compared, and the published data suggest that, at equipotent dosages, the drugs are approxi-mately equal in efficacy with respect to reducing LDL cholesterol.

Effects on Clinical End Points

The benefit of using pravastatin to reduce morbidity and mortality in patients with CAD was first established in the Pravastatin Multinational Study. In this 6-month trial, pravastatin treatment was demonstrated to reduce the incidence of serious cardiovascular events, including myocardial infarction and unsta-ble angina.

Four vascular regression trials using pravastatin have been completed, with the results reported on two of the trials. The First Pravastatin Limitation of Atherosclerosis in the Coronary Arteries (PLAC-I) and Regression Growth Evaluation Statin Study (REGRESS) included patients with CAD to assess by serial angiography the effects of pravastatin on CAD. PLAC-II evaluated the ability of pravastatin to retard the ultrasonographic 3-year progression of extracranial carotid artery in patients with known CAD. The Kuopio Atherosclerosis Study (KAPS) was a 3-year ultrasonographic study that evaluated the effects of pravastatin on the progression of carotid and femoral atheroscleroses.

All the studies were placebo controlled, and pravastatin doses of 20 to 40 mg were used as monotherapy. Patients receiving pravastatin in PLAC-I had a 40% to 50% reduction in the progression of coronary lesions, a 28% reduction in LDL cholesterol, and fewer nonfatal and fatal myocardial infarctions as compared with placebo. In PLAC-II, pravastatin-treated patients showed a 35% reduction of atherosclerosis in the common carotid artery and an 80% reduction in fatal and nonfatal infarctions as compared with placebo. In KAPS, there was a significant reduction in the progression of carotid atherosclerosis as compared with placebo. In REGRESS, there was a significant reduction in the progression of coronary atherosclerosis with pravastatin and a reduced rate of adverse cardiovascular events as compared with placebo, including fewer myocardial infarctions, sudden deaths, strokes, and invasive coronary procedures.

In these four studies, a total of 1891 patients had been evaluated, and although the major objective was to assess regression of atherosclerosis with aggressive lipid lowering with pravastatin, a meta-analysis assessed the impact of treatment on clinical cardiovascular events as compared with placebo. The risk of fatal plus nonfatal myocardial infarctions was reduced by 62%, the risk of stroke was reduced by 62%, and total mortality was reduced by 46%.

In a prospective study of patients with known cardiovascular disease, pravastatin was shown to reduce the level of the inflammatory biomarker C-reactive protein in a largely LDL cholesterol–independent manner, suggesting that statins may have anti-inflammatory in addition to lipid-lowering effects that contribute to their clinical benefit in patients at risk for CAD.

Pravastatin was also shown to have a blood pressure–lowering effect in patients with moderate hypercholesterolemia and hypertension. In addition, the drug improves endothelial function after acute coronary syndromes and decreases thrombus formation.

Pravastatin has been used in one large primary prevention and several secondary prevention studies with reported benefit on clinical cardiovascular outcomes. In the West of Scotland Prevention Study (WOSCOPS), 6595 middle-age men with no history of myocardial infarction and average plasma cholesterol values above 252 mg/dL were randomized to receive placebo or 40 mg of pravastatin and followed for an average of almost 5 years. Pravastatin decreased LDL cholesterol by 26% and increased HDL cholesterol by 5%. Pravastatin treatment also significantly reduced the incidence of myocardial infarction and death from cardiovascular causes by 31% and decreased a variety of other coronary end points without adversely affecting the risk of death from noncardiovascular causes. Total mortality was decreased by 22% (Fig. 15-2).

The Cholesterol and Recurrent Events Study (CARE) assessed whether pravastatin treatment (40 mg daily) could reduce the sum of fatal CAD and nonfatal myocardial infarctions in patients who survived a myocardial infarction yet had a total cholesterol below 240 mg/dL, a population different from that studied in the 4S. Results indicated a significant benefit of pravastatin therapy on cardiovascular outcomes as compared with placebo. The primary

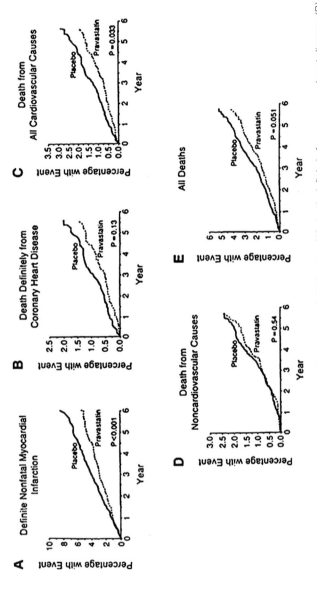

FIG. 15-2 Kaplan-Meier analysis of time to a definite nonfatal myocardial infarction (A), death definitely from coronary heart disease (B), death from all cardiovascular causes (C), death from noncardiovascular causes (D), and death from any cause (E) according to treatment group. (Reproduced with permission from Shepherd J, Cobbe SM, Ford I, et al: Prevention of coronary heart disease with pravastatin in men with hypercholesterolemia. N Engl J Med 333:1301, 1995.)

end point of fatal coronary event or myocardial infarction was reduced 24%, despite this being a population with somewhat lower than average LDL levels (139 mg/dL). Many other coronary end points were significantly reduced, as was stroke. No significant effect on all-cause mortality was detected in this relatively low-risk group. A post hoc subgroup analysis showed that the benefit was confined to those patients having a baseline LDL cholesterol above 125 mg/dL, an observation that led to a period of questioning of the NCEP guidelines target LDL of below 100 mg/dL for patients with know atherosclerotic disease. The NCEP target has been, in the main, supported by the literature and remains the consensus.

The Long-term Intervention with Pravastatin in Ischemic Heart Disease trial (LIPID) was a relatively similar trial that evaluated placebo versus pravastatin, 40 mg, in patients who had an acute myocardial infarction or an unstable angina episode and had cholesterol values of 155 to 271 mg/dL. The study examined the effects of treatment on CAD mortality as the primary end point. Median LDL levels, at 150 mg/dL, were slightly higher. The primary end point was decreased by 24%, there were similar significant effects on other coronary end points, and all-cause mortality was decreased by 22%. In addition, a beneficial effect was seen on the risk of nonhemorrhagic stroke from any cause.

The Pravastatin in Elderly Individuals at Risk of Vascular Disease study was a randomized, double-blind, placebo-controlled trial of 40 mg of pravastatin in elderly men and women (70 to 82 years of age) with a history of vascular disease. Pravastatin given for only 3 years reduced the risk of CAD in selected elderly patients at high risk and those patients with vascular disease. The recent ALLHAT study showed no benefit of pravastatin on cardiovascular outcomes in hypertensive patients older than 65 years when compared with physician-guided therapy. However, the lack of benefit may be related to the 8% difference in LDL cholesterol lowering between the pravastatin and control groups.

Another pravastatin study evaluating the use of HMG-CoA reductase inhibitors with or without vitamin E and marine polyunsaturated fats (fish oil) in 6000 patients with a history of myocardial infarction was stopped early due to the publication of the CARE and LIPID data.

Clinical Use

Pravastatin has a similar approval for treatment of hypercholesterolemia as do other HMG-CoA reductase inhibitors and, in addition, is approved for the primary and secondary prevention of complications related to CAD. The drug is also approved for the secondary prevention of stroke and ischemic attacks and the progression of coronary atherosclerosis. The drug is approved for use in patients with primary hypertriglyceridemia (Fredrickson type IV), primary dyslipoproteinemia (Fredrickson type III), primary hypercholesterolemia (Fredrickson type IIa), and mixed dyslipidemia (Fredrickson type IIa). The recommended starting dose is 10 to 20 mg once daily at bedtime for primary hypercholesterolemia, with a usual dosing range of 10 to 40 mg daily. A 40-mg dose may be necessary to achieve the clinical benefits observed in the primary and secondary prevention trials done with the drug. Recently, a combination package of pravastatin and aspirin has become available for the long-term management to reduce the risk of cardiovascular events in patients with clinically evident coronary disease.

Similar to other HMG-CoA reductase inhibitors, the drug may be combined with other classes of lipid-lowering drugs. When combined with cholestyramine or colestipol, pravastatin should be administered 1 h before or

4 h after the bile acid resin is given. Such precautions appear not to be necessary with colesevelam.

Adverse Effects

The adverse effect profile is similar to those of other HMG-CoA reductase inhibitors in use. Because the drug does not cross the blood–brain barrier, it has been proposed to cause a lower incidence of sleep disturbances than lovastatin or simvastatin. A rare peripheral–neuropathic complication with lovastatin and pravastatin has been described.

As with simvastatin, the low risk of liver enzyme abnormalities and their lack of clinical severity have led to less stringent requirements for liver function testing. The recommendation for liver function testing at 6 weeks has been eliminated, as has the recommendation for semi-annual testing if liver function tests are normal at 12 weeks.

Fluvastatin

Fluvastatin was the first synthetic HMG-CoA reductase inhibitor, and it is structurally distinct from the fungal derivatives lovastatin, simvastatin, and pravastatin. It was approved for clinical use in the United States for the treatment of primary hypercholesterolemia (types IIa and IIb). The drug also received approval as the fourth statin to slow the progression of coronary arteriosclerosis in patients with CAD as part of a treatment to lower total and LDL cholesterol to target rates. With doses of 20 to 40 mg daily in patients with hypercholesterolemia, the drug was shown to reduce LDL cholesterol by 19% to 31%, total cholesterol by 15% to 21%, with small declines in triglycerides of 1% to 12%. The drug raised HDL cholesterol by 2% to 10%. Maximal lipid-lowering effects of a dose are usually seen after 4 weeks of therapy and are sustained long term. On a milligram-to-milligram basis, the drug appears to be less potent in its lipid-lowering effects than other available HMG-CoA reductase inhibitors, and the recommended maximal dose has recently been increased to 80 mg daily in two divided doses.

Fluvastatin is well absorbed after oral administration and, like other HMG-CoA reductase drugs, undergoes extensive first-pass metabolism. Its side effect profile is similar to those of other HMG-CoA reductase inhibitors, and it may cause less myopathy and risk of rhabdomyolysis when used alone or with gemfibrozil, nicotinic acid, cyclosporine, and erythromycin.

The drug has been combined with other lipid-lowering therapies, including cholestyramine, bezafibrate, and nicotinic acid, to achieve greater lipid-lowering effects; it has been used safely in diabetic and hypertensive patients.

Effects on Clinical End Points

Although many patients with known CAD have received fluvastatin, there are no published survival studies with the drug. One study assessed the efficacy of high-dose fluvastatin (80 mg daily) in preventing restenosis after balloon angioplasty; no significant benefit was detected. In another study, known as the Lipoprotein and Coronary Atherosclerosis Study (LCAS), the effects of fluvastatin versus placebo on long-term progression of atherosclerosis were assessed in patients with known CAD by using serial coronary angiography. Results from the LCAS demonstrated a benefit of fluvastatin treatment on the progression and regression of atherosclerosis. Recently, the results of the prospective Lescol Intervention Prevention Study (LIPS) demonstrated that statin therapy initiated soon after successful percutaneous coronary intervention improves clinical outcomes, including recurrent cardiac events and late revascularization procedures. These data support the use of early lipid-lowering therapy in patients with previous percutaneous coronary intervention, regardless of baseline cholesterol level.

Fluvastatin has been evaluated as an anti-ischemic drug in patients immediately after myocardial infarction (Effects of Fluvastatin Administration Immediately After an Acute MI on Myocardial Ischemia: Florida), with no reported benefit as compared with placebo after 1 year. The drug has been shown to lower total and LDL cholesterol levels and dense LDL, a more atherogenic subfraction of LDL.

Clinical Use

Fluvastatin (capsules and an extended-release tablet form of the drug) is indicated as an adjunct to diet to reduce elevated total cholesterol, LDL cholesterol, triglycerides, and apo B levels and to increase HDL cholesterol in patients with primary hypercholesterolemia and mixed dyslipidemia (Fredrickson types IIa and IIb). Both formulations are also indicated to slow the progression of coronary atherosclerosis in patients with CAD as part of a treatment strategy to lower total and LDL cholesterol levels. In addition, fluvastatin is now approved to reduce the risk of undergoing coronary revascularization procedures in patients with CAD.

The recommended starting dose is 40 mg as one capsule or 80 mg as one extended-release tablet administered as a single dose in the evening or 80 mg in divided doses of the 40-mg capsules given twice daily. As in the case of other HMG-CoA reductase inhibitors, it takes at least 4 weeks to achieve the maximal effect. If fluvastatin is combined with cholestyramine, fluvastatin plasma levels drop considerably. Fluvastatin must be given at least 4 h after a cholestyramine dose.

Atorvastatin

Atorvastatin is a newer synthetic HMG-CoA reductase inhibitor with a long half-life (14 h; 20 to 30 h for activity due to the presence of active metabolites) that is similar in structure to fluvastatin. Atorvastatin is twice as potent on a milligram-to-milligram basis as simvastatin and much more potent than fluvastatin in reducing total cholesterol and LDL cholesterol. Early investigations proposed that atorvastatin is unique in its ability to reduce triglycerides. This has been less striking in subsequent studies; if such potency is present at all, the advantage is modest. In 1997, the drug was approved for clinical use in patients with type IIa and IIb hypercholesterolemias and homozygous familial hypercholesterolemia. Its side effect profile appears to be similar to those of other HMG-CoA reductase inhibitors in doses up to 80 mg used once daily.

In the Atherosclerosis Progression in Familial Hypercholesterolemia trial, aggressive therapy with 80 mg of atorvastatin was shown to produce less progression of noninvasively quantitated carotid atherosclerosis than lower-dose therapy with 40 mg of simvastatin. The published long-term clinical experience with atorvastatin remains limited because of its recent introduction, although many trials are ongoing. The clinical end-points evidence base is derived from two large relatively short-term studies. The Myocardial Ischemia Reduction with Aggressive Cholesterol Lowering trial (MIRACL) showed that the administration of atorvastatin, 80 mg, immediately after hospitalization for unstable angina or non–Q-wave myocardial infarction reduces the incidence of recurrent ischemic events over the first 16 weeks. Patients who were treated with simvastatin or pravastatin in the three major secondary prevention statin trials (4S, CARE, and LIPID) or pravastatin or lovastatin in the two major primary prevention trials (WOSCOPS and AFCAPS/TexCAPS) did not show benefit at such an early time point. This result may reflect differences in the biology of acute as opposed to chronic coronary syndromes, increased statistical power due to a high risk of short-term ischemic complications in unstable patients, or particular advantages of the high-dose atorvastatin regimen used. Other trials examining the benefits of initiating high-dose statin therapy soon after an acute coronary event are ongoing. Of note, at high doses, atorvastatin loses some of its effectiveness in raising HDL, an effect not seen with equipotent doses of simvastatin. The clinical significance of this observation is unknown.

To assess the effect of atorvastatin (10 to 80 mg/day) on morbidity and mortality in patients with established CAD, 1600 consecutive patients were randomized to receive the drug or "usual medical care." Long-term treatment with atorvastatin to achieve NCEP lipid targets significantly reduced total and coronary mortality and stroke when compared with the "usual care."

A substudy, the Anglo-Scandinavian Cardiac Outcomes Trial (ASCOT), assessed the effects of atorvastatin (10 mg) and placebo in hypertensive patients receiving blood pressure–lowering treatment who were not dyslipidemic. There were 100 primary events in the atorvastatin group compared with 154 in the placebo group, and over a 3-year period, a relative risk reduction of 36%. Surprisingly, there were no significant treatment effects in the diabetic subgroup.

The Atorvastatin Versus Revascularization Treatment (ADVERT) study examined 341 patients with stable CAD who were referred for percutaneous transluminal coronary angioplasty. Patients were randomly assigned to atorvastatin, 80 mg/day, or to angioplasty followed by usual care, which did not exclude lipid-lowering therapy. Over 18 months of follow-up, the incidence of ischemic events was 36% lower in the atorvastatin group ($P = 0.048$, but not significant after statistical adjustment for interim analyses). The patients who received atorvastatin also had a longer time to the first ischemic event ($P = 0.03$). There was no "usual care" placebo group, and it is unclear to what extent the results in this study reflect the benefit of atorvastatin versus possible disadvantages of angioplasty in the study population.

There have been no primary or secondary CAD prevention trials of lipid-lowering therapy, specifically in a diabetic population. Two studies are currently evaluating the effects of atorvastatin in diabetic patients [Atorvastatin as Prevention of Coronary Heart Disease in Patients with Type II Diabetes (ASPEN) and the Collaborative Atorvastatin Diabetes Study (CARDS)].

Clinical Use

Atorvastatin is approved for reducing elevated total cholesterol, LDL cholesterol, apo B, and triglyceride levels and to increase HDL cholesterol in patients with primary hypercholesterolemia and mixed dyslipidemia. In addition, the drug is approved for use in patients with primary dysbetalipoproteinemia and elevated triglyceride levels.

The recommended starting dose of atorvastatin is 10 mg once daily. The dosage range is 10 to 80 mg once daily. The drug can be administered as a single dose at any time of the day, with or without food.

Atorvastatin, especially at higher doses, may render clopidogrel ineffective at inhibiting platelet aggregation. Clopidogrel and atorvastatin are metabolized in the liver by the cytochrome P450 system and require the same liver enzyme (CYP3A4) for metabolism and activation. Because atorvastatin competitively utilizes the CYP3A4 activity needed for clopidogrel activation, the ability of clopidogrel to convert to its active form is inhibited when both drugs are used concomitantly. Recently, this finding has been questioned, and one study, Interactions of Atorvastatin and Clopidogrel Therapy (INTERACT), has been designed to address this issue by utilizing serial measurements of platelet function.

Rosuvastatin

Rosuvastatin is a highly efficacious HMG-CoA reductase inhibitor that was recently approved for clinical use in doses of 5, 10, 20 and 40 mg, to reduce elevated total cholesterol, LDL, Apo B, non-HDL-cholesterol and triglyceride levels and to increase HDL. It appears to combine a number of the characteristics of the other available statins. Similar to pravastatin, rosuvastatin is liver selective, hydrophilic, and is minimally metabolized via CYP 3A4. Like atorvastatin, rosuvastatin has a prolonged systemic half-life in plasma of about 20 hours, and is quite potent. The maximal 40 mg dose has been shown to reduce LDL by 55%, significantly more than is possible with current monotherapy. Rosuvastatin also produces greater increases in HDL than are seen with high dose atorvastatin. A 10 mg dose of rosuvastatin was shown to reduce LDL by almost 50%. No long-term side effect, clinical endpoint or angiographic data are available. However, large endpoint trials are now in progress, including a study of 15,000 patients with normal cholesterol but high levels of coronary inflammation, to assess whether the drug will reduce coronary risk (JUPITER).

It was observed that Japanese patients residing in Japan and Chinese patients residing in Singapore manifested higher plasma levels of rosuvastatin than Caucasians, Hispanics, Black or Afro-Caribbean subjects. There is also a 3-fold increase in plasma concentrations of rosuvastatin in patients with severe renal impairment (Cl_{Cr} <30 mL/min/1.73 m^2) compared with healthy subjects.

Clinical Use

The dose range of rosuvastatin is 5 to 40 mg once daily. The usual starting dose is 10 mg once daily. Initiation of therapy with 5 mg once daily may be considered for patients requiring less aggressive LDL reductions or who have predisposing factors for myopathy (renal impairment), advanced age, hypothyroidism, combination treatment with fibrates or niacin, or race. Rosuvastatin and other statins should also be temporarily withheld in any patient with an acute, serious condition predisposing to the development of renal failure secondary to rhabdomyolysis (e.g., sepsis, trauma, major surgery, seizures).

NICOTINIC ACID (NIACIN)

Nicotinic acid (pyridine-3 carboxylic acid, or niacin) is a water-soluble B-complex vitamin that is used for the prophylaxis and treatment of pellagra. The substance functions in the body after conversion to either nicotinamide-adenine dinucleotide or nicotinamide-adenine dinucleotide phosphate.

Pharmacokinetics

Nicotinic acid is readily absorbed from the intestinal tract after the oral administration of pharmacologic doses. The level of free nicotinic acid in plasma reaches a peak value between 30 and 60 min after a single dose of 1 g is ingested. Because nicotinic acid is rapidly eliminated, the doses necessary to achieve pharmacologic effects (2 to 8 g daily) are much larger than the amount needed for its physiologic functions as a vitamin. When large doses of the vitamin were given to rats by intraperitoneal injection, the half-life of the compound was found to be approximately 1 h in blood. The half-life of nicotinic acid seems to be determined primarily by the rate of renal clearance of the unchanged compound when given in high doses. At lower doses, it is excreted mainly as its metabolites.

The metabolic fate of nicotinic acid is complex and changes with the dose. Under normal conditions, metabolites of nicotinic acid found in the urine are mainly the products of catabolism of the pyridine nucleotides, the stored forms of the vitamin. The primary route of metabolism is via methylation to N-methyl-nicotinamide, which is further oxidized to N-methyl-2- and -4-pyridone carboxamides. With pharmacologic doses, the excretion of nicotinuric acid, produced by the conjugation of nicotinic acid and glycine, is enhanced and seems to play a role as a detoxification product at these higher doses. Once the dose is large enough to overcome the production rate of nicotinuric acid, nicotinic acid is excreted largely unchanged.

Pharmacology

Nicotinic acid in large doses lowers total plasma cholesterol and has been found to have beneficial effects on the levels of the major serum lipoproteins, including lipoprotein(a). Specifically, it decreases the levels of VLDL triglyceride (VLDL-Tg) and LDL cholesterol and causes an increase in the levels of HDL cholesterol. This lipid-altering activity is not shared by nicotinamide and seems to be unrelated to the role of nicotinic acid as a vitamin in the nicotinamide-adenine dinucleotide and nicotinamide-adenine dinucleotide phosphate coenzyme systems. Pharmacologic doses of nicotinic acid result in a rapid decrease in plasma triglyceride levels, in part by lowering VLDL-Tg concentrations by 20% to greater than 80%. The magnitude of the reduction is related to the initial VLDL levels. Within 1 week of initiation of therapy, concentrations of LDL cholesterol decrease. Typically, a 5% to 10% reduction in LDL cholesterol is observed within 3 to 5 weeks of attaining full dosage. The magnitude of the drop is also related to the dose of nicotinic acid. In addition to these lipid-lowering effects, nicotinic acid raises HDL cholesterol concentrations. Mobilization of cholesterol from peripheral tissues seems to occur after prolonged therapy, as demonstrated by the regression of eruptive, tuberuptive, tuberous, and tendon xanthomas.

There are several mechanisms by which nicotinic acid alters serum lipoprotein levels. The actions of nicotinic acid as an anti-lipolytic agent may be related to its effects on lowering VLDL-Tg concentration. Nicotinic acid has been found to decrease lipolysis in adipose tissue, resulting in decreased levels of plasma free fatty acids. After oral administration of 1 g of nicotinic acid, a significant depression of free fatty acids occurs, as does a reduction in plasma glycerol levels. During fasting, free fatty acids released from adipose tissue serve as the major precursors for the formation of VLDL-Tg, which is synthesized mainly in the liver and serves as the major carrier of endogenous triglyceride. The decrease in the release of free fatty acid from adipose tissue that is induced by nicotinic acid is thought to decrease uptake of free fatty acid by the liver and thereby reduce the hepatic synthesis of VLDL.

Clinical Experience

As outlined above, nicotinic acid has beneficial effects on all plasma lipoprotein fractions, including lipoprotein(a), and was identified as one of the drug choices for the treatment of hypercholesterolemia by the Adult Treatment Panel of the NCEP. Studies of the clinical efficacy of nicotinic acid fall into two main groups: those that examine the use of nicotinic acid in patients with known CAD and those that test its efficacy, often in combination with other lipid-lowering agents, in altering plasma lipoprotein levels in patients with various types of hyperlipoproteinemias.

The Coronary Drug Project, a long-term nationwide, double-blind, placebo-controlled study, examined a number of lipid-altering regimens, including nicotinic acid and clofibrate, in male survivors of myocardial infarction.

Over the follow-up period, nicotinic acid effected mean decreases of 9.9% in total serum cholesterol and 26.1% in total triglycerides. However, the incidence of all deaths in the follow-up period (8.5 years) was insignificantly lower than that in the placebo group (24.4% vs. 25.4%). In contrast to the findings on total mortality, the incidence of definite, nonfatal myocardial infarction over the total follow-up period was 27% lower in the treatment group than in the control group (10.1% vs. 13.9%). Also, during this period, the treatment group showed a 24% lower incidence of fatal or nonfatal cerebrovascular events than did the placebo group. There was also a lower incidence of bypass surgery in the group receiving nicotinic acid (0.9% vs. 2.7%).

Investigators in the Coronary Drug Project conducted a follow-up study nearly 9 years after termination of the original trial. With a mean total follow-up of 15 years, total mortality in the nicotinic acid group was 11% lower than in the placebo group (52% vs. 58.2%). The men in the study had presumably stopped taking the drug after the original mean follow-up of 6.2 years. The decreased mortality was due primarily to a decrease in CAD mortality, with smaller decreases in death due to cerebrovascular causes, other cardiovascular events, cancer, and both noncardiovascular and noncancer causes.

Explanations for this observed late benefit of nicotinic acid on mortality include the early decreases in incidence of nonfatal reinfarction and the cholesterol-lowering effects of nicotinic acid on the coronary arteries. It seems that patients with the largest decreases in cholesterol at 1 year follow-up had lower subsequent mortality than did subjects with increases in cholesterol. Nearly 30% of the men in the nicotinic acid group adhered poorly to the treatment regimen (subjects took less than 60% of the amount of drug called for by the protocol), but there was a significant benefit in 15-year mortality. This observation suggests that less than optimal doses of nicotinic acid may nevertheless result in therapeutic benefits. Of course, statements regarding the efficacy of nicotinic acid as a primary prevention of CAD or whether the administration of nicotinic acid over longer periods would be beneficial or detrimental cannot be made based on the findings of this study.

The effects of combined treatment with nicotinic acid (up to 3 g daily) and clofibrate (2 g daily) in 558 survivors of myocardial infarction randomly assigned to one of two groups 4 months after their acute events were examined. Both groups received advice regarding diet, and the treatment group received both drugs. Subjects in the treatment group exhibited mean reductions of 15% to 20% in total serum cholesterol and 30% in serum triglycerides. Control group subjects showed insignificant reductions in these levels. There were no significant differences between the two groups with regard to total and CAD-related deaths. However, over a 4-year period, the number of nonfatal reinfarctions in the treatment group was reduced by 50% as compared with the control group. In comparison, the Coronary Drug Project reported a 27% reduction in nonfatal reinfarctions in the nicotinic acid group and insignificant reductions in the clofibrate group. Considering the more modest decreases in serum cholesterol and triglycerides (6% and 10%, respectively) in the Coronary Drug Project as compared with those observed in this study, it has been suggested that the rate of nonfatal reinfarction may be related to the degree of serum lipid lowering.

The Cholesterol-Lowering Atherosclerosis Study (CLAS) used a combination of colestipol and nicotinic acid to test the hypothesis that aggressive lowering of LDL cholesterol and raising of HDL cholesterol reverses or retards the progression of atherosclerotic lesions. The subjects, chosen to minimize the effects of other major nonlipid risk factors for atherosclerosis, included 162 normotensive nonsmoking men ages 40 to 59 years with previous coronary bypass surgery and fasting levels of total cholesterol in the range of 4.78 to 9.05 mm/L (185 to 350 mg dL).

The results of angiographic readings showed that the treatment group's score distribution was significantly shifted toward lower scores than that of the control group, indicating less disease progression with the colestipol plus nicotinic acid treatment. In fact, 61% of the treatment group improved or remained the same, and 16.2% showed regression of atherosclerotic lesions at 2 years. These findings differed from the results in the placebo control group, 39% and 2.4%, respectively. With regard to native vessels, treatment reduced the average number of lesions that progressed per subject and the percentage of subjects with new lesions. Similarly, with respect to bypass grafts, the percentage of subjects with new lesions or showing any adverse change in preexisting lesions was significantly lower in the treatment group. Recently reported were the results of a 7-year follow-up of a subpopulation from CLAS. These findings suggested that, after coronary artery bypass surgery, patients should receive intensive interventions to improve blood lipid and lipoprotein levels.

The results of the FATS demonstrated a favorable effect of nicotinic acid plus colestipol on the progression of coronary atherosclerotic disease. With the nicotinic acid plus colestipol combination, 25% of patients showed progression of coronary lesions, 39% showed regression, and only two cardiovascular events occurred. In contrast, 10 cardiovascular events occurred in the control group, 46% of patients showed regional progression, and 11% showed regression of coronary lesions. Patients with disease, a family history of premature cardiovascular events, and elevated levels of apo B (3.23 mm/L or 125 mg/dL) were counseled on diet and assigned to one of three treatment regimens: nicotinic acid, 4 g/day, plus colestipol, 30 g per day; lovastatin, 40 mg/day, plus colestipol; or colestipol alone (control). The combination regimens caused the greatest reductions in LDL and the greatest elevations in HDL. Bimonthly visits spanned 2.5 years between coronary angiograms. Favorable changes in clinical course and lesion severity appeared with the combination regimens.

A blinded, placebo-controlled, larger (160 patients) angiographic regression trial of combination therapy was recently reported. The effects of combination therapy with simvastatin and niacin or of an antioxidant vitamin cocktail (or of both) were evaluated in a population with known CAD and normal LDL levels (mean, 125 mg/dL). The vitamin supplement (vitamin E, vitamin C, β-carotene, and selenium) had no effect on lipid levels but did decrease the susceptibility of LDL to in vitro oxidation. Simvastatin was titrated to obtain an LDL below 90 mg/dL and then slow-release niacin was added in the ultimate dose of 1 g twice a day. Patients whose HDL did not exhibit a desired increase (5 mg/dL at 3 months, 10 mg/dL by 12 months) were switched to crystalline niacin in higher doses. Simvastatin was back-titrated if the LDL fell below 40 mg/dL. Combined antioxidant therapy significantly blunted the benefit of the drug regimen on plasma lipids and on angiographic progression. Proximal coronary stenosis increased by means of 3.9% in the placebo group, 1.8% in the antioxidant group, and 0.7% in the combined therapy group, but it decreased by 0.4% in the group receiving drug therapy alone. In addition, there was a 90% decrease in the incidence of a first cardiovascular event (death, myocardial infarction, stroke, or revascularization) in this group. The end point was reached in 24% of the placebo-treated patients, 21% of the patients given antioxidants alone, 14% of those given both, and 3% of those given simvastatin and niacin alone. These benefits were out of proportion to the LDL lowering achieved (42%), particularly given the limited period of follow-up (38 months), and provide support for the potential value of HDL-raising therapy, in particular using niacin, in the management of coronary risk. The negative effect of combining vitamins with drug therapy cannot be considered established given the modest size and statistical power of this study. However, any benefits of vitamins alone on angiographic disease did not reach statistical significance and were not correlated with any effect on clinical end points.

Clinical Use

Nicotinic acid—through its beneficial effects on VLDL-Tg, LDL, and HDL cholesterol levels—is indicated in most forms of hyperlipoproteinemia and for patients with depressed HDL, including patients with type II, III, IV, and V hyperlipoproteinemias. It is particularly useful in patients who have elevated plasma VLDL-Tg levels as a part of their lipid profile. It is important to remember that a diet low in cholesterol and saturated fats is the foundation of therapy for hyperlipoproteinemia.

Nicotinic acid is available in 100-, 125-, 250-, and 500-mg tablets and in a time-release form. The typical dose is 3 to 7 g daily given in three divided doses. Therapeutic effects of the drug are not usually manifest until the patient reaches a total daily dose of at least 3 g. A greater response may be attained with periodic increases in doses up to a maximum of 7 to 8 g daily, although the incidence of adverse effects also increases with higher doses. In general, it is best to use the lowest dose necessary to achieve the desired alterations in plasma lipoprotein levels. Unfortunately, many patients cannot tolerate therapeutic doses of nicotinic acid, the primary side effects being cutaneous flushing and GI disturbance. However, steps can be taken to minimize these untoward effects.

Nicotinic acid therapy should be initiated with a low-dosage regimen (100 mg daily) that should gradually increase every few days over a period of several weeks until the patient attains a dosage level of 3 g daily given in three divided doses. If, while increasing the dose, the patient develops any adverse effects, the dose should be cut back and then resumed at a more gradual pace. Taking the doses with meals decreases gastric irritation and cutaneous flushing. Further, cutaneous flushing can be reduced or avoided by taking one aspirin tablet daily (more frequent administration is unnecessary, because one tablet will inhibit cyclooxygenase for up to 2 weeks). It is interesting that tachyphylaxis to the flushing phenomenon often occurs within a few days, although the bothersome episodes may recur if the patient misses two or three doses. Once the initial maintenance dose is reached, it is important to evaluate for therapeutic effects by measuring plasma lipoprotein values. If the therapeutic effects are unsatisfactory, the dose should be increased by another 1.0 to 1.5 g/day, with periodic increases to a maximum of 7 to 8 g daily as needed. Usually, when doses of 4 g daily are achieved, another lipid-lowering drug is added. Regardless of the dose, it is important to make several laboratory evaluations for potential adverse effects at regular intervals. These evaluations include assessment of liver function (bilirubin, alkaline phosphatase, and transaminase levels), uric acid levels, and serum glucose levels. Nicotinic acid is contraindicated in patients with active peptic ulcer disease. The drug also may impair glucose tolerance and is contraindicated in patients with diabetes that is difficult to control. Nicotinic acid is also associated with reversible elevations of liver enzymes and uric acid and should not be used in patients with hepatic disease or a history of symptomatic gout.

Various sustained-release preparations of nicotinic acid are available without prescription. Timed-release forms of nicotinic acid were developed after it was noted that the incidence of cutaneous flushing was reduced when the drug was taken with meals, suggesting that this side effect is related to the rate of GI absorption. In fact, patients taking the timed-release preparation do have a lower incidence of flushing than do patients on unmodified nicotinic acid and require less frequent administration. However, this effect is outweighed by the far greater incidence of GI and constitutional symptoms experienced by patients on the timed-release form, including nausea, vomiting, diarrhea, fatigue, and decreased male sexual function. In addition, the timed-release preparations appear to be associated with greater hepatotoxicity, even at low doses, including greater alkaline phosphatase and transaminase elevations. In the doses required for the treatment of hyperlipidemia, these drugs clearly have an increased potential for chemical hepatitis that can be severe.

A proprietary "intermediate-release" formulation of nicotinic acid (Niaspan) that requires a prescription is also suitable for once-daily administration. This preparation also appears to decrease side effects to some extent and is without an increased risk of hepatitis in its recommended dosing range (only up to 2 g daily). Other newer delayed-release preparations are undergoing evaluation for safety and efficacy. A combination of a delayed-release nicotinic acid and lovastatin is now available for clinical use in tablet sizes of 500 and 20 mg, 750 and 20 mg, and 1000 and 20 mg, respectively. The recommended starting dose of this formulation is 500 and 20 mg taken at bedtime with a low-fat snack. At intervals of 4 weeks of longer, the niacin dose may be increased by 500 mg to a maximum of 2000 mg, and the lovastatin dose to a maximum of 40 mg (two 1000-/20-mg tablets). A clinical experience was reported with the use of a new form of nicotinic acid that uses a wax-matrix vehicle for sustained-release drug delivery.

Adverse Effects

Despite the efficacy of nicotinic acid in beneficially altering serum lipoprotein levels, its use is limited by a variety of troublesome and sometimes serious side effects. Some studies have experienced a dropout rate as high as 50% as a result of drug-related side effects.

The Coronary Drug Project, with 1100 subjects on nicotinic acid therapy, reported the common occurrences of cutaneous flushing and pruritus. Other dermatologic side effects include dryness of skin, rash, and acanthosis nigricans, which are reversible with cessation of therapy. The mechanism of the flushing is presumed to be related to the effect of nicotinic acid on vasodilatory prostaglandins and is frequently attenuated by pretreatment with aspirin. This vasodilatory effect in combination with antihypertensive therapy may result in postural hypotension. The Coronary Drug Project also described an increased incidence of atrial fibrillation, and other transient cardiac arrhythmias were noted. In addition, elevations in uric acid levels associated with an increased incidence of acute gouty arthritis were observed.

GI symptoms including diarrhea, nausea, vomiting, and abdominal pain were also frequent complaints encountered in the Coronary Drug Project. Activation of peptic ulcer disease by nicotinic acid is a potential adverse effect, but it was not observed in this large-scale study.

Liver function tests are frequently abnormal during nicotinic acid therapy. In general, there is elevation in alkaline phosphatase and hepatic transaminases. Some studies also have noted elevations in bilirubin, occasionally leading to jaundice. The elevations in transaminases are generally transient and reverse with decrease in dosage or cessation of therapy, and can be minimized by increasing the dosage in gradual increments when therapy is being initiated. Unlike the elevations in hepatic enzymes associated with HMG-CoA reductase inhibitors, the elevations that occur with the use of nicotinic acid may be symptomatic. Several cases of niacin hepatitis progressing to fulminant hepatic failure have been described, most frequently with the time-release formulation, with biochemical, clinical, and histologic evidence of hepatocellular injury. This seems to be a dose-related hepatotoxicity rather than a hypersensitivity, occurring in almost all cases at doses larger than 3 g daily. In most cases, cessation of therapy leads to eventual resolution of abnormalities. Hyperglycemia and impaired glucose tolerance may occur with nicotinic acid therapy and often necessitates adjustments in diet and hypoglycemic therapy in diabetic patients.

The results of a recent study have demonstrated that niacin is an effective treatment for hyperlipidemia in patients with diabetes and that its adverse effects on glycemic control are modest.

The Coronary Drug Project noted a statistically significant increase in CPK levels with nicotinic acid therapy, and there have been reports of associated reversible myopathy. The combination of lovastatin and nicotinic acid has been causally implicated in at least one case of rhabdomyolysis.

CHOLESTEROL TRANSPORT INHIBITORS (EZETIMIBE)

Ezetimibe is the first drug to be approved for clinical use in this novel class of lipid-lowering agents (the 2-azetidinones), known as selective cholesterol absorption inhibitors. Its mechanism of action is not fully elucidated, but it works at the point of enterocyte to selectively inhibit the intestinal transport of cholesterol through the interstitial wall.

Pharmacology

Ezetimibe acts at the brush border of the small intestine and inhibits the uptake of dietary and biliary cholesterol into enterocytes and the delivery of cholesterol to the liver. This action causes a reduction of hepatic cholesterol stores and increase in clearance of cholesterol from the blood. The drug does not affect the absorption of fat-soluble vitamins.

Etezimibe reduces total cholesterol, LDL cholesterol, and apo B and increases HDL cholesterol in patients with hypercholesterolemia. Administration of ezetimibe with statins is effective in improving total cholesterol, LDL cholesterol, apo B, and HDL cholesterol beyond the effects of either treatment alone. After oral administration, ezetimibe is absorbed and extensively conjugated in the small intestine and liver to a pharmacologically active phenolic glucuronide. The drug and its metabolite are highly bound to plasma proteins. Ezetimibde and its metabolite are eliminated slowly from the plasma, with a half-life of approximately 22 hours for both, with their excretion mostly in stool.

Clinical Experience

A randomized, double-blind, 12-week trial in 892 patients with primary hypercholesterolemia found that ezetimibe, 10 mg once daily, as monotherapy lowered LDL cholesterol by 17% and triglycerides by 6% and increased HDL cholesterol by 1.3%, all statistically significant compared with placebo. In a randomized, double-blind, 8-week trial, 769 patients at or above their target LDL cholesterol concentration on monotherapy with various statins received supplementary treatment with placebo or ezetimibe, 10 mg daily. Ezetimibe plus statin lowered mean LDL cholesterol from 138 to 104 mg/dL (25%), whereas placebo plus statin lowered it from 139 to 134 mg/dL (4%). A 12-week study in 668 patients with primary hypercholesterolemia found that ezetimibe at 10 mg daily plus simvastatin at 10, 20, 40 or 80 mg daily, started together, decreased LDL by 44% (10 mg), 45% (20 mg), 53% (40 mg), and 57% (80 mg) as compared with reductions of 27%, 36%, 36% and 44% with simvastatin alone.

Clinical Use

Ezetimibe, administered alone or with statins is approved as adjunctive therapy to diet for the reduction of elevated total cholesterol, LDL cholesterol, and apo B in patients with primary (heterozygous familial and nonfamilial) hypercholesterolemia. The drug is also approved for clinical use in patients with homozygous familial hypercholesterolemia as an adjunct to other lipid-lowering treatments and for patients with homozygous sitosterolemia as adjunctive therapy to diet.

The recommended dose of ezetimibde is 10 mg once daily. The drug can be taken with or without food. The drug can be administered with statins at the same time. It should be taken 22 h before or 74 h after administration of a BAS. The coadministration of ezetimibde with fibrates is not recommended because the safety and effectiveness of this combination has not been established.

Adverse Effects and Contraindications

Ezetimibe is generally well tolerated in contrast to the BASs, which cause constipation and gas and interfere with the absorption of other drugs. In clinical trials, the overall incidence of adverse effects reported with ezetimibe was similar to that reported with placebo, and the discontinuation rate due to adverse effects was similar.

The adverse experience rates were similar between ezetimibe administered with various statins and the statins used alone. However, the frequency of increased transaminases was slightly higher in patients receiving ezetimibe administered with statins than with statins used alone. With combination therapy, it is recommended that liver function tests be performed at the initiation of therapy and according to the recommendations of the particular statin being used. Ezetimibe is not recommended in patients with moderate or severe hepatic insufficiency with and without statins. The drug should not be used in pregnancy. There has been no excess in myopathy or rhabdomyolysis associated with ezetimibe monotherapy or combination with statins.

The drug has no significant effects on medications metabolized by cytochrome P450 and is neither an inhibitor nor an inducer of cytochrome P450. No pharmacokinetic interactions have been observed with warfarin or digoxin. No dose adjustments are necessary in the elderly or for patients with mild renal and hepatic insufficiency. Concomitant cholestyramine administration decreases the plasma levels of ezetimibe by 50%.

HORMONES

T_4 and estrogens have the ability to reduce LDL cholesterol. Many reports have shown possible benefit from estrogen use in preventing CAD in postmenopausal women. In contrast, the Heart and Estrogen/Progestin Replacement Study (HERS), a recent randomized clinical trial, demonstrated that estrogen and progestin therapy do not reduce the overall rate of coronary events in postmenopausal women with established coronary disease, despite reductions in total cholesterol and LDL cholesterol and increases in HDL cholesterol with estrogen.

Several studies, including HERS, have shown increases in plasma triglyceride concentration by estrogen, which can reduce the size of LDL particles. In postmenopausal patients with estrogen-induced hypertriglyceridemia, the resulting reduction in size of LDL particles makes them more susceptible to oxidation, which may counteract the antioxidant effect of estrogen. Future studies are needed to investigate the possible benefit of lowering plasma triglyceride concentrations during hormone replacement therapy on the risk of cardiac events in postmenopausal women with established CAD.

A current question that has yet to be fully answered is whether estrogen is more effective for primary prevention or for treating atherosclerosis once it is already established. According to results in HERS, estrogen may not be effective for secondary prevention of cardiovascular disease. The Estrogen and Prevention of Atherosclerosis Trial (EPAT) is the first randomized clinical trial of estrogen intervention for atherosclerotic disease in postmenopausal women with elevated LDL cholesterol levels but no evidence of coronary disease. The newest data from the EPAT study showed increased carotid wall thickness in the placebo group, as compared with a slight decrease in the estrogen group, suggesting estrogen may be more effective as primary prevention. However, more data from ongoing studies, such as the Women's Health Initiative (WHI), are needed to clarify the role of hormone replacement therapy in lowering lipids. The WHI has shown no benefit of an estrogen plus progestin combination in primary prevention of myocardial infarction and stroke. The safety and efficacy of estrogen used alone in cardiac prevention are being evaluated in the WHI trial.

CONCLUSION

One of the most important breakthroughs in clinical medicine over the past 30 years has been the confirmation of the cholesterol hypothesis by the demonstration that lipid-lowering drug therapy can affect morbidity and mortality from CAD. The drugs also will serve as pharmacologic probes for helping to understand the pathogenesis of atherosclerosis and its major vascular complications.

ADDITIONAL READINGS

Albert MA, Danielson E, Rifai N, et al: Effect of statin therapy on C-reactive protein levels. The Pravastatin Inflammation/CRP Evaluation (PRINCE): A randomized trial and cohort study. *JAMA* 286:64, 2001.

Alderman JD, Pasternak RC, Sacks FM, et al: Effect of a modified, well-tolerated niacin regimen on serum total cholesterol, high density lipoprotein cholesterol and the cholesterol to high density lipoprotein ratio. *Am J Cardiol* 64:725, 1989.

ALLHAT Officers and Coordinators: Major outcomes in moderately hypercholesterolemic patients randomized to pravastatin versus usual care. *JAMA* 288:2998, 2002.

Altschul R, Hoffer A, Stephen JD: Influence of nicotinic acid on serum cholesterol in man. *Arch Biochem* 54:558, 1955.

Arner P, Ostman J: Effect of nicotinic acid on acylglycerol metabolism in human adipose tissue. *Clin Sci* 64:235, 1983.

Athyros VG, Papageorgiou AA, Mercouris BR, et al: Treatment with atorvastatin to the National Cholesterol Educational Program goal versus "usual" care in secondary coronary heart disease prevention. The TREek Atorvastatin and Coronary-Heart Disease Evaluation (GREACE) Study. *Curr Med Res Opin* 18:220, 2002.

Azen SP, Mack WJ, Cashin-Hemphill L, et al: Progression of coronary artery disease predicts clinical coronary events. Long-term follow-up from the Cholesterol Lowering Atherosclerosis Study. *Circulation* 93:34, 1996.

Ballantyne CM, Corsini A, Davidson MH, et al: Risk of myopathy with statin therapy in high-risk patients. *Arch Intern Med* 163: 553, 2003.

Bays HE, Dujovne CA, McGovern ME, et al: Comparison of once-daily, niacin extended-release/lovastatin with standard doses of atorvastatin and simvastatin (The Advicor Versus Other Cholesterol-Modulating Agents Trial Evaluation [ADVOCATE]). *Am J Cardiol* 91:667, 2003.

Beattie MS, Shlipak MG, Liu H, et al: C-reactive protein and ischemia in users and nonusers of β–blockers and statins. Data from the Heart and Soul Study. *Circulation* 107:245, 2003.

Brown G, Albers JJ, Fisher LD, et al: Regression of coronary artery disease as a result of intensive lipid lowering therapy in men with high levels of apolipoprotein B. *N Engl J Med* 323:1289, 1990.

Brown BG, Zhao X-Q, Chait A, et al: Simvastatin and niacin, antioxidant vitamins, or the combination for the prevention of coronary disease. *N Engl J Med* 345:1583, 2001.

Campeau L, Hunninghake DB, Knatterud GL, et al: Aggressive cholesterol lowering delays saphenous vein graft atherosclerosis in women, the elderly, and patients with associated risk factors. NHLBI post coronary artery bypass graft clinical trial. *Circulation* 99:3241, 1999.

Canner PL, Berge KG, Wenger NK, et al: Fifteen year mortality in Coronary Drug Project patients: Long term benefit with niacin. *J Am Coll Cardiol* 8:1245, 1986.

Carlson LA, Danielson M, Ekberg I, et al: Reduction of myocardial reinfarction by the combined treatment with clofibrate and nicotinic acid. *Atherosclerosis* 28:81, 1977.

Cheng-Lai A: Rosurastatin: A new HMG-CoA reductase inhibitor for the treatment of hypercholesterolemia. *Heart Dis* 5:72, 2003.

Chien PC, Frishman WH: Lipid disorders, in Crawford MH (ed): *Current Diagnosis and Treatment in Cardiology,* 2nd ed. New York, McGraw-Hill, 2002, p 17.

Chui MCK, Newby DE, Panarelli M, et al: Association between calcific aortic stenosis and hypercholesterolemia: Is there a need for a randomized controlled trial of cholesterol-lowering therapy? *Clin Cardiol* 24:52, 2001.

Corti R, Fayad ZA, Fuster V, et al: Effects of lipid-lowering by simvastatin on human atherosclerotic lesions. A longitudinal study by high-resolution, noninvasive magnetic resonance imaging. *Circulation* 104:249, 2001.

Corvol J-C, Bouzamondo A, Sirol M, et al: Differential effects of lipid-lowering therapies on stroke prevention. A meta-analysis of randomized trials. *Arch Intern Med* 163:669, 2003.

Crouse JR III, Byington RP, Furberg CD: HMG-CoA reductase inhibitor therapy and stroke risk reduction: an analysis of clinical trials data. *Atherosclerosis* 138:11, 1998.

Crouse JR III, Lukacsko P, Niecestro R, and the Lovastatin Extended-Release Study Group: Dose response, safety and efficacy of an extended-release formulation of lovastatin in adults with hypercholesterolemia. *Am J Cardiol* 89:226, 2002.

Curran MP, Goa KL: Lovastatin extended release: A review of its use in the management of hypercholesterolemia. *Drugs* 63:685, 2003.

Dalton TA, Berry RS: Hepatotoxicity associated with sustained-release niacin. *Am J Med* 93:102, 1992.

Davidson MH, Dillon MA, Gordon B, et al: Colesevelam hydrochloride (Cholestagel). A new, potent bile acid sequestrant associated with a low incidence of gastrointestinal side effects. *Arch Intern Med*159:1893, 1999.

Davidson MH, Lukacsko P, Sun JX, et al: A multiple dose pharmacodynamic, safety and pharmacokinetic comparison of extended- and immediate-release formulations of lovastatin. *Clin Ther* 24:112, 2002.

Diabetes Atherosclerosis Intervention Study (DAIS) Investigators: Effect of fenofibrate on progression of coronary-artery disease in type 2 diabetes. *Lancet* 357:905, 2001.

Downs JR, Clearfield M, Weis S, et al: Primary prevention of acute coronary events with lovastatin in men and women with average cholesterol levels: Results of AFCAPS/TexCAPS. Air Force/Texas Coronary Atherosclerosis Prevention Study. *JAMA* 279:1615, 1998.

Dujovne CA, Ettinger MP, McNeer F, et al: Efficacy and safety of a potent new selective cholesterol absorption inhibitor, ezetimibe, in patients with primary hypercholesterolemia. *Am J Cardiol* 90:1092, 2002.

Dupuis J, Tardif JC, Cernacek P, Theroux P: Cholesterol reduction rapidly improves endothelial function after acute coronary syndromes. The RECIFE (Reduction of Cholesterol in Ischemia and Function of the Endothelium) trial. *Circulation* 99:3227, 1999.

Etchason JA, Miller TD, Squires RW, et al: Niacin-induced hepatitis: A potential side effect with low-dose time-release niacin. *Mayo Clin Proc* 66:23, 1991.

Executive Summary of the Third Report of the National Cholesterol Education Program (NCEP) Expert Panel on Detection, Evaluation and Treatment of High Blood Cholesterol in Adults (Adult Treatment Panel III). *JAMA* 285:2486, 2001.

Faergeman O: Hypertriglyceridemia and the fibrate trials. *Curr Opin Lipidol* 11:609, 2000.

Frishman WH, Choi AY, Guh A: Innovative medical approaches for the treatment of hyperlipidemia, in Frishman WH, Sonnenblick EH, Sica DA (eds): *Cardiovascular Pharmacotherapeutics,* 2nd ed. New York, McGraw Hill, 2003, p 841.

Fumagalli R: Pharmacokinetics of nicotinic acid and some of its derivatives, in Gey KF, Caarlson LA (eds): *Metabolic Effects of Nicotinic Acid and Its Derivatives.* Bern, Hans Huber, 1971, p 33.

Gagne C, Bays HE, Weiss SR, et al: Efficacy and safety of ezetimibe added to ongoing statin therapy for treatment of patients with primary hypercholesterolemia. *Am J Cardiol* 90:1084, 2002.

Goldberg A, Alagona P Jr, Capuzzi DM, et al: Multiple dose efficacy and safety of an extended-release form of niacin in the management of hyperlipidemia. *Am J Cardiol* 85:1100, 2000.

Gotto AM Jr, Farmer JA: Pleiotropic effects of statins: Do they matter? *Curr Opin Lipidol* 12:391, 2001.

Gould AL, Roussouw JE, Santanello NC, et al: Cholesterol reduction yields clinical benefit. Impact of statin trials. *Circulation* 97:946, 1998.

Grundy SM, Vega GL, McGovern ME, et al: Efficacy, safety and tolerability of once-daily niacin for the treatment of dyslipidemia associated with type 2 diabetes: Results of the Assessment of Diabetes Control and Evaluation of the Efficacy of Niaspan Trial. *Arch Intern Med* 162:1568, 2002.

Gupta EK, Ito MK: Lovastatin and extended-release niacin combination product. The first drug combination for the treatment of hyperlipidemia. *Heart Dis* 4:124, 2002.

Gupta EK, Ito MK: Ezetimibe: The first in a novel class of selective cholesterol-absorption inhibitors. *Heart Dis* 4:399, 2002.

Haffner SM, Lehto S, Ronnemaa T, et al: Mortality from coronary heart disease in sub-jects with type 2 diabetes and in nondiabetic subjects with and without prior myocardial infarction. *N Engl J Med* 339:229, 1998

Heart Protection Study Collaborative Group: MRC/BHF Heart Protection Study of cho-lesterol lowering with simvastatin in 20,536 high-risk individuals: a randomised placebo-controlled trial. *Lancet* 360:7, 2002.

Heeschen C, Hamm CW, Laufs U, et al: Withdrawal of statins increases event rates in patients with acute coronary syndromes. *Circulation* 105:1446, 2002.

Horne BD, Mulhestein JB, Carlquist JF, et al: Statin therapy interacts with cytomega-lovirus seropositivity and high C-reactive protein in reducing mortality among patients with angiographically significant coronary disease. *Circulation* 107:258, 2003.

Jones PH, Davidson MH, Stein EA, et al for the STELLAR Study Group: Comparison of the efficacy and safety of rosuvastatin versus atorvastatin, simvastatin, and pravastatin across doses (STELLAR) trial. *Am J Cardiol* 93:152, 2003.

Kidney Disease Outcomes Quality Initiative Clinical Practice Guidelines for Managing Dyslipidemias in Chronic Kidney Disease: II, Assessment of dyslipidemias. *Am J Kidney Dis* 41(suppl 3): S22, 2003.

Kinlay S, Selwyn AP: Effects of statins on inflammation in patients with acute and chronic coronary syndromes. *Am J Cardiol* 91(4A):9B, 2003.

Knapp HH, Schrott H, Ma P, et al: Efficacy and safety of combination simvastatin and colesevelam in patients with primary hypercholesterolemia. *Am J Med* 110:352, 2001.

Knopp RH: Drug treatment of lipid disorders. *N Engl J Med* 341:498, 1999.

Knopp RH, Ginsberg J, Albers JJ, et al: Contrasting effects of unmodified and time-release forms of niacin on lipoproteins in hyperlipidemic Long-Term Intervention with Pravastatin in Ischaemic Disease (LIPID) Study Group: Prevention of cardio-vascular events and death with pravastatin in patients with coronary heart disease and a broad range of initial cholesterol levels. *N Engl J Med* 339:1349, 1998.

Lau WC, Waskell LA, Watkins PB,e t al: Atorvastatin reduces the ability of clopidogrel to inhibit platelet aggregation. A new drug–drug interaction. *Circulation* 107:32, 2003.

Libby P, Aikawa M: Mechanisms of plaque stabilization with statins. *Am J Cardiol* 91(4A):4B, 2003.

Mahley RW, Bersot TP: Drug therapy for hypercholesterolemia and dyslipidemia, in Hardman JG, Limbird LE (eds): *Goodman and Gilman's the Pharmacological Basis of Therapeutics,* 10th ed. New York, McGraw-Hill, 2001, p 971.

Marais AD: Therapeutic modulation of low-density lipoprotein size. *Curr Opin Lipidol* 11:597, 2000.

McTaggart F, Buckett L, Davidson R, et al: Preclinical and clinical pharmacology of rosuvastatin, a new 3-hydroxy-3-methylglutaryl coenzyme A reductase inhibitor. *Am J Cardiol* 87(suppl):28B, 2001.

Newby LK, Kristinsson A, Bhapkar MV, et al: Early statin initiation and outcomes in patients with acute coronary syndromes. *JAMA* 287:3087, 2002.

Pasternak RC, Smith SC Jr, Bairey-Merz CN, et al: ACC/AHA/NHLBT Clinical Advisory on the Use and Safety of Statins. *J Am Coll Cardiol* 40:567, 2002.

Petrack B, Greengard P, Kalinsky H: On the relative efficacy of nicotinamide and nicotinic acid as precursors of nicotinamide adenine dinucleotide. *J Biol Chem* 241:2367, 1966.

Ridker PM, Stampfer MJ, Rifai N: Novel risk factors for systemic atherosclerosis. A comparison of C-reactive protein, fibrinogen, lipoprotein(a), and standard cholesterol screening as predictors of peripheral arterial disease. *JAMA* 285:2481, 2001.

Rubins HB, Davenport J, Babikian V, et al, for the VA-HIT Study Group: Reduction in stroke with gemfibrozil in men with coronary heart disease and low HDL cholesterol. The Veterans Affairs HDL Intervention Trial (VA-HIT). *Circulation* 103:2828, 2001.

Schwartz GG, Olsson AG, Ezekowitz MD, et al: Effects of atorvastatin on early recurrent ischemic events in acute coronary syndromes: The MIRACL study: A randomized controlled trial. *JAMA* 285:1711, 2001.

See M, Hoppichler F, Reavely D, et al: Relation of serum lipoprotein(a) concentration and apolipoprotein(a) phenotype to coronary heart disease in patients with familial hypercholesterolemia. *N Engl J Med* 322:1494, 1990.

Serebruany VL, Steinhubl SR, Hennekens CH: Are antiplatelet effects of clopidogrel inhibited by atorvastatin? A research question formulated but not yet adequately tested. *Circulation* 107:1568, 2003.

Serruys PWJC, deFeyter P, Macaya C, et al, for the Lescol Intervention Prevention Study (LIPS) Investigators: Fluvastatin for prevention of cardiac events following successful first percutaneous coronary intervention. A randomized controlled trial. *JAMA* 287:3215, 2002.

Sever PS, Dahlof B, Poulter NR, et al: Prevention of coronary and stroke events with atorvastatin in hypertensive patients who have average or lower-than-average cholesterol concentrations, in the Anglo Scandinavian Cardiac Outcomes Trial-Lipid Lowering Arm (ASCOT-LLA): a multicentre randomized controlled trial. *Lancet* 361:1149, 2003.

Sharrett AR, Ballantyne CM, Coady SA, et al: Coronary heart disease prediction from lipoprotein cholesterol levels, triglycerides, lipoprotein(a), apolipoproteins A-I and B, and HDL density subfractions: The Atherosclerosis Risk in Communities (ARIC) Study. *Circulation* 104:1108, 2001

Shepherd J, Blauw GJ, Murphy MB, et al, on behalf of PROSPER Study Group: Pravastatin in Elderly Individuals at Risk of Vascular Disease (PROSPER): A randomized controlled trial. *Lancet* 360:1623, 2002.

Smilde TJ, van Wissen S, Wollersheim H, et al: Effect of aggressive versus conventional lipid lowering on atherosclerosis progression in familial hypercholesterolaemia (ASAP): A prospective, randomised, double-blind trial. *Lancet* 357:577, 2001.

Smith SC Jr, Blair SN, Bonow RO, et al: AHA/ACC guidelines for preventing heart attack and death in patients with atherosclerotic cardiovascular disease: 2001 update. *Circulation* 104:1577, 2001.

Staels B, Dallongeville J, Auwerx J, et al: Mechanism of action of fibrates on lipid and lipoprotein metabolism. *Circulation* 98:2088, 1998.

Steinberg D, Gotto AM Jr: Preventing coronary artery disease by lowering cholesterol levels. Fifty years from bench to bedside. *JAMA* 282:2043, 1999.

Stenestrand U, Wallentin L, for the Swedish Register of Cardiac Intensive Care (RIKS-HIA): Early statin treatment following acute myocardial infarction and 1-year survival. *JAMA* 285:430, 2001.

Thompson PD, Clarkson P, Karas RH: Statin-associated myopathy. *JAMA* 289:1681, 2003.

Umans-Eckenhausen MAW, Defesche JC, van Dam MJ, Kastelein JJP: Long-term compliance with lipid-lowering medication after genetic screening for familial hypercholesterolemia. *Arch Intern Med* 163:65, 2003.

Vaugh CL: Prevention of stroke and dementia with statins: Effects beyond lipid lowering. *Am J Cardiol* 91(4A):23B, 2003.

Waldman A, Kritharides L: The pleiotropic effects of HMG-CoA reductase inhibitors. Their role in osteoporosis and dementia. *Drugs* 63:139, 2003.

Warshafsky S, Packard D, Marks SJ, et al: Efficacy of 3-hydroxy-3-methylglutaryl coenzyme A reductase inhibitors for prevention of stroke. *J Gen Intern Med* 14: 763, 1999.

White HD, Simes J, Anderson NE, et al: Pravastatin therapy and the risk of stroke. *N Engl J Med* 343:317, 2000.

Writing Group for the Women's Health Initiative Investigators: Risks and benefits of estrogen plus progestin in healthy postmenopausal women. Principal results from the Women's Health Initiative Randomized Controlled Trial. *JAMA* 288:321, 2002.

Yeung AC, Tsao P: Statin therapy. Beyond cholesterol lowering and anti-inflammatory effects. *Circulation* 105:2937, 2002.

Zimetbaum P, Frishman WH, Kahn S: Effects of gemfibrozil and other fibric acid derivatives on blood lipids and lipoproteins, in Frishman WH (ed): *Medical Management of Lipid Disorders: Focus on Prevention of Coronary Artery Disease.* Mt Kisco, Futura Publishing, 1992, p 125.

Zimetbaum P, Frishman WH, Ooi WL, et al: Plasma lipids and lipoproteins and the incidence of cardiovascular disease in the old: The Bronx Longitudinal Aging Study. *Arteriol Thromb* 12:416, 1992.

16 | Combination Drug Therapy

Michael A. Weber   Joel M. Neutel
William H. Frishman

Almost all major cardiovascular diseases are treated with combination therapy. Conditions such as congestive heart failure and angina pectoris are typically treated with three or more drugs, and there is growing evidence that even prophylactic therapies designed to prevent thrombotic episodes may best be achieved with more than one agent. The main focus of this chapter, however, is to explore the use of combination therapy in systemic hypertension.

The well-established benefits of combination treatment as compared with single-agent treatment include greater efficacy, reduced or attenuated side effects, and convenience. However, new evidence from major hypertension trials with clinical end points has created a new imperative in the management of hypertension: the reduction of blood pressure below aggressive target levels. Current guideline recommendations (see later) have suggested the achievement of blood pressure values below 140/90 mm Hg in hypertensive patients in general; however, for those considered at high risk—including diabetics or those with evidence for renal or other target organ involvement—blood pressure should be 130/85 mm Hg or even lower. In most instances, achieving these goals requires at least two antihypertensive agents and often three or more.

The studies that have helped influence this new attitude include the Hypertension Optimal Treatment study, the United Kingdom Prospective Diabetes Study, and the Modification of Diet in Renal Disease study. These clinical outcomes studies emphasized that the achievement of low blood pressure levels during therapy might be just as important, if not more so, as basing therapy on appropriate pharmacologic agents. One interesting example of this type has been the African American Study of Kidney Disease and Hypertension study, in which progression of renal disease in African American hypertensive patients was substantially slowed by therapy with an angiotensin-converting enzyme (ACE) inhibitor. Even though ACE inhibitors generally have not been highly effective in reducing blood pressure in African American patients, the use of combination therapy in this study achieved appropriate blood pressure goals and allowed these patients to benefit from the selective renal-protective effects of the ACE inhibitor.

Marketing surveys in the antihypertensive area have indicated that physicians in general now understand the value of combination therapy. In particular, fixed combinations of such agents as ACE inhibitors and calcium channel blockers are rapidly growing in use, and fixed combinations of angiotensin receptor blockers (ARBs) with diuretics now account for well over 30% of the use of these newer agents.

PRINCIPLES OF COMBINATION THERAPY

Drug combinations have been used traditionally to treat many cardiovascular conditions such as congestive heart failure, angina pectoris, and hypertension, but the historical development of using multiple medications has differed for each condition. For example, digitalis was used first in the 18th century to provide clinical benefits for patients with congestive heart failure. Then, in the mid-1990s, diuretics were shown to produce symptomatic and functional advantages when used in addition to digitalis. More recently, physicians added an ACE inhibitor to digitalis and diuretic treatment to improve clinical findings and prolong survival, thereby completing a logical triad of drugs, each of which contributed in a separate but meaningful fashion. Most recently, adding beta blockers, spironolactone, and even ARBs to ACE inhibitors has been shown to further enhance outcomes in congestive heart failure, thereby providing a powerful illustration of the potential value of well-fashioned combination therapy.

Hypertension therapy, which is the main focus of this chapter, has almost always required drug combinations. Usually more than one drug was required, because earlier classes of drugs were not effective alone or doses that produced efficacious decreases in blood pressure, unfortunately, also produced unacceptable adverse side effects or events. Indeed, 30 years ago the pooling of low doses of as many as three separate agents into a single fixed-dose product was quite commonplace. SerApEs, for example, brought together reserpine, hydralazine, and hydrochlorothiazide; this fixed-combination product was popular with physicians, reasonably well tolerated by patients, and quite effective for reducing blood pressure.

The first attempt at a systematic method for treating hypertension was termed the *stepped-care* approach. Very simply, it recommended that treatment of all hypertensive patients begin with a diuretic—albeit in higher doses than would be customary at present. If the diuretic was not efficacious, then a second-step drug, typically a sympatholytic agent, could be added. If success was still not achieved, then a third-step drug, usually a vasodilator, would be superimposed on the previous drugs. Yet further agents could be added, as necessary, to bring the blood pressure under control. At each step, the added medication usually would be increased to the maximum dose, often limited by side effects or adverse reactions.

EVOLUTION OF CARE

The stepped-care approach, employing separate drug prescriptions or the use of fixed combinations, became standard practice by the early 1970s. Almost immediately, however, conceptual challenges to this method of treatment began to appear, especially from the volume vasoconstriction hypothesis. It was postulated that essential hypertension is a heterogeneous condition in which each patient has a different combination of volume excess and vasoconstriction as the pathophysiologic cause of the high blood pressure. Thus, ideally, some patients should be treated with diuretics to reduce the volume-excess component, whereas other patients, whose excess vasoconstriction might be due largely to increased activity of the renin-angiotensin system, should be treated with drugs to inhibit renin release or to block the formation of angiotensin II.

It was suggested that a simple measurement of plasma renin activity could guide the selection of a single agent from the drug class most likely to be beneficial. For instance, low plasma renin levels would suggest volume excess (treatable with diuretics), and high plasma renin levels would suggest increased activation of the renin-angiotensin system (treatable with ACE inhibitors or beta blockers). Of course, for the patients whose plasma renin levels fell into the middle range, presumably indicating the presence of volume and vasoconstriction factors, it might be necessary to use a combination of these drugs. Also, at the time, it was reported that patients with different demographic backgrounds had different renin profiles and a tendency to respond preferentially to certain drug types. For example, European American or relatively young patients tended to respond well to such agents as beta blockers, whereas African American patients and the elderly tended to respond well to diuretics.

As diagnostic and therapeutic strategies evolved, innovative new drug classes were created. Later-generation beta blockers, the calcium channel blockers, the ACE inhibitors, and ARBs were effective and produced relatively few adverse events or side effects. For these reasons, the Fourth Joint National Committee (JNC-IV) recommended individualizing therapy and encouraged physicians to search for the single agent that would best suit the needs of each patient. Diuretics, beta blockers, calcium channel blockers, and ACE inhibitors were considered appropriate drugs with which to initiate the treatment of hypertension.

Despite this progress, the overall treatment of hypertension has not progressed satisfactorily. The most recent National Health and Nutrition Examination Survey reported that only 31% of hypertensive patients in the United States had their blood pressures reduced below 140/90 mm Hg. The growing number of drug classes and individual agents for the management of hypertension suggests that, as yet, there are no fully adequate solutions. Drug combinations, therefore, remain a staple of antihypertensive therapy now and for the foreseeable future.

A MATTER OF DEFINITION

Combination therapy involves multiple doses of multiple medications. Most commonly, physicians will start with a single agent and, after making adjustments to its dose, will add additional drugs and adjust the doses as necessary. Most of the discussion in this chapter assumes this approach. However, from the very origins of antihypertensive therapy, manufacturers have made available a variety of fixed combinations. The intent of these products has been to provide a simpler and more convenient way of taking more than one agent. By and large, these fixed-dose combinations have been only moderately successful in the marketplace. For example, it is estimated that fixed formulations of an ACE inhibitor and a diuretic are prescribed only 10% as frequently as the primary ACE inhibitor. The main objection to these products has been that they do not allow physicians to titrate the dose of each drug separately but rather compel them to prescribe the use of the two agents in a prefixed ratio. This objection has been particularly popular in academic medical centers, where physicians usually have not allowed fixed combinations on their formularies. The attitude of the U.S. Food and Drug Administration (FDA) toward these combinations also has not encouraged their use. The regulatory agency has insisted that physicians first titrate each component to an appropriate level and then switch to the combination product only if the doses correspond to an available fixed combination. In reality, these products have gone through rigorous testing to ascertain the optimal doses of each agent within the combination. Apparently, most physicians find this a tedious approach and tend to construct their own multidrug combination regimens.

There have been exceptions to this rule. Combinations of two diuretics, hydrochlorothiazide and triamterene, with the trade names of Dyazide and Maxzide, respectively, have been widely accepted. Likewise, Ziac, which contains a diuretic and a beta blocker, Logimax, which contains a beta blocker and a calcium channel blocker, and Lotrel, Teczem, Lexxel, and Tarka, which contain an ACE inhibitor and a calcium channel blocker, have received attention because of the unusual nature of their dosing or their components.

Manufacturers sometimes have selected names for these fixed combinations that differ totally from those of the individual components to create the impression of what they call "new types of dual-acting single entities." Market research data seem to confirm the success of these strategies. For example, in the United States during the 1993–1994 and 1994–1995 business years, the growth rates of total prescriptions were 6% and 7% for single-agent antihypertensives and 8% and 20% for fixed combinations, respectively.

RATIONALE FOR COMBINATION THERAPY

Treating hypertension with combination therapy provides more opportunity for creative solutions to a number of problems. Five issues in combined therapy—some practical, some speculative—are listed in Table 16-1.

The most obvious benefit of drug combinations is the enhanced efficacy that fosters their continued widespread use. Theoretically, some drug combinations might produce synergistic effects that are greater than would be predicted by summing the efficacies of the component drugs. More commonly, combination therapy achieves a little less than the sum of its component drug efficacies. In contrast, some combinations of drugs produce offsetting interactions that weaken rather than strengthen their antihypertensive effects, as previously seen with agents affecting peripheral and neuronal actions. For instance, guanethidine and reserpine produced this offsetting interaction; however, these agents are now used only rarely, so this issue need not be considered further.

A second benefit of combination therapy concerns the avoidance of adverse effects. When patients are treated with two drugs, each drug can be administered in a lower dose that does not produce unwanted side effects but nonetheless contributes to overall efficacy. A third issue concerns convenience. On the one hand, the multiple drugs of a combination regimen could be confusing and distracting to patients and could lead to poor treatment compliance. On the other hand, a well-designed combination pill that incorporates logical doses of two agents could enhance convenience and improve compliance.

Further potential value of combination treatment may result from the effects that two drugs have on each other's pharmacokinetics. Although this has not been well studied, there might be situations in which the clinical duration of action of the participating drugs becomes longer when used in combination

TABLE 16-1 Rationale for Combination Drug Therapy for Hypertension

Increased antihypertensive efficacy
  Additive effects
  Synergistic effects
Reduced adverse events
  Low-dose strategy
  Drugs with offsetting actions
Enhanced convenience and compliance
Prolonged duration of action
Potential for additive target organ protection

than when they are administered as monotherapies. It is interesting to consider the attributes of such agents as ACE inhibitors, ARBs, and calcium channel blockers that exhibit antigrowth or anti-atherosclerotic actions in addition to their blood pressure-lowering properties. Is it possible that combinations of these newer agents may provide even more powerful protective effects on the circulation? Each of these five potentially important attributes of antihypertensive combination therapy is considered in more detail below.

EFFICACY OF COMBINATION THERAPY

The most common motivation for administering more than one antihypertensive agent is to increase overall efficacy. Most of the time, the effects of the two agents being used are approximately additive, although it is likely—in view of the theories of hypertension heterogeneity reviewed earlier—that one drug plays a predominant role in reducing the blood pressure. Sometimes, a form of synergy can be achieved.

There are data from a study in which each hypertensive patient was treated with three different regimens at different times: the beta blocker metoprolol, 100 to 400 mg daily alone; the diuretic hydrochlorothiazide, 50 mg daily alone; or both drugs in combination. The three active treatment periods were separated by periods of placebo treatment. Metoprolol monotherapy in this predominantly European American group was slightly more effective than the diuretic. The combination in turn clearly was more effective than either of the individual therapies. Of particular note, statistical testing, which used the pooled estimate of the within-sample variance derived from the error sum of squares, confirmed that the lower end of the 95% confidence limits of the decreases in systolic and diastolic blood pressures during combination therapy exceeded the sum of the blood pressure decreases produced by each drug alone. This finding suggested a synergistic effect. In these patients, the 50-mg diuretic dose, high by today's standards, had strong stimulatory effects on the renin-aldosterone axis. In contrast, metoprolol had an inhibitory effect on this axis. Most importantly, the metoprolol appeared to neutralize the renin-stimulating effects of hydrochlorothiazide during the combination therapy, thereby counteracting vasoconstrictor and other reactions to the diuretic. This mechanism appears to explain the excellent efficacy achieved when beta blockers, ACE inhibitors, and other antagonists of the renin axis are combined with a diuretic.

In contrast, another study treated each patient with three different therapies at different times, with placebo periods in between: (1) propranolol, a beta blocker; (2) clonidine, a centrally acting sympatholytic; or (3) propranolol and clonidine combined. Each drug was effective as monotherapy, and the two in combination were slightly better than either monotherapy but not equal to the predicted sum of effects of both drugs. It is noteworthy that each of these agents had inhibitory effects on renin and aldosterone but that their combined use did not potentiate this action. Thus, although these two drugs could be useful when administered together, this combination does not appear to offer the same logic and power of additive or synergistic effects seen when agents with disparate mechanisms are combined.

The principal antihypertensive drug classes in modern use are diuretics, beta blockers, calcium channel blockers, ACE inhibitors, angiotensin II receptor antagonists, selective alpha blockers, centrally acting sympatholytic agents, and direct-acting vasodilators. This wide array of drug classes offers an enormous number of potential combinations. In reality, most fixed-combination products on the market employ a diuretic, mirroring the clinical practice of most physicians. Therefore, the diuretic-containing formulations are discussed and then, briefly, some nondiuretic combinations of interest are reviewed.

COMBINATIONS INVOLVING A DIURETIC

Before considering their role in combination therapy, it is helpful to define the way in which diuretics are used currently. The popularity of this class of agents has increased recently with the results of the Antihypertensive and Lipid-Lowering Treatment to Prevent Heart Attack Trial (ALLHAT) showing their safety and efficacy as monotherapy and in combination with other antihypertensive drug classes. Diuretics are used mostly in doses far lower than when they were first used; 12.5 mg has become quite typical, especially when used as part of a combination, and doses as low as 6.25 mg can be effective when used in combinations. Most of the modern fixed-dose products that include diuretics have used these lower doses.

Combination with ACE Inhibitors

Combining a diuretic with an ACE inhibitor is one of the most logical approaches to the treatment of hypertension. Diuretics work primarily by increasing renal clearance of sodium and water, thereby reducing intravascular volume, at least in the short term. For many patients, a diuretic alone is an effective way to reduce blood pressure. For example, monotherapy with diuretics is often effective in African American patients and in the elderly. The renin-angiotensin system of patients in these two groups often exhibits less of a reactive response to volume depletion and thus generates less compensatory angiotensin-mediated vasoconstriction. In contrast, ACE inhibitors are often effective in European American hypertensive patients and in other settings where renin activity is relatively high. From a clinical perspective, diuretics and ACE inhibitors appear to have complementary properties. These attributes appear to be maximized when the two drug classes are used together, especially as the ACE inhibitors effectively prevent the counterproductive stimulation of the renin-angiotensin system produced by diuretics.

Clinical trials have confirmed that these complementary properties are highly effective. In patients whose blood pressures have responded only partly to initial treatment with an ACE inhibitor, addition of even a very small dose of diuretic is more effective in reducing blood pressure than major increases in the dose of the ACE inhibitor.

Of practical importance, the combination of a diuretic with an ACE inhibitor appears to be effective in as many African American as European American patients. This has strong clinical implications beyond blood pressure itself, as discussed elsewhere in this book. ACE inhibitors are now believed to have powerful renal and cardiovascular protective properties, and the thoughtful use of diuretic and ACE inhibitor combinations will make it possible for African American patients, who are particularly vulnerable to hypertensive renal disease, to benefit from these target organ actions.

It should be stressed that only small doses of diuretics are required in this type of combination treatment. In fact, most currently available fixed-dose combinations of ACE inhibitors and diuretics use a dose of 12.5 mg of hydrochlorothiazide. In addition, ACE inhibitors and diuretics may have off-setting metabolic effects. These are discussed briefly later in this chapter.

A multicenter study of 6105 patients with a history of stroke or transient ischemic attack recently demonstrated that the combination of the diuretic indapamide and the ACE inhibitor perindopril reduce the risk of stroke by one-third when compared with placebo or monotherapy. One of 10 stroke survivors given the combination therapy avoided death, heart attack, or further stroke even without a history of hypertension.

Combination of Diuretics with Angiotensin Receptor Antagonists

Much of the theory underlying the successful pairing of diuretics with ACE inhibitors should apply to diuretics with ARBs. Available agents work by selectively blocking the angiotensin II receptor (AT_1), thereby interrupting most of the known hemodynamic, endocrine, and growth effects of the renin-angiotensin system.

Clinical trials with losartan have shown that the addition of hydrochlorothiazide in a dose of 12.5 mg can increase the antihypertensive response rate from approximately 50% to almost 80%. Clearly, the effects of the AT_1 blocker and the diuretic in combination are additive. An example of this efficacy is shown in Table 16-2. These data show that the addition of 12.5 mg of hydrochlorothiazide in patients receiving placebo or a variety of losartan dosing regimens produces consistent beneficial effects. Indeed, the blood pressure decrements observed when the diuretic is added to the losartan treatments are virtually identical to those observed when the diuretic is added to placebo, suggesting that these two drugs have a true additive effect when given in

TABLE 16-2 Effects on Systolic and Diastolic Blood Pressures of Monotherapy with Placebo or Various Dosages of Losartan Followed by Combination Therapy with Hydrochlorothiazide

Treatment	No. of patients	Systolic/diastolic, mean (SD)		
		Baseline	After 4 wk monotherapy	Additional decrease after 2 wk of combination therapy with HCTZ 12.5 mg/d
Placebo	26	148.5 (14.7)/ 100.5 (3.8)	150.8 (12.9)/ 99.9 (5.9)	8.7 (11.4)/ 4.0 (6.4)
Losartan				
50 mg qd	21	159.3 (16.6)/ 101.0 (4.9)	148.9 (16.5)/ 96.2 (7.9)	5.5 (14.0)/ 5.1 (7.8)
100 mg qd	16	150.9 (14.0)/ 102.3 (4.7)	140.9 (15.7)/ 95.6 (7.6)	6.0 (7.5)/ 4.0 (6.1)
50 mg bid	20	155.2 (13.8)/ 101.7 (4.1)	146.2 (12.6)/ 95.6 (6.4)	7.3 (10.4)/ 4.0 (6.9)

Key: bid, twice daily; HCTZ, hydrochlorothiazide; qd, once daily; SD, standard deviation.
Source: Reproduced with permission from Weber MA, Byyny RL, Pratt JH, et al: Blood pressure effects of the angiotensin II receptor blocker losartan. *Arch Intern Med* 155:405, 1995.

combination. A very low dose of 6.25 mg of hydrochlorothiazide in combination with losartan was tested in one study, and the results indicated that this dose may not be adequate to optimize efficacy.

In clinical trials in patients with essential hypertension, adding hydrochlorothiazide 12.5 or 25 mg/day to valsartan 80 mg/day resulted in a greater blood pressure reduction than did increasing the valsartan dose to 160 mg/day. Similarly, in African American hypertensives, adding 12.5 mg of hydrochlorothiazide to valsartan 160 mg/day resulted in substantially greater blood pressure reduction than that achieved by increasing valsartan from 160 to 320 mg/day or by adding benazepril 20 mg/day. Efficacy of the valsartan and hydrochlorothiazide combination was maintained up to 3 years of treatment. Similar findings have been observed with other diuretic AT_1 blocker combinations (i.e., hydrochlorothiazide/irbesartan, hydrochlorothiazide/telmisartan, and hydrochlorothiazide/candesartan).

Combination of Diuretics with Beta Blockers

The combination of diuretics with beta blockers is highly efficacious and shares mechanisms in common with the ACE inhibitor and diuretic combinations. Earlier we discussed the combination of hydrochlorothiazide with metoprolol and used it as an example of a synergistic relationship between two agents. Although illustrative, that particular example may not be typical of more modern diuretic usage, where doses are lower and stimulation of the renin system is less extreme. Beta blockers, as monotherapy, appear to be effective often in European American patients and the young, although they can be effective in older patients. These agents, however, do not appear to be very effective in low-renin hypertension. In fact, we previously noted a paradoxical increase in blood pressure in low-renin patients treated with propranolol, perhaps reflecting the unmasking of vasoconstrictor alpha-adrenergic activity resulting from the blockade of beta-receptors.

Because beta blockers were introduced into widespread clinical use several years before the ACE inhibitors, most of the experience with beta blocker and diuretic combinations, especially fixed combinations, had been with relatively higher diuretic doses. Typically, hydrochlorothiazide was used in 25-mg doses. There is one unique and exciting recent exception to this rule: the fixed combination of a very low dose of the beta blocker bisoprolol with a dose of only 6.25 mg of hydrochlorothiazide. The implications of this special case are discussed later in this chapter.

Combination of Diuretics with Calcium Channel Blockers

Unlike the ACE inhibitors and the beta blockers, the calcium channel blockers have been theorized to be poor choices for combination with a diuretic. Because the calcium channel blockers and diuretics are thought to work best in similar populations, such as the elderly and African Americans, and to be most effective in low-renin hypertension, they might be too similar to provide additive effects. Acute administration of calcium channel blockers also has been shown to produce measurable natriuresis, further suggesting that these two classes would not have complementary actions. Experience with different states of sodium loading has reinforced these prejudices. Dietary sodium restriction may attenuate the antihypertensive efficacy of calcium channel blocker monotherapy, whereas sodium loading may actually enhance it. In

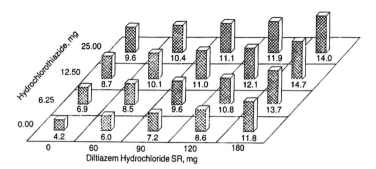

FIG. 16-1   Estimated mean supine diastolic blood pressure reduction (in millimeters of mercury) in response to therapy. Each dose was administered twice a day. SR, slow release. (*Reproduced with permission from Burris JF, Weir MR, Oparil S, et al: An assessment of diltiazem and hydrochlorothiazide in hypertension. Application of factorial trial design to a multicenter clinical trial of combination therapy. JAMA 263: 1507, 1990.*)

experimental rat models, sodium loading has been shown to increase the number of dihydropyridine receptors on cell membranes; under these circumstances, the calcium channel blockers appear to have increased effectiveness in limiting sympathetic stimulation.

However, in practice, the combination of calcium channel blockers and diuretics has worked very well in the clinical setting. All three major types of calcium channel blockers currently available—verapamil, diltiazem, and the dihydropyridines—have been shown to produce additive effects when combined with a diuretic. Indeed, some investigators have shown that the addition of a calcium channel blocker to a diuretic produces antihypertensive effects similar in amplitude to those observed when beta blockers or ACE inhibitors were added to a diuretic.

Some of the pivotal studies of the effects of combining calcium channel blockers and diuretics employed an innovative study design; the efficacies of a matrix of different calcium channel blocker and diuretic doses were compared with each other and with placebo to define the optimal composition of the combinations. The results of a study using this factorial design to evaluate diltiazem and hydrochlorothiazide are shown in Fig. 16-1. Each of the drugs is more efficacious than placebo, and it is clear that their effects are additive when used in combination. It is also interesting that the low 6.25-mg diuretic dose contributes usefully to the combined effect, especially when used with the higher doses of diltiazem. Documentation of the dose–response relationships of the drugs and their combinations can be accomplished by a response surface analysis.

Combination of Diuretics with Sympatholytics

A relatively large array of antihypertensive drugs, especially in the earlier days of antihypertensive drug development, was targeted primarily at the sympathetic nervous system. Some, such as clonidine and alpha-methyldopa, worked centrally to reduce sympathetic outflow. These agents could be effective as monotherapy but were more efficacious when combined with a diuretic. Newer members of this class, most recently, guanfacine, are actually designed to supplement a diuretic. Sympatholytic agents with more peripheral sites of action, including reserpine and guanethidine, benefited similarly from working in combination with a diuretic. It should be remembered that most of these drugs were developed, and became popular, during the era when the stepped-care approach was the standard and when the therapy of most hypertensive patients started with a diuretic. Alpha-methyldopa, clonidine, and reserpine, among others, were formulated in fixed combinations with diuretics and were available as monotherapies. The newer, selective alpha$_1$-blockers—notably prazosin, terazosin, and doxazosin—can also have their efficacy enhanced when combined with a diuretic agent.

Combination of Two Diuretics

It is rarely necessary to prescribe two diuretics at one time. This need usually occurs in the presence of renal insufficiency when refractory fluid retention might not respond adequately to usual or higher doses of a single diuretic. Under those circumstances, a loop diuretic or an agent such as metolazone might be combined with one of the more conventional thiazides.

The use of the combination of hydrochlorothiazide with the potassium-sparing diuretics triamterene, spironolactone, and amiloride has become ubiquitous. The two most common proprietary diuretic formulations in wide use are Dyazide, which contains hydrochlorothiazide 25 mg and triamterene 50 mg, and Maxzide, which contains hydrochlorothiazide 50 mg and triamterene 75 mg. Dyazide is provided as a capsule, whereas Maxzide comes as a tablet that can be halved for a lower dose. These products are so well accepted that they are in effect often considered to be single entities. The confidence of physicians in these formulations may be well placed, for there has been recent evidence that diuretics that are not combined with a potassium-sparing component may be associated with an increased risk of sudden cardiac death in hypertensive patients.

OTHER ANTIHYPERTENSIVE COMBINATIONS

There is almost no limit to the number of ways in which different drug classes and individual agents can be combined effectively in the management of hypertension. Some of the more interesting examples of such combinations are considered below.

Hydralazine, the direct-acting vasodilator, is effective during chronic treatment almost only when used as part of a combination. Although it is a powerful arterial vasodilator, this drug stimulates two powerful reactive mechanisms: it produces marked fluid retention and it causes tachycardia, renin release, and other evidence of sympathetic activation. Therefore, for hydralazine to work effectively, it must be combined with a diuretic and with a sympatholytic agent. For this reason, the stepped-care approach had always listed hydralazine as a third-step drug; it would be futile to administer it without a diuretic and sympatholytic drug already in place. Interestingly, the historical three-part fixed-dose combination SerApEs contained all three of these components: hydrochlorothiazide, reserpine, and hydralazine. This product is no longer available.

The newer drug classes have prompted innovative new combinations, and pharmaceutical manufacturers have been studying formulations pairing two nondiuretic drugs. Three current combination formulations are worth exploring. The first combines calcium channel blockers with beta blockers. Because they have complementary actions, at least in terms of the patient demographics in which they work best, beta blockers and calcium channel blockers should work well together. One combination that has completed pivotal early clinical trials couples felodipine, the calcium blocker, with metoprolol, the beta blocker. This product (brand name Logimax) is significantly more efficacious than either of its component drugs alone. The data indicate that decrements in systolic and diastolic blood pressures are superior with the combination.

The development of Logimax highlights another issue in formulating fixed combinations: because each component drug is formulated to maximize its own constant delivery and duration of action, the marrying of the two agents requires rigorous engineering and testing to ensure that their essential pharmacokinetic properties are maintained.

The second nondiuretic combination to be discussed involves the coupling of a calcium channel blocker with an ACE inhibitor. Fixed combinations of amlodipine and benazepril (Lotrel), verapamil and trandolapril (Tarka), felodipine extended release (ER) and enalapril (Lexxel), and diltiazem and enalapril (Teczem) were released for hypertension therapy and are currently the only available nondiuretic, fixed-dose combination antihypertensives. Their mechanistic logic is similar to that of an ACE inhibitor and diuretic combination. The calcium channel blocker works best in low-renin hypertension and in a large percentage of African Americans and the elderly, and it appears to be effective in blocking actions of the sympathetic nervous system. The ACE inhibitor works best in high-renin hypertension, succeeds in a large percentage of European American patients and the young, and is obviously effective at interrupting the renin-angiotensin system. Moreover, unlike a diuretic, the calcium channel blocker should not cause any unwanted metabolic effects. The effects of amlodipine alone, benazepril alone, their combination, and placebo have been compared. The study employed ambulatory blood pressure monitoring and demonstrated that benazepril and amlodipine each provide consistent antihypertensive efficacy during the 24-h dosing interval. The combination clearly provides additive efficacy throughout the day. The experience obtained during the development of this fixed-dose combination showed that its response rate, defined as a reduction in diastolic blood pressure to less than 90 mm Hg or a decrease of at least 10 mm Hg, exceeded 80% in patients with mild to moderate hypertension.

The third combination, at first sight rather illogical, couples an ACE inhibitor with an angiotensin receptor antagonist. Because each of these agents appears to work primarily by interrupting the renin-angiotensin system, their effects should not be additive. Nevertheless, clinical trials with a combination of an ACE inhibitor and angiotensin receptor antagonist have been completed in patients with systolic and diastolic congestive heart failure, and showed additive benefit and might be expanded to include patients with hypertension. To understand why these drugs might work well together, their respective actions must be delineated in more detail.

ACE inhibitors prevent the conversion of angiotensin I, which is functionally inactive, into angiotensin II, the effector hormone. During chronic treatment with ACE inhibitors, however, it has been observed that plasma concentrations of angiotensin II, which are largely suppressed during the early stages of treatment, tend to rise toward their baseline values after several months. Nevertheless, the ACE inhibitors appear to retain much of their antihypertensive efficacy or, in the case of congestive heart failure, to sustain their beneficial hemodynamic and symptomatic effects and to reduce clinical events such as myocardial infarction. One possible explanation for this apparent discrepancy is that measurements of angiotensin II in the plasma are not an accurate reflection of the overall activity of angiotensin II at its sites of action within the circulation. Alternatively, ACE inhibitors interrupt the action of the kininase enzyme that breaks down kinins; thus, ACE inhibitor treatment results in increased concentrations of bradykinin. Bradykinin has vasodilatory properties and stimulates endothelial nitric oxide, which itself has vasodilatory and antigrowth properties. This stimulation of the brady-kinin pathway may be a crucial part of the ACE inhibitor's efficacy.

In contrast to the ACE inhibitors, angiotensin II antagonists produce powerful and sustained blockade of the effects of angiotensin II at its receptors. For this reason, ACE inhibitors, with their recruitment of kinin and nitric oxide mechanisms, and angiotensin antagonists, with their powerful blockade of the renin-angiotensin system, may produce additive cardiovascular effects.

COMBINATION THERAPY: REDUCTION IN SIDE EFFECTS

For many antihypertensive drugs, there is a difference between their dose and efficacy relationships and their dose and adverse events relationships. In treating hypertension, the dose–response curve for efficacy often flattens early; low doses can achieve a large fraction of the potential maximum effect. However, adverse symptomatic complaints most often become a major problem with doses in the middle to upper end of the range. For this reason, low doses are attractive when they provide a moderate level of efficacy and minimize unwanted effects. If two drugs have additive efficacies, then putting them together at low doses should produce a powerful therapeutic response without inducing adverse effects.

The FDA went so far as to publish an opinion on how this approach could be translated into new therapeutic formulations. In particular, they argued that there could be a basis for approving a low-dose fixed combination for the initial treatment of hypertension. Previously, the FDA had indicated combinations as later-step therapy to be used only after monotherapies had proved inadequate.

To make a first-step approach valid for fixed-dose combination therapy, the FDA required that the two drug components be drawn from classes known to have a dose-dependent increase in side effects and where the use of very low doses thus could be anticipated to provide better-tolerated therapy. By this reasoning, combinations of diuretics and beta blockers would be appropriate; whereas combinations of ACE inhibitors and calcium channel blockers, both of which generally do not have dose-dependent side effects (with the exception of higher dose calcium channel blocker therapy where side effects are more common), would not qualify. A second criterion for approving the low-dose fixed combination was that each of the drugs involved, when tested as monotherapy in its proposed combination dose, should exhibit efficacy that would not differ meaningfully from that of placebo. Thus, a clinically useful

TABLE 16-3 Multifactorial Trial with Bisoprolol, Hydrochlorothiazide, Placebo, and Combination: Mean Reduction (mm Hg) from Baseline Sitting Diastolic Blood Pressure at 3 to 4 Weeks*

HCTZ, mg/d	Bisoprolol, mg/d			
	0	2.5	10	40
0	3.8	8.4	10.9	12.6
6.25	6.4	10.8	13.4	15.2
25	8.4	12.9	15.4	17.2

*Entry criteria: sitting diastolic blood pressure of 95 to 115 mm Hg.
Key: HCTZ, hydrochlorothiazide.
Source: Reproduced with permission from Frishman WH, Bryzinski BS, Coulson LR, et al: A multifactorial trial design to assess combination therapy in hypertension: Treatment with bisoprolol and hydrochlorothiazide. *Arch Intern Med* 154:1461, 1994.

antihypertensive effect would be achieved only if the two drugs were used in combination.

Low-Dose Strategy for Reducing Side Effects

The most successful development of such a combination has been with hydrochlorothiazide, in a dose of 6.25 mg, and bisoprolol, the long-acting cardioselective beta blocker. This combination product has the trade name of Ziac. The data used to justify the approval of this agent are shown in Table 16-3. It is evident that the combinations of the low-dose components produce meaningful decreases in blood pressure, whereas the individual components have only small effects. The JNC-VI and VII guidelines both recommend a low-dose combination treatment as an alternative first-line approach to the management of hypertension.

In another study, this formulation was compared, in double-blind fashion, with full doses of the ACE inhibitor enalapril and the calcium channel blocker amlodipine. The combination decreased blood pressure at least as well as the full-dose monotherapies. Even more important, especially in support of the underlying rationale for this type of formulation, mild and serious clinical adverse events tended to occur less commonly with Ziac than with the other agents. Quality-of-life measurements confirmed that the low-dose combination performed at least as well as enalapril or amlodipine.

Pharmacologic Interactions That Reduce Side Effects

From a practical point of view, most of the adverse effects of antihypertensive treatment can be divided into two main groups: those that cause symptomatic complaints and those that produce metabolic abnormalities in clinical test results—most commonly routine biochemistries. However, during combination therapy, even with full drug doses, it is possible for one agent to modify the adverse metabolic effects produced by the other agent and contribute to overall antihypertensive efficacy.

One of the best examples of complementary metabolic effects is produced when ACE inhibitors are combined with diuretics. The diuretics can produce hypokalemia, hyperuricemia, hyperglycemia, and possibly increased plasma

TABLE 16-4 How Combined Formulations Attenuate the Adverse Effects Produced by Individual Drugs

Adverse experience	Lotrel ($n = 760$)	Amlodipine ($n = 475$)	Benazepril ($n = 554$)	Placebo ($n = 408$)
Edema*	2.1	5.1†	0.9	2.2
Cough	3.3‡	0.4†	1.8	0.2
Headache	2.2	2.9†	3.8	5.6§
Dizziness	1.3	2.3†	1.6	1.5

*Edema refers to all edema, such as dependent edema, angioedema, and facial edema. Adverse experiences were not statistically significant unless noted.
†Statistically significant difference between Lotrel and amlodipine ($P < 0.01$).
‡Statistically significant difference between Lotrel and amlodipine and between Lotrel and placebo ($P < 0.001$).
§Statistically significant difference between Lotrel and placebo ($P < 0.01$).
Source: Reproduced from Ciba-Geigy data on file. Summit, NJ: Geneva Pharmaceuticals.

concentrations of low-density lipoprotein cholesterol. However, concomitant administration of an ACE inhibitor will moderate these changes enough to obviate discontinuing diuretic therapy or introducing additional treatments to manage the unwanted metabolic effects. More recently, the angiotensin receptor antagonist losartan was noted to modify the adverse metabolic consequences of treatment with hydrochlorothiazide.

A good example of how one drug attenuates a clinical finding produced by another is given in Table 16-4. This study with the calcium channel blocker amlodipine and the ACE inhibitor benazepril examined their individual and combined effects on common adverse experiences, most importantly edema. Calcium channel blockers can produce peripheral edema, which for some patients—most frequently women—can be bothersome. It is evident from these data, however, that when patients receive Lotrel, the fixed combination of amlodipine with benazepril, the frequency of edema is no different from that observed with placebo. The ACE inhibitor prevents the edema produced by the calcium channel blocker. The best explanation for this finding is that calcium channel blockers may produce edema because they primarily dilate the arterial side of the circulation. They have minimal venous effects, thereby allowing plasma to pool peripherally. ACE inhibitors dilate the arterial and venous circulations and thus are able to facilitate the central return of peripheral fluid accumulation. It is interesting, therefore, that the combination of a calcium channel blocker with an ACE inhibitor not only enhances efficacy but also has an beneficial effect on the side effect profile.

COMBINATION TREATMENT: CONVENIENCE AND INCONVENIENCE

Persuading patients to continue taking their antihypertensive medications on a long-term basis is one of the more difficult tasks in clinical medicine. Compliance with treatment tends to be poor, and nearly 50% of patients started on drug therapy are lost to follow-up within 1 year. Explanations for this poor outcome include inadequate instructions to the patient, denial and other psychological responses, the side effects of the drugs, the cost of the drugs, and the burden of taking medications on a regular basis—often multiple drugs multiple times a day.

Combination treatment of hypertension, especially where more than two drugs are concerned, might easily have a deleterious effect on patient compliance. Clearly, such an approach may add to cost, complexity, and the likelihood of side effects. Patients find it discouraging to be dependent on this type of regimen when they may not have been taking any medications previously.

Fixed combinations potentially have some advantages. If efficacy can be achieved by two agents that happen to be part of a standard combined formulation, this formulation alone might provide a satisfactory remedy for the hypertension. Combinations that pair an ACE inhibitor or a beta blocker with a diuretic appear to be efficacious in most patients. More innovative products, including the low-dose formulation of bisoprolol with hydrochlorothiazide, the calcium channel blocker and ACE inhibitor combinations, and the formulation of metoprolol ER and felodipine ER may be additional examples of approaches that could enhance treatment compliance. The instructions for using the newly available angiotensin antagonists (losartan, irbesartan, telmisartan, valsartan, olmesartan, candesartan, and eprosartan) also exploit this approach. It is suggested that physicians start treatment with a single 50-mg dose of losartan; if this does not adequately control blood pressure, the recommendation is to switch immediately to the losartan and diuretic combination of Hyzaar. The goal is to facilitate efficacy without intimidating the patient with multiple monotherapy titration steps or a need for multiple drugs. Manufacturers of the fixed combinations have understood that one of the advantages of these formulations is that they can be priced competitively and be made available at a cost only minimally higher than that of the primary monotherapy.

EFFECTS ON DURATION OF ACTION

During the development of new antihypertensive agents or formulations, it is necessary to study pharmacokinetic interactions between the new drug and other drugs that might be used in the same patients. In general, drug–drug interactions among the antihypertensive classes are relatively minimal, and there has been no compelling need to alter doses or frequency of administration of the commonly prescribed agents.

This does not preclude the possibility that coadministration of two agents might sufficiently affect their biological duration of action to justify altering their clinical use. The short-acting ACE inhibitor captopril is a notable example. This drug typically must be given two or three times daily as monotherapy, but adding hydrochlorothiazide changes this. Compared with placebo, the captopril and hydrochlorothiazide combination produced sustained reduction of blood pressure throughout the 24-h dosing interval when administered once daily. Like Ziac, the formulation has been approved as a first-line combination therapy. There was slightly greater efficacy with twice-daily administration, but it is clear that this combination, despite captopril's short duration of action, can provide true day-long efficacy. Indeed, if data in this study are considered only with respect to those patients who were effective responders to the therapy, there is virtually no difference between once-daily and twice-daily treatments.

The mechanism of this prolonged effect is not clear, but captopril may retain sufficient ACE-inhibitory capacity, even with its low serum levels toward the end of the dosing interval, to moderate the diuretic-related stimulation of the renin-angiotensin system. In response to research with this combination, the FDA has granted once-daily labeling for the fixed combination of captopril with hydrochlorothiazide.

Another attempt to exploit this type of relationship was far less successful. A collaboration between the manufacturers of captopril and the calcium channel blocker diltiazem was undertaken to evaluate the efficacy of a fixed combination of the two drugs. At the time this venture was undertaken, diltiazem was made only in its original, immediate-release, short-acting formulation and was typically administered three times daily. There was hope of an interaction between these two short-acting agents that might make their combination effective when administered just once daily. The study results did not support this expectation. Although the formal findings were not published in the medical literature, preliminary data on the efficacy of the combination, as judged by blood pressure reduction at the end of the 24-h dosing interval, demonstrated no differences between combination therapy and monotherapy. Of course, this failure of the combination to demonstrate pharmacokinetic or clinical advantages does not detract from the logic of an ACE inhibitor and calcium channel blocker combination. As discussed earlier, the combined use of long-acting ACE inhibitors and calcium channel blockers offers an example of how this approach to combination therapy can be highly effective.

ADDITIVE VASCULOPROTECTIVE ACTIONS

The chief goals of antihypertensive therapy include preventing coronary events (infarction, arrhythmia, or angina), major cardiovascular episodes, and strokes. Although controlling the blood pressure and reducing other known cardiovascular risk factors are pivotal in achieving these goals, additional strategies are needed to provide optimal protection against cardiovascular disease. A variety of endocrine and paracrine factors—including the renin-angiotensin system, the sympathetic nervous system, and endothelin and other proteins and substances having effects on vascular growth and function—have become the targets of therapeutic intervention.

The ACE inhibitors and the calcium channel blockers have been shown to have strong vasoprotective actions in animal models of atherosclerosis. It is likely that other drug classes already available or in development also will perform in this fashion. It is not yet proven that data from the laboratory will translate into human clinical benefits, but several studies have reported significant reductions in myocardial infarctions when patients with a variety of cardiovascular conditions were treated with ACE inhibitors. Calcium channel blockers also can exhibit anti-atherosclerotic effects in humans, although recent controversies involving the short-acting agents nifedipine and isradipine have raised clinical questions. Experiences with newer, long-acting agents appear more promising.

If each of these drug classes has apparent beneficial actions on the vascular wall, is it possible that their use in combination could provide an additional measure of atherosclerosis prevention? In the same way that combining drugs from two classes produces additive antihypertensive actions, could they also produce additive effects within vascular tissue?

There are current clinical data available demonstrating that combination therapies might produce clinical effects that outweigh those produced with single-agent treatment.

DUAL-ACTING MOLECULES

Traditionally, we have regarded combination therapy as the concomitant use of two or more separate agents, but we have learned that there are some molecules that can produce two separate actions, each of which can complement the other. Currently, there are at least two such agents, labetalol and carvedilol, that have been approved for the treatment of hypertension.

Labetalol is a molecule that possesses alpha- and beta-adrenergic blocking properties. Beta blockade is an effective approach to blood pressure reduction, and agents with this property work particularly well in European American patients, the young, and hypertensives with higher plasma renin values. Alpha blockers are efficacious across all age groups and in African American patients. For this reason, the alpha/beta blocker labetalol has been found to be efficacious in similar numbers of European American and African American patients, whereas the beta blocker propranolol tends to be most effective in European American patients. Of more interest, beta-blocker monotherapy produces a somewhat adverse effect on the lipid profile by decreasing plasma concentrations of high-density lipoprotein cholesterol. In contrast, alpha blockers have a slightly beneficial effect on the lipid profile. During treatment with labetalol, these offsetting actions result in a neutral effect on lipid measurements. Thus, this single molecule provides complementary benefits of alpha and beta blockade on blood pressure reduction and adverse outcomes.

Carvedilol similarly has beta- and alpha-blocking activities. Its clinical effects are weighted more toward the alpha-blocking effect, and the drug appears to produce vasodilatory actions. Like labetalol, this newer agent provides antihypertensive efficacy across all ages, including the elderly, and all racial groups. Moreover, it has clear antianginal properties. Of note, carvedilol appears to provide hemodynamic benefits in patients with congestive heart failure, and it may decrease the incidence of new cardiovascular events in these patients.

Other innovative molecules are currently in development. One of the most visible of these are molecule entities that have been engineered to provide inhibitory effects on neutral endopeptidase (NEP) activity and to function as ACE inhibitors (e.g., omapatrilat). The NEP inhibitory action allows this molecule to interrupt the breakdown of endogenous atrial natriuretic factor (ANF). Because ANF has vasodilatory properties and increases renal sodium and water clearance, NEP inhibition might be a useful treatment for hypertension and congestive heart failure. However, ANF seems to be most effective in low-renin states. Thus, an NEP inhibitor and an ACE inhibitor in combination might be anticipated to have additive and complementary actions. The NEP and ACE inhibitor is designed such that the NEP inhibitory action is carried at one end of the molecule and the ACE inhibitory action is carried at the other. Is this a single agent with true dual actions, or is it simply a clever way of bringing together two separate entities as a hybrid structure? Studies to date do not support a greater advantage from omapatrilat use as compared with ACE inhibitor therapy used alone.

ADDITIONAL READINGS

ALLHAT Officers and Coordinators: Major outcomes in high-risk hypertensive patients randomized to angiotensin converging enzyme inhibitor therapy or calcium channel blocker vs diuretic: The Antihypertensive and Lipid-Lowering Treatment to Prevent Heart Attack Trial (ALLHAT). *JAMA* 288:2981, 2002.

Chobanian AV, Bakris GL, Black HR et al: The Seventh Report of the Joint National Committee on Prevention, Detection, Evaluation and Treatment of High Blood Pressure: The JNC 7 Report. *JAMA* 289:2560, 2003.

Fenichel RR, Lipicky RJ: Combination products as first-line pharmacotherapy. *Arch Intern Med* 54:1429, 1994.

Frishman WH, Bryzinski BS, Coulson LR, et al: A multifactorial trial design to assess combination therapy in hypertension: Treatment with bisoprolol and hydrochlorothiazide. *Arch Intern Med* 154:1461, 1994.

Frishman WH, Cheng-Lai A, Chen J (eds): *Current Cardiovascular Drugs*, 3rd ed. Philadelphia, Current Medicine, 2000.

Gradman AH: Drug combinations, in Izzo JL Jr, Black HR (eds): *Hypertension Primer,* 3rd ed. Dallas, American Heart Association, 2003; p 408.

Guidelines Subcommittee: 1999 World Health Organization-International Society of Hypertension Guidelines for the management of hypertension. *J Hypertens* 17:151, 1999.

Hajjar I, Kotchen TA: Trends in prevalence, awareness, treatment and control of hypertension in the United States, 1988–2000. *JAMA* 90:199, 2003.

Hanson L, Zanchetti A, Carruthers SC, et al: Effects of intensive blood-pressure lowering and low dose aspirin in patients with hypertension: Principal results of the Hypertension Optimal Treatment (HOT) randomized trial. HOT Study Group. *Lancet* 351:1755, 1998.

Heart Outcomes Prevention Evaluation Study Investigators: Effects of an angiotensin-converting-enzyme inhibitor, ramipril, on cardiovascular events and stroke in high-risk patients. *N Engl J Med* 342:145, 2000.

Klahr S, Levey AS, Beck GJ, et al: The effects of dietary protein restriction and blood-pressure control on the progression of chronic renal disease. Modification of Diet in Renal Disease Study Group. *N Engl J Med* 330:877, 1994.

Law MR, Wald NJ, Morris JK, Jordan RE: Value of low dose combination treatment with blood pressure lowering drugs: Analysis of 354 randomised trials. *Br Med J* 326:1427, 2003.

Moser M, Black HR: The role of combination therapy in the treatment of hypertension. *Am J Hypertens* 11:73S, 1998.

Nawarskas JJ, Anderson JR: Omapatrilat: A unique new agent for the treatment of cardiovascular disease. *Heart Dis* 2:266, 2000.

Nawarskas J, Rajan V, Frishman WH: Vasopeptidase inhibitors, neutral endopeptidase inhibitors, and dual inhibitors or angiotensin-converting enzyme and neutral endopeptidase. *Heart Dis* 3:378, 2001.

Neutel JM, Smith DHG, Weber MA: Low-dose combination therapy: An important first-line treatment in the management of hypertension. *Am J Hypertens* 14:286, 2001.

Oparil Z, Aurup P, Snavely D, Goldberg A: Efficacy and safety of losartan/hydrochlorothiazide in patients with severe hypertension. *Am J Cardiol* 87:721, 2001.

Opie LH, Messerli FH (eds): *Combination Drug Therapy for Hypertension*. New York, Lippincott-Raven, 1997.

Packer M, Califf RM, Konstam MA, et al: Comparison of omapatrilat and enalapril in patients with chronic heart failure. The Omapatrilat Versus Enalapril Randomized Trial of Utility in Reducing Events (OVERTURE). *Circulation* 106:920, 2002.

PROGRESS Collaborative Group: Randomised trial of a perindopril-based blood-pressure-lowering regimen among 6105 individuals with previous stroke or transient ischaemic attack. *Lancet* 358:1033, 2001.

Ruzicka M, Leenen FHH: Monotherapy versus combination therapy as first-line treatment of uncomplicated arterial hypertension. *Drugs* 61:943, 2001.

Sica DA: Rationale for fixed-dose combinations in the treatment of hypertension: The cycle repeats. *Drugs* 62:443, 2002.

Sica DA, Elliott WJ: Angiotensin converting enzyme inhibitors and angiotensin receptor blockers in combination: Theory and practice. *J Clin Hypertens* 3:383, 2001.

Sica DA, Gehr TWB: Diuretic combinations in refractory edema states, pharmacokinetic and pharmacodynamic relationships. *Clin Pharmacokin* 30:229, 1996.

United Kingdom Prospective Diabetes Study Group: Tight blood pressure control and risk of macrovascular and microvascular complications in type 2 diabetes: UKPDS 38. *BMJ* 317:703, 1998.

Zanchetti A, Hansson L: Introduction: The role of combination therapy in modern antihypertensive therapy. *J Cardiovasc Pharmacol* 35(suppl 3):S1, 2000.

17 | Selective and Nonselective Dopamine Receptor Agonists

William H. Frishman   Hilary Hotchkiss

Dopamine, the endogenous precursor of norepinephrine and epinephrine, is used predominantly in intensive care unit settings as an intravenous pharmacotherapy for patients with ventricular dysfunction and various forms of shock. Dopamine acts at low doses by stimulating specific peripheral dopaminergic receptors, which are classified into two major subtypes (Fig. 17-1): D_{A1} receptors, which, when stimulated, mediate arterial vasodilation in the coronary, renal, cerebral, and mesenteric arteries and natriuresis and diuresis; and D_{A2} receptors, which are located in presynaptic areas and, when stimulated, mediate the inhibition of norepinephrine release. At still higher doses, dopamine also selectively activates the β_1-adrenergic receptors, leading to a positive inotropic and a chronotropic effect on the heart (see Chapter 8). Next, the α_1- and α_2-adrenergic receptors are activated, leading to an increase in systemic vascular resistance and blood pressure due to vasoconstriction (Table 17-1).

Fenoldopam is an intravenous dopamine agonist that has specificity for the D_1 receptor and has been used in the treatment of congestive heart failure (CHF) and hypertensive crises. The pharmacologic action of fenoldopam is to dilate selected arteries and it has the advantage of maintaining renal perfusion, despite reducing blood pressure. Problems with oral bioavailability have limited the drug's use to parenteral treatment of severe hypertension.

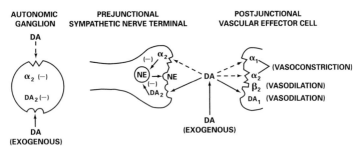

FIG. 17-1   Receptors α_2 and D_2 are located on the autonomic ganglion and prejunctional sympathetic nerve terminal to inhibit release of norepinephrine. Receptors α_1 and α_2 are located on the postjunctional vascular effector cell to cause vasoconstriction. D_1 receptors and β_2-adrenoreceptors are also located on the postjunctional vascular effector cell and induce vasodilation. When dopamine is injected exogenously, it acts on D_1 and D_2 receptors at lower doses and on α_1- and α_2-adrenoreceptors at higher doses. Dopamine has little or no effect on β_2-adrenoreceptors. Dopamine also acts on β_1-adrenoreceptors on myocardial cells to increase cardiac contractility. *(Reprinted with permission from Goldberg LI, Murphy MB: Dopamine, in Messerli FH (ed): Cardiovascular Drug Therapy. Philadelphia, Saunders, 1990, p 1083–1089.)*

TABLE 17-1 Adrenergic and Dopaminergic Receptors:
Locations, Roles, and Agonists

Receptors	Location	Roles	Agonists
α_1	Postsynaptic	↑Vascular contraction and cardiac inotropism	PE, NE, E, EP, DA
α_2	Presynaptic	↑Vascular (vein) contraction	E, NE, EP, DA
	Postsynaptic	↓NE and renin release ↓H_2O, Na^+ reabsorption	
β_1	Postsynaptic	↑Cardiac inotropism and chronotropism ↑Lipolysis	I, NE, EP, DA
β_2	Presynaptic	↑Vasodilation (artery)	I, EP
	Postsynaptic	↑NE and renin release ↑Cardiac chronotropism and inotropism	
D_{A1}	Postsynaptic	↑Vasodilation ↓H_2O, Na^+ reabsorption	Fenoldopam, EP, DA
D_{A2}	Presynaptic	↓Ganglionic transmission ↓NE and aldosterone release	Bromocriptine, EP, DA

Key: ↓, decrease; ↑, increase; DA, dopamine; E, epinephrine; EP, epinine;
I, isoproterenol; NE, norepinephrine; PE, phenylephrine.
Source: Reproduced from Itoh H: Clinical pharmacology of ibopamine. *Am J Med*
90(suppl 5B):36S, 1991.

DOPAMINE RECEPTORS

Molecular pharmacologists have divided the dopaminergic receptors into various subtypes. The peripheral dopaminergic receptors, D_{A1} and D_{A2}, have been the target of various cardiovascular pharmacotherapies that do not cross the blood–brain barrier and therefore do not affect the central nervous system's dopaminergic receptors. Many distinct dopamine receptors in the central nervous system have been found. They have been broken down into two groups: D_1-like and D_2-like. The D_1-like group includes the specific receptors D_{1A}, D_{1B}, and D_5. These are G-protein–linked receptors that stimulate adenylate cyclase, causing an increase in intracellular cyclic adenosine monophosphate (cAMP). The D_2-like group includes D_2, D_3, and D_4. These are also G protein–linked receptors, but they inhibit adenylate cyclase and thus the formation of cAMP. The D_1- and D_2-like receptors are distinct, but they are currently grouped on the basis of their similarities. The peripheral dopamine receptors have a different nomenclature and are classified into two distinct families—D_{A1} and D_{A2} receptors. Recent studies have found the D_{A1} receptors to be similar to the D_1-like central receptors and the D_{A2} receptors to be similar to the D_2-like central receptors. However, additional study is required before a firm conclusion can be made regarding the significance of these similarities. The remainder of this chapter concentrates solely on the peripheral dopamine receptors and their activation.

D_{A1} receptors are located postsynaptically on the smooth muscle cells of the renal, coronary, cerebral, and mesenteric arteries. Their activation results in vasodilation through an increase in cAMP-dependent protein kinase A activity. This causes relaxation of smooth muscle. This vasodilatory effect tends to be strongest in the renal arteries, where blood flow can be increased up to 35% in normal arteries and up to 77% in patients with unilateral renal disease (with dopamine doses of 1 µg/kg per minute). Recent evidence points to additional D_{A1} receptors located in the tubule of the kidney, which seem to be directly responsible for the natriuresis that is also seen with dopamine administration. Although their exact role in renal tubular physiology has not been established, the receptors have been shown to regulate the Na^+/K^+-ATPase pump and the Na^+/H^+ exchanger. It has been demonstrated that dopamine agonists inhibit the Na^+/K^+-ATPase pump; however, Lee recently pointed out the difficulty of dissecting the natriuretic response due to increased blood flow from the natriuretic response secondary to Na^+/K^+-ATPase inhibition. Although the exact mechanism of D_{A1} receptor activation in the kidney remains uncertain, natriuresis associated with dopamine infusion is quite clear. Abnormalities in the renal D_{A1} receptors may, in fact, contribute to the etiology of some cases of systemic hypertension. Based on the combined effects of activated D_{A1} receptors, research on selective D_{A1} agonists has focused on their use as a treatment for systemic hypertension and for hypertensive crises, particularly in patients with impaired renal function. The advantage of this pharmacologic approach over currently available antihypertensive medications would be the maintenance of renal perfusion combined with natriuretic and diuretic effects. In addition, some research on D_1 agonists has focused on the possibility of increased myocardial blood flow with this treatment. Currently available vasodilators often exhibit coronary steal, so a D_{A1} agonist might correct this problem. The potential use of D_{A1} agonists for CHF is attractive based on the observed reduction in afterload caused by their selective vasodilatory ability.

Peripheral D_{A2} receptors are located on presynaptic adrenergic nerve terminals and on sympathetic ganglia; when activated, they inhibit norepinephrine release. They are located on the adrenal cortex, where they inhibit angiotensin II–mediated aldosterone secretion. D_{A2} receptors are also located in the pituitary gland; when stimulated, they can inhibit prolactin release. The D_{A2} receptors in the emetic center of the medulla, when stimulated, can induce nausea and vomiting. D_{A2} receptors are thought to be present in the kidney, although their function is unknown. The consequence of D_2-receptor activation has been experimentally shown to be a reduction in cAMP. The combined effects of inhibiting norepinephrine-induced vasoconstriction and aldosterone release with selective D_{A2} agonists is an attractive approach for the treatments of hypertension and CHF. Many D_{A2} agonists have recently been used to treat hypertension and are discussed below. Presynaptically acting agents are among the few types of drugs that have not been thoroughly researched for the treatment of hypertension. With respect to their use in heart failure, D_{A2} agonists would treat the associated edema by inhibiting aldosterone secretion and could, in theory, reduce afterload through the inhibition of norepinephrine release.

DOPAMINE RECEPTOR AGONISTS

Dopamine

Dopamine, the parent agonist, is given intravenously at different doses to achieve different hemodynamic effects. In the low-dose range (2 to 5 µ/kg per minute), dopamine activates only D_{A1} and D_{A2} receptors. It is used at this dose to improve renal perfusion during acute low cardiac-output situations such as cardiogenic, septic, and hypovolemic shock. Diuresis and natriuresis are also observed at this dose. At a somewhat higher dose (5 to 10 μ/kg per minute), dopamine also activates β_1-receptors for a chronotropic and inotropic effect. Heart rate may actually increase, decrease, or stay the same, depending on the balance of β_1 or D_{A2} receptors found in a particular person. A larger number of β_1-receptors causes an increase in heart rate, whereas a larger number of D_{A2} receptors causes a decrease in heart rate because of the inhibition of nor-epinephrine release. At this dose level, dopamine has been used to treat heart failure, often in combination with vasodilators such as nitroprusside or nitro-glycerin. In addition, if used with dobutamine, a β_1-agonist, the increase in cardiac output can be magnified. Side effects with this dose of dopamine may include arrhythmias and/or tachycardia. At the highest levels of dopamine infusion (10 to 20 μg/kg per minute), α_1- and α_2 vasoconstrictor receptors are activated. Blood pressure and systemic vascular resistance may increase. Because these peripheral effects occur at highly variable doses in different individuals, renal perfusion and blood pressure must be carefully watched dur-ing any dopamine infusion. In addition, potential adverse effects of dopamine may occur at these high doses and can include arrhythmias, myocardial ischemia, and a reduction in blood flow to the limbs. Although these effects are rare, high-dose dopamine must be used with caution and only under close supervision.

   The use of low-dose dopamine as a renal protective agent during acute con-ditions that place patients at risk of impaired renal function is nearly standard practice, despite the lack of strong clinical evidence supporting such use. During recent years, many investigators have questioned the use of "renal dose" dopamine, suggesting that low-dose dopamine does not have the renoprotective effects previously thought. In a multicenter, randomized, dou-ble-blind, placebo-controlled trial of 328 critically ill patients, The effects of low-dose dopamine on renal function in patients with systemic inflammatory response syndrome and early evidence of renal dysfunction were investi-gated. Outcome measures included increase in serum creatinine from base-line, the need for dialysis, duration of stay in the hospital and/or an intensive care unit, and death. These investigators found no significant protection from renal dysfunction conferred by dopamine. In another double-blind, random-ized, controlled trial of 126 patients, Lassnigg and colleagues investigated the renoprotective effects of low-dose dopamine after cardiac surgery. They found no significant difference in the concentration of serum creatinine or the need for dialysis between the groups that received low-dose dopamine or placebo. Whether physicians should continue to use low-dose dopamine in these situations remains to be seen.

Fenoldopam

Fenoldopam is well known as a potent selective D_{A1} agonist. There is also some evidence that fenoldopam has mild α-antagonist activity at the α_2-receptor site. Unlike dopamine, fenoldopam has no significant effects on α_1- or β-adrenergic or D_{A1} receptors. It acts as a vasodilator, being six to nine times as potent as dopamine itself, particularly in the renal bed (Fig. 17-2) It is poorly soluble in lipids and thus does not penetrate the blood–brain barrier and has no central nervous system effects. Fenoldopam is available in an oral formulation; however, its bioavailability is inconsistent (10% to 35%) and particularly poor when it is taken with food. Metabolism is rapid (half-life of about 10 min);

thus, frequent administration is required for a sustained effect. For these reasons, fenoldopam is used primarily via the intravenous route and has been investigated most widely in the treatments of hypertensive emergencies and urgencies.

Hypertensive emergency is a condition that affects 2.4% to 5.2% of hypertensive patients in the United States. This condition—defined as a diastolic blood pressure above 115 mm Hg and/or end-organ damage such as encephalopathy, intracranial hemorrhage, pulmonary edema, dissecting aortic aneurysm, or acute myocardial infarction—requires immediate care. Historically, sodium nitroprusside has been the preferred agent to treat these patients. Nitroprusside is a potent venous and arterial dilator, with a rapid onset of action, a short half-life, a low incidence of tolerance, and a high predictability of response. However, sodium nitroprusside has some disadvantages, including thiocyanate toxicity, a possible deterioration in renal function, and a possible coronary steal due to its potent vasodilation of arteries and veins. Alternative intravenous agents have been used to treat hypertensive emergency, including labetalol, esmolol, nicardipine, and nitroglycerin. Intravenous fenoldopam therapy offers an alternative with potentially fewer side effects and the possible additional advantage of renal protection.

Fenoldopam has been investigated and its effects reported in the literature for more than 20 years. Among the reported clinical trials, there are data from more than 1000 patients who have been treated with fenoldopam for hypertension. Some of these studies have been noncomparative. Of those that are comparative, most compared fenoldopam with sodium nitroprusside. Investigations of fenoldopam in hypertensive adults have demonstrated a clear dose–response relationship in lowering systolic and diastolic blood pressures, in addition to a dose-related reflex tachycardia. Significantly, at doses that reduce the blood pressure into target ranges, little overshoot hypotension is observed.

Ninety four patients were studied in a randomized, double-blind study evaluating 24 h infusions of 1 of 4 different fenoldopam doses (0.01, 0.03, 0.1, or 0.3 μg/kg per min). These patients had a hypertensive emergency defined as diastolic blood pressure above 120 mm Hg and/or target organ damage including new renal dysfunction, hematuria, acute CHF, myocardial ischemia, or grade III or IV retinopathy. The mean times to achieve a 20-mm Hg reduction in diastolic blood pressure were 132.8 ± 15.1, 125 ± 17.0, 89.3 ± 12.6, and 55.2 ± 12.8 min, respectively, illustrating a dose-dependent effect in lowering of blood pressure. At the highest dose (0.3 μg/kg per minute), heart rate increased by an average of 11 beats/min. The investigators reported that two patients in the study developed hypotension, although the dose in these two patients was not specified.

In comparison with nitroprusside, fenoldopam has been shown to have equal efficacy in reducing blood pressure and to produce fewer side effects. Investigators enrolled 183 patients in a randomized prospective trial of fenoldopam versus sodium nitroprusside in hypertensive adults with diastolic blood pressure above 120 mm Hg. The dose of each medication was titrated to achieve a diastolic blood pressure of 95 to 110 mm Hg, or a maximum reduction of 40 mm Hg, and patients remained in the study for at least 6 h. Results of the study showed equivalent antihypertensive efficacy with similar adverse events. Ten patients were withdrawn from the study in the fenoldopam group, five for hypotension and five others for flushing, hypokalemia, tachycardia, and a gastrointestinal bleed. Eleven patients were withdrawn from the nitroprusside group; ten secondary to hypotension and one with palpitations and

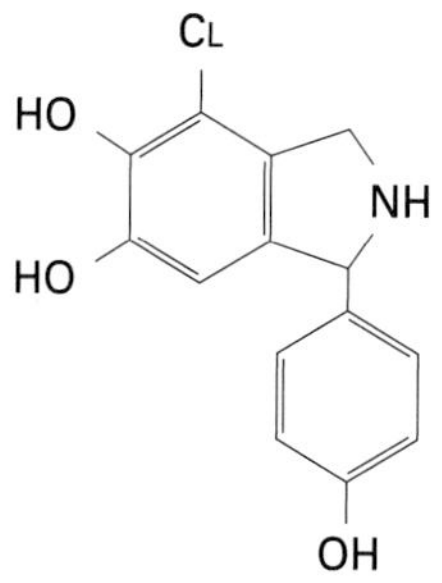

Fenoldopam

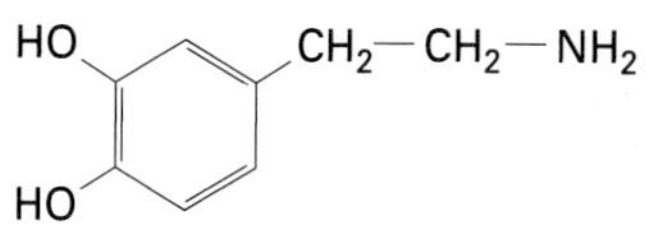

Dopamine

FIG. 17-2 Chemical structure of the dopamine receptor agonist fenoldopam compared with that of dopamine.

dizziness. In a smaller study of 33 patients, others found similar results: equal efficacy for the treatment of severe systemic hypertension with fenoldopam and sodium nitroprusside, with no difference in rate or severity of adverse events. Other studies have reported similar findings. There is limited information comparing the efficacy or safety of fenoldopam with agents other than nitroprusside for the treatment of hypertensive urgencies and emergencies.

The natriuretic and diuretic effects of fenoldopam in hypertensive patients have been studied in smaller trials, including noncomparative and comparative studies with sodium nitroprusside. In a study of 10 patients with hypertension, Murphy and colleagues found that intravenous fenoldopam was associated with a 46% increase in urinary flow rate and a 202% increase in sodium excretion. Glomerular filtration rate increased by 6%. In a study of 22 patients, 11 on fenoldopam and 11 on nitroprusside, a significant increase in creatinine clearance was demonstrated in the fenoldopam group, as well as an increase in natriuresis and diuresis. In addition to natriuresis and diuresis, a significant increase in creatinine clearance was demonstrated in the fenoldopam group. These studies point to additional effects of fenoldopam and illustrate the advantage of fenoldopam over nitroprusside in treating hypertension in patients with chronic renal insufficiency or CHF who would benefit from natriuresis and diuresis.

The adverse effect profile of fenoldopam is similar to that of nitroprusside, including reflex tachycardia and a more moderate risk of hypotension. It has been pointed out that intraocular pressure increases with fenoldopam but not with nitroprusside; thus, it is important to be aware that fenoldopam is contraindicated in patients with glaucoma.

Although most clinical trials with fenoldopam have focused on its use for hypertensive crisis, some researchers are looking at the potential use of fenoldopam for other indications. Kini and coworkers and Tumlin and colleagues suggested that fenoldopam may be a useful adjunct in preventing radiocontrast nephropathy in patients with chronic renal insufficiency who are undergoing cardiac catheterization. Investigators have evaluated the use of fenoldopam in elderly patients undergoing repair of an abdominal aortic aneurysm.

CONCLUSION

Nonselective and selective dopaminergic agonists are available for the treatment of hypertensive crisis and possibly CHF. In addition to intravenous dopamine, a nonselective agonist used for treatment of ventricular dysfunction and for the preservation of renal blood flow in low-output states, newer agents have and continue to be evaluated in clinical trials.

Fenoldopam is a selective D_1 agonist that is used to treat patients with hypertensive emergency. Because of bioavailability problems with the oral formulation, only the intravenous form is in use. Fenoldopam is approved by the U.S. Food and Drug Administration for the treatment of hypertensive emergency and has demonstrated efficacy for this condition.

ADDITIONAL READINGS

Bellomo R, Chapman M, Finfer S, et al: Low dose dopamine in patients with early renal dysfunction: A placebo-controlled randomized trial. Australian and New Zealand Intensive Care Society (ANZICS) Clinical Trials Group. *Lancet* 356:2139, 2000.

Brogden RN, Markham A: Fenodopam. *Drugs* 54: 634, 1997.

Carey RM: Renal dopamine system. Paracrine regulator of sodium homeostasis and blood pressure. *Hypertension* 38:297, 2001.

Cherney D, Straus S: Management of patients with hypertensive urgencies and emergencies: A systematic review of the literature. *J Genl Intern Med* 17:937, 2002.

Frishman WH, Hotchkiss H: Selective and nonselective dopamine-receptor agonists, in Frishman WH, Sonnenblick EH, Sica DA (eds): *Cardiovascular Pharmacotherapeutics,* 2nd ed. New York, McGraw-Hill, 2003, p 443.

Holmes CL, Walley KR: Bad medicine. Low-dose dopamine in the *ICU. Chest* 123:1266, 2003.

Kellum JA, Decker JM: Use of dopamine in acute renal failure: a meta-analysis. *Crit Care Med* 29:1526, 2001.

Kini A, Mitre C, Kamran M, et al: Changing trends in incidence and predictors of radiographic contrast nephropathy after percutaneous coronary intervention with use of fenoldopam. *Am J Cardiol* 89:999, 2002.

Lassnigg A, Donner E, Grubhofer G, et al: Lack of renoprotective effects of dopamine and furosemide during cardiac surgery. *J Am Soc Nephrol* 11:97, 2000.

Mansoor GA, Frishman WH, Comprehensive management of hypertensive emergencies and urgencies. *Heart Dis* 4:358, 2002.

Murphy MB, Murray C, Shorten GD: Fenoldopam: A selective peripheral dopamine receptor agonist. *N Engl J Med* 345:1548, 2001.

Phillips RA, Greenblatt J, Krakoff LR: Hypertensive emergencies: Diagnosis and management. *Prog Cardiovasc Dis* 45:33, 2002.

Post JB, Frishman WH: Fenoldopam: A new dopamine agonist for the treatment of hypertensive urgencies and emergencies. *J Clin Pharmacol* 38:2, 1998.

Tumlin JA, Dunbar LM, Oparil S, et al: Fenoldopam, a dopamine agonist, for hypertensive emergency: A multicenter randomized trial. Fenoldopam Study Group. *Acad Emerg Med* 7:653, 2000.

Tumlin JA, Wang A, Murray PT, Mathur VS: Fenoldopam mesylate blocks reductions in renal plasma flow after radiocontrast dye infusion: A pilot trial in the prevention of contrast nephropathy. *Am Heart J* 143:894, 2002.

18 | Prostacyclin and Its Analogues

William H. Frishman   Masoud Azizad
Yogesh K. Agarwal   Daniel W. Kang

Prostacyclin is found in all tissues and body fluids and is the major metabolite of arachidonic acid in the vasculature. Arachidonic acid is metabolized by cyclooxygenase to prostaglandin (PG) G_2 and then by PG hydroperoxidase into PGH_2. These compounds are converted into prostacyclin by PGI_2 synthetase (Fig. 18-1). Prostacyclin is produced predominantly in the endothelium and also by smooth muscle and has interesting physiologic activity in relation to the cardiovascular system. It is the most potent vasodilator known and affects the pulmonary and the systemic circulations. Relaxation of the blood vessels is caused by increases in intracellular cyclic adenosine monophosphate of vascular smooth muscle. Prostacyclin also has been noted to prevent smooth muscle proliferation. Platelet aggregation and adhesion are inhibited by the increase of intracellular cyclic adenosine monophosphate induced by prostacyclin. An interesting note is that platelet aggregation is inhibited before adhesion. These features have made it and its stable analogues very attractive substances for the treatment of primary pulmonary hypertension (PPH).

EPOPROSTENOL

Epoprostenol is the first synthetic prostacyclin to become commercially available and is currently approved for use in patients with PPH. It has the same structure as prostacyclin and is a very unstable molecule; its in vitro half-life at physiologic pH is approximately 6 min and is noted to be longer in alkaline solutions. It is also degraded by light. The product must be freeze-dried and stored at temperatures between 15°C and 25°C. The drug must be reconstituted just before administration in a glycine buffer with a pH of 10.5 and must be protected from exposure to light during reconstitution and infusion. At room temperature, a single infusion should be completed within 8 h after the medication is reconstituted. Epoprostenol must be administered intravenously, because it is degraded by the gastrointestinal tract before it can be absorbed.

Epoprostenol's in vivo half-life in humans is not measurable. In animal models, the half-life of epoprostenol is 2.7 min. It is hydrolyzed to 6-ketoprostaglandin F_{1a} in vitro, but in vivo, PGI_2 undergoes catalyzed oxidation to 15-*keto*-PGI_2. It has been noted that apolipoprotein A-I, a molecule associated with high-density lipoproteins, can prolong the half-life of prostacyclin.

Clinical Use

Studies done with epoprostenol have usually initiated the infusion rate at a dose ranging from 1 to 2 ng/kg per minute, with increases in the infusion rate at 5- to 15-min increments of 1 to 2 ng/kg per minute until the appearance of side effects or the desired long-term infusion dose is obtained. The manufacturer of the drug recommends initiating the infusion with epoprostenol at

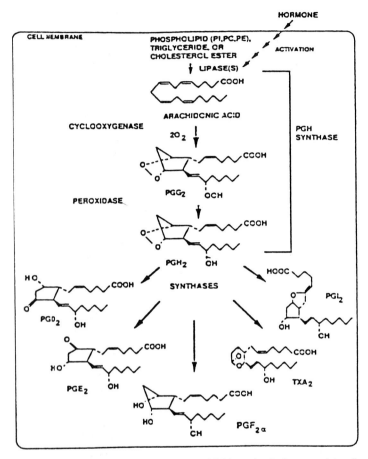

FIG. 18-1 Hormone-activated prostanoid biosynthesis in a model cell. Although all products of "cyclooxygenase pathway" are shown, usually one prostanoid is formed as a major product by a given cell type. PC, phosphatidylcholine; PE, phosphatidylethanolamine; PGG$_2$, PGD$_2$, PGE$_2$, and PGF$_{2a}$, prostaglandins G$_2$, D$_2$, E$_2$, and F$_{2a}$, respectively; PGH, prostaglandin endoperoxide; PGI$_2$, prostacyclin; PI, phosphatidylinositol; TXA$_2$, thromboxane A$_2$. *(Reproduced with permission from Smith WL: Prostanoid biosynthesis and mechanism of action. Am J Physiol 263:F181, 1992.)*

2 ng/kg per minute and increasing it at increments of 2 ng/kg per minute every 15 min. The drug is titrated until the appearance of side effects, including systemic hypotension, or until the desired long-term infusion dose is obtained. The infusion rate can be easily lowered to a dose at which there are no side effects, and, if severe systemic hypotension develops, the infusion can be stopped, with the patient returning to baseline hemodynamic status quickly. This method can be used in acute hemodynamic testing and for long-term infusion. With long-term infusion, the dosage can easily be readjusted to meet the patient's changing needs. Tolerance to prostacyclin has been

observed, but the dose can be down-titrated while preserving its therapeutic activity, especially if a high cardiac output state is observed.

Several side effects are noted with the drug, most commonly flushing, headache, nausea and vomiting, anxiety, and systemic hypotension. Other less common side effects are chest pain, dizziness, bradycardia, abdominal pain, sweating, dyspepsia, hyperesthesia, paresthesia, tachycardia, headache, diarrhea, flulike symptoms, and jaw pain. These unwanted effects are easily reversed by discontinuing the medication.

Most problems with long-term administration of the drug are related to the need for continuous intravenous delivery. These conditions include sepsis, line occlusion secondary to thrombosis, and pump failure—problems that can prove fatal. Long-term studies have shown that most patients are able to reconstitute and properly administer their medication safely at home. In this regard, orally active prostacyclin analogues, such as beraprost sodium, offer some promise in pulmonary hypertension of diverse etiologies.

Primary Pulmonary Hypertension

PPH is an idiopathic disease that is divided into three groups based on pathology: plexogenic arteriopathy, venoocclusive disease, and capillary hemangiomatosis. All three conditions can be complicated by thrombosis in situ. Plexogenic arteriopathy is the most common form and is characterized by abnormalities in the intima and media of precapillary vessels, which can range from mild neointimal proliferation to intimal fibrosis, plexiform lesions, and necrotizing arteritis. Pulmonary venoocclusive disease is less common and is characterized by fibrosis of the endovascular walls of small and medium-size veins. The least common form, pulmonary capillary hemangiomatosis, is characterized by proliferation of the capillary network, leading to changes in the arterial bed.

Although the mechanisms behind the disease are not completely elucidated, there seem to be specific, defining features of the disease process. There is an imbalance of endothelial mediators of vascular tone characterized by an unfavorable balance between thromboxane A and prostacyclin, thereby predisposing the vasculature to thrombosis and constriction. There is also an increase in the production of endothelin by the pulmonary vasculature, a decrease in endothelial clearance, and an increase in circulating endothelin levels in patients with PPH, which causes further vasoconstriction. In addition, plasma serotonin concentrations are raised in PPH patients. There also seems to be a cycle involving vascular injury from an unknown cause in susceptible individuals, which leads to smooth muscle invasion of the endothelium and a further disruption of the normal balance of vascular tone and coagulation mediators, further predisposing the endothelium to thrombosis and obstruction. A defect in K+ channels in the smooth muscle cells of the pulmonary artery may add to vasoconstriction. Intracellular calcium is an important regulator of smooth muscle contraction and proliferation, and the voltage-gated K+ channels that determine cytoplasmic concentrations of free Ca^{2+} may be defective in patients with PPH. Presenting symptoms of the disease are dyspnea on exertion, syncope, and chest pain.

The estimated annual incidence of PPH is one to two cases per million per year, and the mean age at diagnosis is 36 years. The disease has a poor prognosis. The results of a national registry of patients with PPH published in 1991 found that patients had a mean survival of 2.8 years after diagnostic catheterization was performed. In this study, the survival rates were 68% at 1 year, 48% at 3 years, and 34% at 5 years. In this registry, 39% of the patients had been diagnosed with PPH before being entered into the registry, but there was no significant difference between their survival rates and the survival rates of those who had not been previously diagnosed.

Traditionally, this disease has been treated with strong arterial vasodilators, such as calcium channel blockers, anticoagulants, and supplemental oxygen, when needed. Nitrates also have been used as a treatment, and rarely cardiac glycosides and diuretics are used, but only with extreme caution. Recently, the orally active endothelin antagonist bosentan was approved for clinical use in patients with PPH (see Chapter 20). Phosphodiesterase inhibitors are also being studied as possible oral treatments for PPH. There are always a number of patients who fail to respond to medical treatment. Heart and/or lung transplantation have been employed successfully in patients with PPH.

Epoprostenol was approved by the U.S. Food and Drug Administration (FDA) for use in patients with PPH and seems to be useful in two ways. First, epoprostenol use appears to provide a safe method to screen patients with PPH for responsiveness to drug therapy. Second, epoprostenol has been shown to prolong survival in patients with New York Heart Association (NYHA) class III and IV heart failure secondary to PPH.

There are well-defined goals for screening responsiveness to drug therapy in PPH. Not all patients respond to medication, and some have an unfavorable response. An ideal response to administration of medication in patients with PPH would be a 20% decrease in pulmonary vascular resistance (PVR) or a decrease in PVR with a 20% decrease in pulmonary artery pressure (PAP) with or without an increase in cardiac output. An unfavorable response would be the development of symptomatic systemic hypotension or an observed decrease in cardiac output. A nonresponder to therapy would be a person who did not show any significant change in PVR or PAP without the development of adverse side effects.

Epoprostenol seems to be an ideal screening agent for identifying responsiveness to medical therapy in patients with PPH. Advantages of this medication are its easy titratability, its potency, and its short half-life. Other medications used for screening responsiveness to therapy in patients with PPH are acetylcholine, adenosine, nitric oxide, and sublingual nifedipine. Epoprostenol is more potent than acetylcholine, giving it an advantage in this respect. Adenosine causes a decrease in pulmonary pressure, but it is suggested that this result is secondary to its actions on cardiac output and not because of its effects on the pulmonary vasculature. Nitric oxide seems to be comparable to epoprostenol in many of its hemodynamic actions. It has a short half-life and causes a decrease in PVR. A study compared the effects of sequentially administered nitric oxide, PGI_2, and nifedipine in 10 patients with precapillary pulmonary hypertension for screening patient responsiveness to vasodilators. These investigators concluded that nitric oxide inhalation has a predictive ability at least as good or perhaps better than PGI_2 without the associated decrease in systemic vascular resistance, systemic mean arterial pressure, and consequent increases in heart rate and cardiac index. Nitric oxide also does not cause systemic hypotension. However, it is not clear at this time whether nitric oxide will replace epoprostenol as a screening agent for determining responsiveness to medical treatment in PPH. Sublingual nifedipine also has been shown to have effects on the pulmonary and systemic circulations similar to those of epoprostenol. However, the utility of nifedipine is limited by its longer half-life.

If the patient has a favorable drop in PVR with epoprostenol without experiencing systemic hypotension, it is a good indication that the patient will have a favorable response to longer-acting vasodilators such as nifedipine.

The other use for prostacyclin is in severely ill PPH patients who do not seem to be responding to other medical therapy. Recent studies have shown that long-term infusion of epoprostenol can improve survival in patients with PPH.

A small randomized trial examining the effect of epoprostenol in 24 patients with PPH with NYHA class III and IV heart failure for 8 weeks who had not responded to traditional therapy or had adverse reactions to therapy found that patients who received epoprostenol improved symptomatically and had improved hemodynamic function. Acutely, epoprostenol caused no change in PAP, decreased PVR from 27% to 32%, decreased systemic blood pressure, and increased cardiac output by 40%. At 2 months, there were no statistically significant changes in the hemodynamics of either group as compared with the beginning of therapy; however, there was a decrease in PVR from 21.6 to 13.9 U in the epoprostenol group, which approached statistical significance. Perhaps more interesting is that all the epoprostenol patients had an improvement in their NYHA functional class, compared with two patients receiving conventional therapy. Both groups also had improvement in the distance walked during a 6-min walk test, with the epoprostenol group showing a larger increase in distance walked.

Seventeen of these patients were followed from 37 to 69 months in an open, uncontrolled trial. When compared with historical controls, this group showed a decrease in mortality, with a 3-year survival rate of 63.3%, compared with 40.6% in the control group (Fig. 18-2). These patients also had an improvement of approximately 100 m in a 6-min walk test after 6 and 18 months of treatment with epoprostenol, and they showed some improvement in their hemodynamic variables (Table 18-1).

Barst and associates published the results of the largest epoprostenol trial in patients with PPH. In this study, 81 patients were randomized to receive epoprostenol or standard therapy for 12 weeks. There was a dramatic improvement in exercise capacity and a decrease in mortality with epoprostenol. Patients who received epoprostenol were able to walk farther during a 6-min walk test after 12 weeks of epoprostenol infusion. The control group showed a 29-m decrease in the distance walked in 6 min. Functional class improved in 40% of the epoprostenol group in this study. Whereas 48% did not have any change in functional class, 13% worsened. In the control group, 3% improved in functional class, whereas 87% remained unchanged and 10% worsened. It should be noted that only survivors who did not undergo transplant were included in these figures and that there were no deaths in the epoprostenol group and eight among the controls. Cardiac parameters also improved with epoprostenol treatment (Table 18-2). Patients treated with epoprostenol also reported improvement on the Nottingham Health Profile.

Hinderliter and colleagues expanded on this trial by describing the echocardiographic changes associated with long-term epoprostenol therapy. The echocardiographic results showed that patients treated with continuous infusion of epoprostenol for 12 weeks had a lower maximal tricuspid regurgitant jet velocity, less right ventricular dilatation, an improved curvature of the intraventricular septum (during diastole and systole), and a trend toward less tricuspid regurgitation when compared with patients randomized to conventional therapy.

Others studied the long-term effects of continuous epoprostenol therapy (>330 days in 18 patients and 90 to 190 days in 25 patients), demonstrating improved survival rates over 1, 2, and 3 years of 80% ($n = 36$), 75% ($n = 17$), and 49% ($n = 6$), respectively, compared with the historical control subjects at 10, 20, and 30 months of 88% ($n = 31$), 56% ($n = 27$), and 47%

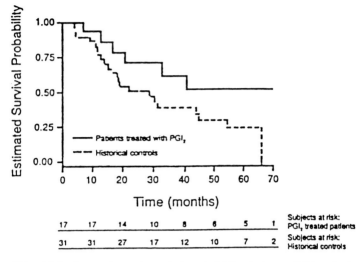

| 17 | 17 | 14 | 10 | 8 | 6 | 5 | 1 | Subjects at risk: PGI, treated patients |
| 31 | 31 | 27 | 17 | 12 | 10 | 7 | 2 | Subjects at risk: Historical controls |

FIG. 18-2 Comparison of survival probabilities between PPH patients treated with prostacyclin and PPH historical controls. Kaplan-Meier observed survival probability curves for NYHA class III and IV patients treated with prostacyclin ($n = 17$) and historical controls from the NIH Registry [NYHA class III and IV patients receiving standard therapy including anticoagulant agents ($n = 31$)]. Survival function was calculated at 6-month intervals for 5 years. Survival was significantly improved in the patients treated with prostacyclin ($P = 0.045$). The 1-, 2-, and 3-year predicted survival rates estimated by the NIH Primary Pulmonary Hypertension Registry equation for the patients treated with prostacyclin were 63.2%, 50.4%, and 41.1%, respectively; for the historical controls, the predicted survival rates were 65.2%, 52.1%, and 42.4%, respectively. NIH, National Institutes of Health; NYHA, New York Heart Association; PPH, primary pulmonary hypertension. (*Reproduced with permission from Barst RJ, Rubin LJ, McGoon MD, et al: Survival in primary pulmonary hypertension with long term continuous intravenous prostacyclin. Ann Intern Med 121: 409, 1994.*)

($n = 17$), respectively. These investigators also described a method for noninvasive long-term follow-up of patients with PPH (see Fig. 18-2).

More recently, McLaughlin and coworkers suggested that the effects of prostacyclin treatment in PPH go beyond those of immediate vasodilation. After establishing baseline hemodynamic variables in 27 patients with severe PPH, the investigators evaluated their response to the administration of adenosine, a vasodilator, and long-term therapy with epoprostenol. When the hemodynamic responses to the two treatments were compared, they found that epoprostenol therapy caused a long-term reduction in PVR that exceeded the short-term reduction achieved with adenosine. Further, long-term epoprostenol therapy also reduced PVR in patients who showed no short-term response to adenosine.

It has also been observed that continuous prostacyclin therapy can also reduce endothelial cell injury, an etiologic factor in the development of PPH. Prostacyclin infusion in patients favorably reduces the plasma levels of P-selectin and increases thrombomodulin levels, markers of endothelial injury, and altered hemostasis. The drug also can improve the balance between endothelin clearance and release, an abnormality seen in patients with PPH.

TABLE 18-1 Hemodynamic Effects of Continuous Epoprostenol Infusion in Patients with Primary Pulmonary Hypertension after 6 and 12 Months of Follow-Up*

	Baseline (n = 18)	6 mo (n = 16)	12 mo (n = 14)
Mean right atrial pressure (mm Hg)	11 ± 7	7 ± 5	8 ± 6
Mean pulmonary arterial pressure (mm Hg)	61 ± 15	55 ± 11	54 ± 16
Mean systemic arterial pressure (mm Hg)	91 ± 13	90 ± 14	84 ± 11
Cardiac index [L/(min•m²)]	1.9 ± 0.6	2.3 ± 0.6	2.5 ± 0.8
Heart rate (beats/min)	81 ± 13	81 ± 13	89 ± 13
Mixed venous saturation (%)	59 ± 12	67 ± 7	64 ± 12
Arterial oxygen saturation (%)	93 ± 6	93 ± 6	92 ± 10
Stroke volume (mL/beat)	41 ± 18	53 ± 18	51 ± 23
Total pulmonary resistance (U)	22 ± 11	15 ± 6	14 ± 6
Total systemic resistance (U)	31 ± 11	25 ± 11	22 ± 10

*Values are presented as mean ± standard deviation.
Source: Reproduced with permission from Barst RJ, Rubin LJ, McGoon MD, et al: Survival in primary pulmonary hypertension with long term continuous intravenous prostacyclin. *Ann Intern Med* 121:409, 1994.

Although epoprostenol does not constitute a cure for PPH, it provides a substantial improvement as a palliative treatment for the disease. Patients with PPH in England were studied since the early 1980s, with a focus on the effect of epoprostenol use on heart and lung transplantation. Their group studied 44 patients, 25 of whom received epoprostenol, and measured the time to transplantation and its success. In this study, they noted that epoprostenol doubled the time on the waiting list for transplant or until death. They also noted that epoprostenol was the one factor that influenced longevity the most. However, it should be noted that only 10 patients were transplanted, and that seven of these patients received epoprostenol.

Secondary Pulmonary Hypertension

Although prostacyclin infusions have been found to be successful in treating patients with PPH, the role of this drug in treating secondary pulmonary hypertension has not been well studied. In an uncontrolled, compassionate-use clinical experience with prostacyclin in 33 patients with secondary pulmonary hypertension associated with congenital heart disease, collagen vascular disease, and peripheral thromboembolic and portopulmonary hypertension, the drug was shown to be of benefit. The drug also was shown to benefit patients with pulmonary hypertension and associated congential heart defects.

Treprostinol

Treprostinol is a prostacyclin analogue with a half-life of 3 h when administered subcutaneously. Studies have suggested that the hemodynamic effects of treprostinol are similar to those of epoprostenol. A phase II study in patients with primary pulmonary hypertension compared the effects of subcutaneous and intravenous treprostinol and demonstrated that both drug delivery methods increased cardiac output and decreased total peripheral vascular resistance and pulmonary artery pressure.

The largest placebo-controlled, randomized study involving pulmonary artery hypertension was an international trial assessing the efficacy of subcuta-

TABLE 18-2 Hemodynamic Effects of Epoprostenol and Conventional Therapy in Patients with Primary Pulmonary Hypertension after 12 Weeks of Follow-Up

Variable	Change from baseline*		Difference between treatments	95% CI†
	E	CT		
Mean pulmonary artery pressure (mm Hg)	−4.8 ± 1.3	1.9 ± 1.6	−6.7	−10.7 to −2.6
Mean right atrial pressure (mm Hg)	−2.2 ± 1.1	0.1 ± 0.9	−2.3	−5.2 to 0.7
Mean systemic artery pressure (mm Hg)	−4.8 ± 1.2	−0.9 ± 1.7	−3.9	−9.6 to 1.7
Mean pulmonary capillary wedge pressure (mm Hg)	0.4 ± 1.2	−1.0 ± 1.6	1.4	−2.5 to 5.3
Cardiac index [L/(min•m²)]	0.3 ± 0.1	−0.2 ± 0.2	0.5	0.2 to 0.9
Heart rate (beats/min)	−0.9 ± 2.5	−1.8 ± 1.5	0.9	−5.2 to 7.2
Systemic arterial oxygen saturation (%)	2.0 ± 1.6	−0.6 ± 1.4	2.6	−1.8 to 7.1
Mixed venous oxygen saturation (%)	1.2 ± 1.8	−2.6 ± 2.0	3.8	−1.6 to 9.2
Stroke volume (mL/beat)	6.6 ± 2.2	−3.5 ± 3.3	10.1	2.5 to 17.8
Pulmonary vascular resistance [mm Hg/(L•min)]	−3.4 ± 0.7	1.5 ± 1.2	−4.9	−7.6 to −2.3
Systemic vascular resistance [mm Hg/(L•min)]	−4.00 ± 1.0	2.1 ± 1.4	−6.1	−9.5 to −2.8

*Values are presented as mean ± standard error.
†The CIs indicate comparisons between treatment groups. A CI that does not contain 0 indicates statistical significance.
Key: CI, confidence interval; CT, conventional therapy; E, epoprostenol.
Source: Reproduced with permission from Barst RJ, Rubin LJ, Long WA, et al: A comparison of continuous epoprostenol (prostacyclin) with conventional therapy for primary pulmonary hypertension. *N Engl J Med* 334:296, 1996.

neously delivered treprostinol in patients with pulmonary artery hypertension, primary or associated with collagen vascular disease, or with congenital systemic-to-pulmonary shunts. The primary end point of this trial was exercise capacity as measured by the 6-min walk distance, which improved in the treprostinol group and was unchanged with placebo. This effect on exercise tolerance appeared to be dose related. Common side effects included headache, diarrhea, nausea, rash, and jaw pain. Eighty-five percent of patients experienced infusion site pain and 83% had erythema or induration at the infusion site; 8% of subjects were withdrawn from the study because of infusion site pain.

Different therapies have been used to control the adverse effects of pain and erythema at the infusion site, including local treatment and anti-inflammatory drugs. More recently, a pharmaceutical transdermal delivery vehicle, Pluronic lecithin organogel, has been compounded with various analgesics and anesthetics for local application to the site.

Because of the longer half-life of treprostinol, interruptions of drug due to dislodgement of the catheter or pump malfunction are less serious than with epoprostenol. The FDA has approved subcutaneous treprostinol for patients with functional class II, III, and IV PAH. Treprostinol should be considered in those patients who are not candidates for or decline therapy with intravenous epoprostenol. In addition, patients who have contraindications to the endothelin blocker bosentan might be candidates for subcutaneous treprostinol.

CONCLUSION

Epoprostenol is now available in the United States and is approved for use in patients with PPH. Although this agent has been used with limited success in other areas, there is a great amount of work to be done with its more stable analogues. Treprostinol, a prostacyclin analogue, recently was approved for subcutaneous use in PPH.

ADDITIONAL READINGS

Barst RJ, McGoon M, McLaughlin V, et al: Beraprost Study Group: Beraprost therapy for pulmonary arterial hypertension. *J Am Coll Cardiol* 41:2119, 2003.

Barst RJ, Rubin LJ, Long WA, et al: A comparison of continuous epoprostenol (prostacyclin) with conventional therapy for primary pulmonary hypertension. *N Engl J Med* 334:296, 1996.

Barst RJ, Rubin LJ, McGoon MD, et al: Survival in primary pulmonary hypertension with long term continuous intravenous prostacyclin. *Ann Intern Med* 121:409, 1994.

Fink AN, Frishman WH, Azizad M, Agarwal Y: Use of prostacyclin and its analogues in the treatment of cardiovascular disease. *Heart Dis* 1:29, 1999.

Frishman WH, Azizad M, Agarwal Y, Kang DW: Use of prostacyclin and its analogues in the treatment of pulmonary hypertension and other cardiovascular diseases, in Frishman WH, Sonnenblick EH, Sica DA (eds): *Cardiovascular Pharmacotherapeutics*, 2nd ed. New York, McGraw-Hill, 2003, p 429.

Gaine S, Lewis R: Primary pulmonary hypertension. *Lancet* 353:719, 1998.

Hinderliter AL, Park WW, Barst RJ, et al: Effects of long-term infusion of prostacyclin (epoprostenol) on echocardiographic measures of right ventricular structure and function in primary pulmonary hypertension. *Circulation* 95:1479, 1997.

Langleben D, Barst RJ, Badesch D, et al: Continuous infusion of epoprostenol improves the net balance between pulmonary endothelin-1 clearance and release in primary pulmonary hypertension. *Circulation* 99:3266, 1999.

Lehrman S, Romano P, Frishman WH, et al: Primary pulmonary hypertension and cor pulmonale. *Cardiol Rev* 10:265, 2002.

McLaughlin VV, Gaine SP, Barst RJ, et al: Efficacy and safety of treprostinol: An epoprostenol analogue for primary pulmonary hypertension. *J Cardiovasc Pharmacol* 41:292, 2003.

McLaughlin VV, Genthner DE, Panella MM, Rich S: Reduction in pulmonary vascular resistance with long-term epoprostenol (prostacyclin) therapy in primary pulmonary hypertension. *N Engl J Med* 338:273, 1998.

McLaughlin VV, Genthner DE, Panella MM, et al: Compassionate use of continuous prostacyclin in the management of secondary pulmonary hypertension: A case series. *Ann Intern Med* 130:740, 1999.

Paramothayan NS, Lasserson TJ, Wells AU, Walters EH: Prostacyclin for pulmonary hypertension. *Cochrane Database Syst Rev* 2:CD002994, 2003.

Reffelmann T, Kloner RA: Therapeutic potential of phosphodiesterase 5 inhibition for cardiovascular disease. *Circulation* 108:239, 2003.

Rich S, McLaughlin VV: The effects of chronic prostacyclin therapy on cardiac output and symptoms in primary pulmonary hypertension. *J Am Coll Cardiol* 34:1184, 1999.

Simmonneau G, Barst RJ, Galie N, et al: Continuous subcutaneous infusion of treprostinil, a prostacyclin analogue, in patients with pulmonary arterial hypertension. *Am J Resp Crit Care Med* 165:800, 2002.

19 | Natriuretic Peptides: Nesiritide

William H. Frishman   Domenic A. Sica
Judy W. M. Cheng

In 1981, de Bold and colleagues infused a homogenized rat extract that triggered a potent natriuresis, diuresis, and a small kaliuresis, thus supporting prior theories suggesting that the heart is more than merely a mechanical pump. This result paved the way for the notion that the heart is also an endocrine organ. Subsequent fractionation and bioassay of rat atrial homogenates confirmed that this natriuretic bioactivity resides in the atrial granules. On the heels of these original observations, several groups isolated atrial natriuretic peptide in a pure form and determined its amino acid sequence. Shortly thereafter, a series of related peptides were isolated, further suggesting the endocrine capabilities of the heart. In 1988, Sudoh and associates discovered a peptide in porcine brain with structural homology and biological properties similar to those of atrial natriuretic peptide. Although subsequent studies showed it to be secreted predominantly by ventricular tissue in the heart, the peptide retained the name *brain natriuretic peptide* (BNP). Soon after the discovery of BNP, C-type natriuretic peptide also was isolated from porcine brain. Although C-type natriuretic peptide production occurs mostly in the central nervous system and vascular endothelium, its structural homology and similarities in metabolism with the other natriuretic peptides led to its inclusion in the same family of peptide hormones. As a result of these findings, there developed an explosive interest in cardiac peptide research, which has led to the heart being recognized as a true endocrine organ.

This chapter reviews the clinical pharmacology of nesiritide, a human form of BNP made by recombinant DNA technology, which is now available for intravenous use in the management of heart failure patients.

PHARMACOLOGY OF NESIRITIDE

The pharmacologic effects of nesiritide are mediated via the same receptor that mediates the actions of other natriuretic peptides. It binds to guanyl cyclase receptors on the cell surface of vascular smooth muscle and endothelial cells. This receptor binding triggers intracellular activation of the secondary messenger cyclic guanosine monophosphate, which in turn causes decreased intracellular concentrations of Ca^{2+}, with subsequent relaxation of smooth muscle and vasodilation.

Nesiritide appears to act in four principal ways to oppose the activity of the renin-angiotensin-aldosterone axis: (a) it causes vasorelaxation; (b) it blocks aldosterone secretion by the adrenal cortex; (c) it inhibits kidney renin secretion; and (d) it opposes the sodium-retaining action of aldosterone. In addition, antagonism of antidiuretic hormone, water intake, and salt intake mediated in the central nervous system amplify the effects of BNP in reducing plasma volume (Fig. 19-1, Table 19-1).

BNP promotes natriuresis and diuresis via a series of mechanisms that are not mutually exclusive of each other, including (a) an increase in glomerular

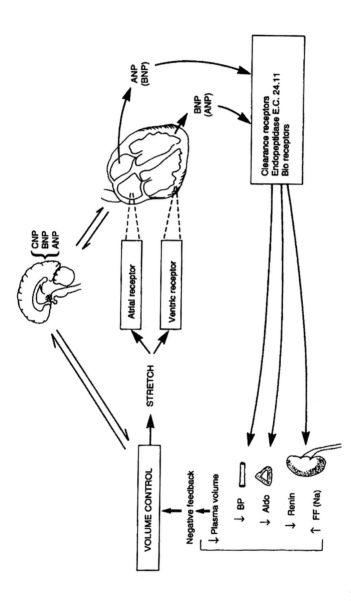

FIG. 19-1 Diagram showing the regulation and actions of natriuretic peptides. Aldo, aldosterone; BP, blood pressure; FF, filtration fraction. (Modified with permission from Espiner EA: Physiology of natriuretic peptides. J Intern Med 235:527, 1994.)

413

TABLE 19-1 Reported Effects of Atrial Natriuretic Peptide in Humans

Vascular effects
Vasodilatation
Hemoconcentration
Hormonal effects
Decrease in plasma renin activity
Decrease in aldosterone, cortisol, ACTH, TSH, and prolactin
Inhibition of vasopressin secretion and/or effects
Induction of pancreatic secretion
Modulation of insulin secretion and/or metabolism
May be endogenous antagonist to angiotensin II
Renal effects
Natriuresis, diuresis with no concomitant kaliuresis
Increase in GFR
Decrease in effective renal plasma flow
Increase in filtration fraction
Increase in renovascular resistance
Increase in urinary volume and electrolytes
Central nervous system effects
Modulation of sympathetic activity
Increase in heart rate
Increase in lipolysis
Effects on blood pressure/volume regulatory regions in the brain
Cardiac effects
Coronary vasodilatation
Left ventricular performance enhancement
Cardiac output reduction
Coronary blood flow (different effects)
Pulmonary effects
Relaxation of vascular smooth-muscle cells
Relaxation of the trachea
Adrenal effects
Blocks release of aldosterone
Pituitary effects
Posterior pituitary: inhibition of ADH production and release
Anterior pituitary: inhibition of ACTH, TSH, and prolactin
Intestinal effects
Effect on fluid movement across intestinal membrane
Growth regulatory effects
Inhibits growth and cell proliferation

Key: ACTH, adrenocorticotrophic hormone; ADH, antidiuretic hormone; ANP, atrial natriuretic peptide; GFR, glomerular filtration rate; TSH, thyroid-stimulating hormone.
Source: Modified from DeZeeuw D, Janssen WM, de Jong PE: Atrial natriuretic factor: its (patho) physiological significance in humans. *Kidney Int* 41:1115, 1992.

filtration rate, which occurs as a consequence of afferent arteriolar vasodilation and efferent arteriolar vasoconstriction, and enhanced Na$^+$ delivery to the medullary collecting duct; (b) inhibition of Na$^+$ reabsorption by medullary collecting ducts secondary to reduction in the effects of aldosterone and/or angiotensin-II; (c) redistribution of blood flow to deeper nephrons with less Na$^+$ reabsorptive capacity; and (d) decreased secretion and/or effect of antidiuretic hormone. On a more primary level, BNP may be an endogenous antagonist to angiotensin II because their binding sites overlap in the brain, kidney, and adrenal cortex. An additional intriguing action of BNP is its ability to induce a natriuresis without a concomitant kaliuresis. When increased potassium (K^+) excretion occurs, it seems to correlate with an enhanced tubular flow rate. BNP inhibits renin release by secondary effects at the macula densa or, less likely, via a direct effect on the juxtaglomerular cells.

Hemodynamic Effects

The hemodynamic effects of nesiritide are characterized by venous and arterial dilation resulting in decreased preload and afterload. A dose of 0.015 µg/kg per minute reduces pulmonary capillary wedge pressure (PCWP) by an average of 6 mm Hg, right atrial pressure by an average of 3 mm Hg, mean pulmonary pressure by an average of 5.5 mm Hg, and systemic vascular resistance by an average of 150 dyn/(s • cm^{-5}). Although nesiritide has no direct positive inotropic effect, the cardiac index also increases by an average of 0.2 L/(min • m^2) secondary to a dose-dependent afterload reduction. After discontinuation of nesiritide, PCWP returns to within 10% of baseline in 2 h, but no rebound increase to levels above baseline state is observed.

Pharmacokinetics

In patients with congestive heart failure (CHF), nesiritide administered intravenously demonstrated biphasic disposition from the plasma. The mean terminal half-life of nesiritide is approximately 18 min, and the mean volume of distribution at steady state is estimated to be 0.19 L/kg. At steady state, plasma BNP levels increase from baseline endogenous levels by approximately three- to sixfold, with nesiritide infusion doses ranging from 0.01 to 0.03 µg/kg per minute.

Human BNP is cleared mainly via binding to cell surface clearance receptors with subsequent cellular internalization and lysosomal proteolysis. BNP clearance also occurs by proteolytic cleavage of the peptide by endopeptidases or by renal filtration. The average total body clearance is approximately 9.2 mL/min per kilogram. Clearance of nesiritide is not affected by age, sex, race or ethnicity, baseline endogenous BNP level, severity of heart failure (HF), or concomitant administration of angiotensin-converting enzyme inhibitors.

Pharmacodynamics

With the recommended nesiritide dose of 2 µg/kg as an intravenous bolus followed by an infusion of 0.01 (µg/kg per minute, 60% of the 3-h effect (the dose of nesiritide is titrated every 3 h; see Dose and Administration) on PCWP reduction is achieved within 15 min after the bolus and reaches 95% of the 3-h effect within 1 h. Approximately 70% of the 3-h effect on systolic blood pressure reduction is reached within 15 min. The pharmacodynamic half-lives of the onset and offset of the hemodynamic effect of nesiritide are somewhat longer than the pharmacokinetic half-life would predict.

CLINICAL TRIALS IN HEART FAILURE

Decompensated HF represents an interaction of hormonal and anatomical responses, including the overactivation of the sympathetic nervous system (elevation of epinephrine and norepinephrine levels and downregulation of β-receptors), leading to vasoconstriction, a decrease in myocardial contractility, and overactivation of the renin-angiotensin-aldosterone system, leading to vasoconstriction and retention of salt and water. Elevation of circulating BNP is another biologic marker of acute HF decompensation.

In HF, the increase in cardiac volume and pressure overload stimulates the production of natriuretic peptides to enhance diuresis and to produce vasodilation to help reduce preload and afterload. Unlike the sympathetic nervous system and renin-angiotensin-aldosterone system, which continue to activate even in chronic and severe HF, the natriuretic peptide system may be overwhelmed in chronic heart failure, leading to a state of relative deficiency.

Colucci and colleagues studied the clinical efficacy of nesiritide and compared its effects with conventional treatment in patients who were admitted with decompensated HF. Patients hospitalized were enrolled to the efficacy trial or the comparative trial. In the efficacy trial, 127 patients were randomized to 6-h infusions of placebo or one of two doses of nesiritide (0.015 or 0.03 μg/kg per minute) preceded by bolus doses of 0.3 and 0.6 μg/kg, respectively. Subsequently, the blind was broken and patients were maintained on open-label treatment for up to 7 days. Most patients had New York Heart Association (NYHA) class III or IV HF and a mean left ventricular ejection fraction of 22%, a mean of PCWP of 28 mm Hg, and a cardiac index of 1.9 L/(min • m^2). Nesiritide caused dose-dependent reduction in PCWP (6 to 9.6 mm Hg) and resulted in 60% and 67% improvement in global clinical status as compared with 14% of those receiving placebo ($P < 0.001$). It also reduced dyspnea in approximately 55% of patients compared with 12% in those receiving placebo ($P < 0.001$). Hypotension resulted in discontinuation of the study drug in one patient who was receiving 0.03 μg/kg per minute. In the comparative trial, 305 patients were randomized to open-label treatment with standard care intravenous agents or double-blind treatment with one of two dose levels of nesiritide (0.015-μg/kg per minute infusion preceded by a 0.3-μg/kg bolus or 0.03-μg/kg per minute infusion preceded by a 0.6-μg/kg bolus). The duration of therapy was based on the usual clinical criteria and ranged up to 7 days. Most patients in the trial had NYHA class III or IV HF. Among 102 patients randomized to standard therapy, 57% were treated with dobutamine, 19% with milrinone, 18% with nitroglycerin, 6% with dopamine, and 1 % with amrinone. End points such as global clinical status and dyspnea were assessed as in the efficacy trials. They were similar to those observed with standard intravenous therapy. The most common adverse event with nesiritide was hypotension, which was symptomatic in 11% and 17% of patients treated with doses of 0.015 and 0.03 μg/kg per minute, respectively, as compared with 4% in patients receiving standard therapy. Other adverse events were similar in frequency in the nesiritide and standard treatment groups, except for the frequency of nonsustained ventricular tachycardia, which decreased with the nesiritide dose of 0.03 μg/kg per minute (1% with 0.03 μg/kg per minute versus 10% with 0.015 μg/kg per minute versus 8% in standard treatment group; $P < 0.02$).

The Vasodilation in the Management of Acute Congestive Heart Failure (VMAC) trial was a multicenter, randomized, double-blind, placebo-controlled study looking at the hemodynamic and clinical effects of nesiritide compared with nitroglycerin therapy for symptomatic decompensated HF. Four hundred eighty-nine patients with dyspnea at rest from HF were randomized to an adjustable dose of nitroglycerin, placebo, fixed-dose nesiritide, or adjustable-dose nesiritide for a 3 h period. At the end of this period, the placebo group was crossed over to a prespecified treatment with nitroglycerin or fixed-dose nesiritide. Duration of treatment after crossover was at the discretion of the investigators. Patients receiving adjustable-dose nesiritide continued on this same regimen. Nesiritide was administered as a 2-μg/kg intravenous bolus followed by a 3-h infusion of 0.01 μg/kg per minute in both the fixed-dose and adjustable-dose groups. After the first 3 h, the adjustable-dose group could have the nesiritide dose increased by administering a 1-μg/kg intravenous bolus followed by an increase of 0.005 μg/kg per minute over the previous infusion rate. The maximum allowable infusion rate was 0.03 μg/kg per minute. The primary end points were change in PCWP and dyspnea at the end of 3 h. Both nesiritide treatment groups (i.e., fixed dose and adjusted dose) were pooled for study analysis. Nesiritide significantly decreased PCWP compared with placebo ($P < 0.001$) nitroglycerin added to standard care ($P < 0.027$) at the 3-h time point. At 24 h, the reduction in PCWP was greater in the nesiritide group than in the nitroglycerin group, but patients reported no significant difference in dyspnea and only modest improvement in global clinical status. The most common adverse effect was headache, which occurred less often in nesiritide-treated patients (8%) then in the nitroglycerin-treated patients (20%; $P = 0.003$). Symptomatic hypotension was similar in frequency (5%) in both groups.

The Prospective, Randomized Evaluation of Cardiac Ectopy with Dobutamine or Natrecor Therapy (PRECEDENT) trial examined the proarrhythmic effects of nesiritide and dobutamine. Two hundred forty-six patients with NYHA class III or IV HF were randomized to one or two doses of nesiritide (0.015 or 0.03 μg/kg per minute) or dobutamine (minimum dose of 5 μg/kg per minute) and underwent Holter monitoring for 24 h before and during treatment. When compared with either dose of nesiritide, dobutamine was associated with significant increases in premature ventricular beats (average change in hourly total premature ventricular beats vs. baseline: dobutamine +69, nesiritide 0.015 μg/kg per minute −13, and nesiritide 0.03 μg/kg per minute −5; $P < 0.002$).

A post hoc analysis combining the long-term mortality results from the comparative trial by Colucci and associates and the PRECEDENT trials (reflecting a total of 507 patients) demonstrated that, compared with treatment with dobutamine, treatment with nesiritide at 0.015 μg/kg per minute was associated with a reduction in cumulative 6-month mortality by 37% (15.8% vs. 25%, $P = 0.03$). This observed mortality difference could not be explained by differences in baseline demographics, severity or etiology of CHF, or other comorbid conditions. However, additional trials are required to confirm this effect and to establish the optimal dose to maximize the effect. In addition, anecdotal reports have appeared that suggest that nesiritide has a demonstrable efficacy in the HF patient with mild-to-moderate renal insufficiency. Interestingly, nesiritide also appears to preserve renal function in some acutely decompensated HF patients (if hypotension does not intervene) who might otherwise experience a significant decline in renal function coincident to the process of diuresis. This latter observation has not been formally studied.

A recent pharmacoeconomic study has also demonstrated an advantage of nesiritide over dobutamine in the treatment of decompensated CHF.

Safety and Drug Interactions

The safety profile of nesiritide was obtained by compiling data from the different randomized clinical trials within the dose range of 0.01 to 0.03 μg/kg per minute. The studied patient population was representative of a compromised chronic HF population, including comorbidities such as significant atrial and ventricular arrhythmias, diabetes, hypertension, significant renal insufficiency, and acute coronary syndromes. The most common side effect of nesiritide was dose-related hypotension (11% to 35%), and approximately 50% of such episodes were symptomatic. The incidence of other side effects was similar to the controlled groups. Nesiritide may affect renal function in patients with severe HF whose renal function may depend on the activity of the renin-angiotensin-aldosterone system. In the VMAC study, when nesiritide was initiated at doses higher than 0.01 µg/kg per minute, serum creatinine levels rose more than that observed with standard therapies, although the rate of acute renal failure and need for dialysis were not increased. To date, a careful prospective look at the change in renal function with nesiritide indexed by blood pressure changes had not been undertaken.

No trial specifically examined potential drug interactions with nesiritide. In addition, there are no long-term studies evaluating the carcinogenic potential of nesiritide.

Dosing and Administration

The recommended dose of nesiritide is an intravenous bolus of 2 µg/kg followed by a continuous infusion at a dose of 0.01 µg/kg per minute. Nesiritide should not be initiated at a dose that is above the recommended dose to prevent excessive hypotension or worsening of renal function. The dose of nesiritide can be adjusted by 0.005 µg/kg per minute (preceded by a bolus of 1 µg/kg) every 3 h up to a maximum of 0.03 µg/kg per minute. There is limited experience with administering nesiritide for longer than 72 h. In the VMAC study, duration of treatment was not specified. The longest infusion was 161 days in a NYHA class IV patient who was poorly responsive to other intravenous therapies while awaiting a cardiac transplant. The patient responded well clinically and tolerated therapy for 161 days. No tolerance or tachyphylaxis was observed.

Nesiritide is physically and chemically incompatible with injectable formulations of heparin, insulin, ethacrynate sodium, bumetanide, enalaprilat, hydralazine, and furosemide. These drugs should not be coadministered with nesiritide through the same intravenous catheter. Injectable drugs that contain sodium metabisulfite as a preservative are also incompatible with nesiritide.

CONCLUSION

The two decades of active natriuretic peptide research have produced tremendous insights into the molecular biology, physiology, and pathophysiology of these hormones and have established the principle that the heart is a pump and a true endocrine organ. In addition, several approaches toward the pharmacologic manipulation of natriuretic peptides in vivo have been developed.

The natriuretic peptides play a fundamental role in the regulation of vascular hemodynamics. They play a crucial role in maintaining vascular fluid homeostasis and act to counterbalance the renin-angiotensin-aldosterone system, endothelin, vasopressin, and various actions of the sympathetic nervous system. In these roles, these peptides are part of the human body's natural system of checks and balances. They perform important protective functions in many acute situations and have proved useful in altering hemodynamics in many studies on CHF.

Nesiritide mimics the actions of endogenous natriuretic peptides. Clinical studies using the intravenous infusion of nesiritide in more than 1700 patients with acute decompensated HF have demonstrated that it exerts dose-related vasodilation that is rapid in onset and sustained for the duration of infusion. Nesiritide reduces PCWP and improves the symptom of dyspnea. These effects compare favorably to nitroglycerin, dobutamine, and other standard treatment of decompensated HF. It decreases preload and afterload and suppresses the renin-angiotensin-aldosterone axis and the release of norepinephrine. Nesiritide also promotes diuresis and seems to have no proarrhythmic property. Nesiritide is a valuable therapeutic option in the treatment of patients hospitalized for decompensated HF. Ongoing studies are examining its beneficial effects in long-term mortality and morbidity and any potential pharmacoeconomic benefits to the entire health care system.

A promising use of these peptides may be as markers for disease. Routine immunoassay of BNP may provide a preliminary test of ventricular function or other abnormalities and may permit physicians to more carefully select patients for further investigation and treatment. The natriuretic peptide field is still in its infancy, and further investigation of the natriuretic peptide family promises to add new insights into their mechanism of action and improved potential clinical uses in the future.

ADDITIONAL READINGS

Abraham WT, Lowes BD, Ferguson DA, et al: Systemic hemodynamic, neurohormonal, and renal effects of a steady-state infusion of human brain natriuretic peptide in patients with hemo-dynamically decompensated heart failure. *J Cardiac Fail* 4:37, 1998.

Achilihu G, Frishman WH, Landau A: Neutral endopeptidase inhibitors and atrial natriuretic peptide. *J Clin Pharmacol* 31:758, 1991.

Bobadilla RV, Oppelt TF, Hirshy TC: Nesiritide treatment of noncardiogenic pulmonary edema. *Ann Pharmacother* 37:530, 2003.

Burger AJ, Aronson D, Horton DP, Burger MR: Comparison of the effects of dobutamine and nesiritide (B-type natriuretic peptide) on ventricular ectopy in acutely decompensated ischemic versus nonischemic cardiomyopathy. *Am J Cardiol* 91: 1370, 2003.

Burger AJ, Horton DP, Elkayam U, et al: Nesiritide is not associated with proarrhythmic effects of dobutamine in the treatment of decompensated CHF: The PRECEDENT Study. *J Cardiac Fail* 5(suppl 1):49, 1999.

Burger AJ, Horton DP, LeJemtel T, et al: Effect of nesiritide (B-type natriuretic peptide) and dobutamine on ventricular arrhythmias in the treatment of patients with acutely decompensated congestive heart failure: The PRECEDENT study. *Am Heart J* 144:1102, 2002.

Cheng JWM: Nesiritide: review of clinical pharmacology and role in heart failure management. *Heart Dis* 4:199, 2002.

Cho Y, Somer BG, Amatya A, et al: Natriuretic peptides and their therapeutic potential. *Heart Dis* 1:305, 1999.

Colucci WS, Elkayam U, Horton DP, et al: Intravenous nesiritide, a natriuretic peptide, in the treatment of decompensated congestive heart failure. Nesiritide Study Group. *N Engl J Med* 343:246, 2000.

Cowie MR, Mendez GF: BNP and congestive heart failure. *Prog Cardiovasc Dis* 44: 293, 2002.

de Bold AJ, Borenstein HB, Veress AT, Sonnenberg H: A rapid and potent natriuretic response to intravenous injection of atrial myocardial extract in rats. *Life Sci* 28:89, 1981.

de Lemos JA, McGuire DK, Drazner MH: B-type natriuretic peptide in cardiovascular disease. *Lancet* 362:316, 2003.

DeLemos JA, Morrow DA, Bentley JH, et al: The prognostic value of B-type natriuretic peptide in patients with acute coronary syndromes. *N Engl J Med* 345:1014, 2001.

Elkayam U, Silver MA, Burger AJ, Horton DP: The effect of short-term therapy with nesiritide (B-type natriuretic peptide) or dobutamine on long-term survival. *J Cardiac Fail* 6(suppl 2):45, 2000.

Frishman W, Sica DA, Cheng JWM, et al: Natriuretic and other vasoactive peptides, in Frishman WH, Sonnenblick EH, Sica DA (eds): *Cardiovascular Pharmacotherapeutics,* 2nd ed. New York, McGraw-Hill, 2003, p 451.

Keating GM, Goa KL: Nesiritide: A review of its use in acute decompensated heart failure. *Drugs* 63:47, 2003.

Koglin J, Pehlivanli S, Schwaiblmair M, et al: Role of brain natriuretic peptide in risk stratification of patients with congestive heart failure. *J Am Coll Cardiol* 38:1934, 2001.

Marcus LS, Hart D, Packer M, et al: Hemodynamic and renal excretory effects of human brain natriuretic peptide infusion in patients with congestive heart failure: A double-blind, placebo-controlled, randomized crossover trial. *Circulation* 94:3184, 1996.

Moazami W, Damiano RJ, Bailey MS, et al: Nesiritide (BNP) in the management of postoperative cardiac patients. *Ann Thorac Surg* 75:1974, 2003.

Silver MA, Horton DP, Ghali JK, Elkayam U: Effect of nesiritide versus dobutamine on short-term outcomes in the treatment of patients with acutely decompensated heart failure. *J Am Coll Cardiol* 39:798, 2002.

Sudoh T, Kangawa K, Minamino N, Matsuo H: A new natriuretic peptide in porcine brain. *Nature* 332:78, 1988.

Stoupakis G, Klapholz M: Natriuretic peptides: Biochemistry, physiology, and therapeutic role in heart failure. *Heart Dis* 5:215, 2003.

VMAC Investigators: Intravenous nesiritide vs nitroglycerin for treatment of decompensated congestive heart failure—A randomized controlled trial. *JAMA* 287:1531, 2002.

20 | Endothelin Inhibitors: Bosentan

William H. Frishman   Judy W. M. Cheng

Endothelin (ET) is a naturally occurring polypeptide substance with potent vasoconstrictor actions. It was originally termed *endotensin* or *endothelial contracting factor* in 1985 by Hickey and colleagues who reported on their finding of a potent, stable vasoconstricting substance produced by cultured endothelial cells. Subsequently, other investigators isolated and purified the substance from the supernatant of cultured porcine aortic and endothelial cells and then went on to prepare its cDNA. This substance was subsequently renamed *endothelin*.

ETs are the most potent vasoconstrictors identified to date. Their chemical structure is closely related to that of certain neurotoxins (sarafotoxins) produced by scorpions and the burrowing asp (*Atractapsis engaddensin*). ETs have now been isolated in various cell lines from multiple organisms. They are considered autocoids or cytokines given their wide distribution, their expression during ontogeny and adult life, their primary role as intracellular factors, and the complexity of their biologic effects.

Bosentan (Tracleer, Actelion Pharmaceuticals) is the first ET receptor antagonist approved for clinical use by the U.S. Food and Drug Administration (FDA). The ET neurohormonal system is activated in several cardiovascular conditions, including pulmonary artery hypertension (PAH), congestive heart failure (CHF), essential hypertension, acute myocardial infarction, and atherosclerosis.

This chapter reviews the biologic effects of ET and its receptors and the experimental and clinical experiences with ET receptor blockers in the treatment of primary pulmonary hypertension.

THE ENDOTHELIN NEUROHORMONAL SYSTEM

The ET family consists of a group of three 21–amino acid peptides with similar structures: ET-1, ET-2, and ET-3. ET-1 is the principal isoform in disease states. It is synthesized and secreted predominantly from the vascular endothelium in response to multiple stimuli, including hypoxia, ischemia, shear stress, growth factors, and other neurohormones, such as angiotensin II and norepinephrine. The development of specific ET receptor agonists and antagonists has led to the identification of two receptor subtypes in mammalian cells, ET_A and ET_B (Fig. 20-1, Table 20-1). ET_A receptors are present on smooth muscle cells and are responsible for the contractile response to ET-1. The vasoconstrictor effect persists even after ET-1 is removed from the receptor, probably due to sustained elevation of intracellular calcium concentration. Nitric oxide (NO) shortens the duration of vasoconstriction by accelerating the decrease of intracellular calcium to its basal concentration. ET_B receptors were first described on endothelial cells. They bind to ET-1 and ET-3 with similar affinity, and their stimulation leads to transient vasodilation, probably caused by increased production of NO and prostacyclin. However, ET_B receptors are also present on vascular smooth muscle cells, where their activation produces vasoconstriction.

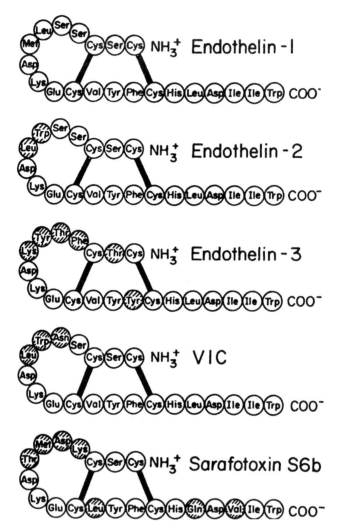

FIG. 20-1   Illustration of amino acid sequences of the three endothelin isoforms: ET1, ET2, and ET3. ET, endothelin. (*Reproduced with permission from Kramer BK, Nishida M, Kelly RA, Smith TW: Endothelins: myocardial actions of a new class of cytokines. Circulation 85: 350, 1992.*)

ET-1 is the most potent endogenous vasoconstrictor identified to date, with its effects persisting for several hours. It is 100 times more potent than norepinephrine and 10 times more potent than angiotensin II on a molar basis. Vasoconstrictive activity of ET-1 has been demonstrated in the pulmonary, coronary, renal, and systemic vasculature beds. In addition, there are clinical and preclinical data available suggesting that ET-1 displays motogenic, pro-

TABLE 20-1 Endothelin Receptors and Their Antagonists

Receptor type	ET_A	ET_B
Affinity	ET-1 > ET-2 >> ET-3	ET-1 = ET-2 = ET-3
Location	VSMC	EC, VSMC
Action	Vasoconstriction	Vasodilation, vasoconstriction
Upregulators	Hypoxia, cAMP	Angiotensin II
Downregulators	ETs, angiotensin II	cAMP
Selective agonist	—	ET-3
Selective antagonist	BQ-123	BQ-788

Key: cAMP, cyclic adenosine monophosphate; EC, endothelial cells; ET, endothelin; VSMC, vascular smooth muscle cells.
Source: Reprinted with permission from Kaur S, Frishman WH, Singh I, et al: Endothelin as a therapeutic target in the treatment of cardiovascular disease. *Heart Dis* 3:176, 2001.

inflammatory, and profibrotic activities in the vasculature and in the myocardium. ET-1 also acts as a potent modulator of the sympathetic nervous and renin-angiotensin-aldosterone systems. These latter actions of ET-1 could have additional deleterious effects in cardiopulmonary disease due to the hypertrophic effects of norepinephrine and angiotensin II and the potential profibrotic properties of aldosterone at the myocardium and in the vasculature. The plasma levels of ET-1 are elevated in CHF, with the magnitude of such elevations associated with disease-state severity and prognosis.

The vascular effect of ET-1 in healthy humans has been investigated by local infusion of the peptide into the brachial artery. ET-1 administration causes a dose-dependent vasoconstriction that is slow in onset and may be prevented by verapamil or nifedipine through blockade of voltage-operated calcium channels. Because of its potent vasoconstrictive effect and long-lasting action, the continuous release of small amounts of ET could contribute to the maintenance of elevated vascular tone. One postulated mechanism for the maintenance of basal tone is the production of vasoactive substances by endothelial cells. ET-induced vascular contraction is effectively antagonized by endothelium-derived vasorelaxant substances, such as prostacyclin and the potent endogenous vasodilator NO. An imbalance between the production of ET and NO could lead to a pathologic state of elevated vascular tone. Moreover, the vasoconstricting property of ET-1 is greatly enhanced in atherosclerotic vessels in which the opposing biological effect of NO is lost. A role of the endothelin system has been postulated in various conditions of disturbed vascular homeostasis, such as hypertension, coronary artery disease, and CHF.

ET of local or circulatory origin significantly contributes to the increased vascular resistance in the renal vasculature characteristic of several disease states. The kidney is considered a major site of endothelin production and an important target organ of this peptide. The highest immunoreactive levels of ET in mammalian cells exist in the renal medulla. However, ET also has been found in the renal cortex. The renal vasculature is preferentially sensitive to the vasoconstrictive effects of ET as compared with other arteries or veins. In contrast to the consistent effects of ET on renal hemodynamics, its effects on the excretion of sodium and water are variable. Systemic infusions of high doses of ET result in anti-natriuretic and antidiuretic effects, probably as a result of a decrease in the renal blood flow and glomerular filtration rate. In contrast, administration of low doses of the peptide induces natriuresis and diuresis. Also, administration of big ET, the precursor of ET, has been shown to have effects similar to those of low doses of ET. This finding supports the hypothesis that local ET acts in an autocrine or paracrine manner on the tubular epithelial cells, where it inhibits sodium reabsorption, thereby enhancing salt and water excretion.

In PAH patients, the expression of ET-1 is substantially increased in the vascular endothelial cells, particularly in the endothelium of elastic and muscular pulmonary arteries, where medial hypertrophy and intimal fibrosis are present. The expression of ET-1 in patients is relatively low in the pulmonary capillaries, veins, and bronchial arteries and is not observed in the systemic vessels of the myocardium or kidneys, suggesting that much of the ET-1 synthesis is localized at the primary site of the disease pathology in these patients. In other studies, plasma ET-1 levels and selective upregulation of ET_B receptor gene expression have been strongly correlated with elevated right atrial pressure in patients with primary PAH.

PHARMACOLOGY AND TOXICOLOGY OF BOSENTAN

Bosentan is a specific and competitive antagonist of ET-1 receptors (ET_A and ET_B). The affinity of bosentan for the ET_A receptor is about 100 times greater than that for the ET_B receptor in cultured cells. Administration of bosentan thus causes vascular smooth muscle relaxation and vasodilation.

Bosentan has been given as a single dose of up to 2400 mg in normal volunteers, or up to 2000 mg/day for 2 months in patients, without major adverse effects. The most common side effect in these situations is headache of mild to moderate intensity. In the Cyclosporin A Interaction Study, in which doses of 500 and 1000 mg twice daily of bosentan were given concomitantly with cyclosporine A, trough plasma concentrations of bosentan increased by 30-fold, resulting in severe headache, nausea, and vomiting, but no other serious adverse events. A mild decrease in blood pressure and increases in heart rate were observed. There is currently no other experience of overdose with bosentan beyond this circumstance. Because bosentan is a vasodilator, it is anticipated that massive overdose may result in pronounced hypotension requiring active cardiovascular support.

STRUCTURE, PHARMACOKINETICS, AND PHARMACODYNAMICS

Structure

Bosentan is a highly substituted pyrimidine derivative, with no chiral centers (Fig. 20-2). Its molecular weight is 569.64. Bosentan is stable in solid state and poorly soluble in water (1 mg/100 mL). It is not hygroscopic and not light sensitive.

Pharmacokinetics

After oral administration, the maximum plasma drug concentration is achieved within 4 to 5 h. The oral bioavailability in healthy subjects is about 50% and is unchanged at steady state. The bioavailability is unaffected by food. Volumes of distribution of bosentan are about 18 L after a single dose and 30 L after multiple dosing. Bosentan is also highly bound to plasma protein (98%), mainly to albumin.

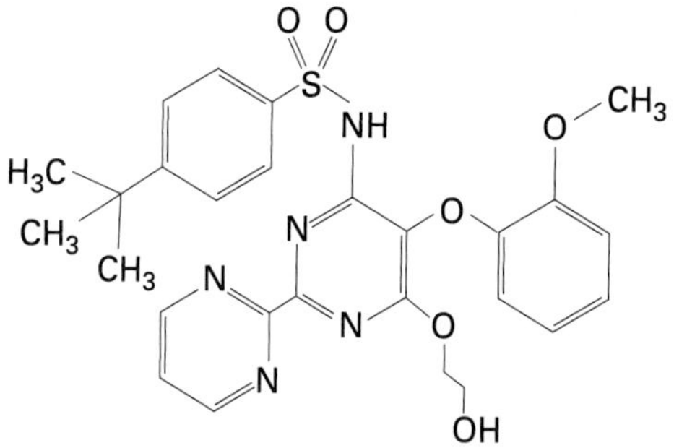

FIG. 20-2 Structure of bosentan.

In the liver, bosentan is metabolized by the cytochrome P450 (CYP) iso-enzymes, CYP3A4 and CYP2C9, to three metabolites, one of which is pharmacologically active. Although plasma levels of these metabolites are low relative to the parent compound, the active metabolite may contribute up to 20% of the pharmacologic effect. Steady-state drug levels are achieved within 3 to 5 days after multiple dosing, at which time plasma levels are approximately 50% lower than those observed after a single dose. This is caused by a twofold increase in clearance, which may be due to an induction of CYP3A4 and CYP2C9 isoenzymes. Bosentan is eliminated primarily by biliary excretion after metabolism in the liver, with less then 3% of an admin-istered oral dose recovered in the urine. The terminal elimination half-life of bosentan is approximately 5 h.

The pharmacokinetics, metabolism, and tolerability of bosentan are similar in healthy subjects and patients with mild liver impairment. Despite the absence of substantive pharmacokinetic changes for bosentan in mild liver dysfunction, caution should be exercised during the use of bosentan in these patients. It should be avoided in patients with moderate or severe liver abnor-malities and/or elevated aminotransferases of greater than the upper limit of normal.

In patients with severe renal impairment (creatinine clearance, 15 to 30 mL/min), plasma concentrations of bosentan were essentially unchanged, and plasma concentrations of the three metabolites were increased about twofold when compared with people with normal renal function. Although one of the metabolites is active, the accumulation of the metabolite does not appear to produce clinically important differences in patient response or inci-dence of side effects.

The pharmacokinetics of bosentan in pediatric patients with PPH and healthy adults are similar. It is not known whether the drug's pharmacokinet-ics are influenced by gender or race.

Pharmacodynamics

In healthy human subjects, the administration of a single oral dose of 600 mg or an intravenous dose of 250 mg of bosentan caused plasma ET-1 concentra-tions to increase maximally by twofold (oral) and threefold (intravenous). This increase with ET-1 was due to the release of ET-1 from the receptor sites and was directly related to bosentan plasma concentrations according to an Emax model. Bosentan reversed the vasoconstrictor effect of ET-1 measured in skin microcirculation. There was a tendency toward decreased blood pressure (approximately 5 mm Hg) and increased pulse rate (approximately 5 beats/min). However, these changes did not appear to be dose dependent. Bosentan is well tolerated orally. Its intravenous use, however, is limited due to local venous irritation. The intravenous form of the drug did not receive FDA approval. Additional pharmacodynamics data in patients with different disease states are discussed in the Clinical Studies section.

CLINICAL STUDIES

Pulmonary Arterial Hypertension

Pulmonary hypertension is characterized by endothelial injury, smooth muscle proliferation, and pulmonary vasoconstriction. ET-1 has been implicated in the pathophysiology of primary and secondary pulmonary hypertension in light of its vasoconstrictor and mitogenic properties. The plasma concentration and the immunoreactivity and expression of mRNA for ET-1 in the endothelial cells of hypertrophied pulmonary vessels are increased in primary and secondary pulmonary hypertension. In the rat model of pulmonary hypertension induced by exposure to a hypoxic environment, pulmonary ET-1 and ET_A and ET_B receptor gene expressions were upregulated. The clearance of ET-1 was thought to be decreased in patients with primary pulmonary hypertension as compared with controls. However, a recent study in which blood was sampled directly from the pulmonary artery has suggested an absence of a transpulmonary gradient for ET-1. ET has been implicated as a plausible contributor in the pathophysiology of pulmonary hypertension seen in patients with varied conditions such as Takayasu's arteritis, fenfluramine use, scleroderma, high-altitude pulmonary edema, and congenital heart disease and in those who have had cardiopulmonary bypass surgery.

In experimental animals, the orally active ET_A and ET_B receptor blocker bosentan and such selective ET -receptor blockers as TA-0201 and CI-1020, have been shown to prevent hypoxia-induced pulmonary hypertension and pulmonary artery remodeling. In another study in rats, combined treatment with an oral ET_A antagonist and an oral prostacyclin analogue was more effective in ameliorating pulmonary hypertension and right ventricular hypertrophy than was either drug alone.

Thirty-two patients with symptomatic, severe, primary PAH or PAH due to scleroderma [World Health Organization (WHO) classes III and IV] were randomized in double-blind fashion to 62.5 mg bosentan twice daily (administered orally) for the first 4 weeks followed by the target dose of 125 mg orally twice daily unless drug-related adverse events occurred (e.g., hypotension) or matching doses of placebo. Patients were allowed to receive other treatment for PAH including digoxin, anticoagulants, diuretics, and vasodilators (calcium channel blockers, angiotensin-converting enzymes inhibitors) but not epoprostenol (prostacyclin). The primary end point of the study was change in exercise capacity, and the secondary end points included changes in cardiopulmonary hemodynamics, dyspnea index, WHO functional class, and withdrawal due to clinical worsening of symptoms. In patients who received bosentan, the 6-min walk distance improved by 70 m at 12 weeks as compared with baseline, whereas in patients receiving placebo, it worsened by 6 m [difference of 76 m; 95% confident interval (CI), 12–139; $P = 0.021$). This improvement was maintained for 20 weeks. The cardiac index in patients receiving bosentan was higher than that in the placebo group by 1 L/(min • m^2) (95% CI, 0.6–1.4; $P < 0.0001$). Pulmonary vascular resistance decreased by 223 dyn-s/cm^5 with bosentan, but increased by 191 dyn-s/cm^5 in patients receiving placebo (difference, –415; 95% CI, –608 to –221; $P = 0.0002$). Patients given bosentan also had a reduced Borg dyspnea index (1.6 lower then placebo; 95% CI, 0–3.1; $P = 0.05$) and an improved WHO functional class as compared with those who received placebo. At baseline, all patients were in functional class III ($P = 0.019$, bosentan vs. placebo). At the end of 12 weeks, 9 of 21 (43%) patients in the bosentan group improved to class II, and none deteriorated to class IV ($P = 0.0039$ vs. baseline within group). With placebo, only 1 of 11 patients (9%) improved to class II, and 2 (18%) deteriorated to class IV ($P = 1.00$ vs. baseline within group). All three patients withdrawn from the study due to clinical worsening were in the placebo group ($P = 0.033$ for number of patients withdrawn, bosentan vs. placebo). The number and nature of adverse events did not differ between the two groups. No hypotension or clinically significant changes in hematologic or biochemical measures were seen in either group. Increases in the concentration of hepatic aminotransferases were seen in 10 patients assigned to bosentan, but these increases were not associated with symptoms, and the concentrations returned to normal without discontinuation or change of dose.

In the Bosentan Randomized Trial of Endothelin Antagonist Therapy Study Group, 213 patients with PAH (primary or associated with connective tissue disease) were randomly assigned to receive bosentan 62.5 mg orally twice daily for 4 weeks, followed by one of two doses of bosentan (125 or 250 mg orally twice daily) for a minimum of 12 weeks, or placebo. The primary end point was the degree of change in exercise capacity. Secondary end points included change in WHO functional class, Borg dyspnea index, and increased time to clinical worsening. At week 16, patients treated with bosentan (both doses) had an improved 6-min walking distance, 44 m more than the placebo group (95% CI, 21–67; $P < 0.001$), whereas a deterioration of 8 m occurred in the placebo group. Although both bosentan doses produced a significant treatment effect, the placebo-corrected improvement was more pronounced for the 250-mg twice-daily dose than for the 125-mg twice-daily dose. However, no dose–response relation for efficacy could be confirmed. Bosentan also improved the Borg dyspnea index (–0.6 in favor of bosentan; 95% CI, –1.2 to –0.1). The placebo-corrected improvement was greater for patients receiving 250 mg twice daily (–0.9, $P = 0.012$) than for those receiving 125 mg (–0.4, $P = 0.42$). At baseline, more than 90% of patients were in WHO functional class III. At the end of the treatment period, in the groups receiving 125 and 250 mg twice daily of bosentan, 38% and 34%, respectively, of patients had improved to class II, and 3% and 1%, respectively, had improved to class I. In contrast, in patients receiving placebo, only 28% improved to class II, and none improved to class I. This resulted in a mean treatment effect of 12% in favor of bosentan (95% CI, –3 to 25).

Another small, open-label, dose-ranging study was performed in seven female patients with primary PAH ($n = 5$) or PAH associated with scleroderma ($n = 2$). Four of these patients were resistant to inhaled NO therapy. Infusions of 50, 150, and 300 mg of bosentan were administered at 2-h intervals, and the hemodynamic responses were measured. Bosentan induced dose-dependent reductions in total pulmonary resistance (–20 ± 11%, $P = 0.01$) and mean pulmonary arterial pressure ($-10.6 \pm 11\%$, $P > 0.05$) compared with baseline. Systemic vascular resistance also was reduced ($-26.2 \pm 12.8\%$, $P < 0.005$), as was mean arterial pressure ($-19.8 \pm 14.4\%$, $P < 0.001$). There was a slight but nonsignificant increase in cardiac index ($15 \pm 12\%$, $P > 0.05$) and a dose-dependent increase in ET-1 level. This study demonstrated that intravenous bosentan is a potent pulmonary vasodilator at the doses tested, even in patients resistant to inhaled NO. However, systemic hypotension and local venous irritation may limit its intravenous use.

There is no current direct comparative trial of bosentan versus epoprostenol therapy.

ADVERSE EFFECTS, DRUG INTERACTION, PRECAUTIONS, AND CONTRAINDICATIONS

Adverse Effects

Safety data on bosentan were obtained from 777 patients in various clinical studies. Doses up to eight times the FDA-approved doses were administered for different durations. The use of bosentan in these trials ranged from 1 day to 4.1 years. In patients using bosentan for PAH, common adverse events that occurred in at least 3% of patients were headache, nasopharyngitis, flushing, liver function abnormalities, lower limb edema, hypotension, palpitation, dyspnea, edema, fatigue, and pruritus. In patients using bosentan for conditions other than PAH (primarily chronic heart failure) in clinical trials, the adverse events that occurred in at least 3% of patients were headache, flushing, abnormal hepatic function, leg edema, and anemia. Of these reported side effects, it is particularly important to pay close attention to hepatic function abnormalities. In clinical studies, the use of bosentan caused at least a threefold upper limit of normal elevation of liver aminotransferases in approximately 11% of patients, accompanied by elevated bilirubin in a small number of cases. The manufacturer currently recommends measurement of liver function test before initiation of therapy and then monthly thereafter. In current clinical trial settings, where close monitoring occurs, all elevations of liver function tests have been reversible within a few days to 9 weeks, spontaneously or after dose reduction or discontinuation, and without sequelae. Bosentan should be avoided in patients with baseline abnormal liver function tests.

Drug Interactions

Bosentan is highly bound to albumin (>98%, mainly to albumin). In vitro displacement studies were undertaken with digoxin, glyburide, phenytoin, tolbutamide, and warfarin. No relevant interactions between bosentan and these agents were observed at the level of protein binding.

Bosentan is metabolized extensively by CYP2C9 and CYP3A4. Inhibition of these isoenzymes may increase the plasma concentration of bosentan. Ketoconazole, a potent inhibitor of CYP3A4, increases maximum concentration and area under the curve of bosentan by 1.6- and 1.8-fold, respectively. There has been no drug-interaction study performed with a pure CYP2C9 inhibitor. In addition, medications that are also metabolized by CYP2C9 and CYP3A4 may compete with bosentan for the isoenzymes and alter each other's plasma concentration. In a study examining the interaction between bosentan and cyclosporin A, trough concentrations of bosentan were increased by about 30-fold. Steady-state bosentan plasma concentrations were three- to fourfold higher than those without cyclosporin A. However, the concentration of cyclosporin A was decreased by approximately 50%. The manufacturer currently contraindicates the coadministration of bosentan and cyclosporin. Bosentan is also an inducer of CYP3A4 and CYP2C9. Therefore, plasma concentrations of drugs metabolized by these two isoenzymes will be decreased when bosentan is coadministered. For example, coadministration of bosentan and glyburide decreased the plasma concentrations of glyburide by approximately 40%. The bosentan concentrations also were decreased by approximately 30%. In addition, an increased risk of elevated liver amino-transferases was observed. For this reason, the manufacturer contraindicates the use of bosentan and glyburide.

Warfarin is metabolized extensively by the liver. In addition, patients with PAH or chronic severe heart failure often receive warfarin for anticoagulation purposes. Therefore, it is anticipated that bosentan and warfarin may be commonly coadministered in clinical practice. In a drug-interaction study between bosentan and warfarin, coadministration of bosentan, 500 mg twice daily for 6 days, decreased the plasma concentrations of S-warfarin (a CYP2C9 substrate) and R-warfarin (a CYP3A4 substrate) by 29% and 38%, respectively. Clinical experience with concomitant administration of bosentan and warfarin in patients with PAH, however, did not show any clinically important changes in the international normalized ratio or the warfarin dose used.

Coadministration of bosentan also has been observed to decrease the plasma concentration of simvastatin (a CYP3A substrate) by approximately 50%. The plasma concentrations of bosentan were not affected. It is also anticipated that similar interactions will exist with other statins that have significant metabolism by CYP3A4, such as lovastatin and atorvastatin.

The manufacturer also studied the interactions between bosentan and digoxin, nimodipine (a CYP3A4 substrate), and losartan (a CYP2C9 substrate). No significant interactions were observed.

Precautions and Contraindications

Bosentan is contraindicated in pregnancy. Animal data have indicated that bosentan is likely to produce major birth defects. Bosentan was teratogenic in rats given oral doses of at least 60 mg/kg per day (twice the maximum recommended for human use based on milligrams per kilogram of body weight). Teratogenic effects observed included malformations of the head, mouth, face, and large blood vessels. Bosentan also increased stillbirths and pup mortality. Pregnancy must be excluded before the initiation of bosentan therapy and avoided after the beginning of therapy. Hormonal contraceptives, including oral, injectable, and implantable, may not be reliable in the presence of bosentan. Although there is no drug interaction study between bosentan and hormonal contraceptives, there is a possibility of reduction of plasma concentration with the coadministration of bosentan, because many of these drugs are metabolized by CYP3A4. Therefore, hormonal contraceptives should not be used as the sole contraceptive method in patients receiving bosentan. Follow-up urine or serum pregnancy tests should be obtained monthly in women of childbearing age receiving bosentan. It is not known whether bosentan is excreted in human breast milk, so the use of bosentan while breast feeding is not recommended.

Treatment with bosentan has been observed to cause a dose-related decrease in hemoglobin and hematocrit. In clinical studies, marked decreases in hemoglobin (>15% decrease from baseline resulting in values <11 g/dL) were observed in 6% of bosentan-treated patients and 3% of placebo-treated patients. Most of these decreases were detected during the first few weeks of bosentan treatment and stabilized at 4 to 12 weeks of treatment. The explanation for the change in hemoglobin is not known, but it does not appear to be related to hemorrhage or hemolysis. The manufacturer recommends that hemoglobin be checked at baseline, 1, and 3 months, and every 3 months after initiation of therapy.

CLINICAL USE

The FDA has approved bosentan (Tracleer) as the first oral drug for the treatment of pulmonary hypertension. The efficacy of bosentan was based on two placebo-controlled studies with symptomatic, severe (WHO class III and IV) primary pulmonary hypertension, or pulmonary hypertension due to scleroderma or other connective tissue diseases or autoimmune diseases. Bosentan was added to current therapy that included vasodilators, anti-coagulants, diuretics, digoxin, or supplemental oxygen. The drug was shown to improve exercise ability and decrease the rate of clinical deterioration.

DOSAGE AND ADMINISTRATION

Bosentan is available for clinical use in tablet form. The drug is not available in pharmacies; it is dispensed via a direct distribution program by the manufacturer. For the treatment of PAH, bosentan should be initiated at a dose of 62.5 mg orally twice daily for 4 weeks and then increased to the maintenance dose of 125 mg twice daily. Doses above 125 mg twice daily do not appear to confer additional benefit. In patients with a body weight below 40 kg but who are older than 12 years, the recommended initial and maintenance dose is 62.5 mg oral twice daily. Tablets should be administered in the morning and evening with or without food. Liver function tests should be performed at baseline, 1 month, 3 months, and every 3 months afterward. If at any point aminotransferase is greater than three but no greater than five times the upper limit of normal, the daily dose should be reduced or treatment should be interrupted. A liver function test should be repeated at least every 2 weeks. If liver function tests return to normal, one may consider continuing or re-introducing the treatment as appropriate. If aminotransferase is five to eight times the upper limit of normal, treatment should be stopped, and a liver function test should be performed at least every 2 weeks. Once the liver function test returns to normal, one may consider re-introducing treatment. If aminotransferase is greater than eight times the upper limit of normal, treatment should be stopped, and re-introduction of treatment should not be considered.

No dosage adjustment is required in renally impaired patients. There are no specific data to guide dosing in hepatically impaired patients. Because bosentan may cause liver injury, caution should be exercised in patients with mildly impaired liver function and generally should be avoided in patients with moderate or severe liver impairment.

There is limited experience with abrupt discontinuation of bosentan. No evidence for acute rebound has been reported. However, to avoid the potential for clinical deterioration, a gradual dose reduction (from 125 mg twice daily to 62.5 mg twice daily for 3 to 7 days before total discontinuation) should be considered.

CONCLUSION

ET, a potent vasoconstrictor and mitogenic agent, plays a role in multiple disease entities involving various organ systems in experimental animals and humans. In the few years since ET's discovery, much progress has been made in the development of specific receptor antagonists. ET antagonists have helped to elucidate the role of ET in normal physiologic processes and in the pathogenetic mechanisms of several conditions; in addition, these agents offer great promise as a new therapeutic intervention.

Bosentan is the first ET receptor antagonist approved by the FDA for the management of PAH. In patients with WHO class III and IV PAH, bosentan has demonstrated improvement of dyspnea and exercise tolerance. ET is a neurohormone that plays an important role in the pathophysiology of different vascular diseases. Although bosentan is currently approved for use in one disease state, its has the potential to alter the outcome of many other diseases such as heart failure, hypertension, ischemic heart disease, renal disease, and cerebrovascular disorders. Due to the rarity and poor prognosis of PAH and to the requirement of close monitoring of bosentan (due to its potential of causing liver dysfunction and its teratogenic effects), bosentan is currently available only through a special access program and distributed by certain selected pharmacies. Patients who are receiving bosentan should be encouraged to recognize early signs and symptoms of liver dysfunction and possible pregnancy. In addition, bosentan is not only a substrate but also an inducer of CYP3A4 and CYP2C9. Therefore, numerous drug interactions might occur. Patients should be advised to consult their physicians or pharmacists should they require other prescription or nonprescription medications.

ADDITIONAL READINGS

Barst RJ, Ivy D, Dingemanse J, et al: Pharmacokinetics, safety, and efficacy of bosentan in pediatric patients with pulmonary arterial hypertension. *Clin Pharmacol Ther* 73:372, 2003.

Bauer M, Wilkens H, Langer F, et al: Selective upregulation of endothelin B receptor gene expression in severe pulmonary hypertension. *Circulation* 105:1034, 2002.

Benigni A, Zoja C, Corna D, et al: A specific endothelin subtype A receptor antagonist protects against injury in renal disease progression. *Kidney Int* 44:440, 1993.

Fattinger K, Funk C, Pantze M, et al: The endothelin antagonist bosentan inhibits the canalicular bile salt export pump: A potential mechanism for hepatic adverse reactions. *Clin Pharmacol Ther* 69:223, 2001.

Frishman WH, Kaur S, Singh I, Tamirisa P: Endothelin as a therapeutic target in the treatment of cardiovascular disease, in Frishman WH, Sonnenblick EH, Sica D (eds): *Cardiovascular Pharmacotherapeutics,* 2nd ed. New York, McGraw-Hill, 2003, p 527.

Giaid A, Yanagisawa M, Langleben D, et al: Expression of endothelin-1 in the lungs of patients with pulmonary hypertension. *N Engl J Med* 328:1732, 1993.

Hickey KA, Rubanyi GM, Paul RJ, Highsmith RF: Characterization of a coronary vasoconstrictor produced by cultured endothelial cells. *Am J Physiol* 248:550, 1985.

Levin E. Endothelins. *N Engl J Med* 333:356, 1995.

Lüscher TF, Barton M: Endothelins and endothelin receptor antagonists. Therapeutic considerations for a novel class of cardiovascular drugs. *Circulation* 102:2434, 2000.

Packer M. ENABLE—the role of bosentan in CHF. American College of Cardiology Meeting, Atlanta, GA. Available at: http://www.acc.org/2002ann_meeting/ssnews/enable.htm. Accessed June 8, 2002.

Rondelet B, Kerbaul F, Motte S, et al: Bosentan for the prevention of overcirculation-induced experimental pulmonary arterial hypertension. *Circulation* 107:1329, 2003.

Rubin LJ, Badesch DB, Barst RJ, et al: Bosentan therapy for pulmonary arterial hypertension. *N Engl J Med* 346:896, 2002.

Sitbon O, Badesch DB, Channick RN, et al: Effects of the dual endothelin receptor antagonist bosentan in patients with pulmonary arterial hypertension: A 1-year follow-up study. *Chest* 124:247, 2003.

Ueno M, Miyauchi T, Sakai S, Goto K: The combined treatment of oral endothelin (ET)–A receptor antagonist and oral prostacyclin (PGI2) analog is more greatly effective in ameliorating pulmonary hypertension (PH) and right ventricular (RV) hypertrophy than each drug alone in rats (abstract). *Circulation* 100(suppl 1):I, 1999.

van Giersbergen PL, Popescu G, Bodin F, Dingemanse J: Influence of mild liver impairment on the pharmacokinetics and metabolism of bosentan, a dual endothelin receptor antagonist. *J Clin Pharmacol* 43:15, 2003.

21 | Cardiovascular Drug Interactions

Lionel H. Opie   William H. Frishman
Domenic A. Sica

Cardiovascular drug interactions are numerous, sometimes unpredictable, and potentially serious to the patient and the physician. Fortunately, serious interactions are relatively uncommon and often avoidable by simple clinical precautions based on a prior knowledge of the properties of the drugs in question. There are two types of drug interactions: pharmacokinetic and pharmacodynamic. *Pharmacokinetic interactions* concern all interactions at any stage of the pharmacokinetic steps that most drugs go through, i.e., absorption, distribution in the blood and binding to plasma proteins, metabolism (often in the liver), and excretion, often in the urine. Active metabolites may have additional interactions. *Pharmacodynamic interactions* result from additive cardiovascular hemodynamic or electrophysiologic effects. An example is added atrioventricular (AV) nodal block from the combination of verapamil and a beta blocker (Fig. 21-1). Although such an interaction could be predicted, its clinical relevance depends on specific unpredictable physiologic or pathologic variations found in the AV node of that particular individual.

The liver is the chief site of pharmacokinetic interactions (Fig. 21-2). An example is increased danger of myopathy with statins during the coadministration of erythromycin or ketoconazole, either of which inhibit the cytochrome P450 (CYP) 3A4 system in which most statins and calcium channel blockers (CCBs) are metabolized. A second example is the decreased rate of hepatic

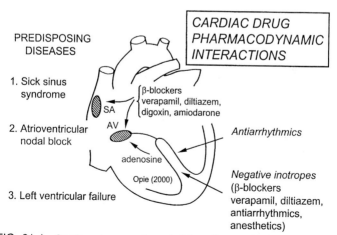

FIG. 21-1 Cardiac pharmacodynamic interactions at the levels of the SA node, AV node, conduction system, and myocardium. The predisposing disease conditions are shown on the left. AV, atrioventricular; SA, sinoatrial. *(Reproduced with permission from Opie LH, 2000.)*

433

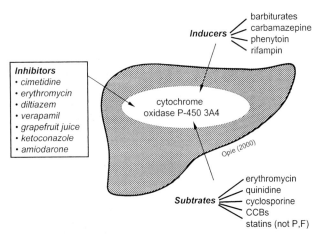

FIG. 21-2 Potential hepatic pharmacokinetic interactions at the level of cytochrome oxidase P450 (isoform CYP3A4). For details of cardiac drugs that might interact, see Table 21-1. CCB, calcium channel blockers; F, fluvastatin; P, pravastatin. *(Reproduced with permission from Opie LH, 2000.)*

metabolism of lidocaine during cimetidine therapy, with possible risk of lidocaine toxicity. A third example of a pharmacokinetic interaction is those drugs that act on the P-glycoprotein, which is the digoxin transmembrane transporter, showing how basic studies can help unravel well-known but poorly understood interactions such as that between quinidine and digoxin (Table 21-1). An example of a pharmacodynamic interaction arises when a CCB is added to β-adrenergic blockade in the therapy of severe angina, sometimes with excess hypotension as a side effect.

This chapter analyzes cardiovascular drug interactions in two ways. First, the *major organ sites* of such interactions are considered, starting with the heart itself, followed by an evaluation of vascular smooth muscle as a site for drug interactions, after which come hepatic and renal interactions. There are only a few interactions at the level of plasma proteins. Second, the major classes of cardiovascular drugs are sequentially considered.

PERSPECTIVE ON DRUG INTERACTIONS: SIDE EFFECTS VERSUS BENEFITS OF COTHERAPY

The existence of a significant interaction does not necessarily mean that the apparently adverse combination must be avoided. Rather, the overall interests of the patient need to be considered. For example, in the case of the combination of amiodarone and beta blocker in post-infarct patients, the combination seems synergistically effective from the point of view of prolonging life. In patients awaiting cardiac transplantation, a nonrandomized study has suggested that the combination improves mortality, albeit at the cost of about 6% of patients requiring a permanent pacemaker. Another example of the risk of the interaction having to be balanced against the expected benefits lies in combination lipid-modifying therapy with statins and fibrates. In some patients with severe lipidemias, the combination brings about the risk of myopathy, albeit relatively low, with a consequent, but even lower, risk of renal failure.

TABLE 21-1 Proposed P-Glycoprotein-Mediated Interactions of Cardiac Drugs: Comparison with Inhibition of Hepatic Cytochrome Isoforms

P-Glycoprotein interaction	Cytochrome inhibition
Antiarrhythmics	
Amiodarone	Inhibits several, including 3A4
Quinidine	Inhibits 2D6
Propafenone	None
Calcium channel blockers	
Verapamil	Inhibits 3A4
Diltiazem (weak)	Inhibits 3A4
Other cardiac agents	
Digoxin	None
Reserpine	None
Spironolactone	None
Other agents	
Cyclosporine	None
Dipyridamole	None
Erythromycin	Inhibits 3A4
HIV protease inhibitors	Inhibit 2D6, 3A4
Ketoconazole	Inhibits 3A4
Phenothiazines	None

Key: HIV, human immunodeficiency virus.
Sources: Abernathy DR, Flockhart DA: Molecular basis of cardiovascular drug metabolism. Implications for predicting clinically important drug interactions. *Circulation* 101:1749, 2000; Opie LH: Adverse cardiovascular drug reactions. *Curr Probl Cardiol* 25:621, 2000.

These risks must be balanced against the expected increase of life duration as a result of the combination achieving the dual aim of reducing the low-density lipoprotein cholesterol, for which statins are very effective, and increasing the high-density lipoprotein cholesterol, for which the fibrates are very effective. It is likely that computer-based decision making will become available to evaluate the exact probability of harm from a drug or drug class versus the expected therapeutic life-prolonging benefit, so that the patient and the doctor can make informed choices rather than relying on shrewd guesses.

THE HEART AS A SITE FOR DRUG INTERACTIONS

Sinoatrial and Atrioventricular Nodes

The sinoatrial (SA) node responds to at least three pacemaker currents, including the inward "funny" sodium current initially described in Purkinje fibers, or I_f; long-acting calcium current, or $I_{Ca(L)}$; and the delayed rectifier, the outward potassium current, I_k. Of these pacemaker currents, two are susceptible to beta blockers and one to CCBs. There are several reasons that the combination of a beta blocker with a CCB does not arrest the heart. First, neither type of drug affects the I_k pacemaker current. Second, the CCB effect is on the $I_{Ca(L)}$. The transient calcium current, $I_{Ca(T)}$, which likely accounts for the initial phases of depolarization in the SA and AV nodes, is not affected by standard CCBs. Third, only CCBs of the verapamil and diltiazem types are effective on the SA node in clinically used therapeutic doses.

Dihydropyridine CCBs (nifedipine, felodipine, isradipine, amlodipine, and others) have a much less marked effect on the SA node. In contrast, SA arrest has been reported when an intravenous bolus of verapamil or diltiazem is given to predisposed patients already receiving a beta blocker. Thus, adverse drug reactions at the level of the SA node causing excess bradycardia, excess tachycardia, or AV block often involve beta blockers, CCBs, or digitalis.

Intraventricular Conduction System

There are many antiarrhythmics that inhibit the intraventricular (His-Purkinje) conduction system. When these are given as co-therapy, they may interact to produce serious additive intraventricular conduction defects.

Proarrhythmic Drug Interactions

There are basically three possible proarrhythmic mechanisms. First, prolongation of the QT interval may occur, especially in the presence of hypokalemia and/or bradycardia (Fig. 21-3). The type of arrhythmia produced by QT prolongation is highly specific, namely torsades de pointes. Second, agents increasing myocardial levels of cyclic adenosine monophosphate or cytosolic calcium levels cause arrhythmias through a different mechanism, namely the precipitation of ventricular tachycardia and/or fibrillation. Third, β-adrenergic stimulants decrease plasma potassium levels, which in turn promote automaticity.

Mood-altering drugs (thioridazine, chlorpromazine, amitriptyline, maprotiline, and nortriptyline) predispose to torsades de pointes, presumably by prolongation of the action potential duration. The complex mechanism may include antimuscarinic, adrenergic, and quinidine-like effects.

Myocardial Contractile Mechanism

Drugs with negative inotropic effects include beta blockers, CCBs, and certain arrhythmic agents. Often, a relatively well-functioning left ventricle is able to withstand co-therapy with these drugs; but when the left ventricle is diseased, then even one of these drugs may precipitate heart failure.

VASCULAR SMOOTH MUSCLE

In vascular smooth muscle, there can be interactions that cause excess vasoconstriction, e.g., the combination of a drug inhibiting the reuptake of norepinephrine from the nerve terminals (such as cocaine) and therapeutic administration of monoamine oxidase inhibitors, which also inhibit the reuptake of norepinephrine in the nerve terminals. The combination of cocaine with these inhibitors theoretically could promote powerful coronary vasoconstriction. When dopamine is infused into a patient receiving monoamine inhibitors, there is a risk of severe hypertension from excess sensitivity to dopamine.

Conversely, there may be a number of drug interactions causing excess vasodilation and hypotension, e.g., the combination of the α_1 blocker prazosin with the powerful calcium antagonist vasodilator, nifedipine.

Vascular smooth muscle also can be the site of drug interactions that lessen the effects of antihypertensive or heart failure therapy.

HEPATIC INTERACTIONS

Pharmacokinetic Interactions

Many cardiovascular drugs are metabolized in the liver, generally via the cytochrome oxidase system involving one of several isoforms (see Fig. 21-2). Of the various isoforms, the CYP3A4 is the site of most hepatic interactions

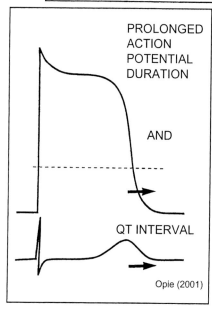

FIG. 21-3 Therapeutic agents, including antiarrhythmics, that may interact by QT prolongation to produce proarrhythmic effects with risk of torsades de pointes. Class III antiarrhythmic agents (amiodarone and sotalol) act chiefly by prolonging the action potential duration. QT prolongation with quinidine may be dose dependent, with a greater effect at relatively low concentrations, whereas with sotalol there is a dose-dependent increase in QT. Diuretics may cause QTu prolongation to precipitate torsades de pointes during co-therapy, e.g., with sotalol. Less commonly, torsades de pointes may develop after initiating antiarrhythmic drug therapy when there is a preexisting QT prolongation. *(For further details, see Opie LH, Gersh BJ: Drugs for the Heart, 5th ed. Philadelphia, WB Saunders, 2001. Reproduced from Opie LH, 2001.)*

of cardiac drugs. A number of interacting drugs, such as phenytoin, barbiturates, and rifampin, and the herbal remedy St. John's wort, can *induce the CYP3A4 isoform.* Accordingly, such drugs accelerate the breakdown of those cardiovascular drugs that are metabolized by this isoform, such as atorvastatin, cerivastatin, cyclosporine, disopyramide, felodipine, lidocaine, lovastatin, nifedipine, nisoldipine, propafenone, and simvastatin. Thus the inducers lessen the blood concentrations of these drugs and their therapeutic efficacy. Conversely, blood levels of these same drugs are increased by those agents that act as *inhibitors of the CYP3A4 isoform.* The prototype inhibitors are cimetidine and erythromycin, with grapefruit juice, the calcium blockers verapamil and diltiazem, and the antifungal agents such as ketoconazole. Thus, in statin-treated patients, excess circulating levels may build up, with a greater risk of adverse effects, including greater risk of myopathy.

There also may be a greater therapeutic effect as result of such drug interactions. For example, the dose of the expensive immunosuppressive cyclosporine can be reduced by co-therapy with verapamil or ketoconazole or high intake of grapefruit juice. Cimetidine inhibits a variety of other isoforms, so it can increase blood levels of a host of drugs, including the antiarrhythmic drugs quinidine, lidocaine, and procainamide; the CCB verapamil; and the beta blocker propranolol. Cimetidine, therefore, increases the blood levels of many of the cardiovascular drugs metabolized in the liver. Ranitidine inhibits fewer isoforms and is less likely to interact in this way.

Pharmacodynamic Interactions

These occur whenever altered hepatic blood flow changes the rate of first-pass liver metabolism. For example, when a beta blocker and lidocaine are given together, as may occur during acute myocardial infarction, the beta blocker reduces the hepatic blood flow to the liver and the rate of hepatic metabolism of lidocaine. The consequence is an increased blood lidocaine level, with the risk of lidocaine toxicity. Conversely, by increasing hepatic blood flow, nifedipine has the opposite effect, so that the breakdown of propranolol is increased, resulting in lower blood levels of propranolol. The combination of nifedipine and atenolol, the latter not being metabolized in the liver at all, therefore seems theoretically better than that of nifedipine and propranolol.

P-Glycoprotein

This newly discovered digoxin transporter operates whenever digoxin crosses the cell membrane (see Table 21-1), e.g., during renal excretion or when being taken up through the gut wall (Fig. 21-4). Inhibition of the transporter explains the major effects of quinidine and verapamil on blood digoxin levels and refutes the previous concept that erythromycin and tetracycline increase digoxin levels by inhibiting the gut flora that break down digoxin. Rather, these agents and especially erythromycin may act at least in part by inhibiting the P-glycoprotein.

RENAL PHARMACOKINETIC INTERACTIONS

Many drugs interact with each other by competing for renal clearance mechanisms by altering the rate of renal clearance of the other drug. For example, the renal clearance of digoxin is decreased by quinidine and by inhibition of the transporter P-glycoprotein, leading to an elevation of blood digoxin levels (see Fig. 21-4). This renal interaction attracted the attention of cardiologists because it explained certain strange aspects of the effects of these two drugs when given in combination. The knowledge of this interaction showed that apparently established properties of a drug might be explained more simply as drug interactions. For example, "quinidine syncope" could be caused by digitalis-induced arrhythmias precipitated by co-therapy with quinidine. Other antiarrhythmics that inhibit the renal excretion of digoxin include verapamil, amiodarone, and propafenone, which act on the same transporter (see Fig. 21-4).

PLASMA PROTEIN BINDING AS A SITE FOR DRUG INTERACTIONS

Sulfinpyrazone powerfully displaces warfarin from protein, so the dose of warfarin required may be dramatically less.

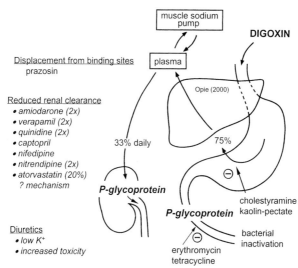

FIG. 21-4   Potential sites of digoxin interactions. Note the importance of reduced renal clearance. Many of the inhibitory effects on digoxin excretion likely are mediated by inhibition of the digoxin transporter, P-glycoprotein (see Table 21-1). 2× indicates that an approximate doubling of digoxin blood levels has been reported. *(Reproduced with permission from Opie LH: Adverse cardiovascular drug reactions. Circulation 25:621, 2000.)*

INTERACTIONS OF β-ADRENERGIC–BLOCKING DRUGS

β-Adrenergic blockers, by their inhibitory effects on the SA and AV nodes, can interact negatively with several other cardioactive drugs, including some of the CCBs (verapamil and diltiazem) and amiodarone (see Fig. 21-1). Otherwise, they have relatively few serious drug interactions (Table 21-2). An example of a pharmacokinetic interaction is that of cimetidine, which reduces hepatic blood flow and therefore increases blood levels of propranolol and metoprolol, both of which are metabolized in the liver. However, there is no interaction of cimetidine with beta blockers such as atenolol, sotalol, and nadolol, which are not metabolized in the liver. Another pharmacokinetic interaction is when verapamil raises blood levels of metoprolol through a hepatic interaction. Presumably other beta blockers metabolized by the liver may be subject to a similar interaction.

Now often used in the acute phase of myocardial infarction, beta blockers may depress hepatic blood flow, thereby decreasing hepatic inactivation of lidocaine. Thus beta blockade increases lidocaine blood levels with enhanced risk of toxicity.

INTERACTIONS OF NITRATES

Pharmacodynamic

The major pharmacodynamic drug interaction of nitrates is with sildenafil (Viagra), both of which are powerful vasodilatory agents. Thus there is risk

TABLE 21-2 Drug Interactions of Beta-Adrenergic-Blocking Agents

Cardiac drug	Interacting drugs	Mechanism	Consequence	Prophylaxis
Hemodynamic interactions				
All beta blockers	Calcium antagonists, especially nifedipine	Added hypotension	Risk of myocardial ischemia	Blood pressure control, adjust doses
	Verapamil or diltiazem; flecainide; most anesthetics	Added negative inotropic effect	Risk of myocardial failure; hypotension	Check for CHF, adjust doses; flecainide levels
Electrophysiologic interactions				
Beta blockers	Verapamil, diltiazem	Added inhibition of SA, AV nodes; added negative inotropic effect	Bradycardia, asystole, complete heart block, hypotension	Exclude "sick-sinus" syndrome, AV nodal disease, LV failure
	Amiodarone	Added nodal inhibition	Bradycardia, heart block	Exclude nodal disease
Hepatic interactions				
All lipid-soluble beta blockers: carvedilol, labetalol metoprolol, propranolol (probably timolol)	Inhibitors of hepatic CYP2D6: cimetidine, ritonavir, quinidine	Decreased hepatic breakdown of the lipid-soluble beta-blocker	Excess beta-blocking effects	Avoid interaction or reduce beta-blocker dose
Antihypertensive interactions				
All beta-blockers	Indomethacin, NSAIDs	Indomethacin inhibits vasodilation	Decreased antihypertensive effect	Omit indomethacin; use alternative drugs
Immune interacting drugs				
Acebutolol	Other drugs altering immune status; procainamide, hydralazine, captopril	Theoretical risk of additive immune effects	Theoretical risk of lupus or neutropenia	Check antinuclear factors and neutrophils; low co-therapy

Key: AV, atrioventricular; CHF, coronary heart failure; LV, left ventricular; NSAIDs, nonsteroidal anti-inflammatory drugs; SA, sinoatrial.
Source: Adapted with permission from Opie LH, Frishman WH: Drug interactions, in Fuster V, Alexander RW, O'Rourke RA, et al (eds): Hurst's the Heart, 10th ed. New York, McGraw-Hill, 2001, p 2251.

of life-threatening hypotension, so the combination is absolutely contraindicated. Other interactions of nitrates are also largely pharmacodynamic (Table 21-3). For example, during triple therapy of angina pectoris (nitrates, beta blockers, calcium antagonists), the efficacy of the combination may be lessened, because each drug can predispose to excess hypotension. Even two components of triple therapy, such as diltiazem and nitrates, may interact adversely to cause significant hypotension. Nonetheless, high doses of diltiazem can improve persistent effort angina when added to maximum doses of propranolol and isosorbide dinitrate, without any report of significant hypotension. Therefore, individual patients differ greatly in their susceptibility to the hypotension of triple therapy.

Other Interactions

Unexpectedly, high doses of intravenous nitrates may induce heparin resistance by altering the activity of antithrombin III. In dogs, nitroglycerin interferes with the therapeutic efficacy of the tissue plasminogen activator, alteplase. There is a beneficial interaction between nitrates and hydralazine, whereby the latter helps to lessen nitrate tolerance. The proposed mechanisms are speculative but may include vasodilation by a different mechanism to overcome the vasoconstriction of nitrate intolerance. Hydralazine also is a free radical scavenger, whereas peroxy nitrite triggers the vasoconstriction.

INTERACTIONS OF CALCIUM CHANNEL BLOCKERS

Many of the interactions of CCBs are *pharmacokinetic*. Hepatic metabolic interactions are especially numerous (Table 21-4). Drugs metabolized by the cytochrome oxidase system, such as nifedipine and verapamil, have their breakdown inhibited by cimetidine but not by ranitidine. Verapamil and diltiazem, which are metabolized by the cytochrome oxidase system in the liver, can inhibit the hepatic oxidation of some other drugs whose blood levels therefore increase. For example, the blood level of cyclosporine may increase during diltiazem therapy, and during verapamil therapy the blood levels of prazosin, theophylline, and quinidine may increase. Diltiazem also can interfere with hepatic nifedipine metabolism, thus potentiating dihydropyridine side effects when the drugs are used together.

In addition, many other interactions of CCBs are *pharmacodynamic*, such as added effects on the SA and AV nodes or on the systemic vascular resistance, with the risk of excess hypotension in predisposed subjects (Table 21-5). Specific examples are verapamil or diltiazem plus beta blockers or excess digoxin (see Fig. 21-1). There may be two important properties of CCBs that distinguish the specific compounds from each other. First, accumulating evidence suggests that short-acting compounds with acute vasodilatory effects induce acute hypotension and repetitive neurohumoral activation and tachycardia. Thus, the long-acting second-generation CCBs, such as amlodipine and nifedipine gastrointestinal therapeutic systems, are less likely to cause acute vasodilatory drug interactions than are shorter-acting compounds. Second, the dihydropyridine CCBs, such as nifedipine, amlodipine, and others, need to be distinguished from the nondihydropyridines, such as verapamil and diltiazem. The dihydropyridines have rather specific vascular dilatory effects, whereas the nondihydropyridines also inhibit the SA and AV

TABLE 21-3 Drug Interactions of Nitrates

Cardiac drug	Interacting drugs	Mechanism	Consequence	Prophylaxis
All nitrates	CCBs	Excess vasodilation	Syncope, dizziness	Monitor BP, caution
	Prazosin; other alpha-blockers	Excess vasodilation	Syncope, dizziness	Check BP, low initial doses
	Sildenafil (Viagra)	Excess hypotension*	Excess hypotension, syncope, myocardial infarction	Before giving nitrates for acute coronary syndrome, question for Viagra use in preceding 24 h
	Alteplase (t-PA)	Decreased t-PA effect	Thrombolytic benefit less	Avoid or reduce nitrate dose, policy not clear

*Viagra is metabolized by the 3A4 isoform so that inhibitors (see Table 21-4) predispose to excess Viagra levels and to nitrate interaction.

Key: BP, blood pressure; CCB, calcium channel blocker; t-PA, tissue-type plasminogen activator.

442

TABLE 21-4 Calcium Channel Blockers: Hepatic Interactions

Hepatic and other interactions of CCBs	Interacting drugs
Inhibitors of CYP3A4 tend to increase blood levels of CCBs	Cimetidine, erythromycin, grapefruit juice, ketoconazole, and related antifungals, amiodarone; St John's wort, a herbal remedy
Inducers of CYP3A4 tend to decrease blood levels of CCB, especially documented for verapamil	Barbiturates, carbamazepine, phenytoin, rifampin
CCBs as inhibitors of CYP3A4: verapamil and diltiazem, which should have similar effects	1. Verapamil increases blood levels of: carbamazepine, prazosin, theophylline, quinidine, cilostazol (expected)
	2. Dilitiazem increases blood levels of: cyclosporine, some HIV protease inhibitors, some statins (lovastatin, atorvastatin, simvastatin), cilostazol
Inhibition of digoxin transport P-glycoprotein	Digoxin blood levels increased by verapamil and nitrendipine

Key: CCBs, calcium channel blockers; HIV, human immunodeficiency virus.

nodes and are more negatively inotropic. Thus, the dihydropyridine CCBs have potentially fewer cardiac pharmacodynamic interactions, whereas the nondihydropyridine CCBs also interact with other nodal inhibitor drugs such as beta blockers and digoxin.

Another pharmacokinetic interaction, in this case at the level of the kidney, occurs between verapamil and digoxin, whereby digoxin clearance is decreased with consequent risk of digoxin toxicity. In the case of nifedipine and diltiazem, such interactions with digoxin appear to be less prominent.

All CCBs are oxidized by the CYP3A4 system, so that inhibition of this isoenzyme by erythromycin or ketoconazole will increase blood levels of CCBs, with increased risks of adverse effects such as hypotension or heart block, depending on the variety of CCB. Amlodipine, weakly metabolized by CYP3A4, is an exception. Thus, amlodipine could be the CCB of choice in those taking known inhibitors of the CYP3A4 system, such as grapefruit juice, cimetidine, erythromycin, or ketoconazole (see Fig. 21-2). In each case, there would be a low, but not zero, probability of an interaction. Grapefruit juice is also an inhibitor of the CYP3A4 system, leading to a doubling of the bioavailability of felodipine and lesser effects on most other dihydropyridine CCBs, with the exception of amlodipine.

INTERACTIONS OF DIURETICS

Thiazide Diuretics

Steroids, estrogens, indomethacin, and other nonsteroidal anti-inflammatory drugs (NSAIDs) lessen the antihypertensive effect of thiazide diuretics and may

TABLE 21-5 Nonhepatic Drug Interactions of Calcium Channel Blockers

Cardiac drug	Interacting drugs	Mechanism	Consequence	Prophylaxis
Verapamil	Beta blockers	SA and AV nodal inhibition; myocardial failure	Added nodal and negative inotropic effects	Care during cotherapy; check ECG, BP, heart size
	Cimetidine	Hepatic metabolic interaction	Blood V increases	Adjust dose
	Digitalis poisoning	Added SA and AV nodal inhibition	Asystole; complete heart block after IV V	Avoid IV V in digitalis poisoning
	Digoxin (D)	Decreased D clearance; inhibition of P-glycoprotein	Risk of D toxicity	Halve D dose; check blood D level
	Disopyramide	Pharmacodynamic	Hypotension, constipation	Check BP, LV function, and gut
	Flecainide (F)	Added negative inotropic effect	Hypotension	Check LV function and F levels
	Prazosin, other alpha-blockers	Hepatic interaction	Excess hypotension	Check BP during cotherapy
	Quinidine (Q)	Added alpha-receptor inhibition; V decreases Q clearance	Hypotension; increased Q levels	Check Q levels and BP
Diltiazem	Beta blockers	Added SA nodal inhibition; negative inotropism	Bradycardia, hypotension	Check ECG and LV function
	Cimetidine	Hepatic metabolism interaction	Increased diltiazem levels	Monitor ECG and LV function
	Cyclosporine (C)	Hepatic metabolism of C inhibited	Increased C levels	Adjust C dose
	Digoxin (D)	Some fall in D clearance	Only in renal failure	Check D levels
	Flecainide (F)	Added negative inotropic effect	Hypotension	Check LV function; monitor F levels
	Cilostazol	Hepatic metabolism of cilostazol inhibited	Increased cilostazol levels	Empirically decrease cilostazol dose
	Simvastatin, lovastatin, atorvastatin	Hepatic metabolism inhibited (less common with atorvastatin)	Increased levels	Decrease dose of respective statin

Nicardipine (see also nifedipine)	Digoxin (D)		Blood D doubles	Decrease D dose; check D levels
Nifedipine (N)	Cyclosporine (C)	Hepatic metabolism of C inhibited	Increased C levels	Adjust C dose
	Beta blockers	Added negative inotropism	Excess hypotension	Check BP, use low initial dose
	Cimetidine	Hepatic metabolic interaction	Blood nifedipine level increases	Halve nifedipine dose
	Digoxin (D)	Minor/modest changes in D	Increased D levels	Check D levels
	Prazosin (PZ), other alpha-blockers	PZ blocks α-reflex to N	Postural hypotension	Low initial dose of N or PZ or other α-blocker
	Propranolol (P)	N and P have opposite effects on blood liver flow	N decreases P levels; P increases N levels	Readjust P and N doses if needed
	Quinidine (Q)	N improves poor LV function; Q clearance faster	Decreased Q effect	Check Q levels
	Diltiazem	Hepatic metabolism of N inhibited	Hypotension	Adjust dose of N and diltiazem

Key: AV, atrioventricular node; BP, blood pressure; ECG, electrocardiogram; IV, intravenous; LV, left ventricle; SA, sinoatrial node.
Source: Adapted with permission from Opie LH, Frishman WH: Drug interactions, in Fuster V, Alexander RW, O'Rourke RA, et al (eds): *Hurst's the Heart,* 10th ed. New York, McGraw-Hill, 2001, p 2251.

worsen congestive heart failure (Table 21-6). Diuretic-induced hypokalemia and/or hypomagnesemia may predispose to ventricular arrhythmias, including torsades de pointes; when that happens, usually an antiarrhythmic agent such as a class III agent, including sotalol, dofetilide, ibutilide, and, probably to a lesser extent, amiodarone, and a class Ia agent, such as quinidine or disopyramide, is administered. The common mechanism of action is prolonging the QT interval, with risk of additional drug interactions (see Fig. 21-3). There is also some suggestion that diuretics may promote torsades independent of hypokalemia. Probenecid interferes with the urinary excretion of thiazide and loop diuretics, so diuretic efficacy is reduced. Diuretics may impair the renal clearance of lithium, thereby increasing the risk of lithium toxicity.

Loop Diuretics

Loop diuretics, given acutely and intravenously, may cause hypokalemia, thereby precipitating digitalis toxicity. Furosemide decreases renal clearance of lithium. Aspirin and certain NSAIDs may antagonize the action of furosemide and other diuretics, particularly in patients with advanced congestive heart failure and cirrhosis. In normal subjects, concurrent captopril therapy can reduce the diuretic effect of furosemide.

Spironolactone and Other Potassium-Retaining Diuretics

Angiotensin-converting enzyme (ACE) inhibitors tend to be potassium retaining and may cause hyperkalemia if combined with other potassium retainers, especially when there is renal failure. In the RALES study, spironolactone was successfully combined with ACE inhibition in the treatment of severe heart failure. However, the serum potassium level had to be between 3.5 and 5.0 mmol/L, and if hyperkalemia developed, the dose of the ACE inhibitor was down titrated. Further, significant renal impairment, which predisposes to hyperkalemia, (initial serum creatinine >2.5 mg/dL) was an exclusion criterion, and medication could be withheld if the value rose above 4.0 mEq/L. With these caveats, serious hypokalemia occurred in 14% and 10% of spironolactone- and placebo-treated subjects, respectively. Less well known is that cyclosporine plus potassium-sparing diuretics may cause hyperkalemia (according to the cyclosporine package insert), presumably via nephrotoxicity of the cyclosporine.

ANGIOTENSIN-CONVERTING ENZYME INHIBITORS AND ANGIOTENSIN RECEPTOR BLOCKERS

In general, ACE inhibitors have few high-dose interactions (Table 21-7). The most feared interaction is with high-dose diuretics, with risk of excess hypotension in over-diuresed patients. The potassium-retaining diuretics or potassium supplements with an ACE inhibitor can cause hyperkalemia. Nonetheless, in the RALES trial, spironolactone was cautiously added in low doses to heart failure patients already receiving an ACE inhibitor, with reduced mortality and no serious hyperkalemia (see previous section); however, in some patients, the dose of the ACE inhibitor had to be reduced. Indomethacin and NSAIDs may decrease the antihypertensive effects of ACE inhibitors (and almost all antihypertensives except for the dihydropyridine CCBs such as nifedipine). Thus, NSAIDs may diminish the benefits of ACE inhibitors in heart failure. Aspirin

TABLE 21-6 Drug Interactions of Diuretics

Cardiac drug	Interacting drugs	Mechanism	Consequence	Prophylaxis
Diuretics: loop and thiazide	Indomethacin and other NSAIDs	Pharmacodynamic	Decreased antihypertensive effect	Adjust diuretic dose or add another agent
	Probenecid	Decreased intratubular secretion of diuretic	Decreased diuretic effect	Increased diuretic dose
	ACE inhibitors, ARBs	Excess diuretics, high renins	Excess hypotension; prerenal uremia	Lower diuretic dose; initial low dose ACE inhibitor or ARB
Loop	Captopril	Possible interference with tubular secretion	Loss of diuretic efficacy of furosemide	Change to another ACE inhibitor
	Aspirin*	Inhibition of acute vasodilator response	Presumed less efficacy in heart failure	Delay aspirin when initiating acute therapy for heart failure
Spironolactone and other Potassium retainers	ACE inhibitors	Both retain potassium	Hyperkalemia	Monitor potassium, reduce ACE inhibitor dose

Key: ACE, angiotensin-converting enzyme; ARBs, angiotensin receptor blockers; NSAIDs, nonsteroidal anti-inflammatory drugs.
*Data from Jhund PS, Davie AP, McMurray JJV: Aspirin inhibits the acute venodilator response to furosemide in patients with chronic heart failure. *J Am Coll Cardiol* 37:1234, 2001.
Source: Adapted with permission from Opie LH, Frishman WH.: Drug interactions, in Fuster V, Alexander RW, O'Rourke RA, et al (eds): *Hurst's the Heart.* 10th ed. New York, McGraw-Hill, 2001, p 2251.

447

TABLE 21-7 Drug Interactions of Angiotensin-Converting Enzyme Inhibitors and Angiotensin Receptor Blockers

Cardiac drug	Interacting drugs	Mechanism	Consequence	Prophylaxis
ACEI (class effect)	Excess diuretics; rare in hypertension	High renin levels in overdiuresed patients; volume depletion	"First" dose hypotension: risk of renal failure	Reduce diuretic dose; correct volume depletion
ACEI (class effect)	Potassium-sparing diuretics; spironolactone	Added potassium retention	Hyperkalemia	Avoid combination or combine with care
ACEI (class effect)	Indomethacin	Less vasodilation	Fewer BP ↓ less anti-failure effects	Avoid, if possible
ACEI (class effect) Captopril	Aspirin, NSAIDs Loop diuretic	Less vasodilation Possible interference with tubular secretion	Fewer heart failure effects Lessened diuretic effect of furosemide	Low-dose aspirin Consider alternate ACEI drug
Captopril (C)	Immunosuppressive drugs, procainamide-hydralazine, possibly acebutolol	Added immune effects	Increased risk of neutropenia	Avoid combination; check neutrophils
	Probenecid (P)	P inhibits tubular secretion of C	Small rise in C levels	Decrease dose of C
ARBs (class effect)	Excess diuretics; rare in hypertension	High renin levels in overdiuresed patients; volume depletion	First dose hypotension; risk of renal failure	Reduce diuretic dose; correct volume depletion
	Potassium-sparing diuretics	Additional potassium retention	Hyperkalemia	Avoid combination or combine with care

Key: ACEI, angiotensin-converting enzyme inhibitor; ARB, angiotensin receptor blocker; NSAIDs, nonsteroidal anti-inflammatory drugs.
Source: Adapted with permission from Opie LH, Frishman WH: Drug interactions, in Fuster V, Alexander RW, O'Rourke RA, et al, (eds): Hurst's the Heart, 10th ed. New York, McGraw-Hill, 2001, p 2251.

also may interact negatively with ACE inhibitors in heart failure. The extent of this interaction is still controversial, and low-dose aspirin may lessen it. Although few clinicians would regard such co-therapy as contraindicated, e.g., in a post-infarct patient with left ventricular dysfunction, common sense would advise using the lowest dose of aspirin thought to be protective.

Captopril

High-dose captopril together with other drugs that alter or impair the immune status (such as hydralazine and procainamide) may predispose to neutropenia. Probenecid inhibits the renal tubular secretion of captopril, thereby potentially increasing blood captopril levels so that doses of captopril may need downward adjustment. Captopril may decrease digoxin clearance by 20% to 30%.

All Other ACE Inhibitors (Including Enalapril)

Drug interactions are similar to those of captopril, except that the immune system is not involved and the risk of neutropenia is much less. Because all these agents (except captopril) have a longer duration of action, adverse hypotensive interactions in diuresed patients are potentially more serious. Perindopril may provide relative protection against first-dose hypotension, although the mechanism behind this effect is poorly understood.

Angiotensin Receptor Blockers

Losartan and irbesartan, but not candesartan, are metabolized by the hepatic 2C9 isoform. Losartan is also metabolized by the 3A4 isoform. The 2C9 isoform is inhibited by fluvastatin. Although sources such as the Georgetown University Web site suggest the potential for an interaction of fluvastatin with losartan, no such interaction was observed in a drug–drug interaction study with fluvastatin and losartan. The hepatic enzymes responsible for candesartan and valsartan breakdown have not been identified but appear not to be part of the P450 isoform superfamily. With regard to pharmacodynamic interactions, blood pressure may drop significantly when these drugs are given to individuals who have been excessively diuresed and/or have a high renin form of hypertension. Hyperkalemia can occur with ACE inhibitor and angiotensin receptor blocker (ARB) therapies, particularly if a patient is predisposed to hyperkalemia. Hyperkalemia risk is highest in renal and/or heart failure patients, although the risk of hyperkalemia is less with ARBs than with ACE inhibitors. When ACE inhibitors and ARBs are used in the management of hypertension, the risk of hyperkalemia is substantially less. Drug interactions are rare for the ARBs, with the possible exception of the ARB telmisartan, whose coadministration with digoxin leads to increases in the serum digoxin level.

INTERACTIONS OF POSITIVE INOTROPIC AGENTS

Digoxin

The best known interaction is *quinidine with digoxin* (Table 21-8). Quinidine approximately doubles the blood digoxin levels, thus decreasing renal and extrarenal clearances. The mechanism is by the inhibition of the digoxin

TABLE 21-8 Interactions of Digitalis and Other Positive Inotropes

Cardiac drug	Interacting drugs	Mechanism	Consequence	Prophylaxis
Digitoxin	Verapamil	Nonrenal clearance of digitoxin falls	Digitoxin levels up by one-third	Check and adjust digitoxin dose
	Other drugs interacting with digitoxin	Altered digitoxin clearance (?)	Digitoxin levels increase (?)	Check and adjust digitoxin dose
Digoxin (D)	Amiodarone	Reduced renal clearance of D; P-glycoprotein*	D level may double	Check D level; halve dose
	Atorvastatin	Not known	D level may rise 20%	Check D level
	Captopril	Reduced D clearance	Blood D increases	Check D dose
	Diltiazem	Variable decrease of D clearance; P-glycoprotein*	Variable blood D increases	Check D level
	Diuretics: potassium-sparing amiloride or triamterene; spironolactone (S)	Reduced extrarenal D clearance; S reduces D clearance, inhibits P-glycoprotein	D levels vary, may rise by 20%; D levels increase, threat of toxicity	Check D level
	Erythromycin	Inhibits P-glycoprotein*	Decreased D loss into bowel; increased D levels, threat of toxicity	Check D levels, reduce dose if needed
	Nifedipine	Variable effect on D clearance	Variable blood D rises	Check D levels

450

	Nitrendipine	Reduced D clearance; mechanism not clear	Blood D Doubles	Check D levels, halve dose
	Prazosin (PZ)	PZ displaces D from binding sites	Blood D rises	Check D level; reduce dose empirically based on level
	Propafenone	P-glycoprotein*	D level increases	Check D level
	Quinidine, quinine	P-glycoprotein*	Blood D doubles	Check D levels, halve dose
	Verapamil	P-glycoprotein*	Blood D doubles or more	Check D levels; halve dose
Sympathomimetic inotropes				
Dobutamine, inamrinone, milrinone	Diuretics, high doses	Additive hypokalemic effects	Arrhythmias	Check blood potassium
Dopamine	MAO inhibitors	Decreased metabolism of dopamine	Increase in vasopressor effect of dopamine	Reduce dopamine dose by 90%
	Ergot derivatives	Additive vasoconstrictor effect	Limb ischemia	Avoid combination use

*See Table 21-1.

Key: MAO, monoamine oxidase.

Source: Adapted with permission from Opie LH, Frishman WH: Drug interactions, in Fuster V, Alexander RW, O'Rourke RA, et al (eds): Hurst's the Heart. 10th ed. New York, McGraw-Hill, 2001, p 2251.

transmembrane transporter, P-glycoprotein. Quinine given for muscle cramps acts likewise. The interaction between *verapamil and digoxin* is equally significant; digoxin levels increase by 60% to 90%. The mechanism is by inhibition of the digoxin transporter. Nitrendipine, not available in the United States but used in Europe, resembles verapamil in approximately doubling the digoxin levels. In the case of administering quinidine, verapamil, or nitrendipine to a patient already receiving digoxin, the previous dose of digoxin should be halved and the plasma digoxin level should be rechecked. The other CCBs, nifedipine and diltiazem, increase digoxin levels much less than does verapamil. Adjustment of the digoxin dose with these agents is usually not necessary, except in the presence of renal failure (which decreases digoxin excretion). Amlodipine does not increase digoxin levels. Hence, there are no simple rules to explain which class of CCBs or which specific agent is likely to increase digoxin levels significantly.

Among antiarrhythmics other than quinidine or verapamil, amiodarone and propafenone also elevate serum digoxin levels. Both inhibit the digoxin P-glycoprotein transporter. Other antiarrhythmics, including procainamide and mexiletine, have no interaction with digoxin except for a relatively small rise of digoxin levels with flecainide. When co-therapy elevates digoxin levels, the features of digitalis toxicity may depend on the agent added. With quinidine, tachyarrhythmias become more likely; whereas amiodarone and verapamil seem to repress the ventricular arrhythmias of digitalis toxicity, so that bradycardia and AV block are more likely.

Diuretics may indirectly precipitate digitalis toxicity by causing hypokalemia, which, when really severe (plasma potassium <3 mEq/L), may limit the tubular secretion of digoxin. Potassium-sparing diuretics (amiloride, triamterene, and spironolactone) and captopril decrease digoxin clearance by about 20% to 30% and may elevate serum potassium levels. When these combinations with digoxin are used in the therapy of congestive heart failure, the blood digoxin level must be watched. Unexpectedly, spironolactone and its metabolite canrenone may decrease features of digitalis toxicity, probably through increased potassium levels resulting from aldosterone inhibition. Nonetheless, the combination of digoxin, quinidine, and spironolactone markedly elevates digoxin levels.

Cholestyramine may cause decreased gastrointestinal absorption of digoxin, probably because of the binding of digoxin to the resin; digoxin therefore should be given several hours before the resin; alternatively, digoxin capsules may be used. Digoxin capsules also decrease interaction with kaolin-pectate, which otherwise reduces digoxin absorption, and with erythromycin and tetracycline. Cancer chemotherapeutic agents may damage intestinal mucosa and depress digoxin absorption.

Increased digoxin bioavailability with erythromycin and tetracycline had been ascribed to changes in the gut flora caused by the antibiotics. An alternative and current explanation is that erythromycin inhibits the P-glycoprotein transporter.

INTERACTION OF SYMPATHOMIMETIC AGENTS

Dopamine

Dopamine is contraindicated during the use of cyclopropane or halogenated hydrocarbon anesthetics (enhanced risk of arrhythmias). Monoamine oxidase inhibitors decrease the rate of dopamine metabolism by the tissues; the dose of dopamine therefore should be cut to one-tenth of the usual dose.

Dobutamine

Dobutamine decreases plasma potassium and should be given with care when given with diuretics, especially intravenous furosemide (see Table 21-8).

Inamrinone and Milrinone

Inamrinone and milrinone are phosphodiesterase inhibitors that also can provoke arrhythmias. During diuretic therapy, plasma K^+ needs monitoring. When these drugs are combined with digitalis, the digoxin level does not change, but digoxin toxicity should be guarded against, because of multiple mechanisms for arrhythmia development.

INTERACTIONS OF VASODILATORS

Nitroprusside and Hydralazine

Nitroprusside and hydralazine (Table 21-9) may decrease digoxin levels, possibly as a result of increased tubular secretion, by improving congestive heart failure and related renal hemodynamics. Hydralazine, by creating hepatic shunts, may substantially increase the blood levels of those beta blockers that undergo hepatic metabolism, such as propranolol and metoprolol. Hydralazine interacts beneficially with nitrates, helping to lessen nitrate tolerance.

Prazosin, Doxazosin, and Terazosin

There is an interaction between prazosin and the CCBs verapamil and nifedipine, resulting in excessive hypotension. In the case of verapamil, part of the effect may be explained by a pharmacokinetic hepatic interaction. Nitrates and prazosin may cause syncope, and these agents should be combined with care. Similar interactions may occur with the other agents in this group. The package insert for terazosin warns of a specific hypotensive interaction with verapamil.

Cilostazol

This is a newly available peripheral vasodilator indicated for intermittent claudication that acts by phosphodiesterase inhibition, a mechanism (with other drugs) associated with an increased mortality in heart failure. It is metabolized by the hepatic CYP3A4 system, so there is a potential interaction with inhibitors of this system, such as verapamil, diltiazem, erythromycin, and ketoconazole, all of which could elevate cilostazol levels with increased risk of adverse effects in heart failure.

INTERACTIONS OF ANTIHYPERTENSIVE DRUGS

Interactions for diuretics, β-adrenergic blockers, CCBs, ACE inhibitors, and vasodilators have already been considered. Note that all vasodilators approved for peripheral vascular disease lower blood pressure, with the exception of cilostazol. In general, NSAIDs interfere with the efficacy of all antihypertensive drugs, with the exception of CCBs. Unlike other NSAIDs, aspirin and sulindac may be spared this interaction. When dihydropyridine CCBs are used as antihypertensives, part of their effect derives from their natriuretic properties, which has led to the suggestion (not borne out by fact) that a diuretic is not additive with a CCB.

TABLE 21-9 Drug Interactions of Vasodilators

Cardiac drug	Interacting drugs	Mechanism	Consequence	Prophylaxis
Hydralazine	BB (hepatically metabolized)	Hepatic shunting	BB metabolism ↓; blood levels ↑	Propranolol, metoprolol dose ↓
	Nitrates (N)	Renal blood flow ↑; added vasodilation; free radicals scavenged	Less N tolerance; risk of excess hypotension	Could be serious interaction with Viagra
Hydralazine/nitroprusside,	Digoxin (D)	Increased renal D excretion	Decreased D levels	Check D levels
Prazosin (Pz), other alpha-blockers	Nifedipine; other dihydropyridine calcium blockers	Pharmacodynamic	Excess hypotension	Start with low dose of of alpha-blocker or dihydropyridine calcium blocker
	Nitrates	Pharmacodynamic	Syncope, hypotension	Decrease PZ dose
	Verapamil	Hepatic metabolism	Synergistic antihypertensive effect	Adjust doses
Cilostazol (C)	Inhibitors of P450 3A4: diltiazem, verapamil, erythromycin, ketoconazole, cyclosporine	↓ Hepatic interaction	Increased C levels, risk of increased mortality in heart failure	Reduce C dose or avoid

Key: BB, beta blocker.
Source: Adapted with permission from Opie LH, Frishman WH: Drug interactions, in Fuster V, Alexander RW, O'Rourke RA, et al (eds): Hurst's the Heart, 10th ed. New York, McGraw-Hill, 2001, p 2251.

INTERACTIONS OF ANTIARRHYTHMIC AGENTS

The emphasis of antiarrhythmic therapy has moved away from agents that do not save lives, such as the class Ia agents quinidine and disopyramide and the class Ic agents such as flecainide and propafenone. All these compounds have potentially proarrhythmic drug interactions (Table 21-10). The new emphasis is on drugs that are known to save lives, such as the beta blockers and amiodarone. Another trend is to intervene in those with serious recurrent supraventricular reentrant tachycardias of the Wolff-Parkinson-White and related syndromes rather than to face prolonged drug therapy. In ventricular tachycardia, the patients at greatest risk are now ideally treated by an implantable cardioverter defibrillator. Thus, lesser importance is attached to some of the numerous drug interactions of these agents, which, nevertheless, must be understood.

The most frequent antiarrhythmic drug interactions are with digoxin (the levels of which increase with quinidine and verapamil due to inhibition of the P-glycoprotein transmembrane transporter for digoxin), with diuretics (there is a risk of QT prolongation with antiarrhythmics, such as quinidine, disopyramide, amiodarone, sotalol, dofetilide, and ibutilide, all of which prolong duration of the action potential), and at the level of hepatic enzyme inhibition. The mechanism whereby quinidine increases blood digoxin levels has only recently been elucidated (see Table 21-1). There is also the risk of antiarrhythmic drug–drug interactions. Thus, amiodarone, when added to quinidine, enhances the risk of QT prolongation (see Fig. 21-3), whereas quinidine levels increase, thus increasing the risk of quinidine toxicity. The combination of antiarrhythmic drugs that depress the sinus node, such as amiodarone and beta blockers, or CCBs occasionally can lead to life-threatening bradycardia that requires a pacemaker (see Amiodarone). Hepatic enzyme inducers can alter the metabolism of agents such as quinidine and other antiarrhythmics that are metabolized in the liver. Cimetidine decreases the hepatic metabolism of these agents, whereas phenytoin, barbiturates, and rifampin have opposite effects (see Fig. 21-2).

Adenosine is used increasingly to terminate supraventricular reentrant tachycardias. Dipyridamole inhibits its breakdown, so the adenosine dose must be markedly reduced, perhaps to about one-eighth, in those receiving dipyridamole. Rarely, in the presence of digoxin or verapamil, adenosine may precipitate ventricular fibrillation (according to the package insert). As an AV nodal inhibitor (see Fig. 21-1), it may have additive inhibitory effects in the presence of digoxin, verapamil, diltiazem, amiodarone, or beta blockade.

INTERACTIONS OF ANTITHROMBOTIC AND THROMBOLYTIC AGENTS

Aspirin

Blood levels of uric acid may be increased by low-dose aspirin and thiazide diuretics, so special care is required in patients with a history of gout. Conversely, aspirin may decrease the uricosuric effects of sulfinpyrazone and probenecid (Table 21-11). Aspirin also reduces the natriuretic effect of spironolactone. Aspirin-induced gastrointestinal bleeding may be a greater hazard in patients receiving other NSAIDs or corticosteroid therapy. Antacids, by altering gastric and urine pH, may decrease plasma salicylate levels.

TABLE 21-10 Drug Interactions of Antiarrhythmic Drugs

Cardiac drug	Interacting drugs	Mechanism	Consequence	Prophylaxis
Class 1a Quinidine (Q)	Amiodarone	Added QT effects; blood Q rises	Torsades de pointes	Check QT levels and potassium
	Antibiotics (some)	Quinidine inhibits muscarinic receptors	Increased antibiotic-induced muscular weakness	Clinical care, drug levels
	Anticholinesterases (Ach)	Quinidine inhibits muscarinic receptors	Decreased ACh efficacy in myasthenia gravis	Avoid Q, if possible
	Antihypertensive agents; beta blockers	Added hypotensive and added SA nodal effects	Hypotension, excess bradycardia	Check BP and ECG
	Cimetidine (C)	C inhibits oxidative metabolism of Q	Increased Q levels, risk of toxicity	Q levels, consider switching to ranitidine
	Warfarin, other coumarin anticoagulants	Hepatic interaction with Q	Bleeding	Check INR
	Digoxin (D)	Decreased D clearance; inhibition of P-glycoprotein	Risk of D toxicity	Check D dose levels
	Diltiazem	Added inhibition of SA node	Excess bradycardia	Check ECG, heart rate
	Disopyramide	Added QT prolongation	Torsades de pointes	Check QT intervals and potassium
	Diuretic, potassium losing	Hypokalemia and QT prolongation	Torsades de pointes	Check QT interval and potassium
	Hepatic enzyme inducers (phenytoin, barbiturates, rifampin)	Increased Q hepatic metabolism by CYP3A4	Decreased	Q levels, dose alterations
	Nifedipine	Increased Q clearance	Decreased Q levels	Q levels, doses
	Class III agents: Sotalol, amiodarone, dofetilide, ibutilide	Added QT prolongation	Torsades de pointes	Check QT interval and potassium
	Verapamil	Decreased Q clearance	Excess bradycardia	Check ECG, Q levels
	Warfarin	Hepatic interaction with Q	Bleeding	Check INR

Drug	Interacting agent	Mechanism	Effect	Recommendation
Procainamide (P)	Cimetidine	Decreased renal P clearance	Prolonged P half-life, excess P effect	Reduce P dose; consider ranitidine
Disopyramide	Agents prolonging APD (quinidine, amiodarone, sotalol)	Added QT prolongation especially if hypokalemia	Torsades de pointes	Check QT interval and potassium
Class1a (all agents)	Drugs inhibiting SA or AV nodes/conduction system (quinidine, beta blockers, methyldopa, digoxin)	Pharmacodynamic additive effects	SA, AV block; conduction block	Check ECG; decrease doses
	Pyridostigmine	Inhibition of cholinesterase activity	Beneficial effect of P on D; harmful effect of D on P	In myasthenia gravis, avoid D
Class 1b				
Lidocaine (L)	Verapamil (V), diltiazem (Di)	Combined negative inotropism	Hypotension	Avoid IV Di or V cotherapy
	Cimetidine	Decreased hepatic metabolism	Increased L levels	Decrease L infusion rate
	Halothane	Decreased hepatic blood flow	Increased L levels	Decrease L infusion rate
	Propranolol	Decreased hepatic blood flow	Increased L levels	Decrease L infusion rate
	Other beta blockers	Decreased hepatic blood flow	Increased L levels	Decrease L infusion rate
Mexiletine (M)	Hepatic enzyme inducers*	Increased hepatic metabolism	Decreased plasma M levels	Increase M dose
Class 1c				
Flecainide (F)	Amiodarone	Unknown	Blood F rises; added effect on nodes, myocardium	Decrease F dose
	Digoxin (D)	Decreased D clearance	Blood D rises slightly	Check D level
	Drugs inhibiting SA or AV nodes, IV conduction, or myocardial function	Pharmacodynamic additive	SA, AV block; conduction block, cardiogenic shock	Avoid combinations, decrease doses
Propafenone	Cimetidine	Decreased hepatic F loss	Blood F rises	Check F dose
	Digoxin (D)	Inhibition of P-glycoprotein	Increased D level	Decrease D dose

(continued)

TABLE 21-10 *(continued)* Drug Interactions of Antiarrhythmic Drugs

Cardiac drug	Interacting drugs	Mechanism	Consequence	Prophylaxis
Class III Amiodarone[†]	Drugs prolonging QT interval (see Fig. 21-2)	Additive effects on repolarization and QT interval	Torsades de pointes	Avoid low potassium; avoid combinations
	Beta blockers	Added nodal depression	Bradycardia; heart block	Cotherapy can be very effective; may need pacemaker
	Quinidine (Q)	CYP 2D6 Inhibition	Blood Q rises	Check Q levels
	Procainamide (P)	Pharmacokinetic	Blood P rises	Check P dose
Sotalol, dofetilide, ibutilide	As for amiodarone and including amiodarone	Hypokalemia plus class III action, as for amiodarone	Torsades de pointes	Exclude low K⁺; use K⁺ retaining diuretic
Class IV Adenosine (Ad)	Dipyridamole (Dp)	Dp inhibits breakdown of Ad	Excess nodal inhibition	Reduce Ad dose to 25% or less
	Theophylline (T)	T blocks Ad receptor	Decrease Ad effect	Carefully adjust Ad dose upward

*See Table 21-4.
†See Table 21-11.
Key: APD, action potential duration; AV, atrioventricular; BP, blood pressure; ECG, electrocardiogram; INR, international normalized ratio; IV, intravenous; SA, sinoatrial.
Source- Adapted with permission from Opie LH, Frishman WH: Drug interactions, in Fuster V, Alexander RW, O'Rourke RA, et al (eds): *Hurst's the Heart,* 10th ed. New York, McGraw-Hill, 2001, p 2251.

TABLE 21-11 Drug Interactions of Antithrombotic Agents

Cardiac drug	Interacting drugs	Mechanism	Consequence	Prophylaxis
Aspirin (A)	ACE inhibitors	Vasodilation	Antifailure effect ↓	Low A dose
	Hepatic enzyme inducers (barbiturates, phenytoin, rifampin)	Increased A metabolism	Decreased A effect	Adjust A dose; check A side effects
	Sulfinpyrazone (S)	A decreases urate excretion	Decreased uricosuric effect of S or P	Increase dose of S or P
	Probenecid (P)			
	Thiazide diuretics	A decreases urate excretion	Hyperuricemia	Check blood urate (no specific treatment for values <12 mg/dL)
Clopidogrel	Warfarin	A is antithrombotic	Excess bleeding	Check INR
	Aspirin	Added platelet inhibition	Excess bleeding	Awareness of risk
	Warfarin (W)	W is antithrombotic	Excess bleeding	Check INR or PT
	Drugs metabolized by CYP2C9	Isozyme inhibition	Excess effects of the other drug	Awareness of risk
Ticlopidine	Aspirin, warfarin	As for clopidogrel	As for clopidogrel	As for clopidogrel
	Cimetidine	Hepatic CYP1A2	Increased levels of ticlopidine	Avoid use of cimetidine
Sulfinpyrazone (S) Warfarin (W)	Warfarin (W)	S displaces W from plasma proteins	Excess bleeding	Check INR
	Potentiating drugs			
	Allopurinol	Mechanism unknown	Excess bleeding	Check INR periodically
	Amiodarone	Mechanism unknown	Sensitizes to W for months	Avoid combination
	Aspirin	Added bleeding tendency	Excess bleeding	Check INR intermittently
	Cimetidine	Decreased W degradation	Excess bleeding	Check INR intermittently
	Quinidine	Hepatic interaction	Excess bleeding	Check INR intermittently
	Statins	Hepatic interaction ?	Excess bleeding	Check INR
	Sulfinpyrazone	Displaces W from plasma proteins	Excess bleeding	Check INR or PT
	Interfering drugs			
	Cholestyramine, Colestipol	Decrease absorption of W	Decreased W effect	Check INR or PT
Alteplase, t-PA	Nitrates	Decreased t-PA effect	Less thrombolytic benefit	Avoid or reduce nitrate dose; increase t-PA dose

Key: ACE, angiotensin-converting enzyme; INR, international normalized ratio; PT, prothrombin time; t-PA, tissue-type plasminogen activator.
Source: Adapted with permission from Opie LH, Frishman WH: Drug interactions, in Fuster V, Alexander RW, O'Rourke RA, et al (eds): *Hurst's the Heart.* 10th ed. New York, McGraw-Hill, 2001, p 2251.

459

Hepatic enzyme inducers of cytochrome P450 (barbiturates, phenytoin, and rifampin) increase aspirin. Aspirin tends to cause hypoglycemia in patients receiving oral hypoglycemics or insulin. Aspirin, especially in high doses, may exaggerate a bleeding tendency and worsen anticoagulant-induced bleeding.

Clopidogrel

The use of this agent will increase in light of positive findings from a large trial in unstable angina in which it was given with aspirin. As expected, the incidence of bleeding, major and minor, was increased without more life-threatening bleeds. The package insert also indicates more gastrointestinal bleeding with NSAIDs, and, by analogy with aspirin, there may be excess bleeding with warfarin. No heparin interaction was found. In general, there are few other documented drug interactions, but at high concentrations, clopidogrel does inhibit the hepatic CYP2C9 that metabolizes carvedilol, cerivastatin, fluvastatin, irbesartan, losartan, torsemide, warfarin, and many NSAIDs. Therefore, there are potential drug interactions that merit consideration during coadministration.

Ticlopidine

This drug inhibits platelet aggregation at the same site as clopidogrel but may cause more serious adverse reactions, such as neutropenia. It similarly interacts with aspirin and NSAIDs, and increased bleeding with warfarin is another risk. It is metabolized by hepatic CYP2C9, with the same potential interactions as clopidogrel, and by CYP1A2, thus explaining why cimetidine, an inducer of this isoenzyme, decreases the clearance of a single dose of ticlopidine by 50%.

Sulfinpyrazone

Sulfinpyrazone is highly bound to plasma proteins (98% to 99%) and may displace warfarin to precipitate bleeding. Like aspirin, sulfinpyrazone may sensitize patients, who are given sulfonylureas and insulin, to hypoglycemia.

Dipyridamole

Dipyridamole is a potent vasodilator, so care is required when it is used in combination with other vasodilators. Dipyridamole inhibits the breakdown of adenosine (see Antiarrhythmics, class IV).

Warfarin

Numerous Drug and Diet–Drug Interactions

Warfarin may be subject to many (up to 80) drug interactions. Further, there is a *diet–drug interaction.* Warfarin's effects are lessened by a diet rich in the precursor of prothrombin, vitamin K, as found in dark, green vegetables and certain plant oils, including those used in margarines and salad dressings. Therefore, to avoid undue fluctuations in the international normalized ratio (INR), a measure of prothrombin time, the dietary intake of these should be constant. Overall, the safest rule is to persuade patients receiving oral anticoagulation to stay on a constant diet and not to use any new or over-the-counter drugs without consultation, while the physician carefully assesses any newly added compounds. More frequent measurements of the INR and dose adjustments are required when potentially interfering drugs, including herbal agents, are added.

Mechanisms

The major known sites of interaction are, first, the plasma proteins, where warfarin is bound while circulating and, second, the hepatic cytochrome P450 system, where warfarin is broken down by the CYP2C9 isoform. For example, with amiodarone, a given dose of warfarin has a greater inhibition of prothrombin, with increased risk of bleeding resulting from the inhibition by amiodarone of the CYP2C9 isoform. It should be recalled that coagulation is a complex process, and any drug impairing platelet function, such as aspirin, ticlopidine, or clopidogrel, may indirectly promote bleeding by warfarin. Very high doses of aspirin (six to eight tablets per day) may act differently by impairing synthesis of clotting factors. Heparin also potentiates the risk of bleeding; there are large individual variations in many of these interactions.

Interfering drugs include those that reduce absorption of vitamin K, warfarin (cholestyramine), or sulfinpyrazone (that displaces warfarin from the plasma protein binding sites) and those that induce hepatic enzymes (barbiturates, phenytoin, and rifampin). The latter drugs and the herbal agent, St. John's wort, increase the rate of warfarin metabolism in the liver. *Potentiating drugs* include those that decrease warfarin degradation by inhibiting the CYP2C9 isoform. These include a variety of antibiotics such as metronidazole (Flagyl) and co-trimoxazole (Bactrim). Other antifungals, such as fluconazole and the vaginal suppository miconazole, also potentiate warfarin. Cimetidine likewise inhibits hepatic degradation; ranitidine does not. Other potentiating drugs include the cardiovascular agents allopurinol, propafenone, quinidine, and amiodarone. Amiodarone is especially dangerous because of its excessively long half-life, so this interaction can occur even after withdrawal of amiodarone. Grapefruit juice does not act on the CYP2C9 but on the CYP3A4; it has no interaction with warfarin. It must be emphasized that sulfinpyrazone powerfully displaces warfarin from blood proteins, so the dose of warfarin may have to be reduced to as low as 1 mg in some patients.

Lipid-Lowering Drugs

Fibrates may markedly potentiate warfarin, whereas the statins in general have little or no effect. The effects of statins are not too surprising because most of them (exceptions: pravastatin and fluvastatin) are metabolized by the CYP3A4 isoform and not through the isoform that metabolizes warfarin. In the case of fluvastatin, the absence of interaction noted in the package insert is surprising because this statin, unlike the others, inhibits the hepatic CYP2C9 according to the Georgetown University Web site data. Nonetheless, caution is advised. In one case, warfarin added to simvastatin precipitated rhabdomyolysis with acute renal failure. The simplest statin to combine with warfarin is pravastatin, because it is metabolized by a route quite different from the cytochrome P450 system.

Heparin

Physically, heparin is incompatible in a water solution with certain substances, including antibiotics, antihistamines, phenothiazines, and hydrocortisone. It is also incompatible with reteplase. However, direct pharmacokinetic or pharmacodynamic interactions have not been described except for a controversial interaction with nitrates.

Tissue-Type Plasminogen Activator

Concurrent use of intravenous nitroglycerin diminishes the efficacy of recombinant tissue-type plasminogen activator (alteplase), possibly because of increased hepatic blood flow and enhanced catabolism of tissue-type plasminogen activator.

INTERACTIONS OF STATINS AND OTHER LIPID-LOWERING AGENTS

Lipid-Lowering Drugs and Warfarin

Many lipid-lowering agents can interact with warfarin (Table 21-12), by decreased absorption (cholestyramine) or by hepatic interference (bezafibrate, fenofibrate, and gemfibrozil). No interaction occurs with niacin. The package inserts for gemfibrozil and fenofibrate, the only two *fibrates* licensed in the United States, include prominent warnings that the warfarin dose should be reduced and the prothrombin time determined more frequently. The exact mechanism is not clear, but inhibition of the hepatic CYP2C9 that breaks down warfarin is possible. There has been a case report of profound hypoprothrombinemia and bleeding 4 weeks after starting gemfibrozil. With fenofibrate, the INR increased after 5 to 10 days.

In general, there appear to be less severe interactions between statins and warfarin than with the fibrates. The package inserts indicate that there have been no interactions detected with fluvastatin, pravastatin, or atorvastatin. There may be a modest increase of the INR with lovastatin and simvastatin. These effects cannot be related directly to the hepatic P450 isoform known to be concerned with the specific statin. For example, fluvastatin is the only statin that is an inhibitor of the CYP2C9 that breaks down warfarin, but no interaction has been noted (package insert).

Other Interactions of the Statins

The 3-hydroxy-3-methylglutaryl coenzyme A reductase inhibitors, such as lovastatin (Mevacor), simvastatin (Zocor), pravastatin (Pravachol), fluvastatin (Lescol), and atorvastatin (Lipitor), ideally should not be combined with the fibrates because of the greater risk of myositis with rhabdomyolysis and possible renal failure. Likewise, concurrent therapy with niacin, cyclosporine, or erythromycin may carry an increased risk of myopathy with the additional risk of rhabdomyolysis. Adding an antifungal azole (a group that includes ketoconazole, which is used in transplantation) has precipitated myolysis in a patient already receiving a statin and niacin. Serum creatine kinase levels should be checked periodically, especially after increasing doses or after starting combination therapy. Nevertheless, sometimes in clinical practice, the advantages of better lipid control with cautiously combined and monitored therapy seems to outweigh these risks, which may have been overestimated. In the case of cerivastatin, the drug had to be withdrawn after more than 50 fatalities, most of which were ascribed to an interaction with gemfibrozil. Pravastatin is not metabolized by the cytochrome P450 system as are all the other statins. Theoretically, this lack of metabolism may avoid many of the drug–drug interactions leading to myopathy. Fluvastatin (Lescol) is

TABLE 21-12 Drug Interactions of Lipid-Lowering Agents

Lipid-lowering drug	Interacting drugs	Mechanism	Consequence	Prophylaxis
Fibric acids (gemfibrozil, clofibrate, bezafibrate, fenofibrate)	Warfarin; statins (see below)	Hepatic interference	Risk of bleeding	Check prothrombin time
Bile acid sequestrants (cholestyramine, colestipol)	Warfarin; many other drugs	Decreased absorption	Decreased warfarin effect; decreased drug effect	Check prothrombin time; space doses
HMG-CoA reductase inhibitors (statins: lovastatin, simvastatin)	Fibrates, inhibitors of, CYP3A4 (erythromycin, antifungal azoles, others*), nicotinic acid, cyclosporine	Added damage to muscle with myositis	Rhabdomyolysis and risk of renal failure; increased cyclosporine levels	Check creatine phosphokinase levels; avoid, if possible
Statins	Warfarin	Hepatic interaction	Increased risk of bleeding	Check INR or prothrombin time
Pravastatin	Cyclosporine	Hepatic interaction; cyclosporine hepatotoxicity	Rhabdomyolysis and risk of renal failure; increased cyclosporine levels	Check creatine phosphokinase levels; avoid, if possible

*See Fig. 21-1.

Key: HMG-CoA, 3-hydroxy-3-methylglutaryl coenzyme A; INR, international normalized ratio.

Source: Adapted with permission from Opie LH, Frishman WH: Drug interactions, in Fuster V, Alexander RW, O'Rourke RA, et al (eds): *Hurst's the Heart.* 10th ed. New York, McGraw-Hill, 2001, p 2251.

metabolized by the CYP2C9 pathway, which distinguishes it from other statins, except for pravastatin (see above), which may explain why it has not been associated with an increased incidence of myopathy during co-therapy with nicotinic acid (according to the package insert).

With regard to statins and digoxin, there is no interaction with lovastatin or pravastatin. A small increase in blood digoxin levels occurs with simvastatin and fluvastatin and a 20% increase occurs with atorvastatin.

INTERACTIONS OF NONCARDIOVASCULAR DRUGS USED IN CARDIAC TRANSPLANTATION

Cyclosporine

Cyclosporine is metabolized without inhibition by the hepatic 3A4 isoform cytochrome system. Thus, the potential interactions are with the inhibitors of this system (see Fig. 21-2). For example, grapefruit juice increases the area under the curve of cyclosporine by approximately 45%. Verapamil and diltiazem increase levels of cyclosporine and may permit a lower dose to be used with cost savings. High levels of cyclosporine increase the risk of renal toxicity and hypertension. It is not clear why cyclosporine predisposes to myopathy with some statins; it does not inhibit the CYP3A4 that breaks down the statins. Presumably cyclosporine hepatotoxicity damages the statin breakdown system. In addition, cyclosporine nephropathy may inhibit that low percentage of the statin that is renally excreted in an intact form. Cyclosporine may predispose to digoxin toxicity by reducing the renal clearance and decreasing its volume of distribution. The mechanism may be by inhibition of the transmembrane digoxin transporter P-glycoprotein.

Ketoconazole

Ketoconazole is an antifungal agent that increases blood cyclosporine levels by inhibition of the 3A4 isoform, so the dose of the more expensive agent, cyclosporine, can be reduced. Its interactions are therefore direct, via inhibition of the breakdown of those many drugs metabolized by this isoform (see Fig. 21-2), and indirect, by increasing blood levels of cyclosporine.

INTERACTIONS OF HERBAL DRUGS

Herbal drugs are now commonly used (see Chapter 23). Often the physician is ignorant of the fact that the patient is taking an herbal drug and, in addition, does not know that such drugs may have harmful interactions. Garlic and ginkgo promote the action of warfarin, perhaps by causing platelet dysfunction. Danshen increases the INR, probably by decreasing the elimination of warfarin. Dong quai increases the INR because it contains coumarin. St. John's wort, a supposed antidepressant, lowers serum warfarin, perhaps by its capacity to stimulate hepatic cytochrome P450. It also decreases the blood digoxin concentration by about one-third.

ADDITIONAL READINGS

Abernethy DR, Flockhart DA: Molecular basis of cardiovascular drug metabolism. Implications for predicting clinically important drug interactions. *Circulation* 101:1749, 2000.

Cheng JWM: Cytochrome P450 mediated cardiovascular drug interactions. *Heart Dis* 2:254, 2000.

Cheitlin MD, Hutter AM Jr, Brindis RG, et al: ACC/AHA Expert Consensus Document: Use of sildenafil (Viagra) in patients with cardiovascular disease. *J Am Coll Cardiol* 33:273, 1999.

Clinicians must remain alert for interactions between herbal medicines and prescribed drugs. *Drug Ther Perspect* 18:17, 2002.

Doucet J, Chassagne P, Trivalle C, et al: Drug–drug interactions related to hospital admissions in older adults: A prospective study of 1000 patients. *J Am Geriatr Soc* 44:944, 1996.

Feinstein RE, Khawaja IS, Nurenberg JR, Frishman WH: Cardiovascular effects of psychotropic drugs. *Curr Probl Cardiol* 27:188, 2002.

Frishman WH, Opie LH, Sica DA: Adverse cardiovascular drug interactions and complications, in Fuster V, Alexander RW, O'Rourke RA, et al (eds): *Hurst's the Heart*, 11th ed. New York, McGraw-Hill, 2003, in press.

Fugh-Berman A: Herb–drug interactions. *Lancet* 355:134, 2000.

Goldberger J, Frishman WH: Clinical utility of nifedipine and diltiazem plasma levels in patients with angina pectoris receiving monotherapy and combination treatment. *J Clin Pharmacol* 29:628, 1989.

Haddad PM, Anderson IM: Antipsychotic-related QTC prolongation, torsade de pointes, and sudden death. *Drugs* 62:1649, 2002.

Jhund PS, Davie AP, McMurray JJV: Aspirin inhibits the acute venodilator response to furosemide in patients with chronic heart failure. *J Am Coll Cardiol* 37:1234, 2001.

Kane GC, Lipsky JJ: Drug–grapefruit juice interactions. *Mayo Clin Proc* 75:933, 2000.

Latini R, Santoro E, Masson S, et al, for the GISSI-3 Investigators: Aspirin does not interact with ACE inhibitors when both are given early after acute myocardial infarction. Results of the GISSI-3 Trial. *Heart Dis* 2:185, 2000.

Leor J, Reicher-Reiss H, Goldbourt U, et al: Aspirin and mortality in patients treated with angiotensin-converting enzyme inhibitors: A cohort study of 11,575 patients with coronary artery disease. *J Am Coll Cardiol* 33:1920, 1999.

Opie LH: Adverse cardiovascular drug reactions. *Curr Prob Cardiol* 25:621, 2000.

Opie LH: Cardiovascular drug interactions, in Frishman WH, Sonnenblick EH, Sica DA (eds): *Cardiovascular Pharmacotherapeutics*, 2nd ed. New York, McGraw-Hill, 2003, p 875.

Opie LH, Gersh BJ: *Drugs for the Heart*, 5th ed. Philadelphia, WB Saunders, 2001.

Sinatra ST, Frishman WH, Peterson SJ, Lin G: Use of alternative/complementary medicine in treating cardiovascular disease, in Frishman WH, Sonnenblick EH, Sica DA (eds): *Cardiovascular Pharmacotherapeutics*, 2nd ed. New York, McGraw-Hill, 2003, p 857.

Sokol SI, Cheng-Lai A, Frishman WH, Kaza CS: Cardiovascular drug therapy in patients with hepatic diseases and patients with congestive heart failure. *J Clin Pharmacol* 40:11, 2000.

Tran C, Knowles SR, Liu BA, Shear NH: Gender differences in adverse drug reactions. *J Clin Pharmacol* 38:1003, 1998.

Yu DK: The contribution of P-glycoprotein to pharmacokinetic drug–drug interactions. *J Clin Pharmacol* 39:1203, 1999.

22 | Drug Treatment of Peripheral Vascular Disease

Robert T. Eberhardt   Jay D. Coffman

Despite intensive investigation over the past several decades, there remains a limited number of clinically useful agents available in the treatment of peripheral vascular disease. In particular, it has been most difficult to find effective drugs for the symptomatic relief of peripheral arterial obstructive disease (PAD). The treatment of PAD has focused on exercise training, modification of risk factors for atherosclerosis, and revascularization for critical limb ischemia. In contrast, treatment of Raynaud's phenomenon has focused primarily on symptomatic relief, with no therapy aimed at altering the underlying problem. The prevention and treatment of deep vein thrombosis (DVT) has evolved with the development and refinement of antithrombotic and thrombolytic therapies. The treatment of vasculitides, particularly those affecting the large vessels, involves suppression of the inflammatory response.

This chapter reviews some of the pharmacotherapeutic armamentarium available in the treatment of these peripheral vascular disorders.

ARTERIOSCLEROSIS OBLITERANS

The manifestations of PAD, typically due to arteriosclerosis obliterans, vary from asymptomatic to critical limb ischemia. However, the most common symptomatic manifestation of PAD is intermittent claudication (IC). Treatment for patients with PAD should focus on relieving symptoms, delaying or preventing disease progression, and reducing morbidity and mortality. There are few agents available for the management of symptomatic PAD (Table 22-1). There are a far larger number of agents useful in the treatment of risk factors for atherosclerosis. In addition, recent findings have provided evidence that an angiotensin-converting enzyme (ACE) inhibitor, ramipril, reduces cardiovascular events in a high-risk group of patients, many with PAD. This cardioprotective benefit was beyond that anticipated simply from a blood pressure–lowering effect. Despite considerable interest in developing new and effective agents for the symptomatic treatment of claudication, few agents have demonstrated a clear benefit. In contrast, the effectiveness of

TABLE 22-1 Drug Therapy and Exercise for Intermittent Claudication

Agent	Dose	Increase in ICD (m)	Increase in ACD (m)
Pentoxifylline	400 mg tid	20–30	45–48
Cilostazol	100 mg bid	28–34	65–90
PLC	2 g qd	31	59
Buflomedil	600 mg qd	75	81
Exercise		139	179

Key: ACD, absolute claudicant distance; bid, twice daily; ICD, initial claudicant distance; PLC, propionyl ʟ-carnitine; qd, daily; tid, thrice daily.
Source: Reproduced with permission from Eberhardt RT, Coffman JD: Drug treatment of peripheral vascular disease. *Heart Dis* 2:62, 2000.

exercise training in the treatment of IC is well established. A recent meta-analysis found that exercise training improved treadmill walking distances with an increase in initial claudicant distance (ICD) of 139 m and absolute claudicant distance (ACD) of 179 m compared with controls. Further, exercise has been shown to improve cardiopulmonary function and functional status during daily activities, with enhanced community-based ambulation.

Pentoxifylline

Pentoxifylline was the first agent approved—and is one of only two agents currently approved—by the U.S. Food and Drug Administration (FDA) for the symptomatic treatment of IC. It is a xanthine derivative that inhibits 3,5-monophosphate diesterase, leading to increased cyclic adenosine monophosphate. The proposed mechanism of action involves decreased whole-blood viscosity due in part to increased erythrocyte deformability, decreased platelet activity, and decreased fibrinogen levels.

Over the past several decades, numerous small studies have evaluated the effect of pentoxifylline for the treatment of IC, with conflicting results. Initial attempts to analyze the aggregate data concluded that a reliable conclusion regarding the drug's efficacy cannot be reached due to inadequate data. Two other recent meta-analyses concluded that pentoxifylline has a modest effect on treadmill walking distance with increases of approximately 20 to 30 m in ICD and 45 to 48 m in ACD when compared with placebo. The clinical relevance of an effect of this magnitude on walking distance has been questioned, but others have concluded that it is highly relevant. This treadmill distance is equivalent to walking 90 m (or longer than one city block) on level ground, which may minimize the disability in these patients, thus enabling engagement in personal and social activities and employment. There is limited (or discouraging) information regarding the impact of pentoxifylline on functional status or quality of life.

Perhaps the greatest benefit of pentoxifylline may be found in those with moderate disease and long duration. It has been suggested that pentoxifylline alters the natural history of PAD. Continuous use of pentoxifylline for 4 months reduced the number of diagnostic and therapeutic procedures within the first year in a small group of patients with IC. The use of pentoxifylline was not associated with a greater cost of PAD-related care and, in fact, was possibly associated with a reduction in hospital costs. The drug also has been used with mechanical compression in the management of venous ulcers and may be effective for patients not receiving compression for this indication.

The dose of pentoxifylline is 400 mg given three times daily, preferably with meals. The most common side effects are gastrointestinal in origin, including dyspepsia, nausea, and vomiting. Pentoxifylline is well tolerated despite these potential side effects, because only 3% of patients are unable to tolerate it. Although there is still uncertainty (and considerable skepticism) regarding the clinical utility of this agent, many vascular clinicians will give a 6- to 12-week trial of pentoxifylline to assess its efficacy after other measures (including exercise) have failed to diminish symptoms.

Cilostazol

Cilostazol is the second agent approved by the FDA for the symptomatic treatment of IC. Cilostazol is a type III phosphodiesterase inhibitor that blocks proteolysis and leads to an increase in intracellular cyclic adenosine monophosphate levels. The proposed mechanisms of therapeutic action are vasodilation, due to direct smooth muscle relaxation and perhaps enhanced effect of prostacyclin, and inhibition of platelet function. In addition, cilostazol appears to favorably influence serum lipids and to have smooth muscle antiproliferative properties.

An extensive clinical development program, with a number of randomized controlled trials, has evaluated the efficacy of cilostazol in the treatment of IC of varying severity. A randomized, double-blind, placebo-controlled trial involving 239 subjects with mild to moderate IC found that cilostazol, at a dose of 100 mg twice daily for 16 weeks, improves walking distance. Cilostazol increased ACD by 62 m (32%) and ICD by 28 m (27%) as compared with placebo ($P < 0.05$) on a variable-grade treadmill protocol. Another trial of cilostazol involving 81 subjects with moderately severe IC found significant improvements in ICD (35%) and ACD (41%) on a fixed-incline treadmill protocol. Several other studies have reported a beneficial effect of cilostazol on walking distance, including a recent trial involving 698 subjects that compared the effectiveness of cilostazol with that of placebo and pentoxifylline. Cilostazol increased ACD significantly more than did pentoxifylline or placebo after 24 weeks of therapy (107 m with cilostazol vs. 64 m with pentoxifylline and 65 m with placebo). The withdrawal of treatment with cilostazol, by crossing over to placebo, worsened the walking distance in subjects with IC who benefited from therapy.

Concomitant with the improved treadmill performance were subjective improvements in walking performance and functional status. There was significant improvement in the Physical Component Scale score of the Medical Outcome Scale Health Survey and walking speed and specific measures of walking difficulty on the Walking Impairment Questionnaire, although there was no change in the perceived walking distance. By using a global therapeutic assessment, more subjects and investigators subjectively judged the claudication symptoms to be improved with cilostazol. More subjects receiving cilostazol rated their outcome as "better" or "much better" when compared with pretreatment. Several trials demonstrated an approximate 9% increase in ankle brachial index with cilostazol; however, the clinical significance of this finding remains uncertain.

The recommended dose of cilostazol is 50 to 150 mg twice daily, with 100 mg twice daily being used most commonly. One study found that 50 mg of cilostazol given twice daily also improved walking distance; however, a dose response was observed, as the standard dose of 100 mg twice daily seemed to provide greater efficacy. Cilostazol is metabolized by cytochrome P450 isoenzymes, especially CYP3A4 and CYP2C19, but does not inhibit their action. It is excreted primarily (~75%) by the kidney; thus plasma levels are increased in renal insufficiency. The plasma levels of cilostazol are also increased by other drugs that use or inhibit the P450 isoenzymes, including erythromycin, omeprazole, diltiazem, ketoconazole, and grapefruit juice.

Most vascular clinicians have found cilostazol to be useful in the treatment of patients with IC. Despite these clear benefits, the use of cilostazol requires some consideration, careful instructions, and close monitoring. Side effects are reported frequently, including gastrointestinal complaints, headaches, and palpitations (>25% of patients). Patients need to be carefully instructed to anticipate side effects, which are often transient and will dissipate with continued use. The use of analgesics is often helpful to palliate symptoms such as headache. Despite the high rate of side effects, the rates of withdrawal among patients taking cilostazol were similar to those among patients receiving placebo or pentoxifylline.

Because cilostazol is a phosphodiesterase inhibitor, it is contraindicated in patients with congestive heart failure of any severity because of detrimental effects observed with other agents in this category in patients with New York Heart Association class III to IV heart failure. It is recommended that patients be screened for a history and for signs or symptoms of congestive heart failure before initiating therapy. Such concerns have led some to recommend regular reassessment of the risk–benefit ratio based on interval ischemic events and close monitoring for tachycardia during initiation of therapy. There are no long-term data available regarding safety; however, experience in the eight U.S. and U.K. phase III trials involving more than 2000 subjects found no increased risk of death or ischemic cardiovascular events during the study period.

Antiplatelet Drugs

Platelets are well known to participate in the development and progression of atherosclerosis and its complications. Activated platelets release a number of vasoactive mediators that also may participate in the pathogenesis of limb ischemia. Inhibition of platelet function provides a potential site for the treatment of claudication. Further, the increase in cardiovascular events among individuals with PAD warrants some form of antiplatelet therapy, given the well-established benefit of these agents in prevention of coronary events (Table 22-2).

Aspirin, the traditional antiplatelet agent, inhibits cyclooxygenase, thereby preventing the formation of thromboxane A_2 and thromboxane-dependent platelet activation. The benefit of antiplatelet therapy (primarily aspirin) in the prevention of cardiovascular events in patients with atherosclerotic vascular disease has been demonstrated in the meta-analysis of studies conducted by the Antiplatelet Trialists' Collaboration. Analysis of the subgroup of patients with IC demonstrated an 18% reduction in cardiovascular events;

TABLE 22-2 Antithrombotic Therapy in Peripheral Arterial Disease

Problem	Agent	Clinical effect
Chronic arterial ischemia	Aspirin	Reduces cardiovascular morbidity and mortality
	Aspirin plus dipyridamole	? Modifies the natural history of limb disease
	Clopidogrel	? Superior to aspirin
Acute arterial occlusion	Heparin	Prevents thrombus propagation
	Thrombolysis	Facilitates recanalization and minimizes need for surgery
Revascularization surgery	Aspirin	Reduces cardiovascular events
Infrainguinal with prosthetic	Aspirin plus dipyridamole	May provide additional benefit
Infrainguinal with high-risk thrombosis	Warfarin ± aspirin	Protects against graft thrombosis

Source: Modified from the recommendations of the 6th American College of Chest Physicians guideline for antithrombotic therapy for the prevention and treatment of thrombosis. *Chest* 119:283S, 2001.

however, this failed to reach statistical significance. This finding has led to various recommendations regarding the use of antiplatelet therapy in patients with PAD. The American College of Chest Physicians' recommended dose of aspirin is 81 to 325 mg daily as life-long therapy in those with PAD in the absence of contraindications. The FDA expert panel found insufficient evidence to approve the labeling of aspirin as indicated for patients with PAD.

There is no evidence to support the use of aspirin for the symptomatic treatment of claudication, but there is some suggestion that it may alter the natural history. The Antiplatelet Trialists' Collaboration found that antiplatelet therapy containing aspirin reduces the risk of graft or vessel occlusion by 43% in those with PAD undergoing revascularization. In the U.S. Physician Health Study, aspirin (325 mg every other day) failed to prevent the development of claudication but decreased the need for peripheral artery surgery.

Aspirin plus dipyridamole may have a modest effect in the treatment of IC. One study involving 54 subjects with IC found that the combination of these two drugs improves resting limb blood flow and ICD when compared with aspirin alone. Two other studies involving 296 and 240 subjects with IC found that aspirin plus dipyridamole improves ankle brachial index and delayed progression of disease, as assessed by serial angiograms. Neither study reported the effect on walking distance or functional status. Thus, aspirin, particularly in combination with dipyridamole, may alter the natural history of lower extremity arterial insufficiency, although larger-scale trials supporting this notion are lacking.

Ticlopidine is an adenosine diphosphate receptor antagonist that prevents adenosine diphosphate-mediated platelet activation and aggregation by inhibiting glycoprotein IIb/IIIa expression on the platelet surface. In 151 subjects with IC, ticlopidine was reported to significantly improve walking distance, with increases in ICD and ACD as compared with placebo. In contrast, another randomized trial involving 169 patients found no effect of ticlopidine on treadmill walking distance. Perhaps a more important finding has been a significant reduction in the combined cardiovascular end points in patients with IC who were treated with ticlopidine. Ticlopidine is dosed at 250 mg twice daily; side effects include bleeding, dyspepsia, diarrhea, nausea, anorexia, rash, and dizziness. The potential for developing severe leukopenia and thrombocytopenia requires regular monitoring of the cell count for at least several months.

Clopidogrel is in the same class of agents as ticlopidine, but the frequency of side effects, including leukopenia and thrombocytopenia, is low. Clopidogrel is given at a dose of 75 mg once daily. The Clopidogrel Versus Aspirin in Patients at Risk of Ischemic Events study demonstrated a benefit of clopidogrel over aspirin in preventing "vascular" events in 19,185 patients with atherosclerotic vascular disease, with a relative risk reduction of 8.7%. The overall incidence of the composite end point of ischemic stroke, myocardial infarction, or vascular death was 5.32% per year in the clopidogrel group versus 5.83% per year in the aspirin group. Subgroup analysis demonstrated that this effect of clopidogrel is most pronounced among the subset of patients with established PAD, with a 23.8% relative risk reduction. Despite the possibility that this result may have been due to chance, this finding has led many to consider clopidogrel as the preferred antiplatelet agent in patients with PAD.

The aggregate data on the use of antiplatelet agents for the symptomatic treatment of IC indicates that they result in, at best, minimal improvement. However, due to the cardioprotective benefit of these drugs, antiplatelet therapy should be part of the medical regimen of nearly every patient with PAD, provided there are no absolute contraindications.

Vasodilators

In theory, vasodilators may be beneficial in the treatment of IC by improving blood flow in muscle and decreasing tissue ischemia. However, there have been no adequate controlled studies to demonstrate the efficacy of vasodilators in the treatment of IC. The lack of benefit may be explained by the failure of these agents to dilate a fixed lesion in the peripheral vessels that limit blood flow in PAD and near maximal dilation of resistance vessels in ischemic limbs. As a result, most vascular specialists agree that there is no role for vasodilators in the treatment of PAD. A single trial suggested a benefit of verapamil in the treatment of IC, with improvements in ICD and ACD of 29% and 49%, respectively, although this represented a small increase in walking distance and testing was performed on level ground.

Thrombolytics

Thrombolytic agents, including streptokinase, urokinase, and tissue plasminogen activator (t-PA), have been evaluated in the management of acute arterial occlusion of the limbs (see Chapter 14). As a group, these agents have been shown to be effective in dissolving thrombus and improving recanalization on angiography. They appear to reduce the need for surgical procedures and improve amputation-free survival.

Randomized trials have compared surgical thrombectomy with thrombolytic therapy in patients with acute arterial occlusion. For example, in a randomized multicenter trial, catheter-guided intraarterial recombinant urokinase was compared with vascular surgery for the management of acute arterial occlusion of the legs. The amputation-free survival rates among patient treated with urokinase was similar to that observed among those treated with surgery at 6 months and at 1 year (71.8% vs. 74.8% at 6 months and 65.0% vs. 69.9% at 1 year).

A comparison of agents is limited and primarily involves open trials. In one such trial, intraarterial recombinant t-PA (rt-PA) was superior to intravenous rt-PA or intraarterial streptokinase, resulting in a rate of 100% for thrombolysis compared with 45% and 80% for intravenous rt-PA and intraarterial streptokinase, respectively. In another trial, rt-PA achieved more rapid thrombolysis than did urokinase; however, there was no significant difference between treatments in success at 30 days.

It is not possible, based on the available data, to make an absolute recommendation on the selection of a specific agent or dose; however, the current clinical practice has favored the use of rt-PA. The preferred route of administration is catheter-guided intraarterial or intrathrombus infusion rather than intravenous administration. Although variable dosing schemes are available, a commonly used regimen for rt-PA is 1 mg/h or 0.05 mg/kg per hour. The common side effects are related to hemorrhagic complications.

Surgical revascularization is still indicated for profound limb-threatening ischemia, with emergent thromboembolectomy for proximal emboli. However, thrombolysis should be considered for acute limb ischemia due to thrombosis or embolus presenting within 24 to 48 h of onset. It is now an acceptable part of a treatment strategy designed to gradually restore blood flow to minimize reperfusion injury. However, successful thrombolysis often will reveal an underlying lesion that requires correction by a percutaneous or a surgical approach. Further, emboli, which may consist of old thrombi and atherosclerotic plaque, may be less amenable to thrombolysis.

Other Agents

α-Tocopherol, the most active form of vitamin E, is a lipid-soluble antioxidant that participates in the defense against oxygen-derived free radicals. Vitamin E has been advocated for the treatment of claudication since the 1950s, when several small studies suggested some improvement. Since that time, the data supporting the use of vitamin E have been limited. In a large cancer-prevention study, α-tocopherol (50 mg daily) did not prevent the development of claudication in male smokers, as assessed by the Rose questionnaire. The results of the Heart Outcome Prevention Evaluation trial regarding the effect of vitamin E use on cardiovascular events in a high-risk group of patients, many with established PAD, were disappointing.

Chelation therapy has been advocated for the treatment of IC and other atherosclerotic disorders. Chelation therapy involves the administration of agents such as ethylenediamine tetraacetic acid, which are theorized to mobilize calcium within atherosclerotic lesions and to promote the regression of existing lesions. There are limited controlled data to suggest a benefit from this type of therapy. A randomized, double-blind, placebo-controlled trial of 153 patients with IC found that chelation therapy does not improve walking distance, angiographic findings, tissue oxygen tension, ankle brachial indices, or subjective assessments of symptoms. Despite its supporters, this type of treatment is of dubious benefit and has significant potential side effects, such as hypocalcemia and renal failure.

Other approaches under investigation include the use of drug-eluting stents using sirolimus for treatment of obstructive superficial femoral artery disease.

RAYNAUD'S PHENOMENON

Raynaud's phenomenon, described by Maurice Raynaud in 1888, is characterized by paroxysmal episodes of digital ischemia resulting from vasospasm of the digital arteries, with subsequent dilation and reperfusion. Clinically it is manifest by episodes of sharply demarcated "color changes" of the skin of the digits, often precipitated by cold exposure or emotional stress. Raynaud's phenomenon is considered primary (or idiopathic) if the symptoms occur in the absence of an associated systemic disorder and secondary if the they occur in association with a disorder such as systemic lupus erythematosus or scleroderma.

Primary Raynaud's phenomenon usually does not require drug therapy; typically, it responds well to conservative measures such as behavior modification and reassurance to the patient that loss of digits will not ensue. Advice about behavior modification would include minimizing cold exposure through the use of mittens (rather than gloves), the use of hand and foot warmers, and—importantly—keeping the entire body warm (to avoid reflex sympathetic vasoconstriction).

Drug therapy becomes necessary if the frequency and severity of vasospastic episodes interfere with daily functioning or quality of life and is often required in patients with secondary Raynaud's phenomenon. Different agents

TABLE 22-3 Drug Therapy for Raynaud's Phenomenon

Agent	Daily dosage	Side effects
Calcium channel blocker		
Nifedipine	30–90 mg	Headache, leg edema, flushing, palpitations
Felodipine	5–10 mg	Same as above
Isradipine	5–20 mg	Same as above
Diltiazem	120–360 mg	Constipation, nausea, headache, flushing
Sympathetic blocking agents		
Prazosin	2–8 mg	Nausea, headache, dizziness, dyspnea, edema, diarrhea
Reserpine	0.25–1 mg	Postural hypotension, bradycardia, lethargy, depression
Angiotensin-enzyme inhibitor*		
Captopril	75–150 mg	Cough, rash, renal, insufficiency, hyperkalemia, angioedema
Angiotensin-blocking agent†		
Losartan	50–100 mg	Same as above

*Comparable dose ranges of any of the available angiotensin-converting enzyme inhibitors can be considered for use.
†Comparable dose ranges of any of the available angiotensin-receptor blockers can be considered for use.

have been evaluated for the treatment of Raynaud's phenomenon; most have potent direct or indirect vasodilator properties (Table 22-3).

Calcium Channel Blockers

Calcium channel blockers are the pharmacologic agents most commonly used for the treatment of Raynaud's phenomenon. As a group, these agents have been shown to reduce the frequency, duration, and severity of attacks. However, calcium channel blockers differ in their vasodilator potencies, with the dihydropyridine class seeming to be the most potent and effective agents.

Nifedipine has been the most intensively investigated of the calcium channel blockers. Several double-blind, placebo-controlled trials have shown it to decrease the frequency and severity of attacks. One such study used a crossover design and found that 60% of patients with Raynaud's phenomenon report moderate to marked improvement in clinical symptoms, with a decreased attack rate while receiving nifedipine, compared with 13% of patients receiving placebo. The largest trial, involving 313 patients with primary Raynaud's phenomenon, found a 66% reduction in vasospastic attacks in the nifedipine-treated subjects as compared with placebo-treated subjects. Although nifedipine is beneficial in patients with primary and secondary Raynaud's phenomena, it is less efficacious in secondary Raynaud's phenomenon, especially in patients with scleroderma.

Despite convincing subjective benefits, confirmation of objective improvement in digital blood flow with nifedipine and other calcium channel blockers have been difficult to substantiate. Early studies reported that nifedipine has variable effects on the peripheral circulation in patients with Raynaud's phenomenon. The drug failed to attenuate cold-induced reduction in digital artery pressure in one study of patients with Raynaud's phenomenon. In contrast, although nifedipine did not significantly increase finger blood flow after acute sublingual administration, it did decrease vascular resistance, indicating that vasodilation of digital vessels had occurred. The largest of these trials, involving 158 patients with primary Raynaud's phenomenon, demonstrated higher digital pressure during cooling in nifedipine-treated patients.

The recommended doses of nifedipine is 10 to 30 mg three times daily for the short-acting preparation and 30 to 90 mg once daily for the long-acting preparations. The long-acting, sustained-release preparations appear to be better tolerated and are probably as effective as the short-acting, immediate-release form. Only 15% of participants discontinued therapy due to adverse effects. Nifedipine may be used intermittently for cold exposure, if it is tolerated. The most common side effects are headache, dizziness, nausea, heartburn, pruritus, palpitations, and peripheral edema. The headache is often mild and transient, lasting for the first several days of use.

Numerous other dihydropyridine calcium channel blockers, including amlodipine, felodipine, isradipine, nicardipine, and nisoldipine, have been shown to have favorable effects in patients with Raynaud's phenomenon. Other types of calcium channel blockers have played a limited role in the treatment of this condition. There is controversy regarding the effect of diltiazem. A reduction in the frequency and severity of attacks was shown with diltiazem, with the most benefit seen among patients with primary Raynaud's. Another study found that diltiazem is ineffective in the treatment of Raynaud's phenomenon associated with connective tissue disease. One trial reported that verapamil is ineffective in patients with severe Raynaud's phenomenon.

Sympathetic Blocking Agents

Sympathetic adrenergic stimulation, especially involving α-adrenergic receptors, of digital arteries plays an important role in the regulation of digital blood flow. A variety of sympatholytic drugs have been used in the treatment of Raynaud's phenomenon, but few controlled trials have been conducted to evaluate their efficacy.

Prazosin is the α_1-adrenoceptor antagonist that has been the best studied of this class of agents for the treatment of patients with Raynaud's phenomenon, in particular Raynaud's phenomenon in progressive systemic sclerosis. Several placebo-controlled studies found a decrease in the frequency, duration, and severity of vasospastic attacks in approximately 66% of patients with Raynaud's after 2 weeks of treatment with prazosin. Its effectiveness, however, appears to decrease with prolonged use, despite titration to the maximally tolerated dose. The recommended dose range is from 2 to 8 mg daily. Side effects, including palpitations, dizziness, fatigue, headache, dyspnea, edema, rash, and diarrhea, may limit its use.

Thymoxamine, another α_1-adrenoceptor antagonist, also has been evaluated in the treatment of Raynaud's phenomenon. In an uncontrolled study, thymoxamine at a dose of 40 mg four times daily resulted in clinical improvement, with a decrease in the frequency of attacks and an improvement in digital perfusion during cold challenge. Side effects are reported to be less frequent than with prazosin; however, experience with this agent is limited and it is not available in the United States.

Although popular two or three decades ago, reserpine and guanethidine are used infrequently in the current treatment of Raynaud's phenomenon. These agents are nonselective adrenoceptor antagonists that have been shown to increase capillary blood flow in patients with primary and secondary Raynaud's phenomena. However, adequate controlled studies have not been performed. In a small study, intraarterial reserpine did not provide benefit over placebo in patients with primary Raynaud's phenomenon. The experience with several other sympatholytic agents, including methyldopa, phenoxybenzamine, and tolazoline, is also limited.

There are limited controlled data to support the routine use of sympatholytic agents in the treatment of Raynaud's phenomenon. In addition, these agents have not been shown to be more effective than calcium channel blockers. They may be considered for patients who do not tolerate calcium channel blockers well or for those with refractory symptoms that do not respond to other measures.

Angiotensin-Blocking Agents

ACE inhibitors and angiotensin-receptor antagonists may have a role in the treatment of Raynaud's phenomenon. These agents may improve local blood flow by blocking the vasoconstrictive action of angiotensin II and, in the case of ACE inhibitors, potentiate the action of bradykinin.

Interest in the use of these agents developed after the report of remarkable improvement in the vasospastic-induced ischemic digital ulceration in a small number of subjects being treated with captopril for scleroderma-associated hypertensive renal crisis. In uncontrolled studies, captopril at a dose of 25 mg three times daily has been reported to decrease the frequency and severity of attacks in patients with primary Raynaud's phenomenon but not in those with Raynaud's phenomenon associated with scleroderma. These subjective benefits were supported by attenuation in the cold-induced vasoconstriction. Similar findings have been observed with the angiotensin-receptor antagonist losartan, which decreased the frequency and severity of attacks in primary Raynaud's phenomenon. However, most vascular clinicians have not found ACE inhibitors to be useful clinically in the prevention or treatment of vasospastic attacks.

Other Agents

A large number of alternative vasodilators has been used in the treatment of severe Raynaud's phenomenon, including minoxidil, hydralazine, and sodium nitroprusside. However, the use of these agents is not recommended, because controlled trials have not been performed and alternative agents are readily available.

Nitroglycerin preparations have been recommended for the treatment of Raynaud's phenomenon for many years, but results of studies evaluating transdermal nitroglycerin have been varied. In one study, nitroglycerin ointment (1%) was beneficial in reducing the frequency and severity of attacks while promoting ulcer healing in patients with secondary Raynaud's phenomenon who were receiving maximally tolerated doses of sympatholytic drugs. There has been limited clinical enthusiasm for using topical nitrates for the treatment of patients with Raynaud's phenomenon.

Pentoxifylline is reported to have some beneficial effects on the peripheral circulation, resulting in an increase in resting digital blood flow and an attenuation of cold-induced vasoconstriction in patients with Raynaud's phenomenon. Despite a suggestion of clinical improvement, double-blind, placebo-controlled studies have not demonstrated convincing beneficial effects of pentoxifylline as opposed to placebo.

Thyroid preparations have been recommended for the treatment of Raynaud's phenomenon since the 1960s. In a more recent double-blind, placebo-controlled, crossover trial of 18 patients with Raynaud's phenomenon, a daily dose of 80 µg of triiodothyronine significantly reduced the frequency, duration, and severity of attacks. However, there was an increase in heart rate, and 33% of patients reported episodic palpitations. The investigators suggested that lower ("physiologic") doses of triiodothyronine should be evaluated.

DEEP VEIN THROMBOSIS

DVT and pulmonary embolus are expressions of venous thromboembolism. DVT, especially involving the proximal lower extremity veins, is the principal source of pulmonary emboli and is a common cause of hospital morbidity and mortality. The goal of therapy for established DVT is to prevent thrombus propagation, recurrent thrombosis, pulmonary embolus, mortality, and the development of late complications. The benefit of anticoagulation in the management of thromboembolic disease is undisputed. Further, prophylactic anticoagulant strategies are an effective means to prevent the development and complications of DVT, particularly in higher-risk patients. A clinical report recently described a reduced frequency of venous thrombosis in patients receiving statin therapy, and there is now a suggestion that atherosclerosis and venous thrombosis may be associated. Atherosclerosis may induce venous thrombosis, or the two conditions may share common risk factors. The American College of Chest Physicians has specific recommendations, based on risk, regarding prevention of thromboembolic complication in various medical and surgical patients (Table 22-4). The evaluation of patients with "idiopathic" or recurrent DVT continues to evolve as knowledge mounts regarding inherited thrombophilias.

Heparin

Unfractionated heparin has been the mainstay of treatment and prevention for DVT. Heparin complexes with antithrombin III, leading to the inactivation of factors IIa, Xa, and IXa and inhibition of factor V and VIII activation by thrombin. The beneficial effects of heparin in the treatment of venous thromboembolism have been known since 1960. For the treatment of established DVT, heparin is usually administered by constant infusion and requires frequent monitoring with dose adjustment. In a randomized trial, patients with proximal DVT treated with continuous intravenous heparin had a lower rate of recurrent thromboembolism than did those treated with subcutaneous heparin (5.2% vs. 19.3% over 6 weeks). The efficacy of heparin was found to be highly dependent on achieving a therapeutic level within the first 24 h of therapy. The use of weight-based nomograms has facilitated the time required to achieve a therapeutic activated partial thromboplastin time (APTT). A therapeutic level of anticoagulation is an APTT of 1.5 to 2.5 times control and corresponds to a heparin blood level of 0.2 to 0.4 IU/mL by protamine sulfate titration assay. Complications of heparin therapy include bleeding, thrombocytopenia (often with paradoxical thrombosis), and osteoporosis.

Unfractionated heparin also has been shown to be effective in the prevention of DVT formation in many higher-risk patient populations. Fixed-dose subcu-

TABLE 22-4 Recommendations for the Prophylaxis
of Venous Thromboembolism

Clinical situation	Suggested prophylaxis
General surgery	
Low risk	Early ambulation
Moderate risk	UH, LMWH, ES, or IPC
Higher risk	UH, LMWM, or IPC
Very high risk	UH or LMWH combined with ES or IPC
Gynecologic surgery	
Brief procedure	Early ambulation
Major procedure	
Benign disease	UH twice daily; alternative: daily LMWH or IPC
Malignant disease	UH thrice daily; alternative: UH plus EC or IPC, or high-dose LMWH
Urologic surgery	
Low risk	Early ambulation
Major procedure	UH, ES, IPC, or LMWH
Highest risk	UH or LMWH plus ES or IPC
Major orthopedic surgery	
Elective hip replacement	LMWH, fondaparinux, or adjusted-dose warfarin
	Alternative: adjusted-dose UH
Elective knee replacement	LMWH, fondaparinux, or adjusted-dose warfarin
	Alternative: IPC; UH not recommended
Hip fracture	LMWH, fondaparinux, or adjusted-dose warfarin
	Alternative: UH
Neurologic surgery	IPC ± ES; alternative UH or LMWH
Trauma	LMWH if no contraindications
	EC ± IPC if delay in starting LMWH
Acute spinal cord injury	LMWH; not UH, ES, or IPC alone
Medical conditions	
Myocardial infarction	SC or IV UH; LMWH*
Ischemic stroke	UH, LMWH, or danaparoid
Others with increased risk	UH or LMWH

*Not mentioned in the American College of Chest Physicians guidelines but
generally accepted for use in acute coronary syndrome.
Key: ES, elastic compression stockings; IPC, intermittent pneumatic compression;
IV, intravenous; LMWH, low-molecular-weight heparin; SC, subcutaneous; UH,
unfractionated heparin.
Source: Modified from recommendations of the 6th American College of Chest
Physicians guideline for antithrombotic therapy for the prevention and treatment
of thrombosis. *Chest* 119:132S, 2001.

taneous heparin (5000 U given 2 h before and every 8 to 12 h after surgery)
reduced the incidences of venous thromboembolism by 70% and fatal pulmonary embolus by 50% after general surgical procedures. Benefits also have
been reported in neurosurgical, general medical, ischemic stroke, and trauma
patients and in those with acute spinal cord injuries and possibly also orthopedic patients. However, the effect in orthopedic patients undergoing knee or hip
surgery was relatively slight and less than that of alternative strategies. Use of
dose-adjusted subcutaneous heparin to keep the APTT in the high normal range
may be more effective but has not been widely tried. One study found that, after

hip arthroplasty, only 5 of 38 patients on adjusted-dose heparin developed a DVT, compared with 16 of 41 patients on fixed-dose heparin. The use of heparin prophylaxis appears to be safe, because the incidence of major bleeding is not increased, although minor wound hematomas may ensue.

Low-Molecular-Weight Heparins

Low-molecular-weight heparins (LMWHs) are currently replacing unfractionated heparin for the prevention and treatment of DVT. The constituents of unfractionated heparin have a molecular weight ranging from 3000 to 30,000 Da, whereas LMWHs have fragments of unfractionated heparin with a mean molecular weight of about 5000 Da. Their mechanism of action is similar to that of unfractionated heparin, although they possess greater relative inhibitory activity against factor Xa than against factor IIa. LMWH is used in fixed and weight-adjusted dosing regimens and is administered subcutaneously once or twice daily. Compared with unfractionated heparin, LMWH has a more predictable anticoagulant response (with no need for routine monitoring), reflecting its better bioavailability, longer half-life, and non–dose-dependent clearance. Additional potential advantages of LMWH include fewer bleeding complications and a lower risk of thrombocytopenia. LMWH may be used in heparin-induced thrombocytopenia; however, there is a significant risk of cross reactivity. The use of LMWH in the prophylaxis and treatment of DVT has been evaluated in numerous randomized, controlled trials and has been the subject of recent meta-analyses. LMWH was more effective than fixed-dose heparin and equivalent (or superior) to adjusted-dose unfractionated heparin in preventing DVT. It has been shown to be effective in many patient populations, including acutely ill medical, general surgical, neurosurgical, and orthopedic surgical patients. Similarly, LMWH appears to be at least as effective and safe as unfractionated heparin for the treatment of DVT, even DVT involving the proximal veins. Several recent meta-analyses found that LMWH is more effective than unfractionated heparin in preventing thrombus propagation, reducing recurrent thromboembolism, and reducing mortality, with a similar or lower rate of major bleeding. An open-label study found that an LMWH is more effective than unfractionated heparin in promoting thrombus regression as assessed by venography. Further, recent studies have supported the feasibility and safety of outpatient treatment of DVT with LWMH in 50% to 75% of patients, which would significantly lower the cost of therapy. This finding has led to suggestions regarding the need for vigilance with the use of home therapy, including the need for appropriate patient selection, adequate resources for clinical services, and documentation of effectiveness of individual centers. In the United States, several agents in this class are currently approved for the prevention and treatment of DVT and for unstable coronary syndromes (Table 22-5).

Warfarin

After the acute phase of DVT treatment with heparin or LMWH, anticoagulation with warfarin is usually continued for 3 to 6 months to prevent recurrent disease and late complications. Warfarin interferes with the action of vitamin K by inhibiting vitamin K epoxide reductase, which leads to impaired function of prothrombin, factor VII, factor IX, and factor X. In patients with proximal DVT, long-term administration of warfarin reduced the recurrence of venous thromboembolism from about 47% to about 2%. Warfarin is dose

TABLE 22-5 Drug Therapy for Deep Venous Thrombosis

Agent	Indication	Typical dose
Unfractionated heparin	Prophylaxis/ treatment	5000 U bid or adjusted for PTT per weight-based nomogram
LMWH		
Enoxaparin	Prophylaxis	30–40 mg qd or bid*
	Treatment	1 mg/kg bid; ?1.5 mg/kg qd
Dalteparin	Prophylaxis	2500–5000 U qd or bid*
	Treatment	100 U/kg bid
Nadroparin	Prophylaxis	3100 U or 40 U/kg qd
	Treatment	90 U/kg bid
Tinzaparin	Prophylaxis	3500 U or 50 U/kg qd
	Treatment	175 U/kg qd
Hirudin	Prophylaxis	1250–2500 U bid
Danaparoid	Prophylaxis	10–20 mg bid
Warfarin	Prophylaxis	Start on day of surgery; adjust dose for INR
	Treatment	Adjust for INR 2.0–3.0
Fondaparinux	Prophylaxis	2.5 mg SC qd
Thrombolytic agents	Treatment	
SK		250,000 IU load; 100,000 IU/h for 48–72 h
UK		4400 IU/kg load; 2200 IU/(kg•h) for 48–72 h
t-PA		0.05 mg/(kg•h) for 8–24 h

*Dose varies according to the risk.
Key: bid, twice daily; INR, international normalized ratio; LMWH, low-molecular weight heparin; PTT, prothrombin time; qd, once daily; SK, streptokinase; t-PA, tissue plasminogen activator; UK, urokinase.
Source: Reproduced with permission from Eberhardt RT, Coffman JD: Drug treatment of peripheral vascular disease. *Heart Dis* 2:62, 2000.

adjusted according to the international normalized ratio (INR), typically to maintain a therapeutic value in the range of 2.0 to 3.0. The INR standardizes the prothrombin time to an international reference thromboplastin to allow for comparison between different laboratories.

Recommendations regarding the duration of treatment with warfarin have been the subject of debate. One study found a marked reduction in the recurrence rate with prolonged therapy for idiopathic DVT as compared with a standard 6 months of therapy (1.3% vs. 27%). Another study found that, after a second DVT, 4 years of therapy with warfarin reduces the recurrence of venous thromboembolism (2.6% vs. 20.7%), although the risk of bleeding significantly increased (8.6% vs. 2.7%). Most recently, it has been shown that long-term low-intensity warfarin therapy (target INR, 1.5 to 2.0) after completion of 3 to 6 months of standard anticoagulant therapy is effective in preventing recurrent venous thrombosis, with a low risk of bleeding.

Despite its delayed onset of action, warfarin was found to be effective in the prevention of DVT after orthopedic surgery, but it has been replaced by LMWH for reasons of efficacy and convenience.

Hirudin

Hirudin is a direct thrombin inhibitor that directly binds to the fibrinogen recognition and catalytic site of thrombin. In addition to the management of acute coronary syndrome, this agent has been evaluated in the prevention of DVT after surgery. In a multicenter, randomized, controlled trial involving

1119 patients undergoing hip surgery, recombinant hirudin was found to be more effective than fixed-dose subcutaneous heparin in preventing DVT formation. In another study involving 2070 patients, subcutaneous recombinant hirudin (desirudin) was compared with enoxaparin in the prevention of DVT after total hip replacement. The rates of all DVTs (18.4% vs. 25.5%) and proximal DVT (4.5% vs. 7.5%) were significantly lower among those receiving hirudin than among those receiving enoxaparin, as assessed by follow-up venography. Recombinant hirudin warrants further investigation and may be useful in heparin-induced thrombocytopenia.

Danaparoid

Danaparoid, a derivative of the intestinal mucosa of the pig after removal of heparin, is a mixture of heparan, dermatan, and chondroitin sulfates. It is an even more selective inhibitor of factor Xa than is LMWH. It is reported to be safe and effective in the prophylaxis of DVT in patients after cancer surgery, hip fracture surgery, or hip replacements and in patients with nonhemorrhagic stroke. In an open-label, randomized, multicenter study, subcutaneous danaparoid was compared with continuous intravenous infusion of unfractionated heparin for the treatment of venous thromboembolism. Danaparoid was more effective in the prevention of thrombus extension or recurrent thromboembolism, with a similar risk of bleeding. Danaparoid has all the advantages of LMWH and has minimal cross reactivity with antibodies generated in heparin-induced thrombocytopenia. Danaparoid is approved for the prevention of DVT in patients undergoing elective hip replacement surgery. The dose of danaparoid is 750 anti–factor Xa units twice per day; side effects include hemorrhage and fever.

Fondaparinux

Fondaparinux, a synthetic pentasaccharide that selectively inhibits factor Xa, is the latest heparin analogue to reach the market in the United States. The drug is an entirely synthetic agent that is structurally related to the antithrombin-binding site of heparin. The drug has been shown to prevent asymptomatic DVT somewhat more effectively than enoxaparin after hip or knee surgery. However, a reduction in symptomatic events has not been demonstrated, and the bleeding risk may be greater with fondaparinux.

The drug is approved for use in the prophylaxis of DVT that could lead to pulmonary embolism in patients undergoing hip fracture surgery, hip replacement surgery, and knee replacement surgery. The recommended dose is 2.5 mg subcutaneously daily for 5 to 9 days.

Thrombolytic Agents

Thrombolytic agents, including streptokinase, urokinase, and t-PA, have been studied in the treatment of DVT. Thrombolytics have been shown to enhance the rate of lysis in peripheral veins, with a greater likelihood of having complete or near complete resolution of the thrombus. In contrast, standard treatment with heparin reduces the extension and embolization of a thrombus but does not appear to effect the rate of lysis.

There remains controversy regarding the benefit of thrombolysis in the treatment of proximal DVT. These agents have not been shown to reduce the subsequent development of pulmonary embolus or to reduce mortality. It appears that their early use may decrease subsequent pain, limb swelling, and loss of venous valves; however, the benefit in reducing the late complications, such as postphlebitic syndrome, remains poorly defined. Further, delayed use of thrombolytics has been less successful, especially if thrombus has been present for longer than 7 days. A recent review of randomized trials using rt-PA in the treatment of lower extremity DVT did not support the routine use of rt-PA. Thrombosis within other venous systems, primarily the subclavian veins, has been treated by direct infusion of thrombolytic agent into the distal vein, which has been successful in preventing surgical thrombectomy. However, this often discloses an anatomic abnormality that led to the development of the thrombus, such as a thoracic outlet syndrome, which then requires surgical correction.

The present recommendations are to consider thrombolysis for massive iliofemoral DVT, typically with marked limb swelling and threatened foot ischemia, if there is a low risk of bleeding. Many have also considered thrombolysis for subclavian vein thrombosis with occlusion. The commonly used dosing regimen of streptokinase is 250,000 IU load followed by an infusion of 100,000 IU/h for 48 h and t-PA 0.05 mg/kg per hour for 8 to 24 h. Successful thrombolytic administration must be followed by systemic antithrombotic therapy and long-term anticoagulation.

VASCULITIS

The vasculitides are a heterogeneous group of disorders characterized by leukocyte infiltration into the vessel wall with reactive damage, leading to tissue ischemia and necrosis. The pattern of vessel involvement, in terms of size and location, varies with the specific disorders. Those involving the large vessels, such as Takayasu's arteritis and giant-cell arteritis, are frequently encountered by the cardiovascular clinician. Takayasu's arteritis primarily affects the aorta and its major branches. The presenting symptoms early in the course of the disease are those of systemic inflammation; whereas the later clinical syndrome is typified by vascular insufficiency. Giant-cell or temporal arteritis most prominently involves the cranial branches of the arteries originating from the aortic arch. The most common presenting symptom is headache, but visual problems, scalp tenderness, malaise, fever, and weight loss are common.

Corticosteroids and immunosuppressive agents are useful in the treatment of most forms of vasculitis, particularly in the acute phase. Systemic vasculitides usually require at least corticosteroid therapy to induce a remission. Rapidly progressive and steroid refractory vasculitides require combination therapy with corticosteroids and cytotoxic drugs such as cyclophosphamide, azathioprine, or methotrexate.

Glucocorticoids

Glucocorticoids are the mainstay of therapy for many vasculitides, including giant-cell arteritis and Takayasu's arteritis. These agents decrease inflammation by suppressing the migration of polymorphonuclear leukocytes and decreasing capillary permeability. There is suppression of the immune system by reducing the activity and volume of the lymphatic system.

Blindness occurred in up to 80% of patients with giant-cell arteritis before the use of steroids. However, remission was induced in nearly all cases with an initial dose of 40 to 60 mg of prednisone in a single or divided daily dose.

Therapy with intravenous pulse methylprednisolone should be initiated in those with recent visual loss. Once a clinical remission has been induced, the dose of steroids are gradually reduced to a minimally suppressive dose. Laboratory evaluations, such as the sedimentation rate or C-reactive protein, are usually monitored to confirm the persistence of the remission. Steroids often are discontinued within a couple of years, because giant-cell arteritis usually runs a self-limited course. However, approximately 50% of all patients will experience a relapse during corticosteroid tapering, and the need for long-term corticosteroid therapy leads to adverse events from the steroids in most patients. Glucocorticoids are used to suppress systemic symptoms and arrest progression of arterial lesions in Takayasu's arteritis. Early in the course of the disease, treatment with corticosteroids may reverse arterial stenoses, even with a restoration of pulses, and can improve ischemic symptoms. The response is diminished once fibrosis or thrombosis has developed within the affected vessels. A commonly accepted initial dose of prednisone for Takayasu's arteritis is 40 to 60 mg/day to induce a remission, but the dose is then gradually tapered to sustain remission. Laboratory markers of systemic inflammation are monitored to confirm the persistence of a remission. As with giant-cell arteritis, many patients with Takayasu's arteritis will experience a relapse during corticosteroid tapering, and complications of long-term corticosteroid therapy are common.

Cytotoxic Drugs

Various cytotoxic agents are used for steroid-resistant disease that has failed to enter remission with corticosteroids. Cytotoxic agents also have been used for their steroid-sparing effects in an attempt to reduce the corticosteroid requirement to keep the disease quiescent. These agents, including cyclophosphamide, azathioprine, and methotrexate, should be handled only by physicians well versed in their use. With the large-vessel vasculitides, the use of methotrexate has been evaluated. The experience with the other agents is very limited.

There is controversy regarding the steroid-sparing effect of methotrexate in giant-cell arteritis. In a recent double-blind, placebo-controlled trial, 42 subjects with new-onset giant-cell arteritis were randomized to weekly methotrexate (at a dose of 10 mg) for 24 months plus prednisone or to placebo plus prednisone. Treatment with methotrexate significantly reduced the proportion of patients who experienced a relapse (45% vs. 84%, $P = 0.02$), reduced the duration of use of prednisone (median times of 29 and 94 weeks, $P < 0.01$), and reduced the mean cumulative dose of prednisone (4.2 vs. 5.5, $P < 0.01$). The rate and severity of side effects were similar in both groups. In contrast, a preliminary report in another placebo-controlled trial found that weekly methotrexate failed to lower the dose of corticosteroids.

The use of methotrexate has been evaluated in the treatment of persistent or recurrent Takayasu's arteritis that is refractory to glucocorticoids. An open-label study evaluated the effect of low-dose methotrexate with glucocorticoids in 18 patients with refractory Takayasu's arteritis; 16 were followed for a mean period of 2.8 years. Weekly administration of methotrexate (mean dose, 17.1 mg) and glucocorticoids induced remission in 81% of patients (13 of 16). However, when the dose of glucocorticoid was tapered, relapse occurred in 44% of patients (7 of 13) requiring retreatment and leading to a remission. There was a sustained remission (with a mean of 18 months) in 50% of patients treated with low-dose weekly methotrexate.

CONCLUSION

Despite years of intense investigation, effective drug therapy for the symptomatic treatment of manifestations of arteriosclerosis obliterans remains elusive. The current focus is on the treatment of modifiable risk factors for atherosclerosis (including smoking cessation) and an exercise regimen. Only two agents, pentoxifylline and cilostazol, are available in the United States for the symptomatic treatment of IC. Antiplatelet agents hold promise in reducing cardiovascular morbidity and mortality among individuals with PAD. Investigational agents involving nitric oxide and carnitine metabolism remain viable therapeutic targets in the management of IC. There was minimal long-term benefit to the use of prostaglandins in the treatment of critical limb ischemia, and angiogenesis is still in the early stages of development. There is a role for catheter-guided thrombolytic therapy in the treatment of acute arterial occlusion of the extremities.

When Raynaud's phenomenon requires drug therapy, dihydropyridine-type calcium channel blockers are effective at decreasing the frequency, duration, and severity of attacks but do not provide complete relief. Alternative vasodilators, such as prazosin, may be tried if calcium channel blockers are ineffective or intolerable. Other agents, including prostaglandins, continue to be evaluated in the treatment of refractory Raynaud's phenomenon to allow wound healing.

Heparin has been the standard agent in the prevention and short-term management of DVT, followed by administration of warfarin for long-term management. The use of weight-based nomograms has facilitated achieving therapeutic anticoagulation with heparin more safely than with the prior regimens. LMWHs are becoming the preferred agents for the prevention and possibly for the treatment of DVT. The ease of administration and fewer side effects with equivalent (or better) efficacy are key to the recent flourishing in the use of LMWH. Heparinoids and direct antithrombin agents, such as danaparoid and hirudin, are emerging as alternative agents in the prevention and perhaps management of DVT. Warfarin should be continued for at least 3 to 6 months to maintain an INR of 2.0 to 3.0 for treatment of DVT, although more prolonged therapy is now being recommended at lower INR levels for idiopathic and recurrent DVT. Thrombolysis may be used selectively for the treatment of proximal DVT, particularly if evidence for limb ischemia is present. Although great strides have been made in the prevention of DVT in high-risk patients, there is a higher than acceptable incidence.

Glucocorticoids and cytoxic agents remain the treatments of choice for managing patients with vasculitis.

ADDITIONAL READINGS

Clopidogrel Versus Aspirin in Patients at Risk of Ischemic Events (CAPRIE) Steering Committee: A randomised, blinded, trial of clopidogrel versus aspirin in patients at risk of ischaemic events (CAPRIE). *Lancet* 348:1329, 1996.

Creager MA: Medical management of peripheral arterial disease. *Cardiol Rev* 9:238, 2002.

Dawson DL, Cutler BS, Hiatt WR, et al: A comparision of cilostazol and pentoxifylline for treating intermittent claudication. *Am J Med* 109:523, 2000.

Eberhardt RT, Coffman JD: Drug treatment of peripheral vascular disease. *Heart Dis* 2:62, 2000.

Eberhardt RT, Coffman JD: Drug treatment of peripheral vascular disease, in Frishman WH, Sonnenblick EH, Sica DA (eds): *Cardiovascular Pharmacotherapeutics,* 2nd ed. New York, McGraw-Hill, 2003, p 919.

Heart Outcome Prevention Evaluation Study Investigators: Effects of an angiotensin-converting-enzyme inhibitor, ramipril, on cardiovascular events in high-risk patients. *N Engl J Med* 342:145, 2000.

Hiatt WR: Medical treatment of peripheral arterial disease and claudication. *N Engl J Med* 344:1608, 2001.

Hirsch AT, Criqui MH, Treat-Jacobson D, et al: Peripheral arterial disease detection, awareness, and treatment in primary care. *JAMA* 286:1317, 2001.

Jull A, Waters J, Arroll B: Pentoxifylline for treatment of venous leg ulcers: A systematic review. *Lancet* 359:1550, 2002.

Kim CK, Schmalfuss CM, Schofield RS, Sheps DS: Pharmacological treatment of patients with peripheral arterial disease. *Drugs* 63:637, 2003.

Prandoni P, Bilora F, Marchiori A, et al: An association between atherosclerosis and venous thrombosis. *N Engl J Med* 348:1435, 2003.

Quriel K: Peripheral arterial disease. *Lancet* 358:1257, 2001.

Radack K, Wyderski RJ: Conservative management of intermittent claudication. *Ann Intern Med* 113:135, 1999.

Ray JG, Mamdani M, Tsuyuki RG, et al: Use of statins and the subsequent development of deep vein thrombosis. *Arch Intern Med* 161:1405, 2001.

Raynaud's Treatment Study Investigators: Comparison of sustained-release nifedipine and temperature biofeedback for treatment of primary Raynaud phenomenon: Results from a randomized clinical trial with 1-year follow-up. *Arch Intern Med* 160:1101, 2000.

Regensteiner JG, Hiatt WR: Current medical therapies for patients with peripheral arterial disease. A critical review. *Am J Med* 112:49, 2002.

Ridker PM, Goldhaber SZ, Danielson E, et al, for the PREVENT Investigators: Long-term, low-intensity warfarin therapy for the prevention of recurrent venous thromboembolism. *N Engl J Med* 348:1425, 2003.

Sixth American College of Chest Physicians guideline for antithrombotic therapy for the prevention and treatment of thrombosis. *Chest* 119:132S, 283S, 2001.

Weyand CM, Goronzy JJ: Medium- and large-vessel vasculitis. *N Engl J Med* 349:160, 2003.

23 | Use of Alternative Medicines in Treating Cardiovascular Disease

Stephen T. Sinatra   *William H. Frishman*
Stephen J. Peterson

For some physicians, complementary therapies as treatment interventions provide a more integrative approach to heart disease. For others, alternative, unconventional, or "unorthodox" medicine is viewed more often as quackery masquerading as legitimate medicine. Nevertheless, alternative medicine has now become a prominent focus for patients and consumers in the orthodox medical system. For example, Americans spent an estimated $15.7 billion on nutritional supplements alone in the year 2000. In six public opinion surveys, researchers analyzed the responses of 1196 people comprising 235 "regular," 381 "sometimes," and 580 "never" users of dietary supplements. The researchers reported that considerable numbers of patients use dietary supplements without proof of efficacy or safety. The appropriate use and need for regulatory guidelines of these products have become controversial issues for patients and physicians. Clearly, modern physicians need to listen to the voice of the public and at least try to become acquainted with alternative methods as part of their continuing medical education. This chapter looks at the scientific revelations and the scientific criticisms on the subject, including an evidence-based review of the existing literature on the use of alternative methods in treating cardiovascular disease.

A decade ago, it was estimated from national survey data that, in a given year, roughly 33% of English-speaking adults in the United States reported using at least one form of alternative medicine, and 33% of these consulted alternative medicine providers. Those who went to providers of alternative medicine averaged 19 visits a year, paying about $27.60 per visit (not including books, herbs, dietary supplements, medical equipment, or other material), with a majority (55%) paying entirely out of pocket. In 1990, there were more visits to alternative medicine providers than to all primary care physicians (general and family practitioners, pediatricians, and specialties of internal medicine) combined.

Demographically, the use of alternative medicine in the United States is more prevalent among college-educated, non–African American persons between 25 and 49 years of age with annual incomes above $35,000 who live in the western United States. Alternative therapies are used most frequently for back problems, anxiety, headaches, chronic pain, and cancer or tumors. Relaxation techniques, chiropractic, and massage therapy are the most frequently used alternative therapies. Although most (83%) of those who have used alternative medicine for a serious medical condition were also being treated by a medical provider for the same condition, most patients (72%) who used alternative therapies did not inform their medical doctors. In 1997, an estimated 4 of 10 adults incorporated some form of alternative therapy, including herbal medicine, massage, and megavitamins. Startling revelations also have indicated that consumers made more visits to alternative medical practitioners—such as chiropractors, naturopaths, and massage therapists—than they did to primary care physicians: an estimated 629 million versus 386 million visits.

Clearly, the use of alternative medicine is far greater than previously reported. Although most alternative therapies are relatively innocuous, some involve the use of pharmacologically active substances (e.g., herbal medicine, megavitamin therapy, and some folk remedies) that could complicate existing medical therapy or even harm patients. Historically, American medical schools did little to educate their students on complementary therapies; but more recently, 64% of American medical schools offered elective courses in this area. Although an increasing number of physicians are becoming more comfortable with alternative medicine, the widespread use of nutritional supplements with potential pharmacologic activities demands that all physicians not only inquire about their patient's use of alternative medicine but also educate themselves and their patients as to the potential harms and benefits of these remedies. The reluctance of patients to disclose their use of complementary medicines stems from fear of disapproval of these interventions by their physicians and from the belief that natural remedies are harmless. Surveys also have indicated that patients fail to discuss the use of dietary supplements with their health care providers because they believe that these practitioners know little or nothing about these products and may even be biased against them.

Rather than dismissing a patient's highly motivated intentions toward health-conscious behaviors or refusing to prescribe for them out of fear of potential drug interactions, it behooves physicians to understand the range of complementary therapies available and when they can be safely integrated into conventional medicine. Thus, they may more effectively counsel their patients in a collaborative and more effective atmosphere of open communication. Physicians' knowledge of nutritional supplement intake is also critical to avoid potentially dangerous interactions with prescribed medication. For example, consider patients taking warfarin who are also ingesting nonprescribed natural blood thinners such as garlic, ginger, fish oil, *Ginkgo biloba,* and even excessive amounts of vitamin E at the same time. Such a combination clearly poses potential risks for the patient and the physician!

This chapter limits its review to some of the pharmacologically active substances most commonly used or that have effects on the cardiovascular system based on the existing scientific literature. Although nonpharmacologic therapies, such as relaxation techniques, biofeedback, and meditation, are known to lower heart rate and blood pressure by decreasing the activity of the sympathetic nervous system, they are not covered because they are beyond the scope of this commentary. This chapter also pays particular attention to medicinal plants, which the authors accept to be pharmacologically active substances in a diluted form; however, two other alternative remedies (vitamins, minerals, and other micronutrient supplements and homeopathy) are also examined briefly, because their mechanisms of action are pharmacologic in nature or beyond the simple central nervous system (CNS) control of the autonomic nervous system.

MEGAVITAMINS AND OTHER MICRONUTRIENT SUPPLEMENTS

Vitamins and minerals are required in trace amounts for normal bodily functioning. Many people have subscribed to the notion that "more is better."

Ingestion of micronutrient supplements (vitamins and minerals) beyond the "recommended daily allowances" is beneficial in certain deficiency states resulting from inadequate intake, disturbed absorption, or increased tissue requirements; however, routine dietary supplementation of micronutrients in the absence of deficiency states and beyond what one can usually obtain from consumption of a well-balanced diet has been shown to be of questionable benefit and in some cases may be harmful. Of course, there are exceptions. This section reviews micronutrient supplements with beneficial and harmful effects on the cardiovascular system.

THE RATIONALE FOR TARGETED NUTRITIONAL SUPPLEMENTS FOR CARDIOVASCULAR HEALTH

The heart, possessing approximately 5000 mitochondria per cell and functioning in a high-oxygen environment, is one of the most susceptible of all organs to free radical oxidative stress. Fortunately, it is also highly responsive to the benefits of targeted nutritional agents, such as phytonutrients, antioxidants, and nutriceuticals. The term *nutriceutical* includes a wide variety of nonprescription nutritional supplements normally found in the body or in natural sources (such as vitamins, amino acids, and herbals). Strong scientific evidence from large and repeated clinical trials have confirmed their efficacy and safety and have developed guidelines for patient selection, dosage, and potential medication interactions. For example, fat-soluble vitamins (K, E, D, and A) are stored to a variable extent in the body and are more likely to cause adverse reactions than are water-soluble vitamins, which are readily excreted in the urine. Excessive vitamin K can cause hemolysis in persons with glucose-6-phosphate dehydrogenase deficiency and anemia (with Heinz bodies), hyperbilirubinemia, and kernicterus in newborns; moreover, vitamin K can counter the effects of oral anticoagulants by conferring biologic activity on prothrombin and factors VII, IX, and X.

Vitamin E

In contrast, high doses of vitamin E may potentiate the effects of oral anticoagulants by antagonizing vitamin K and prolonging prothrombin time. On the benefit side, vitamin E's antioxidant and anticoagulant properties may offer protection against myocardial infarction and thrombotic strokes. A recent extensive review article assessed the preventive effects of vitamin E on the development of atherosclerosis. α-Tocopherols are the key lipid-soluble, chain-breaking antioxidants found in tissues and plasma. Oxidation of unsaturated fatty acids in low-density lipoprotein (LDL) particles, as a pivotal factor in atherogenesis, is widely recognized. Vitamin E, a predominant antioxidant present in the LDL particle, blocks the chain reaction of lipid peroxidation by scavenging intermediate peroxyl radicals. Vitamin E supplementation can reduce lipid peroxidation by as much as 40%. Stabilizing plaque, reducing inflammation, decreasing thrombolytic aggregation, reducing the expression of adhesion molecules on the arterial wall, and enhancing vasodilation are key cardioprotective effects of vitamin E. However, prospective controlled clinical trials have presented a confusing picture.

The Alpha Tocopherol, Beta Carotene (ATBC) Cancer Prevention Study, a randomized, double-blind, placebo-controlled trial involving 29,133 male smokers ages 50 to 69 years, with a median follow-up of 4.7 years, showed a minor but statistically significant decrease in angina pectoris with vitamin E supplementation of 50 mg/day (relative risk, 0.91). A nonsignificant (8%) reduction in mortality rate from coronary artery disease (CAD) was also realized.

In the Cambridge Heart Antioxidant Study (CHAOS), patients with atherosclerosis who received 400 to 800 U of vitamin E daily showed a 77% decrease in the relative risk of nonfatal myocardial infarction (MI); however, there was a nonsignificant increase in death from cardiovascular disease. The Heart Outcomes Prevention Evaluation (HOPE) and the initial Gruppo Italiano per lo Studio della Sopravvivenza nell' Infarto Miocardico (GISSI) Prevenzioni data failed to establish a clear benefit; however, one researcher's reevaluation of GISSI showed a 20% reduced risk of cardiovascular death.

In contrast, in one investigation of patients with a history of MI, mortality was higher when vitamin E was combined with β-carotene. In the most recent review of the major five human trials on vitamin E supplementation—including the ATBC, CHAOS, GISSI, Secondary Prevention with Antioxidants of Cardiovascular Disease in End-Stage Renal Disease (SPACE) and HOPE trials—a statistical reanalysis of the data, including the totality of the evidence, suggested that α-tocopherol supplementation does not have a place in treating patients with preexisting cardiovascular disease. However, it is important to keep in mind that the oxidative modification of LDL cholesterol is only a hypothesis and has yet to be proven, which raises the question of whether or not cardiologists should routinely recommend vitamin E to their patients. In two large prospective Harvard studies (Nurses' Health Study and the Health Professional Study) involving approximately 87,000 women and 40,000 men, investigators attributed reductions in heart disease and stroke to vitamin E rather than to other unidentified factors. In another investigation of men with documented coronary heart disease, 100 U or more of vitamin E per day was correlated with decreased progression of coronary artery lesions as compared with untreated counterparts. In this study of 156 men 40 to 59 years old with a history of coronary artery bypass surgery, supplemental vitamin E intake was associated with angiographically proven reduction in progression of coronary artery lesions.

Considering the many longitudinal epidemiologic studies and prospective randomized trials in which vitamin E consumption was associated with decreased cardiac risk, it is probably safe to say that some vitamin E supplementation could be considered for those individuals at high risk for CAD or with documented CAD, however, there are no definitive data to support such an approach. In addition, the rationale for vitamin E supplementation in healthy individuals is still open to question. In one investigation into the effects of vitamin E on lipid peroxidation in healthy individuals, vitamin E was supplied as D-α-tocopherol capsules. Increased circulating vitamin E levels were not associated with any change in three urinary indices of lipid peroxidation. It would be interesting to note whether administration of a combination of mixed tocopherols and γ-tocopherols could have made any difference in the analysis of lipid peroxidation.

Whenever vitamin E supplements are being considered, γ-tocopherol should be included in the basic formula. α-Tocopherol in the absence of a γ-tocopherol may be ineffective in inhibiting the oxidative damage caused by the reactive peroxynitrite radicals, and, in larger doses, α-tocopherol can displace γ-tocopherol in plasma. γ-Tocopherol also can be obtained in the diet in the form of healthy nuts, such as almonds, sunflower seeds, wheat germ, and wheat germ oil. Vitamin E (α-tocopherol) and mixed tocopherols, including tocotrienols (other derivatives of vitamin E), may be the best combination of tocopherol biochemistry and may play an even larger role in modifying the oxidation of LDL.

Natural, but not synthetic, forms of vitamin E also help to reduce platelet aggregability. In studies examining healthy volunteers, researchers measured how well platelet cells absorb D-α-tocopherol, D-α-tocopherol acetate (both natural forms), and D-L-α-tocopherol (synthetic form). The research showed that platelets effectively absorb D-α-tocopherol acetate and D-α-tocopherol but not synthetic vitamin E. Both forms of natural vitamin E reduced platelet aggregation by more than 50%, whereas no significant change was associated with synthetic vitamin E. The researchers determined that vitamin E's anticoagulant effect was unrelated to its antioxidant properties. Vitamin E's anticoagulant effect appears to result from its inhibition of protein kinase C, an enzyme that facilitates blood clotting.

Vitamin E also has been shown to significantly lower levels of C-reactive protein and monocyte interleukin-6, culprits that can also contribute to atherogenesis. Vitamin E is the least toxic of the fat-soluble vitamins, because it rarely causes adverse reactions even at doses 20 to 80 times the recommended daily requirement taken for extended periods. However, malaise, gastrointestinal (GI) complaints, headache, and even hypertension have been reported, and parenteral vitamin E, which has been withdrawn from the market, has been shown to cause pulmonary deterioration, thrombocytopenia, and liver and renal failure in several premature infants.

Previous investigations also suggested that plasma levels of antioxidants such as vitamins E and C are a more sensitive predictor of unstable angina than of severity of atheroslcerosis. The fact that free radical activity has been noted to influence the degree of coronary ischemia and spasm suggests that the beneficial effects of antioxidants in patients with CAD may result in part from a favorable influence on vascular reactivity rather than from a reduction in atherosclerotic plaque. Results of randomized double-blind, placebo-controlled clinical trials also have indicated that vitamins E and C can prevent nitrate intolerance, a major problem for patients who require long-term treatment with high-dose oral nitrates for relief of anginal symptoms.

Investigational research has suggested that nitrate intolerance is associated with increased vascular production of superoxides. When nitric oxide is released during metabolism of nitroglycerin, it reacts with superoxide anions, resulting in lower levels of cyclic guanosine monophosphate, an important intracellular intermediary that promotes vasorelaxation. There are key vitamins that warrant attention for the prevention of nitrate intolerance, including vitamin E, the main lipid-phase antioxidant, and vitamin C, the main aqueous-phase antioxidant. Supplementation with these nutrients boosts the free radical scavenging ability of the superoxide radical, thus promoting the prevention of nitrate intolerance. As the primary aqueous antioxidant, vitamin C, the major antioxidant in the aqueous phase, acts as the first line of defense against oxidative stress.

Vitamin C

Vitamin C not only is a scavenger antioxidant but also acts synergistically with vitamin E to reduce the peroxyl radical. In addition to blocking lipid peroxidation by trapping peroxyl radicals in the aqueous phase, vitamin C helps normalize endothelial vasodilative function in patients with heart failure by increasing the availability of nitric oxide. Although the evidence linking vitamin C to human cardiovascular disease is still being evaluated, one study did report that vitamin C slows the progression of atherosclerosis in men and women older than 55 years. It is also well known that many groups known to be at an increased risk for CAD have lower blood levels of vitamin C, such as men, the elderly, smokers, patients with diabetes, patients with hypertension, and possibly women taking oral estrogen contraceptives. In a recent large, prospective population study, British researchers evaluated the health of almost 20,000 people ages 45 to 79 over 4 years. They found that men and women consuming about 109 to 113 mg of vitamin C daily had about half the risk of death of those consuming only 51 to 57 mg of vitamin C per day. Higher blood levels of vitamin C were directly and inversely related to death from all causes and specifically to death from ischemic heart disease in men and women. The researchers strongly advocated modest consumption of fruits and vegetables, because their results suggested that the equivalent of one extra serving of vitamin C–rich food reduces the risk of death by 20%. However, carotenoids, flavonoids, magnesium, and other health-promoting nutrients affected these data. Because improved endothelial function has been observed with the administration of vitamin C in patients with hypertension, hypercholesterolemia, and diabetes mellitus, some vitamin C supplementation appears warranted. Vitamin C at daily doses of 500 mg has been shown to increase red cell glutathione by 50%. Glutathione is not only the major antioxidant responsible for inhibiting lipid peroxidation but also a key contributing agent in stabilizing immune function.

Megadose vitamin C (>500 mg/day) in patients who are vulnerable to iron overload states should be avoided. Vitamin C supplements may exacerbate iron toxicity by mobilizing iron reserves. Such patients may accumulate harmful excess iron with higher doses of vitamin C, so caution must be used for those with genetic diseases such as hereditary hemochromatosis, thalassemia major, or other diseases that promote iron overload.

Carotenoids

Serum carotenoids have been studied extensively in the prevention of coronary heart disease. There are approximately 600 carotenoids found in nature, predominantly in fresh fruits and vegetables, with carrots being the primary source of β-carotene and tomatoes being the best source of lycopene. Although lycopene has twice the antioxidant activity of β-carotene, the latter has been the primary focus of study because of its activity as a precursor to vitamin A.

Elevated levels of serum β-carotene have been associated with a lower risk of cancer and overall mortality. However, inconsistent data from randomized clinical trials regarding β-carotene's antioxidant properties on LDL in vitro and its preventive actions on cardiovascular disease cast doubt on the beneficial effects of β-carotene supplementation.

Research has associated a high dietary intake of β-carotene with a reduction in the incidence of cardiovascular disease. One study reported that increased β-carotene stores in subcutaneous fat are correlated with a decreased risk of MI. However, controlled studies have found that excessive supplemental β-carotene do not reduce rates of lung cancer or cardiovascular disease among heavy smokers. An increased incidence of lung cancer was found in the β-Carotene and Retinal Efficacy Trial, which halted the study 21 months early when this alarming cancer rate was observed among smokers and workers exposed to asbestos. Similarly, after the Physician's Health Trial demonstrated that alternate-day administration of 50 mg of β-carotene for 12 years showed no positive effects on coronary heart disease events, the enthusiasm for β-carotene as a preventive intervention for cardiovascular disease declined. The male participants in the Physician's Health Study did benefit from a lower risk of prostate cancer if their β-carotene status was low at the beginning of the study. Researchers suggested that β-carotene in moderate concentrations significantly inhibits the growth of three prostate cancer lines in culture medium.

The use of excess synthetic β-carotene, as done in the ATBC and the β-Carotene and Retinal Efficacy Trials, should be avoided in any high-risk populations because there are as yet unidentified elements that may somehow affect cancer growth in vulnerable individuals. It is safer and more efficacious to take a mixed natural supplement combination of mixed carotenoids including β-carotene, lutein, lycopene, α-carotene, and β-cryptoxanthin. β-Carotene is responsible for an estimated 25% of total serum carotenoid activity. Perhaps the lower mortality associated with higher levels of baseline serum β-carotene had more to do with long-term dietary habits of individuals who eat more fruits and vegetables containing multiple carotenoids than with artificial elevation of serum β-carotenes with supplementation. Excessive carotene ingestion is relatively innocuous and results in yellowing of the skin, particularly on the palms and soles, but sparing the sclerae. Hypothyroid patients are more susceptible to carotenemia.

The other carotenoids, such as lutein, that enter the LDL and high-density lipoprotein particles may retard CAD by their favorable effects on LDL oxidation. In the Toulouse Study, those participants with greater lutein activity in their blood had a lower incidence of CAD. Some researchers consider the lutein found in a diet rich in green and yellow fruits and vegetables to be more responsible for the inhibition of CAD than the red wine benefit referred to as the "French paradox."

Flavonoids

Residents of France—whose diet is steeped in high-fat cheeses, rich sauces, gravies, patés, and other highly saturated fats—have a lower incidence of coronary heart disease than their American counterparts. This paradoxical situation challenges the belief that a low-fat diet is protective against heart disease. Offsetting the "risk" that we see in the typical French diet is the routine consumption of fresh fruits and vegetables that contain vital phytonutrients, including tocopherols, carotenoids (especially lutein), flavonoids (quercetin), phenols, catechins, and other phytonutrients that may effectively reduce peroxidative tendencies and retard the varied interactions involved in atherogenesis and thrombosis. Red wine consumption could be another factor.

The serum antioxidant activity of red wine was addressed in a small study of volunteers; the results indicated that two glasses of red wind consumed before a meal offer considerable antioxidant protection for at least 4 h. Red wine increased antioxidant activity through a flavonoid–polyphenol effect. In another small investigation performed in the Netherlands, the use of dietary bioflavonoids, phenolic acids, and quercetin showed a reduction in the incidence of heart attack and sudden death. The findings in 64- to 85-year-old men showed an inverse relation between the amount of quercetin ingested and mortality. Quercetin-rich black tea, apples, and onions were the best foods evaluated, because they contain polyphenols in amounts similar to those found in the red grapes used in making wine and grape juice.

A recent study with grape juice in normal volunteers demonstrated favorable effects on platelet aggregation, platelet-derived nitric oxide release, and free oxygen–derived free radical production. Short- and long-term consumptions of black tea were shown to reverse endothelial vasomotor dysfunction in patients with CAD.

Oligomeric proanthocyanidins, such as carotenoids, are found predominantly in brightly colored fruits and vegetables and represent a safe source of polyphenols and quercetin, which are believed to be the most active protective ingredients in preventing the oxidation of LDL. Oligomeric proanthocyanidins are significant free radical scavengers that inhibit lipid peroxidation and exhibit anti-inflammatory and antiallergenic properties.

Magnesium

Magnesium has a profound influence on coronary vascular tone and reactivity; deficiencies have been shown to produce spasm of the coronary vasculature, pointing to the low magnesium state as a possible risk factor in nonocclusive MI (see Chapter 7). Hypomagnesemia can result in progressive vasoconstriction, coronary spasm, and even sudden death. In anginal episodes due to coronary artery spasm, treatment with magnesium has been shown to be considerably efficacious.

Magnesium deficiency, which is better detected by mononuclear blood cell magnesium than by the standard serum level performed at most hospitals, predisposes to excessive mortality and morbidity in patients with acute MI. Several studies have shown an association between intravenous magnesium supplementation during the first hour of admission for MI and reductions in morbidity and mortality. Although other trials of magnesium therapy in patients with acute MI have produced inconsistent results, the most efficacious use of magnesium, like thrombolytics, occurs with the earliest administration. Multiple cardioprotective and physiologic activities of magnesium include antiarrhythmic effects, calcium channel blocking effects, improvement in nitric oxide release from coronary endothelium, and the ability to help prevent serum coagulation, to name a few.

Research into the inhibition of platelet-dependent thrombosis has indicated that magnesium may have a positive preventive role for patients with CAD. In one double-blind, placebo-controlled study of 42 patients, median platelet-dependent thrombosis was reduced by 35% in 75% of patients receiving oral administration of magnesium oxide tablets (800 to 1200 mg daily) for 3 months. This antithrombotic effect occurred despite the use of aspirin therapy in the study population.

Magnesium also has shown considerable efficacy in relieving symptoms of mitral valve prolapse (MVP). In a double-blind study of 181 participants, serum magnesium levels were assessed in 141 patients with symptomatic MVP and compared with those of 40 healthy control subjects; decreased serum magnesium levels were identified in 60% of the patients with MVP, whereas only 5% of control subjects showed similar decreases. The second arm of the study investigated response to treatment. Subjective results in the magnesium group were dramatic, with significant reductions noted in weakness, chest pain, shortness of breath, palpitations, and even anxiety. Lower levels of epinephrine metabolites also were found in the urine. For patients with MVP, magnesium supplementation offers a reduction in symptomatology and improvement in quality of life. Blood pressure lowering with magnesium, especially when combined with calcium and potassium, also has been reported. Supplemental magnesium and potassium should be avoided in patients with renal insufficiency, unless a true deficiency state exists.

Trace Minerals and the Heart

Cobaltous chloride is sometimes used in the treatment of iron deficiency and chronic renal failure. Excessive cobalt intake may cause cardiomyopathy and congestive heart failure (CHF), with pericardial effusions due to deposition of cobalt–lipoic acid complexes in the heart. High cobalt consumption also has been implicated in thyroid enlargement, polycythemia, neurologic abnormalities, and interference with pyruvate and fatty acid metabolism. Rarely, excessive iron ingestion may cause cardiomyopathy, CHF, and cardiac arrhythmias from hemochromatosis.

Chromium assists in glucose and lipid metabolism. It may bring about regression of cholesterol-induced atherosclerosis. In a double-blind study involving 34 male athletes with elevated cholesterol levels, supplementation with 200 µg of elemental chromium (chromium as a niacin-bound chromium complex) significantly lowered serum cholesterol by an average of 14%. In a more recent study of 40 hypercholesterolemic patients (total cholesterol, 210 to 300 mg/dL), a combination of 200 µg of chromium polynicotinate (Cr) and (proanthocyanidin) grape-seed extract, 100 mg twice daily, resulted in profound lowering of LDL and total cholesterol. However, there was no significant change in high-density lipoprotein or triglyceride levels in the treatment or the placebo group. Because insulin resistance may be a major factor in disturbed lipid metabolism, chromium's favorable action on glucose and insulin metabolism may be the key factor in lowering cholesterol. Although no significant adverse reactions from chromium polynicotinate have been observed at the dose of 400 µg/day, massive ingestion of chromium has been associated with renal failure.

Selenium is an antioxidant with immune-enhancing and cancer-fighting properties. In some areas of the world, soil deficiencies in selenium have produced Keshan disease, a disorder of cardiac muscle characterized by multifocal myocardial necrosis that causes cardiomyopathy, CHF, and cardiac arrhythmias. Men with low levels of serum selenium (<1.4 µmol/L) demonstrated increased thickness in the intima and media of the common carotid arteries. Selenium, when combined with coenzyme Q10, also may offer cardioprotective benefits in patients after MI. In one study of 61 patients admitted for acute MI, 32 subjects in the experimental group received 100 mg of coenzyme Q10 with 500 µg of selenium in the first 24 h of hospitalization, followed by daily doses of 100 mg of coenzyme Q10, 100 µg of selenium, 15 mg of zinc, 1 mg of vitamin A, 2 mg of vitamin B_6, 90 mg of vitamin C, and 15 mg of vitamin E for 1 year. The control group (29 patients) received placebo for the same period. During their hospital stay, none of the participants in the experimental group showed prolongation of the QT interval, compared with 40% of the control subjects, whose corrected QT increased 440 ms (about a 10% increase). Although there were no significant differences in early complications between the two groups, six (21%) patients in the control group died of recurrent MI, whereas only one patient in the study group (3%) died a noncardiac death. Although selenium is quite safe at levels below 200 μg, excessive selenium can result in alopecia, abnormal nails, emotional lability, lassitude, and a garlic odor to the breath. Skin lesions and polyneuritis have been reported in people taking selenium from health food stores.

Copper is a pro-oxidant that oxidizes LDL and may contribute to the development of atherosclerosis. Men with high serum copper (>17.6 μmol/L) demonstrate increased thickening in the intima and media of the common carotid arteries. Excessive oral intake of copper may cause nausea, vomiting, diarrhea, and hemolytic anemia. Even higher doses can result in renal and hepatic toxicity and CNS disturbances similar to those of Wilson's disease. Any multivitamin with higher than the recommended daily allowance level of copper (2 mg) should be avoided. Excessive levels of copper in drinking water, especially noted in homes with copper pipes, can contribute to elevated serum copper levels.

B Vitamins

Clinical cardiologists must be familiar with B vitamin support for their patients. B vitamin depletion commonly occurs as a result of high-dose diuretic therapy used in the treatment of CHF and should be considered in any patient with refractory CHF that is unresponsive to high-dose diuretic therapy. The nocturnal leg cramps associated with diuretic therapy are a hallmark symptom of B vitamin depletion. The involuntary, painful contraction of the calf muscles and other areas of the leg can be alleviated with B vitamin support, resulting in an improved quality of life. A randomized, placebo-controlled, double-blind study validated the efficacy of B complex supplementation in the treatment of nocturnal cramps. Of 28 elderly patients, 86% taking vitamin B complex reported remission of prominent symptoms, compared with no benefit in the placebo group.

Most cardiologists are now familiar with the clinical significance of providing B vitamin supplementation to lower hyperhomocysteinemia. In 1969, the homocysteine hypothesis was first proposed, which identified accelerated vascular pathology as a sequela to homocystinuria, a rare autosomal recessive disease caused by a deficiency in cystathionine B-synthetase. Several investigations have confirmed the proposed connection between high plasma homocysteine levels and occlusive arterial disease, including atherosclerosis, peripheral vascular disease, and CAD. An increased plasma homocysteine level has also been shown to increase the risk of developing CHF in adults with prior MI.

Hyperhomocysteinemia may be even more detrimental in women. In one study, women with coronary disease had higher homocysteine levels than did matched control subjects. In a study comparing men and women with high homocysteine levels, women demonstrated greater carotid thickening ratios than did their male counterparts. In another study involving postmenopausal women, high homocysteine levels in combination with hypertension resulted in an alarming 25 times higher incidence of stroke.

The actual mechanism of action in homocysteine-associated endothelial damage remains unclear. The fact that the injury may be inhibited by the addition of catalase suggests that the process may be the result of free radical oxidative stress. This theory is strengthened by the fact that free radical hydrogen peroxide is generated during the oxidation of homocysteine. Homocysteine also enhances thromboxane A_2 and platelet aggregation and increases the binding of lipoprotein Lp(a) and fibrin. Because the association between homocysteine and atherothrombotic vascular events has been shown to be consistent regardless of other factors, high levels of homocysteine are a significant marker for atherothrombotic vascular disease. The relation between high homocysteine and degree of myocardial injury was studied in 390 consecutive patients who presented with acute coronary syndromes, 205 with MI and 185 with unstable angina. In a multivariate analysis, a homocysteine level in the top quintile (>15.7 µg/L) was an excellent predictor of possible peak cardiac protein troponin T level in patients with acute coronary syndromes and an even stronger predictor in those with unstable angina. The researchers suggested that homocysteine has a causal prothrombotic effect and indicated that further study is needed to assess homocysteine-lowering therapy. Because enzymatic deficiencies occur in as many as 5% of the population and 28% of patients with premature vascular disease have high blood levels of homocysteine, screening for this lethal risk factor should be considered. Should future randomized trials correlate homocysteine lowering with a significant reduction in vascular events, supplementation with B complex therapy must be strongly considered for patients with elevated homocysteine levels.

Certainly, administration of B vitamins at the recommended daily allowance levels (folic acid, 400 µg; B_6, 2 mg; B_{12}, 6 µg) is safe and can be recommended routinely. Research has shown a dose-dependent relationship between higher homocysteine levels and lower serum levels of B vitamins, so much higher doses must be administered to those patients with severe hyperhomocysteinemia and documented CAD. It is also encouraging to note that the U.S. Food and Drug Administration (FDA) has required that enriched grains be fortified with folic acid at a concentration that provides the average individual with an extra 100 µg of folic acid per day.

A potential hazard of folic acid therapy is subacute degeneration of the spinal cord with a subclinical vitamin B_{12} deficiency; folic acid may mask the development of hematologic manifestations in these patients. This situation can be avoided by ruling out B_{12} deficiency before initiating folic acid therapy or by supplementing folic acid with vitamin B_{12}.

High-dose niacin (vitamin B_3) is used in the treatment of hyperlipidemia and hypercholesterolemia (see Chapter 15) and helps curb the development of atherosclerosis. Side effects include cutaneous flushing, pruritus, GI disturbances, exacerbation of asthma, and even acanthosis nigricans. Very high doses can cause liver toxicity. Vasodilation and flushing, the most common side effect of niacin, may help patients who suffer from Raynaud's phenomenon.

Coenzyme Q10

Coenzyme Q10, present in most foods, especially organ meats and fish, facilitates electron transport in oxidative metabolism. Its reduced form, ubiquinol, protects membrane phospholipids and serum LDLs from lipid peroxidation and mitochondrial membrane proteins and DNA from free radical–induced oxidative damage. Ubiquinol's antioxidant effects on membrane phospholipids and LDL directly antagonize the atherogenesis process. Vitamin E regeneration is significantly improved by the addition of coenzyme Q10 because of the ability of coenzyme Q10 to recycle the oxidized form of vitamin E back to its reduced form. Coenzyme Q10 also prevents the pro-oxidant effect of α-tocopherols.

Supplemental coenzyme Q also may improve use of oxygen at the cellular level, hence benefiting patients with coronary insufficiency.

Perhaps coenzyme Q10's most remarkable effects involve tissue protection in the setting of myocardial ischemia and reperfusion. The results of a controlled study of patients with acute MI demonstrated reduction in free radical indices, infarct size, arrhythmia, and cardiac death in those patients receiving coenzyme Q10. Although side effects of coenzyme Q10, such as nausea and abdominal discomfort, are rare, it is not suggested for healthy pregnant or lactating women, because the unborn and the newborn produce sufficient quantities of the compound.

However, statin drugs cause profound deficiencies in coenzyme Q10, because 3-hydroxy-3-methylglutaryl coenzyme A reductase inhibitors (statins) block the endogenous production of coenzyme Q10. Coenzyme Q10 treatment has been used occasionally to counteract the side effect of myalgia associated with statin therapy.

L-Carnitine

L-Carnitine has a synergistic relationship with coenzyme Q10, because it also penetrates the inner mitochondrial membrane. As a trimethylated amino acid, L-carnitine's primary function is in the oxidation of fatty acids. Supplemental L-carnitine has a wide application in cardiovascular disease.

Omega-3 Fatty Acids

Omega-3 fatty acids, such as eicosapentaenoic acid (EPA) and docosa-hexaenoic acid (DHA), are found in fish oils. They stimulate the production of nitric oxide, which relaxes vascular smooth muscle. Their actions can counteract the impairment of nitric oxide production that is caused by atherosclerotic plaques. In addition, consumption of EPA stimulates the production of prostaglandin I_3, an antithrombotic and anti–platelet-aggregating agent similar to prostacyclin. As an anticoagulant, omega-3 fatty acids can increase bleeding time, inhibit platelet adhesiveness, decrease platelet count, and reduce serum thromboxane levels. Omega-3 fatty acids also can blunt the vasopressor effects of angiotensin II and norepinephrine and may reduce blood pressure.

In one recent placebo-controlled trial, an average systolic reduction of 5 mm Hg and a mean diastolic decrease of 3 mm Hg were realized in those participants taking DHA. The triglyceride-lowering effect of these fish oil components may be one of many factors that inhibit the progression of atherosclerosis. There are conflicting data from studies regarding the role of omega-3 fatty acids in the reduction of arterial restenosis after coronary angioplasty.

In a recent landmark decision, the FDA reported that it would allow products containing omega-3 fatty acids to claim heart health benefits. The FDA based its decision on the wealth of scientific evidence suggesting a correlation between omega-3 fatty acids such as EPA and DHA and a reduced risk of CAD. In the GISSI Prevenzione trial, Italian investigators reported overwhelming health benefits for participants who were placed on 1 g of omega-3 essential fatty acids a day. After the initial study had been reevaluated, participants on the omega-3 program experienced a 20% reduction in all-cause mortality and a 45% decrease in sudden cardiac death. One case-controlled study showed that those participants eating the equivalent of one fish meal a week had a 50% less chance of sudden cardiac death as compared with their counterparts whose daily menus did not contain these vital fish oils.

A recent National Institutes of Health (NIH) conference on fatty acids concluded that there is now sufficient evidence of the importance of omega-3 in the diet to recommend 220 mg of DHA per day as an adequate intake for adults and 300 mg/day for pregnant and lactating women. Attaining this proposed recommendation will require an approximate fourfold increase in omega-3 fatty acid consumption in the United States. Although side effects of fish oils are mostly abdominal upset or burping, excessive intake (>6 g daily of omega-3 fatty acids) may interfere with the effects of oral anticoagulants.

Homeopathy

Homeopathy is a healing system dating to the 18th century that was created by Samuel Christian Hahnemann, a German physician who lost faith in conventional allopathic medicine. He began his investigation around 1785 and by 1810 was 45 years old and practicing homeopathic medicine. Hahnemann based homeopathy on three laws: (a) the law of similars, (b) the law of infinitesimals, and (c) the law of chronic suppressions or law of chronic disease. The law of similars states that a substance that induces complaints in a healthy person resembling the symptoms of the patient can be used to cure the patient. A similar concept is employed in allopathic medicine in the form of vaccination and allergy desensitization. The law of chronic suppressions or chronic disease suggests that, in a chronic patient, only his or her disease or syndrome is treated instead of the whole patient. If the treatment of the disease or syndrome is successful, it often happens that a more profound and vital organ may start showing evidence of disease. Diseases that are refractory to therapy are a result of conditions that have been driven deep into the body by allopathic medicine. This concept is difficult to prove and has generated much controversy, even among homeopaths.

However, the most difficult notion for allopathic physicians to accept is the law of infinitesimals. It states that the more dilute the remedy, the stronger and more potent it becomes when it is combined with a certain shaking technique. Dilutions above 10^{-24} are unlikely to contain even a single molecule of the original substance. Nevertheless, many homeopathic remedies start near 10^{-24} dilution and many solutions go far beyond, even as great as $10^{-20,000}$.

Thus, even though homeopathic medicine prepares its medicine by starting initially with a substance, the final product may contain little, if any, trace of the original substance. Homeopaths concede that many of their medicines may contain no molecules of the original substance but say that their method of succussion (this being the combination of shaking and dilution) leaves some sort of "imprint" on the solvent. Existing physical and chemical laws dictate that a substance diluted beyond 10^{-24} is no more active than placebo. To accept homeopathic theory as the truth would require scientists and physicians to revise long-established laws of physics and chemistry—something most allopathic physicians are unwilling to do.

Numerous controlled trials have been conducted on homeopathic remedies and reported positive (significant difference between drug and placebo) and negative (no significant difference between drug and placebo) results. One study performed a meta-analysis of 107 controlled trials and weighed them on the basis of scientific methodology. The result showed a positive trend in favor of homeopathy, although the review may have been complicated by the publication bias of certain journals to trials with positive results. In a subsequent analysis combining the data of 89 studies, the investigators felt that, although there was insufficient evidence that homeopathy is effective for any single clinical situation, the evidence was "not compatible with the hypothesis that the clinical effects are completely due to placebo." In an updated review, two of the same investigators examined 32 trials and continued to conclude that, although their methodologic quality was still variable, the case of homeopathy was less convincing. However, overall, homeopathy was statistically significant in relation to placebo. If homeopathic remedies actually do work better than placebos, their pharmacologic mechanisms are unknown.

HERBAL MEDICINE

Since the beginning of human civilization, herbs have been an integral part of society, valued for their culinary and medicinal properties. However, with the development of patent medicines in the early part of the 20th century, herbal medicine lost ground to new synthetic medicines touted by scientists and physicians to be more effective and reliable. Nevertheless, about 3% of English-speaking adults in the United States report having used herbal remedies in the preceding year. This figure is probably higher among non–English-speaking Americans. The term *herbal medicine* refers to the use of plant structures, known as phytomedicinals or phytopharmaceuticals. Herbal medicine has become an increasing presence and area of interest to pharmacists and other health care professionals with the advent of the German commissioned E monographs reporting extensive information about the safety and efficacy of herbal preparations.

Herbal medicine has made many contributions to current commercial drug preparations, including ephedrine from *Ephedra sinica* (ma-huang), digitoxin from *Digitalis purpurea* (foxglove), salicin (the source of aspirin) from *Salix alba* (willow bark), and reserpine from *Rauwolfia serpentina* (snakeroot), to name just a few. The discovery of the antineoplastic agent paclitaxel (Taxol) from *Taxus brevifolia* (the Pacific yew tree) stresses the role of plants as a continuing resource for modern medicine.

Regulations in the United States

There are many laws in the United States affecting the sale and marketing of drugs, including the Food and Drug Act (1906) with its Sherley amendment (1912) and the Federal Food, Drug, and Cosmetic Act (1938) with its many amendments. The amendments passed in 1962, also known as the Kefauver-Harris amendments, required that all drugs marketed in the United States be proved safe and effective. To evaluate the safety and efficacy of drugs, the FDA turned to the Division of Medical Sciences of the National Academy of Sciences, National Research Council, which then organized a "drug efficacy study" based on reviews of in vitro tests and clinical trials on patients, usually supplied by the companies interested in marketing the drugs. At the time, very few herbs had their active ingredients isolated and even fewer had undergone clinical trials. Hence, only a small number of herbs were evaluated and only for specific indications.

In 1990, the results of the FDA's study on over-the-counter (OTC) medications, which included many herbs and herbal products, were released to the public. A few plant products, such as *Plantago psyllium* (plantago seed),

Cascara sagrada (cascara bark, *Rhamnus purshiana*), and *Cassia acutifolia* (senna leaf, *Senna alexandrina*), were judged to be "both safe and effective" (category I) for their laxative actions. However, 142 herbs and herbal products were deemed "unsafe or ineffective" (category II), and there was "insufficient evidence to evaluate" (category III) another 116 herbs. Many herbs and herbal products in categories II and III had been grandfathered by the 1938 act and 1962 amendments, because they were already covered in the 1906 act. Thus, they were not subject to the requirements of proving safety and efficacy to be out on the market. However, to deal with these grandfathered OTC products, the FDA declared that any grandfathered drug with claims of efficacy on the package or in the package insert that did not concur with the FDA's OTC study would be considered misbranded and subject to confiscation.

Unfortunately for the herbal industry, complying with the new FDA regulations meant having to remove all but the names of the herbal products from their labels and marketing them as nutritional supplements or food additives. Therefore, consumers who wish to obtain factual information regarding the therapeutic use or potential harm of herbal remedies would have to obtain them from books and pamphlets, most of which based their information on traditional reputation rather than on existing scientific research. Another major problem is that the marketing of herbal products under their common names, which is usually the case in health food stores, does not allow for proper identification, because there may be many species of herbs with the same common name. Another problem is the lack of dose standardization with herbal medicinals having active pharmacologic ingredients. These problems will remain until herbal medicinals are recognized as the drugs that they are.

One may wonder why the herbal industry never chose simply to prove their products safe and effective with more in vitro tests or clinical trials. The answer is primarily economic. With the cost and time of developing a new drug estimated at $231 million over 12 years (based on a 1990 report from the Center for the Study of Drug Development at Tufts University), most members of the herbal and pharmaceutical industries shy away from such endeavors, especially with the slim chance of obtaining patent protection for the many herbs that have been in use for centuries. Without financial sponsorship from pharmaceutical companies, there is very little financial incentive for doing research to evaluate the merits of herbal remedies, resulting in the paucity of scientific data from the United States. One step in the right direction was the decision by the NIH to allocate $2 million each for 1992 and 1993 and $2.4 million in 2000 for research to validate alternative medical practices; however, if these amounts are compared with the estimated cost of developing a single new drug, this grant allocation is clearly inadequate.

Effects of Herbal Remedies on the Cardiovascular System

The use of herbal medicine has skyrocketed over the past 5 years. Out-of-pocket therapy is estimated at more than $5 billion in the United States alone. The following review of herbal medicinals affecting the cardiovascular system is based on information gleaned from the scientific literature. These herbs are roughly categorized under the primary diseases they are used treat (Table 23-1). Note that most herbal medicinals have multiple cardiovascular effects and that the purpose of this organization is to simplify, not pigeonhole, herbs under specific diseases. In general, the dilution of active components in herbal medicinals results in fewer side effects and toxicities in comparison with the con-

TABLE 23-1 Some Conditions in Which Herbal Medicines
Are Used as Cardiovascular Treatments

Conditions	Examples of herbs used
Congestive heart failure	*Digitalis purpurea*
	Digitalis lanata
Systolic hypertension	*Rauwolfia serpentina*
	Stephania tetrandra
	Veratrum alkaloids
Angina pectoris	*Crataegus* species
	Panax notoginseng
	Salvia miltiorrhiza
Atherosclerosis	Garlic
Cerebral insufficiency	*Ginkgo biloba*
	Rosmarinus officinalis
Venous insufficiency	*Aesculus hippocastanum*
	Ruscus aculeatus

centration of active components in the allopathic medicines. However, cardiovascular disease is a serious health hazard, and no one should attempt to self-medicate with herbal remedies without first consulting a physician.

Congestive Heart Failure

Cardiac Glycosides

Many herbs contain potent cardioactive glycosides that have positive inotropic effects on the heart. The drugs digitoxin, derived from *Digitalis purpurea* (foxglove) or *Digitalis lanata,* and digoxin, derived from *D. lanata* alone, have been used in the treatment of CHF for many decades. Cardiac glycosides have a low therapeutic index, and the dose must be adjusted to the needs of each patient. The only way to control dosage is to use standardized powdered digitalis, digitoxin, or digoxin. Treating CHF with nonstandardized herbal agents would be dangerous and foolhardy. Accidental poisonings due to cardiac glycosides in herbal remedies are abundant in the medical literature. Some common plant sources of cardiac glycosides are *D. purpurea* (foxglove, already mentioned), *Adonis microcarpa* and *Adonis vernalis* (Adonis), *Apocynum cannabinum* (black Indian hemp), *Asclepias curassavica* (redheaded cotton bush), *Asclepias fruticosa* (balloon cotton), *Calotropis precera* (king's crown), *Carissa acokanthera* (bushman's poison), *Carissa spectabilis* (wintersweet), *Cerbera manghas* (sea mango), *Cheiranthus cheiri* (wallflower), *Convallaria majalis* (lily of the valley, convallaria), *Cryptostegia grandiflora* (rubber vine), *Helleborus niger* (black hellebore), *Helleborus viridus, Nerium oleander* (oleander), *Plumeria rubra* (frangipani), *Selenicereus grandiflorus* (cactus grandiflorus), *Strophanthus hispidus* and *Strophanthus kombé* (strophanthus), *Thevetia peruviana* (yellow oleander), and *Urginea maritime* (squill). Even the venom glands of the *Bufo marinus* (cane toad) contain cardiac glycosides. Health providers should be aware of the cross reactivity of cardiac glycosides from herbal sources with the digoxin radioimmunoassay. Treatment of intoxication with these substances is directed at controlling arrhythmias and hyperkalemia, which are the usual causes of fatalities. The effects and treatment of digitalis toxicity are reviewed in Chapter 8.

Berberine

Berberine is an example of an alkaloid that is distributed widely in nature and used in the Orient for the treatment of CHF. It is reported to also have anti-hypertensive and antiarrhythmic actions. In a recent placebo-controlled trial, patients with heart failure and significant ventricular ectopy on standard therapy received berberine 1.2 to 2.0 mg/day for up to 24 months. Compared to placebo, there was a reduction in mortality and ventricular ectopy, with an improvement in quality of life.

Hypertension

Rauwolfia serpentina

The root of *Rauwolfia serpentina* (snakeroot), the natural source of the alkaloid reserpine, has been a Hindu Ayurvedic remedy since ancient times. In 1931, the Indian literature first described the use of *R. serpentina* root for the treatment of hypertension and psychoses; however, the use of rauwolfia alkaloids in western medicine did not begin until the mid-1940s. Standardized whole-root preparations of *R. serpentina* and its reserpine alkaloid are officially monographed in the *United States Pharmacopeia*. A 200- to 300-mg dose of powdered whole root taken orally is equivalent to 0.5 mg of reserpine.

Reserpine was one of the first drugs used on a large scale to treat systemic hypertension. It acts by irreversibly blocking the uptake of biogenic amines (norepinephrine, dopamine, and serotonin) in the storage vesicles of central and peripheral adrenergic neurons, thus leaving the catecholamines to be destroyed by the intraneuronal monoamine oxidase in the cytoplasm. The depletion of catecholamines accounts for reserpine's sympatholytic and anti-hypertensive actions.

Reserpine's effects are long-lasting because recovery of sympathetic function requires synthesis of new storage vesicles, which takes days to weeks. Reserpine lowers blood pressure by decreasing cardiac output, peripheral vascular resistance, heart rate, and renin secretion. With the introduction of other antihypertensive drugs with fewer CNS side effects, the use of reserpine has diminished. The daily oral dose of reserpine should be 0.25 mg or less and as little as 0.05 mg if given with a diuretic. When using the whole root, the usual adult dose is 50 to 200 mg/day administered once daily or in two divided doses.

Rauwolfia alkaloids are contraindicated for use in patients with previously demonstrated hypersensitivity to these substances, in patients with a history of mental depression (especially with suicidal tendencies) or an active peptic ulcer or ulcerative colitis, and in those receiving electroconvulsive therapy. The most common side effects are sedation and inability to concentrate and perform complex tasks. Reserpine may cause mental depression, sometimes resulting in suicide, and must be discontinued at the first sign of depression. Reserpine's sympatholytic effect and its enhancement of parasympathetic actions account for its other well-described side effects: nasal congestion, increased secretion of gastric acid, and mild diarrhea.

Stephania tetrandra

Stephania tetrandra is an herb sometimes used in Traditional Chinese Medicine (TCM) to treat hypertension. Tetrandrine, an alkaloid extract of *S. tetrandra,* has been shown to be a calcium channel antagonist paralleling the effects of verapamil. Tetrandrine inhibits T and L calcium channels, interferes with the binding of diltiazem and methoxy verapamil at calcium-associated sites, and suppresses aldosterone production. A parenteral dose (15 mg/kg) of tetrandrine in conscious rats decreased mean, systolic, and diastolic blood pressures for longer than 30 min; however, an intravenous dose of 40 mg/kg killed the rats by myocardial depression. In stroke-prone hypertensive rats, an oral dose of 25 or 50 mg/kg produced a gradual and sustained hypotensive effect after 48 h without affecting plasma renin activity. In addition to its cardiovascular actions, tetrandrine has reported antineoplastic, immunosuppressive, and mutagenic effects.

Tetrandrine is 90% protein bound with an elimination half-life of 88 min according to dog studies; however, rat studies have shown a sustained hypotensive effect for longer than 48 h after a 25- or 50-mg oral dose. Tetrandrine caused liver necrosis in dogs orally administered 40 mg/kg of tetrandrine thrice weekly for 2 months, reversible swelling of liver cells at a 20-mg/kg dose, and no observable changes at a 10-mg/kg dose. Given the evidence of hepatotoxicity, many more studies are necessary to establish a safe dosage of tetrandrine in humans, if such a dose even exists.

Lingusticum wallichii

The root of *Lingusticum wallichii* (chuan-xiong, chuan-hsiung) is used in TCM as a circulatory stimulant, hypotensive agent, and sedative. Tetramethyl pyrazine, the active constituent extracted from *L. wallichii,* inhibits platelet aggregation in vitro and lowers blood pressure by vasodilation in dogs. With its actions independent of the endothelium, tetramethyl pyrazine's vasodilatory effect is mediated by calcium antagonism and nonselective antagonism of α-adrenoreceptors. Some evidence has suggested that tetramethyl pyrazine can selectively act on the pulmonary vasculature. Currently, there is insufficient information to evaluate the safety and efficacy of this herbal medicinal.

Uncaria rhynchophylla

Uncaria rhynchophylla (gou-teng) is sometimes used in TCM to treat hypertension. Its indole alkaloids, rhynchophylline and hirsutine, are thought to be the active principals of *U. rhynchophylla*'s vasodilatory effect. The mechanism of *U. rhynchophylla*'s actions is unclear. Some studies have pointed to an alteration in calcium flux in response to activation, whereas others have pointed to hirsutine's inhibition of nicotine-induced dopamine release. One in vitro study has shown that *U. rhynchophylla* extract relaxes norepinephrine-precontracted rat aorta through endothelium-dependent and -independent mechanisms. For the endothelium-dependent component, *U. rhynchophylla* extract appears to stimulate endothelium-derived relaxing factor and nitric oxide release without involving muscarinic receptors. Also, in vitro and in vivo studies have shown that rhynchophylline can inhibit platelet aggregation and reduce platelet thromboses induced by collagen or adenosine diphosphate plus epinephrine. The safety and efficacy of this agent cannot be evaluated at present owing to a lack of clinical data.

Veratrum

Veratrum (hellebore) is a perennial herb growing in many parts of the world. Varieties include *V. viride* from Canada and the eastern United States, *V. californicum* from the western United States, *V. album* from Alaska and Europe, and *V. japonicum* from Asia. All *Veratrum* plants contain poisonous veratrum alkaloids, which are known to cause vomiting, bradycardia, and hypotension.

Most cases of *Veratrum* poisoning are due to misidentification with other plants. Although once a treatment for hypertension, the use of *Veratrum* alkaloids has lost favor owing to a low therapeutic index, unacceptable toxicity, and the introduction of safer antihypertensive drug alternatives.

Veratrum alkaloids enhance nerve and muscle excitability by increasing sodium conductivity. They act on the posterior wall of the left ventricle and the coronary sinus baroreceptors, causing a reflex hypotension and bradycardia via the vagus nerve (Bezold-Jarisch reflex). Nausea and vomiting are secondary to the alkaloids' actions on the nodose ganglion.

The diagnosis of *Veratrum* toxicity is established by history, identification of the plant, and strong clinical suspicion. Treatment is mainly supportive and directed at controlling bradycardia and hypotension. *Veratrum*-induced bradycardia usually responds to treatment with atropine; however, the blood pressure response to atropine is more variable and may require the addition of pressors. Electrocardiographic changes may or may be reversible with atropine. Seizures are a rare complication and may be treated with conventional anticonvulsants. For patients with preexisting cardiac disease, the use of β-agonists or pacing may be necessary. Nausea may be controlled with phenothiazine antiemetics. Recovery is usually within 24 to 48 h.

Angina Pectoris

Crataegus

Hawthorn, a name encompassing many *Crataegus* species (such as *C. oxyacantha* and *C. monogyna* in the West and *C. pinnatifida* in China), has acquired the reputation in the modern herbal literature as an important tonic for the cardiovascular system, particularly useful for angina. *Crataegus* leaves, flowers, and fruits contain a number of biologically active substances such as oligomeric procyanidins, flavonoids, and catechins. From current studies, *Crataegus* extract appears to have antioxidant properties and can inhibit the formation of thromboxane A_2. Also, *Crataegus* extract antagonizes the increases in cholesterol, triglycerides, and phospholipids in LDL and very LDL in rats fed a hyperlipidemic diet; thus, it may inhibit the progression of atherosclerosis. According to one study, *Crataegus* extract in high concentrations had a cardioprotective effect on the ischemic reperfused heart without an increase in coronary blood flow. However, oral and parenteral administrations of oligomeric procyanins of *Crataegus* leads to an increase in coronary blood flow in cats and dogs. Double-blind clinical trials have demonstrated simultaneous cardiotropic and vasodilatory actions of *Crataegus*. In essence, *Crataegus* increases coronary perfusion, has a mild hypotensive effect, antagonizes atherosclerosis, has positive inotropic and negative chronotropic actions, and improves CHF. *Crataegus* lowers blood pressure due to its action in lowering peripheral vascular resistance. Animal studies also have indicated that peripheral and coronary blood flows increase, whereas arterial blood pressure decreases. Hawthorn is relatively devoid of side effects, and appears to have no pharmacokinetic interaction when combined with digoxin. It is currently being evaluated as an adjunctive treatment for CHF. To that end, the Survival and Prognosis Investigation of *Crataegus* Extract-WS1442 (SPICE) trial is enrolling approximately 2300 patients from 120 international centers to evaluate the long-term effects of a standard preparation of hawthorn extract as compared with placebo on hospitalizations and mortality in patients with moderate heart failure receiving an established medical regimen.

Panax notoginseng

Because of its resemblance to *Panax ginseng* (Asian ginseng), *Panax noto-ginseng* (pseudo-ginseng; san-qui) has acquired the common name of *pseudo-ginseng,* especially because it is often an adulterant of *P. ginseng* preparations. In TCM, the root of *P. notoginseng* is used for analgesia and hemostasis. It is also often used in the treatment of patients with angina and CAD.

Although clinical trials are lacking, in vitro studies using *P. notoginseng* do suggest possible cardiovascular effects. One study that used purified notoginsenoside R1, extracted from *P. notoginseng,* on human umbilical vein endothelial cells showed dose- and time-dependent syntheses of tissue-type plasminogen activator without affecting the synthesis of plasminogen-activating inhibitor type 1, thus enhancing fibrinolytic parameters.

Another study has suggested that *P. notoginseng* saponins inhibit atherogen-esis by interfering with the proliferation of smooth muscle cells. In vitro and in vivo studies using rats and rabbits have demonstrated that *P. notoginseng* may be useful as an antianginal agent, because it dilates coronary arteries in all con-centrations. The role of *P. notoginseng* in the treatment of hypertension is less certain, because it causes vasodilation or vasoconstriction, depending on con-centration and the target vessel. The results of these in vitro and in vivo studies are encouraging; however, clinical trials will be necessary to enable more informed decisions regarding the use of *P. notoginseng.* The most common side effects reported with ginseng were insomnia, diarrhea, and skin reactions.

Salvia miltiorrhiza

Salvia miltiorrhiza (dan-shen), a relative of the Western sage *S. officinalis,* is native to China. In TCM, the root of *S. miltiorrhiza* is used as a circulatory stimulant, sedative, and cooling agent. *Salvia miltiorrhiza* may be useful as an antianginal agent because, like *P. notoginseng,* it has been shown to dilate coronary arteries in all concentrations. Also, *S. miltiorrhiza* has variable action on other vessels, depending on its concentration, so it may not be as helpful in treating hypertension. In vitro, *S. miltiorrhiza,* in a dose-dependent fashion, inhibits platelet aggregation and serotonin release induced by adenosine diphosphate or epinephrine, which is thought to be mediated by an increase in platelet cyclic adenosine monophosphate caused by *S. miltiorrhiz*'s inhibition of cyclic adenosine monophosphate phosphodiesterase. *Salvia miltiorrhiza* appears to have a protective effect on ischemic myocardium by enhancing the recovery of contractile force upon reoxygenation. Qualitatively and quantita-tively, a decoction of *S. miltiorrhiza* was as efficacious as the more expensive isolated tanshinones. Clinical trials will be necessary to further evaluate the safety and efficacy of *S. miltiorrhiza.*

Atherosclerosis

Allium sativum

In addition to its use in the culinary arts, *Allium sativum* (garlic) has been val-ued for centuries in many cultures for its medicinal properties. In recent decades, animal and human data have focused on garlic's use in treating ath-erosclerosis and hypertension. Many studies have demonstrated garlic's effects, which include lowering blood pressure, reducing serum cholesterol and triglycerides, enhancing fibrinolytic activity, and inhibiting platelet aggregation. However, some investigators have been hesitant to endorse the routine use of garlic for cardiovascular disease outright despite positive evidence, because many of the published studies had methodologic shortcomings. For example, in one of the largest collective reviews of randomized controlled trials of garlic lasting 4 weeks or longer, the researchers concluded that the effects of garlic treatment are tainted by an inadequate definition of active constituents in the study preparations. The pharmacologic properties of garlic are extremely complex, comprising a variety of sulfur-containing compounds that include allicin, alliin, diallyl disulfide, ajoene, s-allylcysteines, and γ-glutamyl peptides, to mention a few. Many of the previous controlled trials of garlic used different preparations containing all or some of these active pharmacologic factors. This may be the major reason for the variability and confusion found in the research. The definition and delineation of the major active garlic ingredients and their specific mechanisms of action are absolutely necessary before future trials are planned and conducted.

Intact cells of garlic bulbs contain an odorless, sulfur-containing amino acid derivative known as *alliin*. When garlic is crushed, alliin comes into contact with alliinase, which converts alliin to allicin. Allicin has potent antibacterial properties but is also highly odoriferous and unstable. Ajoenes, self-condensation products of allicin, appear to be responsible for garlic's antithrombotic activity. Most authorities now agree that allicin and its derivatives are the active constituents of garlic's physiologic activity. Fresh garlic releases allicin in the mouth during the chewing process. Dried garlic preparations lack allicin but do contain alliin and alliinase. Because alliinase is inactivated by acids in the stomach, dried garlic preparations should be enterically coated so that they pass through the stomach into the small intestine, where alliin can be enzymatically converted to allicin. Few commercial garlic preparations are standardized for their allicin yield based on alliin content, thus making their effectiveness less certain. However, one double-blind, placebo-controlled study over 4 months involving 261 patients using one 800-mg tablet of garlic powder daily, standardized to 1.3% alliin content, demonstrated significant reductions in total cholesterol (12%) and triglycerides (17%). In studies using garlic supplements containing no allicin or poorly bioavailable allicin, no lipid lowering was realized. Consumption of large quantities of fresh garlic (0.25 to 1 g/kg body weight or about 5 to 20 average-size 4-g cloves in a 175-lb person) does appear to produce beneficial effects. However, in a meta-analysis, it was demonstrated that garlic, in an amount approximating one-half to one clove per day, decreased total serum cholesterol by about 9% in the patients studied. The allicin yield of each 800-mg garlic tablet is equivalent to 2.8 g of fresh garlic—less than one average-size 4-g clove; in other words, therapeutic effectiveness may be seen in doses much lower than five cloves of garlic. In 11 large databases collected from January 1966 through February 2000, various garlic preparations did produce small reductions in total cholesterol, LDL, and triglyceride, but no statistically significant changes were noted in high-density lipoproteins. Significant reductions in platelet aggregation and insignificant effects on blood pressure outcomes also were observed.

Aside from a garlic odor on the breath and body, moderate garlic consumption causes few adverse effects. Consumption in excess of five cloves daily may result in heartburn, flatulence, and other GI disturbances. Case reports have also described bleeding in patients ingesting large doses of garlic (average of four cloves per day). Because of its antithrombotic activity, garlic also should be used with caution in people taking oral anticoagulants. Some individuals have reported allergic reactions to garlic.

Cerebral and Peripheral Vascular Diseases

Ginkgo biloba

More than 200 million years ago, *Ginkgo biloba* (maidenhair tree) apparently was saved from extinction by human intervention, surviving in Far Eastern temple gardens but disappearing for centuries in the West. It was reintroduced to Europe in 1730 and became a favorite ornamental tree. Although the root and kernels of *G. biloba* have long been used in TCM, *Ginkgo* gained attention in the West during the 20th century for its medicinal value after a concentrated extract of *G. biloba* leaves was developed in the 1960s. At least two groups of substances within *G. biloba* extract have demonstrated beneficial pharmacologic actions. The flavonoids reduce capillary permeability and fragility and serve as free radical scavengers. The terpenes (i.e., ginkgolides) inhibit platelet-activating factor, decrease vascular resistance, and improve circulatory flow without appreciably affecting blood pressure. Continuing research appears to support the primary use of *G. biloba* extract for treating cerebral insufficiency and its secondary effects on vertigo, tinnitus, memory, and mood. In a study evaluating 327 demented patients, 120 mg of *G. biloba* extract produced improvements in dementia, similar to other studies with donepezil and tacrine. However, a more recent study showed no benefit of *G. biloba* on cognitive functioning. In addition, *G. biloba* extract appears to be useful for treating peripheral vascular disease, including intermittent claudication and diabetic retinopathy.

Although approved as a drug in Europe, *Ginkgo* is not approved in the United States and is instead marketed as a food supplement, usually supplied as 40-mg tablets of extract. Because most investigations examining the efficacy of *G. biloba* extracts have used preparations such as EGb 761 or LI 1370, the bioequivalence of other *G. biloba* extract products has not been established. The recommended dose in Europe is one 40-mg tablet taken three times daily with meals (120 mg daily). Adverse effects of *G. biloba* extract are rare but can include GI disturbances, headache, and skin rash. Several case reports of bleeding, including subarachnoid hemorrhage, intracranial hemorrhage, and subdural hematoma, have been associated with *G. biloba*. *Ginkgo biloba* should not be used in combination with analgesic agents such as aspirin, ticlopidine, and clopidogrel or anticoagulants such as warfarin, because it undermines the effect of the platelet-inhibiting factor.

Rosmarinus officinalis

Known mostly as a culinary spice and flavoring agent, *Rosmarinus officinalis* (rosemary) is listed in many herbal sources as a tonic and all-around stimulant. Traditionally, rosemary leaves are said to enhance circulation, aid digestion, elevate mood, and boost energy. When applied externally, the volatile oils are supposedly useful for arthritic conditions and baldness.

Although research on rosemary is scanty, some studies have focused on antioxidant effects of diterpenoids, especially carnosic acid and carnosol, isolated from rosemary leaves. In addition to having antineoplastic effects (especially skin), antioxidants in rosemary have been credited with stabilizing erythrocyte membranes and inhibiting superoxide generation and lipid peroxidation. Essential oils of rosemary have demonstrated antimicrobial, hyperglycemic, and insulin-inhibiting properties. Rosemary leaves contain large amounts of salicylates, and its flavonoid pigment diosmin is reported to decrease capillary permeability and fragility.

Despite the conclusions derived from in vitro and animal studies, the therapeutic use of rosemary for cardiovascular disorders remains questionable, because few, if any, clinical trials have been conducted using rosemary. Due to lack of studies, no conclusions can be reached regarding the use of the antioxidants of rosemary in inhibiting atherosclerosis. Although external application may cause cutaneous vasodilatation from the counterirritant properties of rosemary's essential oils, there is no evidence to support any prolonged improvement in peripheral circulation. Although rosemary does have some carminative properties, it may also cause GI and kidney disturbances in large doses. Until more studies are done, rosemary probably should be limited to its use as a culinary spice and flavoring agent rather than as a medicine.

Venous Insufficiency

Aesculus hippocastanum

The seeds of *Aesculus hippocastanum* (horse chestnut) have long been used in Europe to treat venous disorders such as varicose veins. The medicinal qualities of horse chestnut reside mostly in its large seeds, which resemble edible chestnuts. The seeds contain a complex mixture of saponins, glycosides, and several other active ingredients. The grouping of most interest is called *aesculic acid* or *aescin*. In addition to a high level of flavonoids, horse chestnuts contain several minerals including magnesium, manganese, cobalt, and iodine.

The saponin glycoside aescin from horse chestnut extract (HCE) inhibits the activity of lysosomal enzymes, which are thought to contribute to varicose veins by weakening vessel walls and increasing permeability, resulting in dilated veins and edema. In animal studies, HCE, in a dose-dependent fashion, increased venous tone, venous flow, and lymphatic flow. HCE also antagonizes capillary hyperpermeability induced by histamine, serotonin, or chloroform. HCE decreases edema formation of lymphatic and inflammatory origin. HCE has anti-exudative properties suppressing experimentally induced pleurisy and peritonitis by inhibiting plasma extravasation and leukocyte emigration. HCE's dose-dependent antioxidant properties can inhibit in vitro lipid peroxidation. Randomized, double-blind, placebo-controlled trials using HCE showed a statistically significant reduction in edema, as measured by plethysmography. Although still controversial, prophylactic use of HCE does not appear to decrease the incidence of thromboembolic complications of gynecologic surgery.

Standardized HCE is prepared as an aqueous alcohol extract of 16% to 21% of triterpene glycosides, calculated as aescin. The usual initial dose is 90 to 150 mg of aescin daily, which may be reduced to 35 to 70 mg daily after improvement. Standardized HCE preparations are not available in the United States, but nonstandardized products may be available.

Some manufacturers promote the use of topical preparations of HCE for treatment of varicose veins and hemorrhoids; however, at least one study has demonstrated very poor aescin distribution at sites other than the skin and muscle tissues underlying the application site. Moreover, the involvement of arterioles and veins in the pathophysiology of hemorrhoids makes the effectiveness of HCE doubtful, because HCE has no known effects on the arterial circulation. For now, research studies have yet to confirm any clinical effectiveness of topical HCE preparations.

Although side effects are uncommon, HCE may cause GI irritation and facial rash. Parenteral aescin has produced isolated cases of anaphylactic reactions in addition to hepatic and renal toxicity. In the event of toxicity, aescin is completely dialyzable.

Ruscus aculeatus

Like *A. hippocastanum, Ruscus aculeatus* (butcher's broom) is known for its use in treating venous insufficiency. *Ruscus aculeatus* is a short evergreen shrub found commonly in the Mediterranean region. Two steroidal saponins, ruscogenin and neurogenin, extracted from the rhizomes of *R. aculeatus* are thought to be its active components. In vivo studies on hamster cheek pouch have shown that topical *Ruscus* extract dose-dependently antagonizes a histamine-induced increase in vascular permeability. Moreover, topical *Ruscus* extract causes dose-dependent constriction on venules without appreciably affecting arterioles. Topical *Ruscus* extract's vascular effects are also temperature dependent and appear to counter the sympathetic nervous system's temperature-sensitive vascular regulation: Venules dilate at a lower temperature (25°C), constrict at near-physiologic temperature (36.5°C), and further constrict at a higher temperature (40°C); arterioles dilate at 25°C, are unaffected at 36.5°C, and remain unaffected or constricted at 40°C depending on *Ruscus* concentration. Based on the influences of prazosin, diltiazem, and rauwolscine, the peripheral vascular effects of *Ruscus* extract appear to be selectively mediated by effects on calcium channels and α-adrenergic receptors.

Several small clinical trials using topical *Ruscus* extract have supported its role in treating venous insufficiency. One randomized, double-blind, placebo-controlled trial involving 18 volunteers showed a statistically significant decrease in femoral vein diameter (median decrease, 1.25 mm) by using duplex B-scan ultrasonography 2.5 h after applying 4 to 6 g of a cream containing 64 to 96 mg of *Ruscus* extract. Another small trial ($n = 18$) showed that topical *Ruscus* extract may be helpful in reducing venous dilatation during pregnancy. Oral agents may be as useful as topical agents for venous insufficiency, although the evidence is less convincing.

Although capsule, tablet, ointment, and suppository (for hemorrhoids) preparations of *Ruscus* extract are available in Europe, only capsules are available in the United States. These capsules contain 75 mg of *Ruscus* extract and 2 mg of rosemary oil. Aside from occasional nausea and gastritis, side effects from using *R. aculeatus* have rarely been reported, even at high doses. Nevertheless, one should be wary of any drug that has not been thoroughly tested. Although there is ample evidence to support the pharmacologic activity of *R. aculeatus,* there is a relative deficiency of clinical data to establish its actual safety and efficacy. Until more studies are completed, no recommendations regarding dosage can be offered.

NONCARDIOVASCULAR HERBS WITH NOTEWORTHY CARDIOVASCULAR EFFECTS

For the following noncardiovascular herbs, only cardiovascular actions are emphasized (Table 23-2).

Tussilago farfara

Tussilago farfara (coltsfoot, kuan-dong-hua) is a perennial herb that is grown in many parts of northern China, Europe, Africa, Siberia, and North America.

TABLE 23-2 Adverse Cardiovascular Reactions Observed with Herbal Medicines Used for Other Indications

Examples	Herbal medicines
Antithrombotic actions that could potentiate the effects of warfarin	Garlic
Hypertension	*Tussilago farfara*
	Ephedra sinica
Hypotension	*Aconitum* species
Digitalis toxicity	More than 20 herbal substances with activity to digitalis radioimmunoassay
Bradycardia	*Aconitum* species
	Jin-bu-huan

Over the years, *T. farfara* has acquired a reputation as a demulcent antitussive agent due to a throat-soothing mucilage within the herb. Recently, the use of *T. farfara* has lost favor due to several studies that found senkirkine, a pyrrolizidine alkaloid known to cause hepatotoxicity, in all parts of the herb. In addition, rats fed a diet containing *T. farfara* had a high risk of developing hemangioendothelial sarcoma of the liver.

A diterpene isolated from *T. farfara,* named *tussilagone,* is a potent respiratory and cardiovascular stimulant. Administered intravenously, tussilagone produces a dose-dependent increase in the peripheral vascular resistance of dogs, cats, and rats without much effect on ventricular inotropy and chronotropy. The median lethal dose in mice with an acute intravenous administration of tussilagone is 28.9 mg/kg.

Ephedra sinica

Ephedra sinica (joint fir, ma-huang), the natural source of the alkaloid ephedrine, has been used in TCM for more than 5000 years as an antiasthmatic and decongestant. *Ephedra* has gained recent notoriety stemming from several fatalities of youths who took an excess of *Ephedra,* which is promoted by some as a "legal high," "weight-loss aid," "energy booster," and "aphrodisiac." In a study involving a review of 140 adverse case reports submitted to the FDA between 1997 and 1999, *Ephedra* alkaloids in dietary supplements caused 10 deaths and 13 permanent disabilities. Most of these tragic events were cardiovascular (e.g., cardiac arrest, arrhythmia) or neurologic (e.g., stroke, seizure).

Ephedrine acts by releasing stored catecholamines from synaptic neurons and nonselectively stimulates α- and β-adrenergic receptors. Ephedrine increases mean, systolic, and diastolic blood pressures by vasoconstriction and cardiac stimulation. Ephedrine's bronchodilating actions may be helpful for the chronic treatment of asthma. Ephedrine enhances the contractility of skeletal muscle. It penetrates the CNS and can produce nervousness, excitability, and insomnia. Patients taking monoamine oxidase inhibitors or guanethidine should not be receiving any product containing ephedrine alkaloids. Patients with preexisting CAD, hypertension, and severe glaucoma also should avoid ephedrine alkaloids. The FDA recently raised concerns about the safety of Ephedra when used as a weight-reducing supplement.

Commercially synthesized ephedrine in the United States is identical with the alkaloid derived from *Ephedra.* Oral preparations of ephedrine sulfate are supplied as capsules and syrups. The usual adult dose is 25 to 50 mg every 6 h; for children, the dose is 3 mg/kg every 24 h in four divided doses.

Aconitum

The roots of *Aconitum* species, such as *A. kusnezoffii* (cao-wu) and *A. carmichaeli* (chuan-wa), are sometimes used in TCM to treat rheumatism, arthritis, bruises, and fractures. In Europe, *A. napellus* (monkshood, wolfsbane) grows in the wild and is sometime cultivated as an ornamental.

Plant parts of *Aconitum* species contain diterpenoid ester alkaloids, including aconitine, which have been linked to several deaths in Hong Kong and Australia. Death usually results from cardiovascular collapse and ventricular tachyarrhythmias induced by aconite alkaloids. These alkaloids activate sodium channels and cause widespread membrane excitation in cardiac, neural, and muscular tissues. Characteristic manifestations of aconite intoxication include nausea, vomiting, diarrhea, hypersalivation, and generalized paresthesias (especially circumoral numbness). Muscarinic activation may cause hypotension and bradyarrhythmias. Transmembrane enhancement of sodium flux during the plateau phase prolongs repolarization and induces afterdepolarizations and triggered automaticity in cardiac myocytes. Aconite-induced cardiac arrhythmias also can lead to cardiac failure from as soon as 5 min to as long as 4 days.

Management of aconite intoxication consists of symptomatic relief, because no specific antidote exists. Amiodarone and flecainide may be used as antiarrhythmic agents. Intragastric charcoal can decrease alkaloid absorption. A fatal dose can be as small as 5 mL of aconite tincture, 2 mg of pure aconite, or 1 g of plant. Considering their low therapeutic index and unacceptable toxicity, *Aconitum* and its products are not recommended, even in therapeutic doses, because an erroneous dose can be fatal.

Jin-Bu-Huan

Often misidentified as a derivative of *Polygala chinensis,* jin-bu-huan most likely is derived from the *Stephania* genus. This herbal remedy contains an active alkaloid known as *levotetrahydropalmatine,* which is a potent neuroactive substance that produces sedation, naloxone-resistant analgesia, and dopamine receptor antagonism in animals. Jin-bu-huan is used as an analgesic, sedative, hypnotic, and antispasmodic agent and as a dietary supplement. It is associated with significant cardiorespiratory toxicity, including respiratory failure and bradycardia requiring endotracheal intubation. There is no specific antidote for the treatment of acute jin-bu-huan overdose. Several cases of hepatitis have been associated with long-term ingestion of jin-bu-huan. Although it is now banned in the United States, jin-bu-huan is still being imported illegally as jin bu huan anodyne tablets.

CONCLUSION

With the widespread use of alternative medicine in the United States, health practitioners, in taking clinical histories, should remember to ask patients about their alternative health practices and stay informed regarding the beneficial or harmful effects of these treatments. Continuing research is elucidating the pharmacologic activities of many alternative medicines and may stimulate future pharmaceutical development; however, such research is lacking in the United States and may require support from government agencies. Legal surveillance of alternative medicine practices with low safety margins should be instituted for the sake of public health. As more information becomes available regarding the safety and efficacy of alternative medicines, research-supported claims may one day appear on the labels of alternative medicinals.

The integration of proven complementary therapies with conventional treatments in heart disease will allow cardiologists to offer many additional options to their patients. An open mind and a willingness to support conventional methodology while investigating alternatives can improve quality of life and reduce human suffering. Choosing from the best conventional and complementary options is the only logical and ethical thing to do.

ADDITIONAL READINGS

Blendon RJ, DesRoches CM, Benson JM, et al: Americans' views on the use and regulation of dietary supplements. *Arch Intern Med* 161:805, 2001.

Frishman WH, Kruger NA, Nayak DU, Vakili BA: Antioxidant vitamins and enzymatic and synthetic oxygen-derived free-radical scavengers in the prevention and treatment of cardiovascular disease, in Frishman WH, Sonnenblick EH, Sica DA (eds): *Cardiovascular Pharmacotherapeutics,* 2nd ed. New York, McGraw-Hill, 2003, p 407.

Goldman P: Herbal medicines today and the roots of modern pharmacology. *Ann Intern Med* 135:594, 2001.

Haller CA, Benowitz NL: Adverse cardiovascular and central nervous system events associated with dietary supplements containing ephedra alkaloids. *N Engl J Med* 343:1833, 2000.

Harris WS, Park Y, Isley WL: Cardiovascular disease and long-chain omega-3 fatty acids. *Curr Opin Lipidol* 14:9, 2003.

Kinsel JF, Straus SE: Complementary and alternative therapeutics: Rigorous research is needed to support claims. *Ann Rev Pharmacol Toxicol* 43:463, 2003.

Kruger NA, Frishman WH, Hussain J: Fish oils, the B vitamins and folic acid as cardiovascular protective agents, in Frishman WH, Sonnenblick EH, Sica DA (eds): *Cardiovascular Pharmacotherapeutics,* 2nd ed. New York, McGraw-Hill, 2003, p 381.

Lin MC, Nahin R, Gershwin E, et al: State of complementary and alternative medicine in cardiovascular, lung, and blood research. Executive summary of a workshop. *Circulation* 103:2038, 2001.

Pittler MH, Schmidt K, Ernst E: Hawthorne extract for treating chronic heart failure: Meta-analysis of randomized trials. *Am J Med* 114:665, 2003.

Salonen RM, Nyyssonen K, Kaikkonen J, et al: Six-year effect of combined Vitamin C and E supplementation on atherosclerotic progression. The Antioxidant Supplementation in Atherosclerosis Prevention (ASAP) Study. *Circulation* 107:947, 2003.

Shekelle PG, Hardy ML, Morton SC, et al: Efficacy and safety of ephedra and ephedrine for weight loss and athletic performance: A meta-analysis. *JAMA* 289:1537, 2003.

Sinatra ST, Frishman WH, Peterson SJ, Lin G: Use of alternative/complementary medicine in treating cardiovascular disease, in Frishman WH, Sonnenblick EH, Sica DA (eds): *Cardiovascular Pharmacotherapeutics,* 2nd ed. New York, McGraw-Hill, 2003, p 857.

Stein CM: Are herbal products dietary supplements or drugs? An important question for public safety. *Clin Pharmacol Ther* 71:411, 2002.

Tankanow R, Tamer HR, Streetman DS, et al: Interaction study between digoxin and a preparation of hawthorn (*Crataegus oxyacantha*). *J Clin Pharmacol* 43:637, 2003.

Thies F, Garry JMC, Yaqoob P, et al: Association of n-3 polyunsaturated acids with stability of atherosclerotic plaques: A randomized conrtolled trial. *Lancet* 361:477, 2003.

Vandenbroucke JP, de Craen AJM: Alternative medicine: A "mirror image" for scientific reasoning in conventional medicine. *Ann Intern Med* 135:507, 2001.

Wong SS, Nahin RL: National Center for Complementary and Alternative Medicine perspectives for complementary and alternative medicine research in cardiovascular diseases. *Cardiol Rev* 11:94, 2003.

Wood MJ, Stewart RL, Merry H, et al: Use of complementary and alternative medical therapies in patients with cardiovascular disease. *Am Heart J* 145:806, 2003.

Vasan RS, Beiser A, D'Agostino RB, et al: Plasma homocysteine and risk for congestive heart failure in adults without prior myocardial infarction. *JAMA* 289:1251, 2003.

Zeng X-H, Zeng X-J, Li Y-Y: Efficacy and safety of berberine for congestive heart failure secondary to ischemic or idiopathis dilated cardiomyopathy. *Am J Cardiol* 92:173, 2003.

24 | Pediatric Cardiovascular Pharmacology

Michael H. Gewitz   Paul Woolf
William H. Frishman   Joyce Wu

Increasingly, infants and children with cardiovascular disorders, even those with severe illnesses, are living through childhood into their adult years. The quality of life, with growth, development, and successful psychologic maturation as markers, continues to steadily improve for these patients. Much of this success is related to better refinement of pharmacologic supports, which has developed through increased understanding of the interplay of developing biologic systems and pharmacotherapeutics. This chapter reviews several important issues relating to the treatment of cardiovascular problems in infants and children with the broadening spectrum of agents available to the clinician. In many instances, pharmacologic treatments reflect modification of approaches learned from practice in the adult population. In others, novel approaches have been developed specifically for the unique problems encountered in children as a result of their primary disorder or as a result of its partial palliation. In all circumstances, documented differences in gastrointestinal physiology, in volumes of distribution, in receptor physiology, and in other key elements of metabolic and circulatory dynamics, exist, which affect cardiovascular pharmacotherapeutics. Many of these important differences are reviewed in this chapter. Recognition of the fact that, with regard to pharmacotherapeutics, important differences exist between infants and children as compared with adults has led to an important initiative on the part of the U.S. Food and Drug Administration (FDA) and the pharmaceutical industry to understand how these differences affect the use of specific pharmaceuticals. However, given the large amount of information still to be developed, the overall view should be one of a work in progress, as each day more and more agents become officially approved for use in children with attendant modification and alteration. This chapter also builds on the information developed in the pediatric chapter in the first edition of this text, reiterating important points made in that original effort, amplifying them where appropriate, and updating them as new information becomes available.

There are many conditions that overlap between the adult and pediatric populations, and we start with a review of the pharmacotherapeutics of these problems.

CONGESTIVE HEART FAILURE

Table 24-1 reviews the causes of congestive heart failure (CHF) in childhood. Most of these problems are amenable to surgical correction or to substantial palliation of the underlying anatomic disorder. An important proportion of CHF is related to inherited or acquired problems of cardiac muscle mechanics. Survival in this population is generally increasing, although recovery can require an extended period, even as long as 2 years. Thus, medical therapy has become increasingly important in the childhood management of CHF for several reasons: (a) to allow underlying reparative mechanisms to develop

513

TABLE 24-1 Etiologic Considerations for Congestive Heart Failure

Congenital heart disease	Acquired heart disease	Endocrine/metabolic	Other
Pressure overload	Myocarditis	Electrolyte disturbances	Ingestions/toxins
Left ventricular outflow obstruction	Viral infections	Hypoglycemia	Cardiac toxins (e.g., digitalis)
(e.g., aortic stenosis, severe coarctation)	Kawasaki disease	Hypothyroidism	Arrhythmogenics (e.g.,
Left ventricular inflow obstruction	Collagen–vascular disease	Calcium or magnesium	tricyclic antidepressants)
(e.g., cor triatriatum)	Cardiomyopathy	disorders	Chemotherapy agents
Volume overload	Chronic anemia (e.g., thalassemia major)	Lipid disorders	(e.g., Adriamycin)
Left-to-right shunts	Nutritional disorders	Carnitine deficiency	
(e.g., ventricular septal defect)	Acquired immunodeficiency syndrome	Carbolic acid disorders	
Anomalous pulmonary	Pericardial disease	Fatty acid disorders	
Venous return	Rheumatic heart disease	Storage diseases	
Valvular regurgitation	Cor pulmonale		
(e.g., aortic insufficiency)	Acute (e.g., upper airway obstruction)		
Arteriovenous fistulae	Cystic fibrosis		
Other structural disease	Neuropathies		
Anomalous coronary artery	Endocarditis		
Traumatic injury			
Rhythm disturbance			
Supraventricular tachycardia			
Complete heart block			
Postoperative heart disease			
Malfunctioning prosthetic valve			

Source: Reprinted with permission from Gewitz MH, Vetter VL: Cardiac emergencies, in Fleisher G, Ludwig S (eds): *Textbook of Pediatric Emergency Medicine,* 4th ed. Phildelphia, Lippincott Williams & Willkins, 2000, p 665.

after acquired or iatrogenic acute insults to cardiac muscle; (b) to enable chronic survival while awaiting extreme interventions, such as orthotopic transplantation or longer-term mechanical supports; and (c) to improve lifestyle quality after surgical intervention for complete repair or for palliation.

Inotropes and Vasopressors

Digoxin

In the pediatric population, digoxin is the most extensively used digitalis glycoside and essentially the only inotropic agent available for oral administration. The desired effects of digoxin are mechanical and electrical, i.e., improve contractility of the failing heart and prolong the refractory period of the atrioventricular (AV) node, respectively (see Chapter 8). Inhibition of the sarcolemmal Na^+/K^+-ATPase pump and an associated increase in available intracellular calcium result in digoxin's positive inotropic effect. It slows conduction velocity and increases refractoriness at the AV node, mediated mostly through its vagal effect. In canine studies, the electrophysiologic effects of digoxin were less pronounced in neonatal Purkinje fibers than in human adult myocardium. This difference may be related in part to the increased concentrations of Na^+/K^+-ATPase (the enzyme inhibited by digoxin) in the neonatal myocardium.

Digoxin is used in a variety of circumstances causing CHF. In infants with large left-to-right shunts or with severe valvular regurgitation, surgical correction is preferred; when not feasible, digoxin may help with the accommodation to large-volume loads. This has been a controversial indication because, in many of these situations, normal or even increased myocardial contractility is present. In this circumstance, the effect of digoxin on sympathetic tone is probably key because it helps to counter the catabolic effects of increased catecholamine output in these babies. The classic indication for digoxin involves diminished myocardial performance, when it is used in conjunction with diuretics and afterload reducing agents.

Digoxin toxicity is relatively common because of the drug's narrow therapeutic window. As in adults, digoxin toxicity in children includes sinus bradycardia, sinus arrest, complete AV block, and ventricular arrhythmias. Other effects include anorexia in older children and vomiting in infants, in addition to central nervous system (CNS) disturbances. A variety of drugs may predispose to digoxin toxicity, especially antiarrhythmic medications such as quinidine, verapamil, and amiodarone, although the effects of quinidine on digoxin in childhood may differ from those seen in adults. It is well established that quinidine increases serum digoxin levels in adult patients on a stable dose of digoxin. However, quinidine has no effect on the serum digoxin level of neonatal dogs, but quinidine does result in higher levels of digoxin in the brain. In one pediatric study, no relation was observed between quinidine and digoxin levels. In fact, infants younger than 2 months showed no increase in digoxin levels. In adult patients taking maintenance digoxin, amiodarone is reported to cause significant elevation of serum digoxin levels. After the initiation of amiodarone therapy, significant increases of digoxin levels, associated with prolongation of the digoxin half-life, have been observed in children. Verapamil, like quinidine, inhibits the renal elimination of digoxin without changing the glomerular filtration rate (GFR) and thereby increases plasma digoxin concentrations. Hence, in settings where it is accepted practice to use verapamil and digoxin simultaneously, such as therapy for a variety of arrhythmias in children, frequent measurements of serum digoxin levels should be done. It is recommended that, when starting quinidine or amiodarone in children on maintenance digoxin, the serum digoxin level should be measured and the digoxin dose reduced by 40% to 50%. Serial digoxin levels should then be measured and the digoxin dose titrated upward.

Because digoxin is eliminated primarily by the kidneys, any drug given simultaneously that causes renal impairment may change the pharmacokinetics of digoxin. This is particularly true when digoxin is used in combination with vasodilators (see below) such as enalapril and diuretics. Potassium loss also can potentiate toxicity, and potassium monitoring is required whenever these drugs are used together. There is no specific correlation of higher serum levels and enhanced digoxin effect. Therefore, current recommendations suggest a serum level of 1 to 2 ng/mL as an appropriate target for maintenance therapy. In neonates, endogenous "digoxin-like" substances can interfere with digoxin level interpretation.

Newborns, in particular premature neonates, present a problem with regard to loading dosages, specifically the commonly prescribed method of initiating treatment with digoxin because of the large volume of distribution. Thus, reductions in loading dose regimens have been devised that take into account gestational age and weight to decrease the risk for toxicity, as noted in Table 24-2.

Dopamine

Dopamine is an endogenous catecholamine and the precursor of norepinephrine. In adults, it is particularly useful for the treatment of heart failure associated with hypotension and poor renal perfusion because of the

TABLE 24-2 Digitalization with Digoxin

	Weight (g)	Dose (TDD)*
Usual doses (IM or oral)		
Premature infants	500–1000	20 µg/kg or 0.02 mg/kg
	1000–1500	20–30 µg/kg or 0.02–0.03 mg/kg
	1500–2000	30 µg/kg or 0.03 mg/kg
	2000–2500	30–40 µg/kg or 0.03–0.04 mg/kg
Term to 12 y		40–60 µg/kg or 0.04–0.06 mg/kg (No dose >1.5 mg TDD)
Alterations in usual doses		
Lower if renal function is impaired		
Lower with poor myocardial function (cardiomyopathy, myocarditis)		
Lower with metabolic imbalance (electrolyte abnormalities, hypoxia, acidosis)		
IV dose is 75% of oral or IM dose		

*The digitalizing regimen usually given as the initial dose is one-half of TDD; the second dose is one-fourth of TDD at 8 to 12 h; the third dose is final one-fourth TDD at 8 to 12 h after the second dose. Maintenance is then started as one-eighth TDD every 12 h. The parenteral preparation contains 100 µg/mL, and the oral preparation contains 50 µg/mL.
Key: IM, intramuscular; IV, intravenous; TDD, total digitalizing dose.
Source: Reprinted with permission from Gewitz MH, Vetter VL: Cardiac emergencies, in Fleisher G, Ludwig S (eds): *Textbook of Pediatric Emergency Medicine,* 4th ed. Philadelphia, Lippincott Williams & Wilkins, 2000, p 665.

unusual, dose-dependent combination of actions that it exerts (see also Chapters 8 and 17). At low doses (0.5 to 2 µg/kg per minute), it interacts primarily with D_1 dopaminergic receptors, which are distributed in the renal and mesenteric vascular beds. Their stimulation causes local vasodilation and augments renal blood and GFR, thereby facilitating diuresis. Moderate doses of dopamine (2 to 5 µg/kg per minute) directly increase contractility by stimulation of cardiac β_1-receptors and indirectly by causing the release of nor-epinephrine from sympathetic nerve terminals. At high doses (5 to 10 µg/kg per minute), dopamine stimulates the systemic α-adrenergic receptors, thereby causing potent vasoconstriction and an elevation in systemic vascular resistance (SVR).

It is often stated that infants display reduced sensitivity to dopamine, but the evidence is far from conclusive. In support of reduced sensitivity, it has been found that, in critically ill neonates, infusion rates of 50 µg/kg per minute do not impair cutaneous or renal perfusion. There is also some experimental evidence for diminished sensitivity to dopamine in infants, but this is limited to studies in immature animals. An opposing observation was made when cardiac output (CO) was measured in a group of infants and it was found that mean blood pressure increased at doses of 0.5 to 1 µg/kg per minute, whereas heart rate increased with doses beyond 2 to 3 µg/kg per minute. CO (and stroke volume) increased before heart rate, and SVR did not change within the range of dopamine infusion rates (0.5 to 8 µg/kg per minute). The dose–response relationship is best described by a threshold model: below a threshold level of drug concentration, no clinical response is seen, and beyond that level, a log-linear dose–response relationship is seen. The threshold values obtained were 14 ± 3.5 ng/mL for increase in mean blood pressure, 18 ± 4.5 ng/mL for increase in systolic blood pressure, and 35 ± 5 ng/mL for increase in heart rate. Steady-state concentration reached at infusion rates between 1 and 2 µg/kg per minute was 16.5 ± 3.4 ng/mL. Thus, newborns may exhibit clinical response when using doses as low as 0.5 to 1 µg/kg per minute. This is good evidence against the concept that newborns are relatively insensitive to dopamine.

Low infusion rates of dopamine are used frequently to augment renal function during critical illness. Although there is evidence that this may promote salt excretion and urine flow rate, there are no adequate data to conclude that the chances of renal failure are thereby made lower.

Plasma dopamine clearance ranges from 60 to 80 mL/kg per minute in normal adults. The half-life has not been reliably determined but likely is in the range of 2 to 4 min. Clearance is lower in patients with renal or hepatic disease. Age has a striking effect on clearance of dopamine, and clearance in children younger than 2 years is approximately twice as rapid as it is in older children (82 vs. 46 mL/kg per minute). This observation has been confirmed in a study by Allen and associates demonstrating that, during the first 20 months of age, the clearance of infused dopamine decreases by almost 50%, with an additional 50% decrease at ages 1 to 12 years. This pharmacokinetic difference, rather than a difference in receptors or myocardial sensitivity, may account for the observation that infants tolerate higher infusion rates.

In clinical practice, dopamine is an effective inotropic and vasopressor agent in neonates and infants with a variety of conditions associated with circulatory failure, including hyaline membrane disease, asphyxia, sepsis syndrome, and cyanotic congenital heart disease. Although there are surprisingly few formal data concerning use of dopamine in critically ill children, clinicians use dopamine to enhance renal function and to exploit its inotropic and vaso-pressor properties. Dopamine is less likely to produce severe tachycardia or dysrhythmias than is epinephrine or isoproterenol.

After volume depletion, dopamine is indicated in the context of moderately severe degrees of distributive shock (sepsis and hypoxia-ischemia) and cardiogenic shock. It is also indicated in the absence of hypotension, when clinical signs or hemodynamic measurements suggest a state of compensated shock or inadequate peripheral perfusion. Dopamine is not the agent of choice when hemodynamic measurements show an elevated CO in the context of a markedly reduced SVR and profound hypotension. This pattern is commonly observed in septic shock and suggests judicious use of a vasopressor such as norepinephrine (see below). Dopamine also is not the drug of choice to treat hypotension associated with major reductions in cardiac index [e.g., < 2 to 2.5 L/(min • m^2)]. Epinephrine is more appropriate. Children with primary myocardial disease not complicated by frank hypotension will benefit from a more selective inotropic agent such as dobutamine. Infusion rates of dopamine needed to improve signs of severe myocardial dysfunction may be associated with troublesome tachycardia or dysrhythmia and may increase myocardial oxygen consumption disproportionately to myocardial perfusion. Although dopamine is used extensively after cardiac surgery, there are reports that dopamine is less effective after cardiac surgery in infants than it is in older children or adults. Lang and colleagues treated five children with dopamine after cardiac surgery. For the group as a whole, hemodynamic improvement did not occur at infusion rates of less than 15 μg/kg per minute. When CO did increase, it was attributed to an increase in heart rate rather than to improved stroke volume. More recently, one study indicated that, after cardiac surgery, dopamine and dobutamine have similar inotropic efficacies, but that dopamine is associated with pulmonary vasoconstriction at doses larger than 7 μg/kg per minute.

To treat shock associated with hypotension, therapy is initiated with an infusion rate of 5 to 10 μg/kg per minute. The rate of infusion is increased in increments of 2 to 6 μg/kg per minute, guided by evidence of improved blood flow (skin temperature, capillary refill, sensorium, and urine output) and by restoration of a blood pressure appropriate for age. Infusion rates greater than 25 to 30 μg/kg per minute of dopamine are not customary, even if they maintain a "normal" blood pressure. At infusion rates at this dose, the effect on blood pressure is likely to represent an increase in SVR (α-adrenergic activation) rather than CO. Although infusion rates of this magnitude or higher have been proposed, a requirement for a dopamine infusion at this high dose suggests that the physician reexamine the physiologic diagnosis or select a different agent, such as epinephrine or norepinephrine.

Dopamine can produce cardiovascular toxicity, including tachycardia, hypertension, and dysrhythmia. With the possible exception of the byperidines all inotropes increase myocardial oxygen consumption because they increase myocardial work. If the resulting increase in oxygen consumption is balanced by improved coronary blood flow, the net effect on oxygen balance is beneficial. When shock is caused by or complicated by myocardial disease, then improved myocardial contractility may reduce preload and afterload (decrease oxygen consumption), improve coronary perfusion pressure (increase oxygen supply), and prolong diastolic coronary perfusion by reducing heart rate. If the same drug is administered to a patient with normal myocardial contractility, then the result may be an increase in cardiac oxygen consumption without an increase in oxygen delivery to the myocardium. Tachycardia, by increasing oxygen consumption and shortening diastole, is a particular burden. Thus, the effect of dopamine on myocardial oxygen balance is better than that for isoproterenol, but not as good as for dobutamine, inamrinone, and milrinone.

Dopamine depresses the ventilatory response to hypoxemia and hypercarbia by as much as 60%. Dopamine (and other β-agonists) can decrease the partial pressure of oxygen by interfering with hypoxic vasoconstriction. In one study, dopamine increased intrapulmonary shunting in patients with adult respiratory distress syndrome from 27% to 40%. Dopamine can cause or worsen limb ischemia and gangrene of distal parts and entire extremities and result in extensive loss of skin. Infusion rates as low as 1.5 µg/kg per minute have been associated with limb loss. The presence of an arterial catheter also increases the possibility of limb ischemia. Because dopamine promotes release of norepinephrine from synaptic terminals (and is converted to norepinephrine in vivo), it is associated more often with limb ischemia than are other adrenergic compounds. Extravasation of dopamine should be treated immediately by local infiltration with a solution of phentolamine (5 to 10 mg in 15 mL of normal saline) administered with a fine hypodermic needle. Dopamine should not be administered by mixing with sodium bicarbonate because alkaline solutions inactivate this agent.

Dobutamine

Dobutamine is a synthetic analogue of dopamine that stimulates β_1-, β_2-, and α-adrenergic receptors (see Chapter 8). It increases cardiac contractility via its β_1 effect and may not significantly alter SVR because of the balance between α_1-mediated vasoconstriction and β_2-mediated vasodilation. Unlike dopamine, dobutamine does not stimulate dopaminergic receptors (it is not a renal vasodilator) and it does not facilitate the release of norepinephrine from peripheral nerve endings.

In adults with CHF, dobutamine produces a 50% to 80% increase in CO, which is almost entirely due to improvement in stroke volume. Left atrial pressure falls, and SVR decreases or remains the same. Heart rate increases little, if at all. Although renal function is not directly affected by dobutamine, renal function and urine output may improve because the increase in CO fosters relaxation of sympathetic tone and improved perfusion. Dobutamine is a dilator of the pulmonary vasculature.

A threshold model with a log-linear dose–response relationship above the threshold has been demonstrated in critically ill term and preterm neonates and in children between 2 and 168 months of age. In one small study, dobutamine infusion (10 µg/kg per minute) was associated with increases in CO (30%), blood pressure (17%), and heart rate (7%). The thresholds for these increases were 13, 23, and 65 ng/mL, respectively, demonstrating that dobutamine is a relatively selective inotrope with little effect on heart rate at customary infusion rates. Somewhat greater thresholds for improved CO were observed in another group of children and in infants, but in all studies, dobutamine improved cardiac contractility without substantially altering heart rate unless high infusion rates were used.

The half-life is about 2 min in adults and the volume of distribution is 0.2 L/kg. CHF increases the volume of distribution. In adults, clearance is about 2 L/m² per minute. Typical clearance values in children are 70 to 100 mL/kg per minute. Infusions in the range used clinically yield plasma dobutamine concentrations from approximately 50 ng/mL to 160 to 190 ng/mL in children and in adults. The principal route of elimination is methylation by catechol methyltransferase, followed by hepatic glucuronidation and excretion into urine and bile. Dobutamine is also cleared from the plasma by nonneuronal uptake. Some investigators have reported nonlinear elimination kinetics, but other data have suggested that dobutamine's kinetics can be adequately described by a simple first-order (linear) model.

Several studies in infants and children have demonstrated that dobutamine improves myocardial function in a variety of settings. Stroke volume and cardiac index improve without a substantial increase in cardiac rate. SVR and pulmonary vascular resistance (PVR) may decrease toward normal.

Dobutamine has been evaluated in children after cardiac surgery with cardiopulmonary bypass. In one study, dobutamine enhanced CO by increasing heart rate. Indeed, tachycardia prompted discontinuation of the infusion in several patients. The expected fall in SVR was not observed in children receiving the drug after cardiopulmonary bypass. These investigators found no benefit over isoproterenol or dopamine. These differences between adults and children may be due to the fact that myocardial dysfunction and CHF are not characteristic of the circulatory status of many children undergoing repair of congenital heart disease. Unlike adults, indication for operation involves abnormalities in ventricular architecture or abnormal circulatory anatomy. It was found that children undergoing operations for mitral valve disease responded to dobutamine with an increase in stroke volume; children having repair of tetralogy of Fallot did not, and their CO increased only through higher heart rate. A more recent report by the same group indicated that, after repair of the tetralogy of Fallot, dobutamine enhances CO when combined with atrial pacing to increase heart rate. Isoproterenol without pacing provided a higher CO than did dobutamine alone or dobutamine in combination with pacing at therapeutic doses.

Specific indications for prescribing dobutamine in the pediatric age group include those conditions associated with a low CO and normal to moderately decreased blood pressure. Typical examples include viral myocarditis, cardiomyopathy associated with use of anthracyclines, cyclophosphamide or hemochromatosis (related to hypertransfusion therapy), or myocardial infarction (Kawasaki disease). Patients with CHF who have a normal or slightly low blood pressure may benefit by combining dobutamine with a left ventricular afterload-reducing agent. For rapid titration in the unstable patient, nitroprusside is available. When rapid adjustment is not necessary, angiotensin-converting enzyme (ACE) inhibitors such as captopril or enalapril (see below) can be used for this purpose. A decrease in afterload improves stroke volume and may enhance CO at a lower cost of oxygen consumption than use of an inotropic agent alone.

Dobutamine is not a first-line agent to treat low output states caused by intracardiac shunting. Dobutamine is indicated after corrective or palliative cardiovascular surgery in the child; however, in this context, its use should be limited to occasions in which demonstrated or suspected myocardial dysfunction exists.

Dobutamine may be of adjunctive value in treating myocardial dysfunction that complicates a primary condition such as adult respiratory distress syndrome (ARDS) or septic shock. Rarely, however, is it appropriate to use dobutamine as the sole agent to treat hemodynamic compromise associated with sepsis, ARDS, or shock after an episode of severe hypoxia-ischemia.

Dobutamine can be useful when combined with other adrenergic agonists such as norepinephrine to treat myocardial dysfunction associated with so-called "hyperdynamic" shock. For example, the child with anthracycline cardiotoxicity who develops septic shock may be a candidate for this type of combined therapy.

Dobutamine usually increases myocardial oxygen demand. In subjects with myocardial dysfunction, coronary blood flow and oxygen supply improve with the increase in demand. However, if dobutamine is used when myocardial contractility is normal, oxygen balance will be adversely affected. Tachycardia greatly increases oxygen use by the heart and should prompt a reduction in the dose of dobutamine (or an alternate agent).

Although less likely than other catecholamines to induce serious atrial and ventricular dysrhythmias, these do occur in patients receiving dobutamine, particularly in the context of myocarditis, electrolyte imbalance, or high infusion rates. Dobutamine and other inotropes should be administered cautiously, if at all, to patients with dynamic left ventricular outflow obstruction (hypertrophic subaortic stenosis).

Isoproterenol

Isoproterenol is an intravenously administered, synthetic catecholamine. As a nonselective β-agonist, it augments myocardial contractility, increases heart rate, reduces afterload, and dilates the bronchial tree. It is useful for the treatment of bradycardia in all age groups and for life-threatening reactive airway disease in young children. The dosage varies with clinical indication. Dosages required for the treatment of bradyarrhythmias are lower than those needed for bronchial hyperreactivity. In the neonate, isoproterenol produces a greater increase in heart rate than does dopamine or dobutamine.

In the past, isoproterenol was used for a variety of indications, including septic shock and cardiogenic shock associated with myocardial infarction. Other agents, such as dopamine and dobutamine, and a more subtle understanding of the pathophysiology of shock have limited the use of isoproterenol to very few specific indications. Isoproterenol may be used to treat hemodynamically significant bradycardia. However, an epinephrine infusion is probably preferable. When bradycardia results from heart block, then atropine is the initial urgent form of drug therapy, and placement of a pacemaker is definitive treatment. Bradycardia due to anoxia is treated by administering oxygen and improving gas exchange, but isoproterenol may be a useful adjunct in this setting.

Some clinicians prefer isoproterenol as a first-time agent for infants after cardiac surgery with cardiopulmonary bypass. Although this indication is not well explored in the literature, the agent may be effective in improving CO by combining inotropic and chronotropic activity with a capacity for pulmonary and systemic vasodilations. Isoproterenol may provide greater improvement in CO than atrial pacing or atrial pacing combined with dobutamine.

The main concerns regarding the use of isoproterenol include sinus tachycardia, which can be counterproductive to ventricular filling and to myocardial oxygen debt burden, and induction of arrhythmias, especially ventricular extrasystoles. Patients must be monitored closely for this latter complication when receiving isoproterenol.

Epinephrine

Epinephrine is an endogenous catecholamine that acts on α- and β-adrenergic receptors resulting in an increase in heart rate, contractility, and SVR. These actions make it especially useful under circumstances of severe myocardial dysfunction associated with hypotension.

A wide interindividual variation in epinephrine clearance is observed in healthy adults. In critically ill children receiving epinephrine at doses from 0.03 to 0.2 μg/kg per minute, plasma concentrations at steady state ranged from 0.67 to 8.5 ng/mL and were linearly related to dose.

Epinephrine is used to treat shock associated with myocardial dysfunction. Thus, it may be an appropriate drug for treatment of cardiogenic shock unresponsive to dopamine or after open cardiac surgery.

The septic patient who does not improve adequately after intravascular volume repletion and treatment with dopamine or dobutamine may benefit from infusion of epinephrine. Epinephrine is most likely to be useful when hypotension exists in the context of a low cardiac index and stroke index. At modest infusion rates (0.05 to 0.1 μg/kg per minute), SVR decreases slightly; heart rate, CO, and systolic blood pressure increase somewhat. At intermediate infusion rates, α_1-adrenergic activation becomes important but is balanced by the improved CO and activation of vascular β_2-receptors. Even though epinephrine constricts renal and cutaneous arterioles, renal function and skin perfusion may improve. Very high infusion rates (>1 to 2 μg/kg per minute) are associated with significant α_1-adrenergic–mediated vasoconstriction; blood flow to individual organs will be compromised, and the associated increase in afterload may further impair myocardial function. Epinephrine by infusion is also the agent of choice for hypotension or shock after successful treatment of cardiac arrest. Shock after an episode of hypoxemia or ischemia is usually cardiogenic and may respond to epinephrine infusion.

Bolus injections of epinephrine are used to treat asystole and other nonperfusing rhythms. The recommended initial dose (American Heart Association) is 0.01 mg/kg (10 μg/kg or 0.1 mL/kg of the 1:10,000 solution). Subsequent doses are 10-fold greater ("high-dose epinephrine"): 0.1 mg/kg (100 μ/kg or 0.1 mL/kg of a 1:1000 solution). Although initial studies using high-dose epinephrine were encouraging, published reports have indicated no improvement in return of spontaneous circulation or survival after high-dose epinephrine following out-of-hospital cardiac arrest in children. Epinephrine also may be given by endotracheal tube (dose, 100 μg/kg). Intraosseous administration is appropriate for bolus and continuous administrations of epinephrine. The dose is the same as that for intravenous injection. The intraosseous route is effective in briskly achieving high plasma levels of epinephrine and other catecholamines when direct vascular access is difficult.

Epinephrine has the potential to cause multiple adverse reactions. The drug produces CNS excitation manifested as anxiety, dread, nausea, and dyspnea. Enhanced automaticity and increased oxygen consumption are the main serious toxicities of epinephrine. Extreme tachycardia carries a substantial oxygen penalty, as does hypertension. A severe imbalance of myocardial oxygen delivery and oxygen consumption produces characteristic electrocardiographic changes of ischemia. A sub-ischemic, but persistently unfavorable, ratio of oxygen delivery to consumption also may be harmful to the myocardium.

Epinephrine produces tachycardia, and increases in infusion rate lead to successively more serious events, including atrial and ventricular extrasystoles, atrial and ventricular tachycardia, and, ultimately, ventricular fibrillation. Ventricular dysrhythmias in children are not frequent but may occur in the presence of myocarditis, hypokalemia, or hypoxemia.

Epinephrine overdose is serious. Several neonates have died when inadvertently subjected to oral administration of huge amounts of epinephrine. The syndrome mimicked an epidemic of neonatal sepsis with shock and metabolic acidosis. Intraaortic injection in infants (per umbilical artery) produces tachycardia, hypertension, and renal failure. Intravenous overdosage of epinephrine is immediately life-threatening. Manifestations include myocardial infarction, ventricular tachycardia, extreme hypertension, cerebral hemorrhage, seizures, renal failure, and pulmonary edema. Paradoxically, bradycardia has also been observed.

Manifestations of acute overdosage are treated symptomatically. β-Receptor antagonists, such as propranolol, are contraindicated. Hypertension is treated with short-acting antihypertensives (i.e., nitroprusside).

Hypokalemia can be produced during epinephrine infusion due to stimulation of β_2-adrenergic receptors, which are linked to sodium-potassium-ATPase located in skeletal muscle. Hyperglycemia results from α-adrenergic–mediated suppression of insulin release. Other metabolic abnormalities include hyperlactemia and hypophosphatemia.

Epinephrine is an α_1-adrenergic agonist, and infiltration into local tissues or intraarterial injection can produce severe vasospasm and tissue injury. Concurrent activation of β_2-receptors by epinephrine limits vasospasm, and local injury to tissue is less frequent than with norepinephrine or dopamine.

Norepinephrine

Norepinephrine is an endogenous catecholamine that stimulates β_1- and α-adrenergic receptors, thereby increasing contractility and SVR. Its ultimate effect on heart rate is variable and is the net result of opposing forces. Some of its inotropic activity may result from α_1-receptor stimulation and β-receptor agonism. Whereas its direct cardiac β_1 effect favors an increase in heart rate, its peripheral α-adrenergic effect, which leads to activation of the baroreceptor reflex, favors a decrease in heart rate. Published pediatric data in infants and children are quite limited, but the observed hemodynamic response to norepinephrine seems to resemble that seen in adults. Its use, for the most part, is reserved for the persistently hypotensive patient, such as the child in whom hypotension persists despite being given doses as high as 20 μg/kg per minute of dopamine. It should not be used as a positive inotrope in the context of depressed myocardial contractile function unaccompanied by hypotension, because its marked vasoconstrictive effects may result in an extremely high SVR with reduced renal blood flow. Its adverse effects profile is similar to that of epinephrine.

Norepinephrine improves perfusion in children with low blood pressure and a normal or elevated cardiac index, as occurs in septic shock. Norepinephrine is administered only after intravascular volume repletion and is best guided by knowledge of CO and SVR. There is very little published experience on the use of norepinephrine to treat distributive shock in children; however, a randomized study (in adults) has indicated that norepinephrine is superior to dopamine for treating hypotension and other hemodynamic abnormalities associated with hyperdynamic septic shock. In this study, the average infusion rate for norepinephrine was 1.5 μg/kg per minute, although others have reported that somewhat lower average doses (0.4 μg/kg per minute) are effective in adults with sepsis. Thus, titration is important and may entail fairly rapid escalation of dosage.

Norepinephrine produces increases in SVR, arterial blood pressure, and urine flow. It is most valuable in the context of tachycardia, because infusion of the drug does not produce significant elevation of heart rate and may even lower heart rate through reflex mechanisms.

The usual starting dose is an infusion of 0.1 μg/kg per minute. The goal is to elevate perfusion pressure so that the flow to vital organs is above the threshold needed to meet metabolic requirements. The lowest infusion rate that improves perfusion should be used, as judged by skin color and temperature, mental status, urine flow, and reduction in plasma lactate level. Other causes of distributive shock (e.g., vasodilator ingestion, intoxication with CNS depressants) also should respond to norepinephrine infusion when the predominant hemodynamic problems are low SVR and blood pressure.

The net effect of norepinephrine infusion on oxygen balance varies. The increase in afterload that it produces should increase myocardial oxygen consumption, but norepinephrine also decreases heart rate, which should reduce oxygen consumption and improve diastolic coronary perfusion. Injudicious use of norepinephrine will lead to compromised organ blood flow. Norepinephrine infusion may elevate blood pressure but not improve clinical indices of perfusion.

Phosphodiesterase Inhibitors

Inamrinone and milrinone are intravenously administered nondigitalis, non-catecholamine, byperidine derivatives that exert their positive inotropic effects by inhibiting cyclic adenosine monophosphate (cAMP) phosphodiesterase in cardiac myocytes (see Chapter 8). Increased levels of cAMP, by inhibition of its breakdown, promote Ca^{2+} entry into the cell, thereby increasing contractility. These drugs may cause adverse effects, including ventricular arrhythmias.

Inamrinone, a phosphodiesterase inhibitor, thereby prevents the degradation of cAMP. It is used as an adjunct to dopamine or dobutamine in the intensive care unit. In adults, inamrinone acts as a positive inotropic agent and as a vasodilator. The cardiovascular effects of inamrinone and milrinone appear to be markedly age dependent. Studies have shown a lack of responsiveness to inamrinone or milrinone in the newborn dog and rabbit. Nevertheless, by 2 weeks of age, the response of rabbit myocardium to milrinone exceeds that of an adult. Inamrinone in the treatment of children with cor pulmonale has been reported to have beneficial effects on the pulmonary vasculature.

Compared with dobutamine, milrinone produces a greater reduction in SVR for a given degree of improvement in inotropic status. Blood pressure is well maintained, even in the face of reduced SVR, because of the associated improvement in contractility and stroke volume. However, when inamrinone is administered to patients who are intravascularly volume depleted or in whom the expected improvement in CO does not occur, hypotension may result. In patients with CHF, amelioration in global hemodynamic function is associated with an improvement in the ratio of myocardial oxygen delivery to consumption. Inamrinone may improve contractility in patients who have failed to respond to catecholamines and may further increase cardiac index even in patients who have responded to dobutamine.

Inamrinone reduces pulmonary artery pressure and resistance in children with intracardiac left-to-right shunts. In one study, children with elevated PVR showed a 47% reduction in PVR with infusion of inamrinone. The

PVR/SVR ratio decreased by 45%. In these children, pulmonary blood flow and left-to-right shunt increased. In children with normal pulmonary pressure, inamrinone infusion was associated with a decrease in SVR but not in PVR. Inamrinone may be undesirable in children with an elevated pulmonary artery pressure associated with a high-flow left-to-right shunt but normal PVR. Conversely, inamrinone (and probably milrinone) may be effective adjunctive therapy in the child with elevated pulmonary vascular resistance and reduced pulmonary blood flow.

Milrinone was licensed for use in the United States in 1992. A derivative of inamrinone, it shares the same mechanism of action and pharmacodynamic profile. The major advantage of milrinone is that, unlike inamrinone, it does not appear to evoke thrombocytopenia. It is eliminated through the kidneys. In adults, milrinone acts as an inotrope and vasodilator. In adults with CHF, milrinone causes a much greater change in left and right filling pressures and SVR than does dobutamine, even at equivalent increases in contractility. It has been used extensively after cardiac surgery and in adults with CHF, where it increases cardiac index and reduces SVR, filling pressure, and, often, systemic blood pressure. Reports have indicated that use of milrinone is increasing in pediatric intensive care units, and there are now data with which to evaluate this practice. One early study evaluated treatment of neonates after congenital heart disease repair. In this study, a loading dose of 50 μg/kg followed by a continuous infusion of 0.5 μg/kg per minute was associated with mild tachycardia and a slight decrease in systemic blood pressure. Cardiac index increased from 2.1 to approximately 3.1 L/(min • m^2), whereas the SVR index decreased from approximately 2100 to 1300 dyne-s/(cm^5 • m^2). The PVR index also decreased from approximately 488 to 360 dyne-s/(cm^5 • m^2), as did right and left atrial mean pressures. More recent studies have shown equally efficacious results.

Inamrinone is metabolized by *N*-acetyl transferase. In addition, up to 40% is eliminated unchanged in the urine. In healthy adults, the half-lives of inamrinone are 4.4 h in slow acetylators and 2 h in fast acetylators. It is not known whether this difference is clinically important. Protein binding is not extensive. The rate of elimination of inamrinone appears to be reduced in CHF. There is little pharmacokinetic information available regarding the use of inamrinone in children and virtually no information derived from children with organ system failure. One study of children younger than 1 year after cardiopulmonary bypass found that the half-life is prolonged in those younger than 4 weeks and that volume of distribution (1.7 to 1.8 L/kg) is threefold greater than others have reported in adults. A second study found wide interpatient variability in pharmacokinetic measurements. Beyond 1 month of age, there was no relation between age and any measured pharmacokinetic parameter. The average clearance was approximately 2 mL/kg per minute, which is similar to that recorded in adults, and was associated with a mean half-life of about 5.5 h. There are limited published pharmacokinetic data for milrinone in infants or children. In adults, the volume of distribution of milrinone is 0.5 L/kg and the clearance is 0.11 to 0.1 L/kg per hour. The half-life is approximately 2 h in adults with CHF. Typically, the plasma level during therapy is in the range of 80 to 120 ng/mL.

In adults with CHF, inamrinone and milrinone are safe and effective, and their clinical place in short-term management of patients with refractory heart failure is clearly established. The byperidines are most useful in management of children and adolescents with isolated cardiac dysfunction, particularly when it is due to myocardial failure. They provide inotropic and afterload reduction and may be an alternative to coadministration of dobutamine and an afterload-reducing agent.

Inamrinone should not have a major role in management of critically ill children in whom the primary disturbance is other than myocardial failure. The relatively long half-life and the observation that clearance is depressed in patients with cardiac or hepatic dysfunction are important limitations in the patient with multiple organ system failure. It is likely that these precautions also should be applied to milrinone. For example, in patients with septic shock or ARDS, inamrinone or milrinone should be reserved for the individual with impaired myocardial performance who has not responded adequately to aggressive support with other agents, such as dobutamine, dopamine, or epinephrine.

Inamrinone produces reversible dose-dependent thrombocytopenia (incidence, 2.4%), which is more common during prolonged therapy. This was not seen in the largest published pediatric study, but anecdotal reports have suggested that it does occur in children. Supraventricular and ventricular dysrhythmias have occurred during infusion of inamrinone, but these may have been related to the underlying condition of the patient. Overdosage has been fatal in a child. Progressive hypotension developed and peritoneal dialysis was not effective in removing drug. This case involved excessive administration due to a computing error.

A rapid infusion of inamrinone or milrinone during the loading dose can produce hypotension. This problem is exacerbated in volume-depleted patients.

Diuretics

These drugs, which reduce central congestion and pulmonary edema directly, remain key to the treatment of volume overload states (see Chapter 6). In pediatrics, diuretics are a more common treatment for CHF than for hypertension. Traditionally, these agents are classified by principal sites of action in the kidney.

Loop Diuretics

Loop diuretics, which act by inhibiting the Na-K-2Cl transporter in the thick ascending limb of the nephron's loop of Henle, are widely used in pediatric patients.

Furosemide is the most commonly used agent of this type. This drug also has effects mediated through renal prostaglandin agonist action. It increases renal blood flow, reduces renal vascular resistance, and stimulates renin release. There also may be beneficial pulmonary nondiuretic effects from furosemide, making it a useful agent in children with combined cardiopulmonary disorders, such as bronchopulmonary dysplasia. In general, it is used for acute and chronic management of congestive circulatory states and for promoting a diuresis after cardiac surgery. In the treatment of infants with CHF, the existing hyperaldosteronism may decrease the patient's response to furosemide. The addition of an aldosterone antagonist such as spironolactone is then indicated to combat aldosterone's influence and to help reduce potassium loss. Furosemide may be administered orally or parenterally. With intravenous use in a newborn, 55% of the dose is excreted unchanged into the tubular lumen. For a given plasma level of furosemide, neonates exhibit higher urinary drug excretion due to lower protein-binding of the drug, and plasma clearance has been shown to increase with age. In the neonate, more of the unchanged drug appears in the urine because less biotransformation via glucuronidation occurs in its undeveloped renal epithelial cell. Hence, in infants with immature renal function and in patients with renal failure, the dosage must be carefully adjusted as per clinical need.

Adverse effects at all ages include hypovolemia and electrolyte disturbances. Hypokalemia is a relatively common side effect that is usually not of clinical significance in children during chronic therapy unless they also are taking digoxin. However, at high doses of furosemide, potassium supplementation may be necessary. Hypochloremic metabolic alkalosis is also a well-documented side effect with chronic therapy and, if severe, may necessitate chloride supplementation. In infants with bronchopulmonary dysplasia, chloride depletion has been implicated as a cause of increased mortality. Hyponatremia may occur, and, in the setting of CHF, furosemide may worsen existing hyponatremia.

Ototoxicity also may occur. There is an increased prevalence of ototoxicity in premature infants that may be due to an immature barrier to the inner ear. Whereas the risk of ototoxicity is minimal with standard dosages in patients with normal renal function, the risk of ototoxicity is higher in patients with renal dysfunction. In addition, the risk increases in those patients receiving other ototoxic drugs.

Ethacrynic acid is used in patients refractory to furosemide therapy, and the drug is sometimes used in the acute management of volume overload. Although the pharmacokinetics in adults are similar to those observed with furosemide, in newborns and children this has yet to be determined. Limited data are available for bumetanide, a newer loop diuretic, in the pediatric age group. Hence, its use is generally reserved for those patients in whom conventional diuretic therapy has failed. Bumetanide differs from furosemide in that it is partly metabolized in the liver and about 50% is excreted unchanged in the urine. Further, in neonates and children, it is many times more potent than furosemide and must be administered carefully.

Bumetanide and metolazone (see below) may be particularly valuable in children with right heart failure, such as those post repair of tetralogy of Fallot or in children who have undergone the Fontan operation or its variants. More data are needed before the utility of this combination can be definitively established.

Thiazide Diuretics

Hydrochlorothiazide (HCTZ) and chlorothiazide, structural analogues, are the primary thiazide diuretics used in pediatric patients with cardiovascular disease. Their diuretic effect is mediated primarily by inhibition of sodium and chloride transport in the nephron's distal convoluted tubule. Thiazides are effective until the GFR drops below 50% of normal, at which point a loop diuretic should be started instead. Thiazides are used in the chronic outpatient management of congestive circulatory states. In addition, they are used in the treatment of hypertension in older children and adolescents. Whereas the mechanism of action, diuretic efficacy, and adverse effects of HCTZ and chlorothiazide are similar, their pharmacokinetics differ. Among its adverse effects are electrolyte imbalance, including hypokalemia and hypercalcemia, and hyperuricemia. In addition, it may negatively alter the lipid profile in the short term and may cause carbohydrate intolerance.

Metolazone

Metolazone is a sulfonamide derivative whose site and mechanism of action are similar to those of thiazides. It is used in the short-term treatment of edematous states refractory to loop and thiazide diuretic therapies. Furosemide is commonly administered with a more distally acting diuretic, such as metolazone, because, if given alone, the unaffected distal tubule compensates for the disabled loop of the Henle. It is administered once a day or every other day. The major adverse effects are severe electrolyte disturbances (hypokalemia) and significant volume depletion.

Potassium-Sparing Diuretics

Spironolactone, the most commonly used potassium-sparing diuretic, is reserved for long-term therapy, because it is administered only orally. It exerts its diuretic effect by competitively inhibiting aldosterone at the distal tubule. It is weaker than loop or thiazide diuretics and thus is mostly used in combination with either. Its major adverse effects are hyperkalemia and hyperchloremic metabolic acidosis, and patients with existing renal and/or hepatic dysfunction are at greatest risk. Concomitant potassium supplementation and ACE inhibitor coadministration should occur with extreme care. Gynecomastia and menstrual abnormalities have been reported in adults. Data regarding the use of other potassium-sparing diuretics, such as triamterene, eplerenone, and amiloride, in pediatrics are limited, and recommendations cannot be made currently.

Spironolactone has other, nondiuretic benefits for the patient with CHF. Recently, the findings of direct myocardial function enhancement, of inhibition of the collagen production and fibrosis stimulated by aldosterone, and of additive effects when combined with ACE inhibition (see below) have focused new attention on the use of spironolactone. The Randomized Aldactone Evaluation Study supported such findings and was interrupted early because morbidity and mortality benefits of spironolactone ethically precluded continuation of the trial.

Eplerenone is a new potassium-sparing diuretic that has been shown to be useful in adult patients with hypertension and heart failure. There are no reported experiences using this diuretic in children.

Osmotic Diuretics

Mannitol is the most commonly used drug in this class used in pediatrics. Mannitol's cardiovascular use is reserved for the acute treatment of severe circulatory congestion in the face of limited renal output, i.e., prerenal failure and azotemia. The primary site of action is the proximal tubule, and mannitol will maintain high rates of tubular flow to prevent obstruction. More of the total salt and water reabsorptions occur in the distal tubule in neonates than in older patients. Hence, mannitol as a proximally acting agent is less effective than more distally acting agents in neonates. Adverse effects are hemodynamic: immediately after its administration, mannitol may temporarily increase intravascular volume and the risk of electrolyte disturbances increases with the level of diuresis.

Vasodilators

Vasodilator therapy has become central to the management of impaired circulatory status in infants and children. With the tremendous development of the basic science knowledge base in microcirculatory function, particularly the factors involved with control of vasomotor tone, a growing armamentarium of agents has become available. When vasodilators are combined with other agents, such as the inotropes reviewed above, efficacy is enhanced beyond the use of either class of agents alone.

For acute usage, particularly in the intensive care unit, the nitrovasodilators have become agents of choice. These drugs have rapid onset of action and exceedingly short duration of action, making them especially suitable for the acutely ill patient. Principally, but not entirely, these are venoactive agents that work through nitric oxide activation and consequent cyclic guanosine monophosphate mediation of regulatory proteins involved with smooth muscle contraction. In pediatric usage, nitroprusside is used most frequently, although nitroglycerin is used in the postoperative cardiac surgery patient.

Nitroprusside

This drug has venous and arteriolar activities and is the most widely used acute intravenous vasodilator in the pediatric population. Similar to nitroglycerin, it was used originally for pediatric patients after cardiac surgery during the immediate postoperative period. With doses ranging from 1.5 to 12 μg/kg per minute, there is a decline in filling pressures, an increase in CO, and no change in heart rate. Nitroprusside is effective in pediatric patients with left ventricular dysfunction or mitral regurgitation. Pulmonary and systemic vascular resistances and atrial pressures are reduced, causing a net increase in CO. Heart rate may be unaffected or increase slightly. Its effects in neonates are comparable to those in older children. One neonatal study showed that 40% had improved systemic perfusion, and almost all the infants had improved urine output after initiation of therapy. Nitroprusside must be administered parenterally by continuous infusion because it is metabolized so rapidly.

Nitroprusside's safety and efficacy have been demonstrated in neonates. In hypoxemic neonatal and juvenile lambs, in contrast, nitroprusside decreased PVR in the juvenile but not in the neonatal group. Moreover, the newborn lambs were not able to hemodynamically tolerate the nitroprusside-induced decrease in preload. These age-related differences in vascular response suggest that nitroprusside should be used with extra caution in neonates.

Nitroprusside's metabolite, cyanide, is toxic. Symptoms of toxicity include headache, disorientation, fatigue, vomiting, anorexia, tachypnea, and tachycardia. In patients being given long-term or high-dose therapy, the meaningfulness of periodic red blood cell cyanide and plasma thiocyanate measurements are uncertain; clinical evidence of toxicity has not been shown to correlate well with specific cyanide and thiocyanate concentrations.

Nitroglycerin

In pediatrics, nitroglycerin is used most commonly after cardiac surgery in the immediate postoperative period, with several studies demonstrating its beneficial effect in this setting. It is used most commonly in patients with increased preload and symptoms of systemic and/or pulmonary venous congestion. Nitroglycerin has been demonstrated to be beneficial in newborns with low CO due to congenital heart disease, asphyxia, and sepsis. Although nitroglycerin can affect all smooth-muscle sites, its predominant action is to relax venous vascular smooth muscle and thus reduce left ventricular preload. Nitroglycerin reduces pulmonary venous and arterial pressures.

The hemodynamic actions of nitroglycerin appear to be dose related. At doses lower than 2 μg/kg per minute, a venodilation effect predominates. Doses from 3 to 5 μg/kg per minute result in progressive arteriolar dilatation with a decrease in SVR and a resultant rise in CO. Higher than conventional doses may cause hypotension and reflex tachycardia. Conventional pediatric doses, such as a mean nitroglycerin dose of 20 μg/kg per minute used in one study, may not significantly alter the mean arterial pressure in children, but similar doses produce hypotension in adults. In children with pulmonary hypertension, a decrease in PVR is noted.

Nitroglycerin can be administered sublingually, intradermally, or intravenously, but not orally, because it undergoes extensive first-pass hepatic metabolism. When given intravenously, it must be given by continuous infusion because of its short serum half-life. Recommendations for chronic management in pediatric patients cannot be made because of insufficient data. Patients must be monitored for (a) the possibility of further reduction of CO secondary to even lower filling pressures than desired, and (b) hypotension accompanied by tachycardia and hypoxemia secondary to overdosage.

Nitric Oxide

Much recent attention has focused on nitric oxide and its role in modulating vascular smooth muscle vasomotor tone, as noted in the discussion of therapeutic infused nitrovasodilators. Use of nitric oxide as a pharmaceutical in its inhaled form to effect pulmonary vasodilation has become more widely accepted. As an inhaled agent with little systemic action, nitric oxide causes selective and prolonged reduction in pulmonary artery pressure in a variety of clinical settings with consequent beneficial effects on right ventricular mechanics and relief of cor pulmonale. The most recent use for this therapy has been for modulating pulmonary vasomotor tone in the newborn with congenital heart or lung disease or a combination of both. Use in other forms of pulmonary hypertension and right heart failure has been more limited, but some studies have suggested a possible role in the treatment of ARDS.

Peripheral α_1-Adrenergic Receptor Blockers

Prazosin

Prazosin is an α_1-selective blocker that can reduce SVR and mean arterial pressure. Its selectivity for the α_1-receptor explains its ability to produce less reflex tachycardia than nonselective agents. It exerts an effect on arteriolar and venous capacitance vessels. Prazosin has been used in pediatric patients with CHF due to systolic dysfunction. The drug is administered orally, and its peak effect occurs within 2 to 3 h. Although its serum half-life is 2.5 to 4 h, prazosin's duration of action lasts for about 12 h. Prazosin is generally tolerated well, with only minor side effects. However, the "first-dose phenomenon," characterized by dizziness, hypotension, and syncope, may occur within approximately 0.5 to 1.5 h after initiation of therapy. It also may occur after an increase in dosage. This effect can be avoided by giving the patient the drug at bedtime. It is unclear whether the tendency in adults with CHF to develop drug tachyphylaxis also applies to children. There is little pediatric experience with other similar drugs, terazosin or doxazosin, two newer, long-acting congeners.

Phentolamine

Phentolamine is a nonselective α blocker. Unlike the selective α_1 blockers such as prazosin, phentolamine is more likely to cause tachycardia and arrhythmias by virtue of its α_2-blocking effect. It has been used in children with CHF after cardiac surgery to reduce ventricular afterload and augment CO. The published pediatric experience to date with regard to short-term parenteral therapy is limited.

Angiotensin-Converting Enzyme Inhibitors

In the past several years, use of ACE inhibition therapy has become integral to the management of chronic left ventricular dysfunction in children and adults. These agents act as vasodilators through a decrease in the production of the potent vasoconstrictor, angiotensin II (see Chapter 5). In addition, they enhance the vasodilator action of bradykinin by decreasing its degradation and may inhibit norepinephrine release from sympathetic nerve endings. These actions result in reduced SVR and blood pressure, resulting in decreased afterload and increased CO.

In the pediatric population, most of the published experience is with captopril and enalapril. Many other ACE inhibitors are now available (fosinopril, lisinopril, ramipril, trandolapril, benazepril, quinapril, perindopril, and moexipril), but captopril and enalapril continue to be used most frequently in children. Clinical trials with other ACE inhibitors are now underway at pediatric centers.

Captopril

The use of captopril has been studied in children of all ages and has proved to be an effective antihypertensive agent. Initial pediatric experience with captopril was for the treatment of systemic hypertension in infants and children. Dose–response studies in older children have shown similar responses to 0.5, 1.0, and 2.0 mg/kg per dose; hence, the lowest dose of 0.5 mg/kg is recommended when therapy is initiated in children older than 6 months. If the desired effect is not achieved with that low dose, then the dose should be increased to 1.0 mg/kg; an additional increase most likely would not result in better control, and another agent should be used. Captopril is given orally. Although twice-daily dosing has been successful, captopril is generally administered three times daily. In premature infants, reductions in blood pressure levels as great as 60% were achieved with doses of 0.3 mg/kg; oliguria also was reported. Normotensive blood pressures have been achieved in premature and full-term infants with doses as low as 0.01 mg/kg. Captopril's absorption is inhibited by food in the stomach, so the drug should be given on an empty stomach. Peak plasma concentrations are reached within 1 to 2 h after an oral dose, and effects generally last for 6 to 8 h. In young infants and newborns, captopril is more potent and its duration of action is longer than in older children. Approximately half of the drug is excreted in the urine unchanged. Drug clearance is positively correlated with renal function, so dosage should be reduced in renal disease. Side effects of captopril described in adults, including hypotension, hyperkalemia, renal insufficiency, and dry cough, are less common in children. However, in neonates, idiosyncratic side effects, including significant hypotension, oliguria, and neurologic complications, have occurred. Hence, it is obligatory to monitor blood pressure closely during the use of captopril. Increases in serum urea nitrogen and creatinine also must be monitored when using this drug.

Captopril has been used successfully in children with large left-to-right shunts and elevated SVR to reduce the magnitude of the left-to-right shunting. In addition, in patients with dilated cardiomyopathies or paradoxical hypertension after coarctation surgery, captopril appears to be beneficial.

Patients with ventricular volume loading associated with chronic aortic or mitral regurgitation also have derived benefit from captopril. Recently, clinical practice has focused on the use of captopril and other agents of this group as prophylactic therapies in those at risk for declining ventricular function, such as post–cancer chemotherapy patients or patients with single ventricle conditions, such as those who have undergone Fontan's operation or its variations. Multicenter clinical trials are needed to objectively verify the value of such prophylaxis.

Enalapril

Enalapril, the second commercially available ACE inhibitor in the United States, is also effective in the treatment of children with systemic hypertension and CHF. It is a prodrug that must be de-esterified in the liver to the active form. (Enalaprilat is the only ACE inhibitor available for intravenous administration.) Enalapril differs from captopril in two significant ways: (a) its molecular structure contains no sulfhydryl group, postulated to be an etiologic factor in the development of some side effects, and (b) its half-life is longer. In general, enalapril's side effects are similar to those of captopril but may occur somewhat less frequently.

Lisinopril

Lisinopril, another long-acting ACE inhibitor, was evaluated in 115 hypertensive children (aged 6 to 16 years) and found to lower blood pressure in a dose-dependent manner. A starting dose of 0.07 mg/kg was appropriate, and the drug was well tolerated.

β-Adrenergic Blockers

Although much experience in pediatric patients has been accumulated for β blockers in the treatment of hypertension and arrhythmias, only recently were these drugs found to be useful in heart failure. First- and second-generation drugs of this group are reviewed under Arrhythmia Treatment. In several important trials and reports on adult CHF patients, carvedilol, bisoprolol, and metoprolol appear to have important clinical benefit. Their efficacy relates to interference with the deleterious effects of excess sympathetic activity in chronic heart failure and in pediatric patients, particularly to those with nonischemic cardiomyopathy.

Bisoprolol and metoprolol are β_1-selective blockers. Carvedilol, a nonselective β blocker, is also an α-adrenergic antagonist with antioxidant capability.

In pediatrics, a few favorable original studies with small numbers of patients have been supported by the recently published multicenter carvedilol trial demonstrating the value of this agent in patients deemed severe enough to warrant heart transplantation, and by randomized studies. As more information is developed, it seems likely that these drugs will secure an important a place in the management of pediatric patients with CHF, as they currently have in adults.

ANTIHYPERTENSIVE AGENTS

In pediatrics, antihypertensive pharmacotherapy is used primarily to treat secondary forms of hypertension. In more than 80% of children younger than 10 years, the cause of hypertension is likely to be a disease of the kidney, the cardiovascular system, or the endocrine system. The prevalence of essential hypertension in the first decade of life is significantly less than 1% of this age group. During the second decade of life, the prevalence increases, but the percentage of teenagers with essential hypertension continues to be extremely low. An aggressive approach to therapy with multidrug regimens is often necessary for adequate control of secondary hypertension because it is generally more resistant to therapy than is essential hypertension. Repeated measurements exceeding the 95th percentile for age and sex, as defined by the Second Task Force on Blood Pressure Control in Children, necessitates the initiation of drug therapy.

Hypertensive Emergencies

Hypertension accompanied by clinical evidence of end-organ injury is an emergency and requires immediate pharmacotherapy. Signs and symptoms such as retinal hemorrhages or papilledema, seventh nerve palsy, diplopia, symptoms of encephalopathy (headache, vomiting, altered mental status, or seizures), CHF, or renal insufficiency reflect end-organ injury due to malignant hypertension. The patient's blood pressure must not be reduced too rapidly because it may lead to hypotension, obtundation, or other disabling adverse effects.

Nifedipine

Nifedipine, the most potent vasodilator of the calcium channel blockers, has been used to treat hypertension in children with hypertensive emergencies. Its rapid onset of action and relatively short duration of action make it ideal for this purpose. It also has been used to treat infants with hypertrophic cardiomyopathy, primary pulmonary hypertension, and ventricular septal defect with pulmonary hypertension. It is supplied as an encapsulated liquid that must be swallowed and not taken sublingually, because very little absorption occurs via the latter route. Rectal administration of perforated nifedipine capsules may be a reliable way to acutely treat young children with severe hypertension. Pediatric patients appear to tolerate nifedipine better than do adult patients, with infrequent and mild side effects. However, cardiovascular collapse and cardiac arrest after ingesting an extraordinary large dose of nifedipine can reflect nifedipine poisoning in which the antihypertensive effect is not maintained.

Diazoxide

Diazoxide, a nondiuretic thiazide derivative, is a potent arteriolar dilator. Its antihypertensive effect is rapid in onset, and it has been used safely in children. One may avoid an abrupt decrease in blood pressure and its associated complications (see above) by administering diazoxide as a slow, rather than as a rapid infusion, as was done in one adult study, which demonstrated the efficacy of the slower infusion. Adverse effects of diazoxide include fluid retention and hypertrichosis, especially with frequent administration.

Labetalol

Labetalol acts as a nonselective beta blocker. It also has α-adrenergic blocking properties and direct vasodilating activity. Its β-blocking properties, however, are about eight times as potent as its α-blocking ability. It is well absorbed after an oral dose and undergoes extensive first-pass hepatic metabolism. The intravenous use of labetalol was recently reported in children. Bunchman and colleagues noted that the intravenous infusion of labetalol in children with severe hypertension or in those with uncontrollable hypertension is effective in controlling blood pressure when oral medication cannot be tolerated.

Labetalol's antihypertensive effect was observed within 1 h after a starting dose of 0.2 to 1.0 mg/kg. Its effect was sustained with a continuous parenteral infusion of 0.25 to 1.5 mg/kg per hour. Side effects were rare, and the response to labetalol was independent of kidney function. Labetalol is particularly useful in treating the hypertensive crisis of chronic renal failure.

Hydralazine

Hydralazine's primary action is to relax precapillary arteriolar vascular smooth muscle. It reduces SVR and therefore afterload, which permits increased ventricular muscle fiber shortening during systole. This results in an enhanced stroke volume at any given end-diastolic volume. In infants and children, hydralazine has been shown to be effective in the treatment of ventricular systolic dysfunction. It also may decrease shunt magnitude and increase systemic output by decreasing SVR to a greater degree than PVR in infants with left-to-right shunts.

Hydralazine can be given orally and parenterally. After an oral dose, the drug undergoes extensive first-pass metabolism by acetylation, which limits its bioavailability. Hemodynamic effects occur within 30 to 60 min and last for as long as 8 h. Unlike adults to whom hydralazine has been given by continuous infusion, infants and children should be given hydralazine by bolus infusions. After intravenous administration, hemodynamic responses are apparent after approximately 5 to 10 min, peak by approximately 30 min, and last for 2 to 4 h. Its rapid onset of action makes intravenous hydralazine useful for treating hypertensive urgencies.

At present, the incidence of adverse effects in infants and children is not well delineated. The most common adverse effects seen in adults include headache, dizziness, nausea, vomiting, postural hypotension, and tachycardia. About 10% of adult patients on long-term hydralazine therapy develop a generally reversible lupus-like syndrome. Without clinical suspicion of a lupus-like syndrome, routine monitoring of antinuclear antibody is not justified, because only some of the patients in whom antinuclear antibodies are present will subsequently develop clinical features of lupus. For a given dose, slow acetylators achieve higher plasma concentrations and are at increased risk for adverse effects. It is unclear whether tolerance to long-term hydralazine therapy, as demonstrated in adults, will occur in pediatric patients.

Chronic Hypertension Management

Calcium Channel Blockers

Chronic drug therapy in hypertensive children is predicated on the expectation that reduction of high pressure will result in decreased long-term morbidity and mortality, which has been proved with at least some antihypertensive agents in adults. In fact, there is mounting evidence, as suggested by the Bogalusa Heart Study, that hypertension in childhood may herald the development of essential hypertension later in life. Chronic antihypertensive drug therapy in children has been modified in recent years to include initially an ACE inhibitor or a calcium channel blocker. Their once-a-day dosages and favorable side effect profile have tended to improve compliance, a major issue in childhood and adolescence.

Calcium channel blockers reduce the influx of calcium responsible for cardiac and vascular smooth-muscle contractions. These agents are divided into two groups based on their molecular structure and clinical application. Type I agents are characterized by a tertiary amine structure similar to that of verapamil. They are used primarily to treat cardiac arrhythmias and are discussed under Antiarrhythmic Therapy. Type II agents have a dihydropyridine nucleus, similar to that of nifedipine. These agents exhibit less antiarrhythmic activity but are more potent vasodilators and are used in pediatrics to treat hypertension.

The effects of nitrendipine, a dihydropyridine compound, were studied in 25 hypertensive children (ages 6 months to 16 years) who had systolic and diastolic blood pressures consistently exceeding the 95th percentile for age and sex. Significant reductions in blood pressures (mean decrease from 148/99 to 128/77 mm Hg after 1 day and to 121/75 mm Hg after 2 weeks) were observed within 24 h, and the effects were sustained through 3 months of treatment with a dose of 0.25 to 0.50 mg/kg given every 6 to 12 h. It was apparently safe. The duration of action and the long-term clinical response to nitrendipine were believed to be substantially better than those to nifedipine.

Amlodipine, another long-acting dihydropyridine calcium channel blocker, was evaluated in an international, placebo-controlled study of 268 hypertensive children 1 to 17 years of age and found to be safe and effective. Headache was the most common adverse effect.

β Blockers

β Blockers act at the β-adrenergic receptor. Although they share this common characteristic, they differ from each other with regard to the presence or absence of β_1-selectivity, lipid solubility, intrinsic sympathomimetic activity, membrane stabilization, and potency (see Chapter 2). These drugs' high therapeutic index has been confirmed by reports in children. The antihypertensive effect is poorly correlated with plasma concentrations and surpasses the anticipated duration of action based on plasma half-life. Hence, even preparations with short half-lives generally can be given on a twice-daily basis and possibly even once a day. The reported incidence of side effects to β blockers in children is exceptionally low. Administration of any of the β-blocking agents, which can inhibit β_2-receptor bronchodilation, to children with obstructive forms of lung disease such as asthma should be strongly discouraged. CNS side effects in children are more likely to present in the form of sleep disturbances as opposed to the depression, dreams, confusion, and agitation seen in adults. Glucose and lipid profiles can be adversely affected.

The most extensive published clinical pediatric experience with β blockers has been with propranolol. Ninety-five patients with persistent hypertension, defined as greater than the 90th percentile for blood pressure over a 4-month interval, were randomized to a drug-treatment group consisting of low-dose propranolol and chlorthalidone therapy or to a control group. Both groups were exposed to an educational program oriented toward the treatment of hypertension by diet and exercise. Those in the drug-treatment group, after 30 months of follow-up, had significantly lower mean systolic and diastolic blood pressures, with minimal side effects. In a study of nine children with hypertension secondary to renal disease associated with high plasma renin levels who had failed pharmacotherapy with diuretics, hydralazine, and methyldopa, one patient developed resting bradycardia. A 1-year-old male with Wilms' tumor and elevated plasma renin activity was successfully treated with propranolol doses as high as 24 mg/kg per day. Another investigation reported a need for higher plasma propranolol levels to achieve therapeutic results in those patients with secondary hypertension due to renal parenchymal disease or hypoplastic abdominal aorta than in those patients with essential hypertension (140 vs. 111 ng/mL). In a single-blind, 8-month, crossover trial that compared propranolol with placebo in 10 patients (14 to 17 years of age) with essential hypertension, systolic and diastolic pressures were significantly reduced with propranolol. None of the patients developed adverse effects severe enough to require cessation of propranolol therapy. Three of 10 patients did, however, experience fatigue after exercise, bradycardia, and transient Raynaud's phenomenon. A prospective study on the effect of propranolol (1.0 to 9.0 mg/kg per day) in 13 post–kidney transplant, high-renin, hypertensive children was conducted in which some of the patients were concomitantly administered diuretics, methyldopa, and hydralazine. There was a mean reduction of blood pressure from 139/94 to 127/84 mm Hg. Two of the 13 patients did not improve with propranolol therapy, and there was no correlation between change in renin levels and change in blood pressure. Propranolol also has been shown to be effective preoperatively in children with coarctation of the aorta. One study addressed the question of whether preoperative administration of propranolol could prevent paradoxical hypertension noted in children after surgery for coarctation of the aorta. The investigators found that propanolol effectively decreased postoperative rises in blood pressure and plasma renin activity. Others have confirmed the effectiveness of propranolol in this regard in a randomized, controlled, double-blind trial.

In previously noted pediatric studies, β blockade caused a fall in serum renin activity, but there was no relation between that reduction and an antihypertensive response. Falkner and associates reported adequate blood pressure control with metoprolol and a blunted change in the systolic pressure and heart rate response to aerobic exercise and mental stress. At maximum exercise, patients were able to increase their heart rate to expected maximal levels, without limitation in endurance capacity (as measured by exercise stress testing), suggesting that metoprolol may be useful in diabetics who fail propranolol therapy. In addition, metoprolol had no short-term adverse effect on glucose levels and insulin requirements. Propranolol therapy, particularly in infants and children, diabetic or not, has been associated with hypoglycemia, especially during fasting, as in preparation for surgery.

Central α₂-Adrenergic Agonists

These agents, including clonidine and guanabenz, act centrally by stimulating α_2-mediated inhibition of sympathetic outflow, which results in decreased SVR (see Chapter 10). These drugs are used primarily in the treatment of hypertension. Abrupt discontinuation of therapy may result in rebound hypertension. Other side effects are sedation and dry mouth. Published pediatric experience with these agents is limited.

Minoxidil

Minoxidil results in arteriolar vasodilation without significant venous vasodilation, similar to hydralazine. Its use is reserved primarily for children with severe drug-resistant hypertension. Side effects of minoxidil include hypotension, tachycardia, hypertrichosis, and fluid retention.

TREATMENT OF LIPID DISORDERS

Increasingly, evidence is accumulating that links atherosclerosis in adults with a juvenile onset. In addition, there are primary lipid disorders with marked elevation of cholesterol and its congeners, which exist in childhood in their own right. As a result, over the past decade, increasing attention has focused on developing strategies of pharmacologic management of lipoprotein metabolism in childhood.

There is considerable experience with anti-lipid pharmacotherapy in children with familial hypercholesterolemia (FH), the most commonly recognized and best understood disorder of lipoprotein metabolism in childhood. In FH heterozygotes (1 of 500), the plasma cholesterol [total and low-density lipoproteins (LDLs)] are elevated approximately two- to threefold; FH homozygotes (1 of 1,000,000) have cholesterol levels that are elevated five- to sixfold. The published studies have been small in size, making it difficult to thoroughly assess the potential adverse side effects of anti-lipid drug therapy. Further, therapeutic approaches studied in FH may not have broad-based applicability to other types of childhood dyslipidemias. In addition, in these studies, therapy for the most part has been oriented toward the reduction of serum total cholesterol and LDL cholesterol without addressing other constituents of the serum lipid profile, which may have prognostic and therapeutic significance.

In children with dyslipidemias, it may be reasonably assumed that atherosclerosis is developing at an accelerated rate. The treatment of dyslipidemic children hinges on the assumption that modifying the serum lipoprotein concentrations will reduce the rate of atherogenesis. The use of combined diet and drug intervention has been shown to arrest the progression of arteriographically defined coronary atherosclerosis and to reduce cardiovascular disease risk in middle-age men, although such data are not available in children.

As in adults, initial medical intervention for dyslipidemias in childhood is generally nonpharmacologic. On average, the LDL cholesterol will decrease approximately 10% to 15% with diet therapy. In some children, however, diet therapy alone will not suffice. The National Cholesterol Education Program (NCEP) Expert Panel on Blood Cholesterol Levels in Children and Adolescents selected cutoff points for initiation of pharmacotherapy. According to those guidelines, in children 10 years and older, drug therapy should be initiated after a 6- to 12-month trial of diet if (a) serum LDL cholesterol is greater than 190 mg/dL or (b) serum LDL cholesterol is greater than 160 mg/dL in addition to a positive family history of premature coronary artery disease or two or more other risk factors that remain present after vigorous attempts have been made to control them. In children younger than 10 years, clinical judgment of the physician must dictate treatment.

Another set of recommendations has been issued by the American Academy of Pediatrics Committee on Nutrition. Although specific levels for screening algorithms differ to a limited extent, there is consensus agreement that indications for pharmacotherapy include a 190 mg/dL value of LDL cholesterol in children 10 years or older who have attempted diet modification or an LDL greater than 160 mg/dL if there is a family history of premature cardiovascular disease or other risk factors are present, assuming a strong attempt at dietary control. In addition, there are advocates for beginning treatment at even younger ages, although the value of this approach remains to be tested in large population samples.

Approved medication options for use in the pediatric population are limited. The most widespread experience is with the bile acid sequestrants colestipol and cholestyramine. However, other drugs, including various statins, niacin, and fenofibrate, also reduce total cholesterol.

Bile Acid–Binding Resins

Cholestyramine and Colestipol

The NCEP recommends only the use of the bile acid sequestrants. These agents have been used successfully to lower LDL cholesterol in children over long intervals, apparently with relatively few side effects. Doses are not related to the body weight of the child but to the post–dietary LDL cholesterol levels. These drugs are the safest to use because they are not absorbed systemically. Cholestyramine and colestipol have been used for up to 8 years in children, without evidence of fat-soluble vitamin deficiencies, steatorrhea, calcium, or vitamin D metabolic disturbances or erythrocyte folate deficiency. However, no placebo-controlled, double-blind, prospective study of the safety and efficacy of these agents, particularly with regard to long-term growth and development, has been done.

The dose range frequently recommended is 2 to 16 g/day. Most common side effects include flatulence, nausea, and constipation. Approximately a 15% to 20% reduction in LDL cholesterol values can be achieved, on average, over the long-term, although greater reductions have been reported in selected circumstances.

Statins

3-Hydroxy-3-methylglutaryl coenzyme A reductase inhibitors have not been approved by the FDA for use in patients younger than 10 years. Nevertheless, many recent studies have indicated a promising role for these agents based on the encouraging work that has been amassed in adults. In the past several years, placebo-controlled, double-blind, clinical trials have demonstrated reductions in LDL cholesterol in children when using statins and diet, with and without concomitant bile acid sequestrant therapy. Only limited side effects have been reported in these studies, involving pravastatin, lovastatin, or simvastatin in doses ranging from 5 to 40 mg/day, depending on the particular study. Some children were treated for as long as 12 months. Reductions in mean LDL cholesterol ranged from as high as 21% to 36% in one study to 17% to 27% in another, with similar reductions found in other trials. As with adults, monitoring of creatine kinase and liver function studies is required, as is accurate reporting of muscle cramping, rash, and fatigue. Importantly, statin use in these trials has not had adverse effects on growth or maturation in males. The caveat against their use in the pubertal female remains because there are no data proving safety in this group for the patient or a prospective fetus. Long-term studies are needed, perhaps spanning decades, for obtaining secure data concerning the impact of such treatment in children on the development of cardiovascular complications in adults with lipid disorders.

Niacin

Niacin functions by suppressing hepatic production and secretion of LDL and very LDLs. There are descriptions of the use of niacin in childhood, but its clinical use is limited by well-documented adverse effects. The most worrisome is its potential hepatotoxicity at therapeutic doses, as suggested by elevation of liver enzymes. Common adverse effects include "niacin flush," which can be prevented by taking aspirin (dose is age dependent) 20 to 30 min before the niacin dose. Less commonly, itching, dry skin, headaches, nausea, vomiting, diarrhea, and increased liver function tests may occur.

Usually, niacin is recommended to be used in combination with diet therapy plus bile acid sequestrants in doses of 1 to 1.5 g/day.

Ezetimibe

Ezetimibe is in a class of lipid-lowering drugs that selectively inhibit the intestinal absorption of cholesterol and related phytosterols. It can be used as a monotherapy or in combination with statins in patients with FH and sitosterolemia. There are limited clinical data with the use of ezetimibe in the pediatric population, however, there appear to be no pharmacokinetic differences between adolescents and adults. Pharmacokinetic data in the pediatric population under 10 years of age are not available.

ANTIARRHYTHMIC DRUGS

Arrhythmias are encountered much less frequently in children than in adults but remain important reasons for pharmacotherapy in childhood. Arrhythmia therapy differs from that in adults because of the spectrum of arrhythmias most frequently encountered in children and the differences in pharmacokinetics and specific effects of antiarrhythmic drugs between children and adults. In addition, the strategy for fetal arrhythmia drug therapy given via the mother and the cardiac electrophysiologic effects of commonly used psychotropic medications in childhood make discussion of this topic in childhood unique.

Children without congenital structural heart disease most frequently have supraventricular tachycardia and, rarely, ventricular tachycardia. After corrective surgery for congenital heart defects, supraventricular tachycardia, atrial flutter, atrial fibrillation, and ventricular tachycardia can occur. Children with complex congenital heart disease are living longer postoperatively with an increasing incidence of arrhythmias with increasing age. Investigators recently extensively reviewed evidence-based drug therapy of arrhythmias in children and adults.

Overview of Diagnoses in Children

Supraventricular Arrhythmias

Supraventricular tachycardia (SVT) is the most frequent significant arrhythmia in children, with an estimated incidence of 1 in 250 to 1 in 1000. The most common electrophysiologic mechanisms are AV and AV nodal reentry. In the hemodynamically unstable patient, electrical cardioversion is indicated. If the patient with SVT is hemodynamically stable after a trial of vagal maneuvers, intravenous adenosine is the drug of choice for acute conversion to sinus rhythm. Intravenous procainamide or amiodarone has been shown to be effective in children and may be used if adenosine is unsuccessful or unavailable. Intravenous verapamil may be used, but not in patients younger than 1 year because of reported cardiovascular collapse. For prevention of subsequent episodes, digoxin, propranolol, atenolol, verapamil, flecainide, and amiodarone may have roles. In the presence of preexcitation (Wolff-Parkinson-White syndrome), digoxin should be avoided because it can accelerate conduction along the bypass tract. Transcatheter radiofrequency ablation, however, has become an increasingly popular alternative to chronic pharmacologic therapy.

Atrial flutter and atrial fibrillation occur infrequently in infants without structural heart disease and in children with surgical repairs involving extensive atrial suturing (Mustard, Senning, Fontan, or TAPVR repair). Electrical cardioversion is the definitive therapy and indicated for hemodynamic instability, although care must be taken to follow anticoagulation guidelines to prevent thromboembolic complications. For pharmacologic rate control or conversion to sinus rhythm, β blockers, calcium channel blockers, digoxin, amiodarone, procainamide, flecainide, and sotalol may be effective. Therapy is determined by the presence or absence of preexcitation and the hemodynamic status. Junctional tachycardia may be encountered after open heart surgery and may be treated by intravenous amiodarone, procainamide, or propafenone.

Ventricular Tachycardia

In children, ventricular tachycardia is encountered much less frequently than are supraventricular arrhythmias, but it does occur in certain settings, including the long QT syndrome and after cardiac surgery involving ventricular suturing (e.g., tetralogy of Fallot repair). Hemodynamically unstable ventricular tachycardia warrants electrical cardioversion. In the hemodynamically stable child, effective acute drug therapy for monomorphic ventricular tachycardia includes intravenous amiodarone, procainamide, or lidocaine. Polymorphic ventricular tachycardia, i.e., torsades de pointes, may be treated by intravenous magnesium, pacing, β blockers, or isoproterenol. Other polymorphic ventricular tachycardias may be treated by intravenous lidocaine, amiodarone, procainamide, sotalol, β blockers, or phenytoin. Pulseless ventricular tachycardia and ventricular fibrillation are electrically cardioverted; but if refractory to electroshock, the arrhythmias can be treated with epinephrine, intravenous amiodarone, lidocaine, procainamide, or magnesium.

Chronic therapy for ventricular tachycardia may include β blockers, mexiletine, amiodarone, or phenytoin. In the presence of long QT syndrome, β blockade is the mainstay of therapy.

Prolonged QT Syndrome

It has been suggested that 10% of the 7000 annual crib deaths are the result of unrecognized cardiac causes—notably concealed cardiac arrhythmias, including those related to a prolonged QT interval. In 80% of untreated patients with prolonged QT syndrome, ventricular tachycardia occurs, especially torsade de pointes. Although many cases are sporadic, there is a clear genetic pattern in the Romano-Ward (autosomal dominant) and Jervell-Lange-Nielsen (autosomal recessive) syndromes. The dominant disorder has no clinical marker aside from the arrhythmia, whereas the recessive syndrome is associated with hereditary neurosensory deafness. The congenital long QT syndrome is familial in 60% of cases. The current understanding of the pathogenetic mechanism of the long QT syndrome involves the sympathetic nervous system as the primary defect (sympathetic imbalance hypothesis) or as an intracardiac abnormality probably related to the control of potassium currents. Recent findings of specific mutations on specific genes that determine specific abnormalities in cardiac ion channels leading to different forms of long QT syndrome will determine precise therapies for each type of ion channel disorder, allowing for more effective pharmacologic therapy.

Whereas the length of QT intervals in infants deemed to be at high risk for crib death do not strictly correlate with the likelihood of sudden death, corrected QT intervals lasting for longer than 500 ms appear to confer the greatest risk to patients.

Therapy is oriented toward the prevention of sudden death by acutely terminating torsade de pointes and its immediate re-initiation and chronically preventing its recurrence. Because bradycardia or long pauses may potentiate the tachycardia and are important risk factors, ventricular pacing and isoproterenol infusion have been studied. Lidocaine infusion has variable results. In vitro, magnesium inhibits early afterdepolarizations and may play a role in suppressing re-initiation of torsade de pointes. Experimental data have suggested that calcium channel blockers may be of some acute benefit.

β Blockade with propranolol has been the mainstay for chronic therapy of long QT syndrome because it has proven effective in 75% to 80% of patients. In some patients, antiarrhythmic agents, such as tocainide and mexiletine, have been used effectively. However, despite full-dose β blockers, 20% to 25% of patients continue to have syncopal episodes and remain at a high risk for sudden cardiac death. For those unresponsive patients, high thoracic left sympathectomy has been used. Recently, an international prospective study has provided evidence that left cardiac sympathetic denervation is a very effective therapy.

The treatment of asymptomatic children with long QT syndrome remains controversial. Garson and colleagues recommended that asymptomatic children with a corrected QT interval longer than 0.44 and a positive family history of the long QT syndrome should be treated because a cardiac arrest may be the first symptom (9% presented with a cardiac arrest). This differs from adults where the majority of patients have syncopal episodes before a cardiac arrest. They noted that ineffective treatment, particularly for symptoms, was a predictor for late symptoms and sudden death. In addition, ineffective treatment with one agent likely predicted ineffective therapy with other pharmacologic agents. Hence, lack of clinical response to even one drug should prompt the clinician to consider alternative therapies, including pacing or left cardiac sympathetic denervation.

Propranolol is equal to other β blockers in providing effective treatment for symptoms and ventricular arrhythmias and is similar in terms of incidence of late sudden death. The sudden death risk was not related to the type of other β blocker used.

Specific Antiarrhythmic Drugs

When the pediatric cardiologist is challenged with the task of selecting an appropriate antiarrhythmic drug and finding pediatric drug dosing guidelines for antiarrhythmics, one discovers the relative lack of information available. Antiarrhythmic medications can have pharmacokinetics and effects in children different from those in adults. Use of antiarrhythmia medications in children are based mostly on studies in adults, although pediatric data likely will be collected in the near future. In fact, digoxin is the only agent that is officially approved by the FDA for use in children with cardiac arrhythmias. In the following discussion, the Vaughan Williams classification of antiarrhythmics is used. The electrophysiologic actions of the drugs are summarized in Chapter 12.

Class Ia Agents

Quinidine

Quinidine can be used for the treatment of supraventricular and ventricular tachycardias in children. Animal studies have suggested that the effects of quinidine are less pronounced in the immature than in the mature heart. Whereas quinidine's direct electrophysiologic effect tends to be antiarrhythmic, its indirect anticholinergic effect tends to be proarrhythmic. Quinidine will increase the sinoatrial (SA) node's rate of discharge and, at the AV node, indirectly augment conduction through its anticholinergic action. Quinidine also can act as an α-adrenergic blocker.

The clinician must attempt to ensure that the resulting in vivo effect of quinidine is the desired one. For example, in patients with atrial fibrillation or flutter, enhanced AV nodal conduction due to the anticholinergic effect may translate into an inappropriately accelerated ventricular rate. This can be avoided by combining quinidine with an agent that will combat quinidine's effect at the AV node, such as digoxin, which slows AV nodal conduction.

Quinidine usually is prescribed orally but may be slowly given parenterally in the gluconate or sulfate form. Quinidine gluconate is absorbed more slowly and takes longer to reach its peak concentration than does quinidine sulfate, allowing for the less frequent dosing of every 8 h. Significant age-related differences in protein binding have been shown—63% in newborns versus 86% in older children, approximating the 90% protein binding seen in adults. Similarly, in the presence of cyanotic heart disease, changes in protein binding have been demonstrated. Quinidine is metabolized primarily by the liver; 20% is excreted unmetabolized in the urine with its metabolites. The elimination half-life of quinidine is shorter in children (about 4 h) than in adults (about 6 h). The dose of quinidine in children is correspondingly higher than that for adults. Dosage for quinidine gluconate is generally 20% higher.

The dreaded cardiovascular complication of quinidine therapy is excessive prolongation of the QT interval associated with a potentially fatal ventricular arrhythmia, torsade de pointes. In children, an association between "quinidine syncope" and the presence of structural heart disease and/or hypokalemia has been noted. In adults, syncope usually occurs within 5 days of initiation of therapy. In children, however, syncope may occur as late as 2 weeks after treatment initiation. Further, the likelihood of syncope to occur does not appear to correlate with serum quinidine levels. Hence, in such patients, it is advisable to initiate quinidine therapy only in the hospital. Hypotension, especially with parenteral administration, also may occur due to α-adrenergic blockade. Other adverse effects are gastrointestinal (diarrhea, nausea, vomiting) and hematologic (antibody-mediated thrombocytopenia). Importantly, quinidine can raise serum digoxin levels, as discussed earlier in this chapter.

Procainamide

Procainamide has indications similar to those of quinidine. It does not prolong the action potential and QT interval as much as quinidine. It also has weaker autonomic effects, which include less anticholinergic activity and no α-adrenergic blocking action. Procainamide does act as a mild ganglionic blocker and, hence, may cause peripheral vasodilation and a negative chronotropic effect. Animal studies have shown that, like quinidine, in neonates, higher concentrations of procainamide are necessary to produce effects similar to those on adult myocardium.

Procainamide may be used intravenously. It is rapidly absorbed after oral administration, with peak plasma concentrations achieved in about 75 min. Unlike quinidine, only 20% of procainamide is protein bound. Conventional and sustained-release forms are available. More than 50% of the drug is excreted unmetabolized in the urine. The rest undergoes *N*-acetylation to form *N*-acetyl procainamide (NAPA), which is then excreted in the urine. The rate of metabolism corresponds to a genetically determined acetylator phenotype. NAPA itself displays class III antiarrhythmic properties. Whereas NAPA's parent drug exerts its effect on the duration and the upstroke of the action potential, NAPA's electrophysiologic effect is limited to its ability to prolong the action potential.

Procainamide has a significantly shorter elimination half-life in children (1.7 h) than in adults. Its cardiovascular adverse effects in children are similar to those of quinidine. However, torsade de pointes is less frequent and appears to be dose related. Gastrointestinal effects occur less often than with quinidine. Approximately 33% of patients can develop a lupus-like syndrome with fever, rash, and thrombocytopenia after 6 months of therapy, and up to 70% of patients will develop antinuclear antibodies, conditions that are reversible with cessation of therapy. Slow acetylators carry an increased risk for developing adverse effects from treatment. Amiodarone may increase plasma levels of procainamide.

Disopyramide

Not only does disopyramide exert class Ia antiarrhythmic effects, but it also exhibits a pronounced negative inotropic effect. In recently has been used successfully in children with hypertrophic obstructive cardiomyopathy to reduce outflow tract gradients. In addition, it exhibits much greater anticholinergic activity than do the other class Ia agents. It is administered orally, is well absorbed, and is subject to first-pass hepatic metabolism. Apparent age-related differences in the ability of pediatric patients to maintain therapeutic disopyramide serum levels have been noted. Whereas older children may achieve satisfactory levels after being given 5 to 15 mg/kg per day, children younger than 2 years may require as much as 30 mg/kg per day to obtain the same levels. The cardiovascular adverse effects are similar to those of quinidine. It also may precipitate CHF due to its negative inotropic actions. Gastrointestinal side effects occur less frequently than with the other class Ia agents. Anticholinergic side effects do occur, and the drug does not increase serum digoxin levels.

Class Ib Agents

Lidocaine

Lidocaine is useful in suppressing delayed afterdepolarizations and has little benefit for supraventricular tachycardias. Canine studies have shown that neonatal fibers require greater lidocaine concentrations to achieve the same effects on the action potential as that seen in adult dogs. Lidocaine is less effective in reducing conduction velocity in young, as compared with adult, Purkinje fibers, and the time constant of recovery from rate-dependent conduction delay in the intact newborn canine heart is notably shorter than that in the adult heart. Lidocaine is not administered orally because it undergoes extensive first-pass hepatic metabolism. Its half-life, which is related to hepatic blood flow, is approximately 3.2 h in neonates versus 1.8 in adults. Adverse effects appear to be dose related and may occur at plasma levels as low as 5 µg/mL. Most commonly, CNS symptoms (confusion, dizziness, seizures) occur, which can be avoided by reducing the infusion rate and by monitoring drug serum levels. With serum levels exceeding 9 µg/mL, even more serious reactions have been seen, including hypotension, low CO, muscle twitching, and respiratory arrest. Lidocaine may exacerbate preexisting electrophysiologic abnormalities (AV block, sinus node dysfunction).

Other Ib Agents

In children, phenytoin is used as an antiarrhythmic agent for chronic therapy of ventricular arrhythmias after cardiac surgery and for treating digoxin-induced arrhythmias. Mexiletine and tocainide are used for chronic oral treatment of ventricular tachycardia that had previously responded to intravenous lidocaine.

Class Ic Agents

Flecainide

Some of flecainide's electrophysiologic effects appear to be less pronounced in the neonatal than in the adult myocardium. Flecainide has been used in children to treat supraventricular tachycardias, atrial flutter, and ventricular arrhythmias. However, the adult CAST trial raised concern about the safety of flecainide and prompted the review of the use of flecainide in children. The pediatric patient with ventricular arrhythmias and structural heart disease most closely parallels the profile implicated in the CAST trial, namely the adult with ventricular arrhythmias after myocardial infarction. In their comprehensive review of the use of flecainide in children, Perry and Garson concluded that, in pediatric patients with supraventricular tachycardia (excluding atrial flutter) and normal hearts, flecainide appears to be effective and safe (no deaths with usual oral dosing and fewer than 1% with serious proarrhythmia). In patients with atrial flutter or ventricular arrhythmias with structurally abnormal hearts, flecainide may not be safe. However, for those patients with ventricular arrhythmias and structurally normal hearts, the safety of flecainide has yet to be established.

The elimination half-life of flecainide manifests age dependence. Although children between 1 and 12 years of age have a mean elimination half-life of 8 h, pediatric patients outside that age range have a longer elimination half-life of 11 to 12 h. The therapeutic flecainide dose is 100 to 200 mg/m^2 per day, or 1 to 8 mg/kg per day. The risk of toxicity is increased in patients who require high doses of flecainide because of persistently low plasma trough levels and in those patients whose diets are changed to include fewer milk products because milk can increase flecainide absorption.

Propafenone

In addition to possessing the electrophysiologic properties of flecainide, propafenone exerts a mild β-blocking and calcium channel blocking effects. In children, intravenous propafenone has been used to treat postoperative junctional ectopic tachycardia and congenital junctional ectopic tachycardia. It appears to be effective for treating children with supraventricular tachycardias, particularly those arising from an ectopic site. It can be given orally or intravenously. The use of oral propafenone (mean dose, 353 mg/m^2 per day divided into three doses) effectively controlled supraventricular tachyarrhythmias in 41 of 47 (87%) patients studied, most of whom were infants. This report provided dosing guidelines (200 to 600 mg/m^2 per day divided into three doses) for oral propafenone use. The investigators also suggested that, for monitoring drug effect, measuring QRS duration is preferred over measuring drug plasma levels. Because of propafenone's interaction with digoxin, it has been recommended that the digoxin maintenance dosage should be halved when initiating propafenone therapy in a child already taking digoxin.

Class II Agents

β-Adrenergic Blockers

β Blockers have been used for years in children to treat supraventricular arrhythmias and ventricular arrhythmias. Propranolol can significantly inhibit SA node automaticity in children with normal SA node function and has had little, if any, effect on SA conduction. The usefulness of β blockade in the treatment of children with supraventricular tachycardias has been elucidated in several studies, and are briefly summarized here. In one study, in three of six children with supraventricular tachycardia in whom digoxin treatment failed, propranolol (1 to 3 mg/kg per day) restored normal sinus rhythm. Another report demonstrated the usefulness of digoxin plus propranolol in suppressing supraventricular tachycardia in a 4-month-old female and illustrated propranolol's adverse effects of bronchospasm and sleep disturbances, which necessitated its discontinuation. The substitution of propranolol with metoprolol (2 mg/kg per day) produced effective arrhythmia suppression, which was devoid of side effects over the next 7 months. Investigators described five of five patients who had supraventricular tachycardia inadequately controlled by digitalis, who were free of arrhythmias for up to 2 years with propranolol dosed at 7 to 14 mg/kg per day, and who maintained peak serum drug levels between 118 and 250 ng/mL. Others reported beneficial effect in seven of nine children who failed to respond to other therapy (digoxin and/or quinidine and/or cardioversion) but did respond to propranolol in doses of 0.5 to 4.0 mg/kg per day. The side effects that led to dosage reduction were sinus bradycardia, feeding difficulties, and worsening of ketotic hypoglycemia. Still others described five patients with chronic supraventricular tachycardia who were refractory to digitalis alone and were successfully treated, without adverse effects, by using the combination of digitalis and propranolol at doses of 20 to 120 mg/day.

The efficacy of β blockade for the treatment of ventricular tachycardia also has been documented. Propranolol has been used for the acute termination of ventricular tachycardia and chronically for the prevention of its recurrence. For chronic management, for the most part, β-blocking agents have not been effective when given alone but have been effective when combined with another drug such as procainamide or another therapeutic modality such as electrical pacing. However, successful acute treatment and chronic suppression of ventricular tachycardia after 1.5 years of follow-up was reported in an infant born to a heroin addict, with continued doses of 1 mg/kg of propranolol used alone.

Because of its once-a-day and twice-a-day dosing, atenolol, a β-selective blocker, has gained popularity for the treatment of older children and adolescents with arrhythmias, but a high incidence of side effects limits its usefulness. Esmolol, an ultrashort-acting β blocker, is helpful in slowing an incessant supraventricular tachycardia in children while other long-term agents are being titrated. Hypotension is a serious limitation with esmolol, especially if ventricular dysfunction already exists as a result of an incessant arrhythmia. The pharmacokinetics of esmolol in children have been reviewed recently, and the investigators suggested using pediatric dosing guidelines, since the dose of esmolol required for β-blockade is considerably higher than that typically used in adults.

Class III Agents

Amiodarone

As in adults, amiodarone exhibits a broad spectrum of antiarrhythmic efficacy that includes the termination of supraventricular and ventricular tachycardias. However, its use is limited due to its multiple, serious adverse effects, including a tendency to be proarrhythmic. A recent report described the successful treatment of SVT-induced cardiomyopathy in a neonate with amiodarone. Another reported on oral amiodarone's safety and efficacy in 17 infants. Oral amiodarone was successful in relieving arrhythmias in 10 of 17 patients (59%). In three infants with primary atrial tachycardias, the combination of amiodarone with a class Ic antiarrhythmic agent was effective. In two infants, amiodarone was found to be proarrhythmic because they developed "incessant episodes" of reentrant supraventricular tachycardia soon after the initiation of treatment. Those who "failed" amiodarone therapy were considered to have reentrant supraventricular tachycardias and were sent for ablative therapy. The use of intravenous bolus amiodarone for life-threatening tachyarrhythmias in 10 pediatric patients was well tolerated, devoid of significant adverse effects, and effective in terminating rapid tachyarrhythmias in 6 of 10 patients. Among those who responded was one patient with postoperative junctional ectopic tachycardia. Fifty infants treated with amiodarone for supraventricular arrhythmias demonstrated a low incidence of adverse effects. The corrected QT interval increased during drug loading, but no ventricular arrhythmias were encountered. There were increases in alanine and aspartate aminotransferases and in thyroid-stimulating hormone, but no clinical abnormalities in liver or thyroid function.

Other Class III Agents

Ibutilide is a class III antiarrhythmic drug with an FDA indication for the rapid conversion of atrial fibrillation and atrial flutter to sinus rhythm. The dosage is 0.01 mg/kg intravenously over 10 min. The safety and efficacy of ibutilide in children has been studied in a limited fashion, and its safety is not firmly established. Dofetilide is a similar agent that can be used orally, but there is no published experience with the drug in children.

Intravenous bretylium use is reserved for patients with recurrent or refractory ventricular fibrillation. Significant hypotension may follow its administration because of the drug's antiadrenergic properties. Sotalol, similar to ibutilide, is a β blocker that possesses class III rather than class II antiarrhythmic properties. It appears to be effective in the treatment of supraventricular tachycardia.

Class IV Agents

Class IV antiarrhythmic drugs exert their electrophysiologic effects by blockade of the slow calcium channels.

Verapamil

Verapamil has been used in the initial treatment of supraventricular tachycardia in older children. Whereas the drug lengthens the action potential of mature Purkinje fibers, it shortens it in the neonatal myocardium. Further, verapamil's negative inotropic effect is greater on neonatal than on adult ventricular myocardium, and the drug should not be used in conjunction with β blockers. Pediatric pharmacokinetic studies have shown that verapamil can have slower and faster elimination half-lives than in adults. Although as many as 44% of children develop adverse effects while on chronic oral verapamil therapy, fewer than 10% of those reactions are severe enough to necessitate discontinuation of the drug. Verapamil is contraindicated in infants younger than 1 year, however, because it may reduce CO and produce hypotension and cardiac arrest.

Miscellaneous Antiarrhythmics

Adenosine

Adenosine has emerged as the drug of choice for the acute termination of supraventricular tachycardia in the hemodynamically stable infant or child in whom the use of nonpharmacologic vagal maneuvers have failed. It is an endogenous nucleoside with a very short half-life (10 s). Its net electrophysiologic effect is to slow the SA node firing rate and to decrease AV nodal conduction. It has a rapid onset of action and minimal effects on cardiac contractility. Intravenous adenosine was used in 24 patients and achieved the desired AV block in 21 (88%). The investigators demonstrated the diagnostic and therapeutic utilities of causing AV block with intravenous adenosine. In 11 patients, AV block terminated the reentrant tachycardia; in the remaining 10 patients, AV block allowed for proper diagnosis of the enduring atrial arrhythmias. In a recent review of the use of adenosine in children in the emergency room, the most effective dose was found to be between 0.1 and 0.3 mg/kg (maximum, 12 mg) by rapid intravenous push. No major adverse effects, including bronchospasm and sinus arrest, were reported. Minor adverse effects, including nausea, vomiting, headache, flushing, and chest pain, were found to occur with an incidence of 22%.

Digoxin

Digoxin was described earlier in this chapter. It is commonly used for the long-term therapy of supraventricular tachycardia. In atrial flutter and fibrillation, it is used to lessen the ventricular response.

Fetal Arrhythmias

Currently, the most common indication for cardiovascular drug therapy for the fetus is for intrauterine SVT. In 1969, supraventricular tachycardia was first implicated as a cause of fetal heart failure. In 1980, the first report of in utero treatment of SVT appeared. Soon after, in the mid-1980s, with the advent of new fetal echocardiographic techniques that facilitated the detection and diagnosis of fetal arrhythmias, the treatment of fetal arrhythmias became more common.

The mother will be affected by any therapy for the fetus, and maternal drug toxicity often limits the effective employment of commonly used antiarrhythmic agents for treating fetal arrhythmias. Likewise, difficulties in controlling fetal arrhythmias stem from difficulties in maintaining adequately high drug concentrations in the mother to provide an effective concentration in the fetus. Some newer, technically more demanding approaches for fetal drug delivery, which bypass the placenta, have been used but may present greater risk to the fetus.

Most fetuses found to have an arrhythmia have unsustained, isolated ectopy, and this rhythm constitutes about 80% of all fetal arrhythmias detected by echocardiography, most of these being premature atrial contractions (PACs), isolated ventricular ectopy, and variable AV block. These arrhythmias are of little clinical significance, because only 1% of fetuses will have underlying structural congenital heart disease and only 0.5% will go on to develop sustained supraventricular tachycardia. In the absence of structural heart disease, the arrhythmias are generally benign and do not necessitate drug therapy.

SVT, usually generated by a reentrant mechanism, is by far the most commonly treated fetal arrhythmia. It was postulated that atrial septal aneurysms, found in 78% of those fetuses with persistent arrhythmia, may serve as a nidus for PACs and subsequent supraventricular tachycardias. For the viable, near-term, nonhydropic fetus developing a sustained tachyarrhythmia, delivery is the treatment. For the immature fetus who exhibits pulmonary immaturity or who displays signs of CHF, pharmacotherapy should be initiated. Atrial flutter or fibrillation with variable AV block and ventricular response is less commonly treated. Digoxin is the drug of choice for the treatment of fetal supraventricular tachycardia. It may be more effective to load the mother with digoxin intravenously rather than orally. In the hydropic fetus who may display increased resistance to drug therapy, it may be necessary to administer digoxin directly, i.e., intraperitoneally or via the umbilical vein. For the fetal supraventricular tachycardia patient refractory to digoxin alone, a class Ia antiarrhythmic agent such as quinidine or procainamide may be added to the maternally administered regimen. Although verapamil has been used, it is advocated against in view of more recent findings, which demonstrate the fetus's greater dependence on calcium influx to support myocardial contractility than later in life.

Bradyarrhythmias account for about only 5% of all fetal arrhythmias. Etiologies include sinus bradycardia, nonconducted PACs, and complete heart block. In and of itself, sustained fetal bradycardia is not an indication for therapeutic intervention, and the fetus should be monitored for fetal distress. However, in combination with fetal distress, such as hydrops fetalis, sustained bradycardia may herald demise. Sustained bradycardia in a fetus with structural heart disease renders the fetus a dismal prognosis. The fetus should be delivered early and paced. Unfortunately, in utero pacing is not yet a widely available therapeutic option.

Arrhythmias and Psychotropic Drugs in Children

Psychotropic drugs are used with increasing frequency in children with a variety of disorders, including attention deficit disorder, hyperactivity, depression, and a number of other psychiatric disorders. There are reports of arrhythmias and sudden death related to the cardiac and, specifically, the cardiac electrophysiologic effects of these medications. In 1999, the American Heart Association issued recommendations for cardiac monitoring of children being treated with certain drugs of this type based on knowledge of their cardiac electrophysiologic effects. Tricyclic antidepressants can cause prolonged corrected QT, QRS, and PR intervals. Phenothiazines, butyrophenones, and diphenylbutylpiperidines have been reported to prolong the corrected QT. Phenothiazines and tricyclic antidepressants also have been reported to cause sinus tachycardia. Clinical and electrocardiographic monitorings have been recommended for these medications.

SPECIAL PHARMACOLOGIC APPROACHES

Patent Ductus Arteriosus

Pharmacologic manipulation of the ductus arteriosus has become central to the treatment of neonates with congenital heart disease and to the management of premature newborns, even those with structurally normal hearts.

The ductus arteriosus is a physiologically vital channel required for normal development of fetal circulation. It is found normally in all mammalian fetuses. As lung blood flow in the fetus amounts to only less than 10% of the right ventricular output, and the right ventricle ejects approximately 65% of the combined ventricular output, the ductus arteriosus carries 55% to 60% of the combined ventricular output of the fetus. After birth, as the transition from fetal to normal postnatal circulation develops, the ductus arteriosus closes, first functionally and then anatomically. Functional closure occurs by 24, 48, and 96 h in 10%, 82%, and 100%, respectively, of term infants. Anatomic closure is usually finished by age 2 to 3 weeks. In about 0.04% of term infants, however, the ductus fails to close and remains patent.

Different factors are contributory to the initial closure process. These factors include oxygen, calcium, endogenous catecholamines, and other vasoactive compounds. The most important substances involved are the prostaglandins: prostacyclin produced by the ductus arteriosus and prostaglandin $E_2(PGE_2)$. Although prostacyclin is produced more vigorously, PGE_2 is much more potent as a ductus relaxer. Because PGE_2 metabolism by the lung is limited in the fetus and the placenta also is a source of this hormone, relatively high circulating levels are maintained. After birth, PGE_2 levels decline substantially, and ductal relaxation is less well maintained, thus allowing oxygen and other vasoconstrictors to become dominant. The effects and countereffects of these substances differ at different postnatal gestational ages, another factor relevant for clinical pharmacotherapeutics. In less mature infants, the ductus is more sensitive to dilating prostaglandins. In as many as 40% of infants born weighing less than 2000 g and as many as 80% of infants weighing less than 1200 g, the ductus remains patent after birth. In addition, even in term infants, any lowering of arterial partial pressure of oxygen, as with pulmonary disease or asphyxia, can result in delayed normal closure. These physiologic relationships underlie the development of pharmacologic strategies to modulate tone of the ductus. There are two distinct strategies necessitated by the importance to augment or to reduce pulmonary blood flow in the newborn infant.

Indomethacin, as an example of a cyclooxygenase inhibitor, is currently the most widely used medication to effect closure of the ductus. Indomethacin is most useful in the preterm infant in whom a patent ductus arteriosus may complicate other problems of prematurity by causing circulatory overload and even CHF. Dosage varies based on weight and age and regimens differ from center to center. Table 24-3 outlines a typical regimen.

Indomethacin also has vasoconstrictive action in other vascular beds. In humans, these actions include renal and cerebral artery vasoconstriction. Gut perfusion also may be affected. In view of this activity, the preferred route of administration is by slow intravenous infusion. In particular, this approach reduces cerebral blood flow alteration. A similar salutary effect on renal blood flow also results from continuous infusion. Although control of fluid volume, including the use of diuretics, had been advocated in the past, vigorous diuresis, such as with furosemide, is no longer thought to be useful because furosemide may enhance release of PGE_1 and, hence, promote ductal dilation. The patent ductus arteriosus, even when treated with cyclooxygenase inhibition, can re-dilate, and this reopening has been linked to increasing dilator prostaglandin levels.

Complications from indomethacin affect not only renal, cerebral, and mesenteric blood flow but also platelet and neutrophil functions. In addition, bilirubin metabolism must be monitored, because indomethacin can displace bilirubin from albumin-binding sites and may influence serum bilirubin levels. Some interest has been shown in the use of other prostaglandin synthesis inhibitors, such as ibuprofen, mefenamic acid, and others, but use of these agents is not widespread in the United States.

Pharmacologic manipulation of the ductus to maintain patency, instead of promoting closure, has become a mainstay of the management of the newborn with certain forms of congenital heart disease. In this circumstance, the aim of therapy is to overcome the physiologic cascade that normally results in a decline in circulating dilating prostaglandins shortly after term birth. PGE_1 has become the agent of choice for this purpose. Dosages of 0.05 to 0.1 mg/kg per minute are usual, and the drug must be given by continuous intravenous infusion because greater than 80% is metabolized on transhepatic and transpulmonary passage. Side effects include apnea, bradycardia, rash, seizures, hypotension, and hyperthermia. Maintenance intravenous infusion can be extended for a prolonged period until surgery is possible for more permanent palliation. However, oral PGE_1 administration

TABLE 24-3 Indomethacin Dosing Regimen (mg)*

Age/weight	Time (h)		
	0	12	24–36
<48 h/all weights	0.2	0.1	0.1
2–7 d/<1250 g	0.2	0.1	0.1
2–7 d/>1250 g	0.2	0.2	0.2
>7 d/all weights	0.2	0.2	0.2

*Most infants should receive the third dose 24 h after the first dose; infants with poor renal function, most commonly those weighing less than 1000 g, should be given the third dose 36 h after the first dose. The same schedule is used for the second course unless it is begun within 24 h of the last dose, in which case, 0.1 mg/kg × 3 is used. An alternate schedule for infants weighing less than 1000 g, especially if treatment is initiated after 3 to 4 days of life, is to give 0.1 mg/kg every 24 h × 7 d.

Source: Reprinted with permission from Gewitz MH: Patent ductus arteriosus, in Burg FD, Ingelfinger JR, Wald ER, et al (eds): *Gellis and Kagan's Current Pediatric Therapy,* 16th ed. Philadelphia, WB Saunders, 1999, p 354.

is not efficacious for long-term treatment, because the drug has a very short half-life and absorption from the gastrointestinal tract can be unpredictable. If prolonged intravenous therapy is required (usually in the preterm or low–birth-weight infant), electrolyte depletion, metabolic alkalosis, and delayed wound healing can complicate management. In addition, during prolonged PGE_1 usage, the unique x-ray findings of periosteal calcification and cortical hyperostosis involving long bones, ribs, and clavicles can develop. Fortunately, this appears to be a reversible phenomenon once PGE_1 is discontinued.

Cyanotic Spells

In certain types of physiologic abnormalities, infants and young children can be predisposed to the rapid onset of extreme arterial desaturation, the so called hypoxemic attack or cyanotic spell. These circumstances involve dynamic right ventricular outflow obstruction in the setting of baseline, pre-existing pulmonary, or subpulmonary stenosis. An associated intracardiac shunt also is present, which allows egress of desaturated blood into the systemic circulation. The typical condition with this anatomic and physiologic arrangement is tetralogy of Fallot. Components of the tetrad include (a) right ventricular outflow obstruction, usually at the pulmonary valve and subvalvular levels; (b) "malalignment" ventricular septal defect, which allows right ventricular blood access to the aorta; (c) dextroposition of the aortic root, which accepts blood flow from right and left ventricles; and (d) right ventricular hypertrophy.

Although definitive therapy for tetralogy of Fallot is surgical repair, pharmacologic management of the acute hypercyanotic episode can be critically important to allow the child to reach surgery in the first place.

The initial trigger for an episode of sudden extreme cyanosis has not been defined conclusively but probably involves decreased systemic vascular resistance, excess endogenous catecholamine release, or both. Changes in cardiac rhythm, such as tachyarrhythmias, and peripheral vascular pooling, such as occurs with prolonged recumbent position, can precipitate an event. Similarly, sudden or sharp pain or prolonged agitation can lead to a hypercyanotic episode. Medications, such as isoproterenol, also can induce an episode.

If an acute intervention is required to ameliorate a cyanotic "spell," morphine sulfate (0.1 mg/kg) has been demonstrated over many years to be an effective remedy. Morphine has primary sedating effects to interfere with catecholamine production and secondary effects to slow heart rate and respiratory rate, thus favorably effecting right ventricular filling. This drug, when used in combination with positional changes to augment systemic vascular resistance, is often singularly effective to improve oxygenation. Administration of oxygen, by raising the pulmonary-to-systemic vascular resistance ratio, also can be helpful as long as the net right-to-left intracardiac shunt is reduced. On occasion, more direct pharmacologic manipulation of systemic vascular resistance is required. For this purpose, infusion of phenylephrine, an α-agonist, at 2 to 10 µg/kg per minute, is of value. When a hypercyanotic spell is persistent despite these maneuvers, general anesthesia may be required and surgical augmentation of pulmonary blood should follow quickly.

Long-term pharmacologic palliation of tetralogy of Fallot and its variations is less common, coincident with advances in surgical techniques and perioperative management. Combined surgical and interventional cardiologic approaches have made treatment available to many more children with even marked pulmonary arterial bed anomalies. However, there are occasional indications for extended medical management. Because positive inotropy may result in a hypercontractile right ventricular outflow tract ("infundibular") and promote intracardiac right-to-left shunting with resultant systemic cyanosis, agents that decrease contractility can be beneficial. β Blockers, specifically propranolol, are particularly useful in this context. In the 1980s, several major studies documented the usefulness of propranolol for long-term palliation (several months' duration), thus confirming suggestions first raised 15 years previously. Potential complications, including bronchospasm, hypoglycemia, and bradycardia, must be monitored for once this therapy is initiated. Most clinicians continue β-blocker therapy until shortly before surgery, but there is controversy in this regard because β blockers may adversely affect myocardial recovery after cardiopulmonary bypass.

CONCLUSION

Cardiovascular drugs evaluated in adults for clinical approval are frequently used to treat disorders in children with few therapeutic guidelines. Although most experiences with pediatric drug use are favorable, carefully done clinical trials need to be conducted to guide physicians in the future drug management of cardiovascular disorders in children.

ADDITIONAL READINGS

Blumer JL: Labeling antihypertensive agents for children. *Curr Ther Res Clin Exp* 62:281, 2001.

Bruns LA, Chrisant MK, Lamour JM, et al: Carvedilol as therapy in pediatric heart failure: An initial multicenter experience. *J Pediatr* 138:457, 2001.

Chobanian AV, Bakris GL, Black HR, et al: The Seventh Report of the Joint National Committee on Prevention, Detection, Evaluation, and Treatment of High Blood Pressure. The JNC 7 Report. *JAMA* 289:2560, 2003.

Friedman AL: Approach to the treatment of hypertension in children. *Heart Dis* 4:47, 2002.

Gewitz MH, Vetter VL: Cardiac emergencies, in: Fleisher G, Ludwig S (eds): *Textbook of Pediatric Emergency Medicine,* 4th ed. Philadelphia, Lippincott Williams & Wilkins, 2000, p 665.

Gewitz M, Woolf P, Frishman WH, Wu J: Pediatric cardiovascular pharmacology, in Frishman WH, Sonnenblick EH, Sica DA (eds): *Cardiovascular Pharmacotherapeutics,* 2nd ed. New York, McGraw-Hill, 2003, p 893.

Golombek SG: The use of inhaled nitric oxide in newborn medicine. *Heart Dis* 2:342, 2000.

Gow RM, Bohn D, Koren G, et al: Cardiovascular pharmacology, in Radde IC, MacLeod SM (eds): *Pediatric Pharmacology and Therapeutics,* 2nd ed. St Louis, Mosby Year Book, 1993, p 197.

Gutgesell H, Atkins D, et al: Cardiovascular monitoring of children and adolescents receiving psychotropic drugs. *Circulation* 99:979, 1999.

Hoffman TM, Wernovsky G, Atz AM, et al: Efficacy and safety of milrinone in preventing low cardiac output syndrome in infants and children after corrective surgery for congenital heart disease. *Circulation* 107:996, 2003.

Ivy D: Diagnosis and treatment of severe pediatric pulmonary hypertension. *Cardiol Rev* 9:227, 2001.

Kay JD, Colan SD, Graham TP Jr: Congestive heart failure in pediatric patients. *Am Heart J* 142:923. 2001.

Kronn, DF, Sapru, A, Satou, GM: Management of hypercholesterolemia in childhood and adolescence. *Heart Dis* 2:348, 2000.

Liberthson RR: Current concepts: Sudden death from cardiac causes in children and young adults. *N Engl J Med* 334:1039, 1996.

Pasquali SR, Sanders SP, Li JS: Oral antihypertensive trial design and analysis under the pediatric exclusivity provision. *Am Heart J* 144:608, 2002.

Pitt B, Remme W, Zannad F, et al, for the Eplerenone Post-Acute Myocardial Infarction Heart Failure Efficacy and Survival Study Investigators: Eplerenone, a selective aldosterone blocker, in patients with left ventricular dysfunction after myocardial infarction. *N Engl J Med* 348:1309, 2003.

Shaddy RE, Curtin L, Sower B, et al: The pediatric randomized carvedilol trial in children with chronic heart failure: Rationale and design. *Am Heart* J 144:383, 2002.

Sonnenblick EH, LeJemtel TH, Frishman WH: Inotropic agents, in Frishman WH, Sonnenblick EH, Sica DA (eds): *Cardiovascular Pharmacotherapeutics,* 2nd ed. New York, McGraw-Hill, 2003, p 191.

Stein EH, Illingworth DR, Kwiterovich PO Jr, et al: Efficacy and safety of lovastatin in adolescent males with heterozygous familial hypercholesterolemia: A randomized controlled trial *JAMA* 281:37, 1999.

Stier CT, Koenig S, Lee DY, et al: Aldosterone and aldosterone antagonism in cardiovascular disease: Focus on eplerenone. *Heart Dis* 5:102, 2003.

25 | Infective Endocarditis and Rheumatic Fever

William H. Frishman   Ronald L. Shazer
Nauman Naseer   Michael H. Gewitz

Infective endocarditis (IE) is a disease with protean manifestations resulting from an endovascular infection within the heart. The location of infection is usually the heart valves; however, the chordae tendineae, mural endocardium, or septal defects or other sites may be involved. The initial event in the pathogenesis of IE is endothelial damage at a site of turbulent blood flow. Fibrin, leukocytes, and platelets are deposited on the abnormal endothelial surface, forming a sterile vegetation referred to as *nonbacterial thrombotic endocarditis.* Pathogenic organisms gaining access to the bloodstream may become incorporated in the fibrin–platelet network, resulting in an infected vegetation, the pathologic hallmark of IE. Continued deposition of fibrin and platelets protects microorganisms from cellular defense mechanisms and, perhaps, from contact with antimicrobials and allows the density of organisms to reach high levels. Virulent bacteria such as *Staphylococcus aureus* or *Streptococcus pneumoniae,* with the capacity to adhere to less severely damaged endothelium, may cause infection on apparently normal heart valves.

Embolization, one of the dreaded complications of the disease, occurs when portions of friable vegetation are lost in the circulation. Vegetations on the left side of the heart give rise to systemic emboli, leading to organ and limb infarction, including stroke or coronary artery occlusion. Right-side heart vegetations embolize to the lungs. Rarely, in the setting of a septal defect with elevated right atrial pressures, such as a patent foramen ovale, paradoxical emboli to the systemic circulation occur with right-side valvular lesions. Emboli from either side of the heart may be septic or noninfected.

From the vegetation, infection and inflammation may spread locally to damage the valve itself or its supporting structures. The valvular incompetence that ensues can result in hemodynamic compromise and congestive heart failure. Invasion of the myocardium, through direct spread or embolization, may cause abscesses that can lead to myocardial dysfunction, continued sepsis, and conduction abnormalities, including complete heart block. In the absence of effective therapy, the vegetation is a source of continuous bacteremia, leading to peripheral foci of infection and eventually death. Some of the more subtle manifestations of the disorder are caused by the immunologic response to the persistent bacteremia, including glomerulonephritis, arthritis, Osler nodes, Janeway lesions, and Roth spots.

DIAGNOSIS

The Duke Criteria

The diagnosis of IE is established with unequivocal certainty only when vegetations obtained at cardiac surgery, at autopsy, or from an artery (an embolus) are examined histologically and microbiologically. Nevertheless, a highly sensitive and specific diagnostic ischemia, known as the *Duke crite-*

ria, has been developed on the basis of clinical, laboratory, and echocardiographic findings (Table 25-1). Documentation of two major criteria, of one major and three minor criteria, or of five minor criteria allows for a clinical diagnosis of definite endocarditis to be made. The diagnosis of endocarditis is rejected if an alternative diagnosis is established, if symptoms resolve and do not recur within 4 days of antibiotic therapy, or if surgery or autopsy after 4 days of antimicrobial therapy yields no histologic evidence of endocarditis. The specificity of the initially proposed criteria (the ability to reject the diagnosis correctly) is high (0.99, with a 95% confidence interval of 0.97–1.0), and the negative predictive value is greater than 92%. Also, in a retrospective study of 410 patients with diagnosed endocarditis, the Duke criteria were found to have good agreement (72% to 90%) with clinical assessment by infectious disease experts. Most discrepancies occurred when the experts rejected cases categorized as "possible" endocarditis according to the criteria. A modified version of the Duke criteria has recently been proposed (see Table 25-1).

Echocardiography

Transthoracic echocardiography (TTE) is rapid and noninvasive and has excellent specificity for vegetations (98%). However, TTE may be technically inadequate in up to 20% of adult patients because of obesity, chronic obstructive pulmonary disease, or chest wall deformities; the overall sensitivity for vegetations may be less than 60% to 70%. Transesophageal echocardiography (TEE) is more costly and invasive but increases the sensitivity for detecting vegetations to 75% to 95% and maintains a specificity of 85% to 98%.

The appropriate use of echocardiography depends on the prior probability of IE. If this probability is less than 4%, a negative TTE is cost effective and clinically satisfactory in ruling out IE. For patients whose prior probability of IE is 4% to 60%, initial use of TEE is more cost effective and diagnostically efficient than initial use of TTE, which, if negative, is followed by TEE. This category of intermediate prior probability includes patients with unexplained bacteremia with a gram-positive coccus, those with catheter-associated *S. aureus* bacteremia, and those admitted with fever or bacteremia in the setting of recent injection drug use.

THERAPY

In the absence of antibacterial and antifungal chemotherapies, bacterial endocarditis is a uniformly fatal disease; host defense mechanisms alone are inadequate. Further, therapy of bacterial endocarditis generally requires the use of bactericidal agents. The goals of therapy are the eradication of all organisms within the vegetation and the prevention of embolic and immunologic phenomena and valve destruction. Several factors make this vegetation particularly difficult to treat. Because it is endovascular, white blood cells alone are ineffective in eliminating the infection. Antibiotic therapy is problematic because (a) the inner layers of the vegetation may be exposed to very low concentrations of antibiotic because of poor penetrability; (b) those antibacterial agents that require active growth for killing (most cell wall active agents) are relatively ineffective against the slow growing organisms found deep within the vegetation; and (c) high density

TABLE 25-1 Modified Duke Criteria for the Diagnosis of Infective Endocarditis

Criteria*	Comments
Major criteria	
Microbiologic	
Typical microorganism isolated from 2 separate blood cultures: *Viridans streptococci, Streptococcus bovis,* HACEK group, *Staphylococcus aureus,* or community-acquired enterococcal bacteremia without a primary focus	In patients with possible IE, at least 2 sets of cultures of blood collected by separate venipunctures should be obtained within the first 1–2 h of presentation; patients with cardiovascular collapse should have 3 cultures of blood obtained at 5- to 10-min intervals and thereafter receive empirical antibiotic therapy
or	
Microorganism consistent with IE isolated from persistently positive blood cultures	
or	
Single positive blood culture for *Coxiella burnetii* or phase I IgG antibody titer to *C. burnetii* >1:800	*C. burnetii* is not readily cultivated in most clinical microbiology laboratories
Evidence of endocardial involvement	
New valvular regurgitation (increase or change in preexisting murmur not sufficient)	
or	
Positive echocardiogram (TEE recommended in patients who have a prosthetic valve, who are rated as having at least possible IE by clinical criteria, or who have complicated IE	Three echocardiographic findings qualify as major criteria: a discrete, echogenic, oscillating intracardiac mass at the site of endocardial injury; a periannular abscess; and a new dehiscence of a prosthetic valve

Minor criteria

Predisposition to IE that includes certain cardiac conditions and injection drug use	Cardiac abnormalities that are associated with IE are classified into 3 groups: High-risk conditions: previous IE, aortic valve disease, rheumatic heart disease, prosthetic heart valve, coarctation of the aorta, and complex cyanotic congenital heart diseases Moderate-risk conditions: mitral valve prolapse with valvular regurgitation or leaflet thickening, isolated mitral stenosis, tricuspid valve disease, pulmonary stenosis, and hypertrophic cardiomyopathy Low- or no-risk conditions: secundum atrial septal defect, ischemic heart disease, previous coronary artery bypass graft surgery, and mitral valve prolapse with thin leaflets in the absence of regurgitation
Fever	Temperature >38°C (100.4°F)
Vascular phenomena	Petechiae and splinter hemorrhages are excluded
Immunologic phenomena	Presence of rheumatoid factor, glomerulonephritis, Osler's nodes, or Roth spots
Microbiologic findings	Serologic evidence of active infection: single isolates of coagulase-negative staphylococci and organisms that very rarely cause IE are excluded from this category

*Cases are defined clinically as definite if they fulfill two major criteria, one major criterion plus three minor criteria, or five minor criteria. They are defined as possible if they fulfill one major and one minor criterion or three minor criteria.

Key: HACEK, *Haemophilus* species (*Hemophilus parainfluenza, H. aphrophilus, H. paraphrophilus*), *Actinobacillus actinomycetemcomitans, Cardiobacterium hominis, Eikenella corrodens,* and *Kingella kinga*; IE, infective endocarditis; IgG, immunoglobulin G; TEE, transesophageal echocardiography.

Source: Adapted from Li JS, Sexton DJ, Mick N, et al: Proposed modifications to the Duke criteria for the diagnosis of infective endocarditis. *Clin Infect Dis* 30:633, 2000.

of bacteria in a vegetation may produce exceedingly high local levels of antibiotic-modifying enzymes.

For these reasons, the therapy of IE customarily has required high doses of bactericidal agents for prolonged periods. A controversial issue has been the usefulness of serum inhibitory and bactericidal levels in monitoring therapy of endocarditis. The trough serum inhibitory concentration is determined by serially diluting the patient's serum obtained just before the next dose of antibiotic and testing the ability of these dilutions to inhibit the growth of a standard inoculum of the patient's bacterial isolate. The highest serum dilution to inhibit growth is the serum inhibitory concentration. The serum bactericidal concentration (SBC) is determined by subculturing those tubes with inhibited growth onto fresh agar and demonstrating killing of the initial inoculum. The highest serum dilution to accomplish this degree of killing is the SBC. The same determinations can be made for peak inhibitory and bactericidal levels by drawing serum shortly after administration of an antibiotic dose.

Although the American Heart Association (AHA) previously recommended that the peak SBC be maintained at 1:8 or higher in the treatment of viridans streptococcal endocarditis, clinical experience has not supported an association between these levels and clinical outcome. Current AHA guidelines do not recommend the use of serum bactericidal titers in most cases of IE. These levels may be helpful in circumstances in which response to antimicrobial therapy is poor, in disease due to unusual organisms, and in therapy with unconventional agents.

Current guidelines suggest value for measuring the minimum inhibitory concentration (MIC) as a means for assessing organism sensitivity to an antibiotic regimen.

The first sign of successful therapy often is the patient's increased sense of well-being. In uncomplicated IE, fever generally resolves over days to a week or more, and the patient remains afebrile. Immune complex nephritis and arthritis generally parallel the course of the infection, although some patients may be left with residual impairment of renal function. In IE caused by *S. aureus,* blood cultures may remain positive after 1 week. Many patients are cured with medical therapy. Persistently positive cultures, however, usually imply failure to eradicate the initial focus of infection, spread of infection to the myocardium, or metastasis to a distant focus. Persistent fever may be caused by one of these factors, superinfection, or drug fever. It often is difficult in any one patient to identify with certainty the etiology of persistent or recurrent fever. Repeated examination of the patient, preferably by the same observer, is of paramount importance. The development of a new murmur, a pericardial friction rub, heart failure, or embolic phenomena in such a patient suggests continued active endocarditis. Complaints of bone or joint pain, abdominal pain, or persistent bacteriuria should direct attention to a new focus.

The timing of initial therapy depends on the patient's presentation. In a patient with subacute illness, antibiotic therapy should be withheld until the diagnosis is made securely. In the patient with suspected acute IE, blood cultures should be obtained and empiric antibiotic therapy begun immediately. Isolation of the causative microorganism from blood cultures is critical not only for diagnosis but also for determination of antimicrobial susceptibility and planning of treatment. In the absence of prior antibiotic therapy, a total of three blood culture sets, ideally with the first separated from the last by at least 1 h, should be obtained from different venipuncture sites over 24 h. If the cultures remain negative after 48 to 72 h, two or three additional blood cultures, including a lysis-centrifugation culture, should be obtained, and the laboratory should be asked to pursue fastidious microorganisms by prolonging incubation time and performing special subcultures. Infectious disease expert consultation can be extremely helpful in these circumstances.

Patients with an acute presentation of IE (often injection drug users) require empiric therapy before culture results. For the treatment of native valve endocarditis (NVE), empiric treatment while awaiting culture results is based on common microbiologic isolates, i.e., staphylococci (20% to 35%) and streptococci (viridans, 30% to 40%; other, 15% to 25%; and enterococci, 5% to 18%), with occasional cases due to gram-negative bacilli. The combination of penicillin, a penicillinase-resistant penicillin, and an aminoglycoside will provide effective empiric coverage for a majority of cases. The antibiotics nafcillin plus oxacillin and aminoglycosides, e.g., gentamicin, may not be adequate coverage for enterococci, hence the addition of penicillin G pending culture results. Vancomycin should be an alternate drug in situations in which community-acquired methicillin-resistant *S. aureus* (MRSA) IE occurs in at least 10% to 15% of cases and for those allergic to penicillin.

Once the infecting organism is isolated and antimicrobial susceptibility is determined, the antibiotic regimen should be adjusted accordingly. Discussion of therapeutic approaches to the treatment of the more common bacterial isolates follows.

Nonenterococcal Streptococcal Endocarditis

Approximately 30% to 55% of all cases of IE are caused by penicillin-susceptible streptococci. *Viridans streptococci,* a heterogeneous group of organisms, accounts for the majority, with the remainder caused by group G, nonenterococcal group D, and other streptococci. For these patients, there are several recommended regimens (Table 25-2). For most patients with highly sensitive streptococci (MIC for penicillin, <0.1 μg/mL), single drug therapy for 4 weeks or a combination of penicillin and gentamicin for 2 weeks has replaced 4 weeks of penicillin given with streptomycin for 2 weeks as the conventional therapy. Regimens containing β-lactam antibiotics achieve cure in at least 98% of cases. Vancomycin appears to be as effective as penicillin when given for 4 weeks in viridans streptococcal IE.

Gentamicin is now preferred to streptomycin in combined regimens because of its broad clinical use, approved intravenous or intramuscular route of administration, and the widespread availability of serum drug levels. Also, streptomycin is becoming less and less available for general use. In vitro and clinical data have demonstrated the efficacy of gentamicin combined with penicillin in streptococcal IE. Some authorities continue to recommend penicillin for 4 weeks with gentamicin for the initial 2 weeks for sensitive *S. viridans* IE if the course is complicated or the duration of disease is longer than 3 months. Consideration of a patient's age, renal status, eighth cranial nerve function, and drug allergy guide the choice of therapy. Outpatient treatment, for all or part of therapy, has become feasible with current regimens. The largest experience with outpatient therapy is with ceftriaxone for sensitive viridans streptococcal endocarditis; however, staphylococcal, enterococcal, and some gram-negative diseases may be suitable for outpatient therapy with a variety of antibiotics. Therapy with ceftriaxone and netilmicin is synergistic against susceptible *S. viridans* and is more effective than either agent alone in an animal model of IE,

TABLE 25-2 Antibiotic Regimens for Treatment of Infective Endocarditis

Anatomic site, diagnosis, modifying circumstances	Etiologies (usual)	Suggested regimens		Adjunct diagnostic or therapeutic measures and comments
		Primary	Alternative	

Infective endocarditis—Native valve—empirical rx awaiting cultures NOTE: Diagnostic criteria include evidence of continuous bacteremia (multiple positive blood cultures), new murmur (worsening of old murmur) of valvular insufficiency, definite emboli, and echocardiographic (transthoracic or transesophageal) evidence of valvular vegetations. Review: *NEJM* 345:1318, 2001.

Anatomic site, diagnosis, modifying circumstances	Etiologies (usual)	Primary	Alternative	Adjunct diagnostic or therapeutic measures and comments
Valvular or congenital heart disease including mitral valve prolapse but no modifying circumstances	Viridans strep 30–40%, "other" strep 15–25%, enterococci 5–18%, staphylococci 20–35%	[(Pen G 20 mU qd IV, continuous or div. q4h) or (AMP 12 gm qd IV, continuous or div. q4h) + (nafcillin or oxacillin 2.0 gm q4h IV) + gentamicin 1.0 mg/kg q8h IM or IV, not once daily dosing)]	Vanco 15 mg/kg* q12h IV (not to exceed 2 gm qd unless serum levels monitored) + gentamicin 1.0 mg/kg* q8h IM or IV	If patient not acutely ill and not in heart failure, we prefer to wait for blood culture results. If initial 3 blood cultures neg. after 24–48 hrs, obtain 2–3 more blood cultures before empiric rx started. Nafcillin/oxacillin + gentamicin may not be adequate coverage of enterococci; hence addition of penicillin G pending cultures. When blood cultures +, modify regimen from empiric to specific based on organism, in vitro susceptibilities, clinical experience.

Infective endocarditis—Native valve—culture positive (Consensus opinion on treatment by organism: *JAMA* 274:1706, 1995) (Review: *NEJM* 345:1318, 2001)

Anatomic site, diagnosis, modifying circumstances	Etiologies (usual)	Primary	Alternative	Adjunct diagnostic or therapeutic measures and comments
S. viridans, S. bovis with penicillin G MIC ≤ 0.1 μg/mL	*S. viridans, S. bovis*	[(Pen G 12–18 mU/d IV, continuous or q4h ×2 wks) PLUS (gentamicin IV 1 mg/kg q8h IV ×2 wks)] OR (Pen G 12–18 mU/d	(Ceftriaxone 2.0 gm qd IV + gentamicin 1 mg/kg IV q8h both×2 wks) If allergy pen G or ceftriax, use vanco 30 mg/kg/d	Also effective: (ceftriaxone 2.0 gm qd) + (netilmicin[NUS] 4 mg/kg qd) ×2 wks (*CID 21:1406, 1995*) Target gent levels: peak 3 μg/mL, trough <1 μg/mL. If very obese pt, recommend consultation for dosage adjustment.

	IV, continuous or q4h ×4 wks) OR (ceftriaxone 2.0 gm qd IV ×4 wks)	in 2 div. doses to 2 gm/d max unless serum levels measured ×4 wks	Infuse vanco over ≥1 hr to avoid "red man" syndrome. *S. bovis* suggests occult bowel pathology. Since relapse rate may be greater in pts ill for >3 mos. prior to start of rx, the penicillin-gentamicin synergism theoretically may be advantageous in this group.
S. viridans, S. bovis with penicillin G MIC >0.1 to <0.5 µg/mL	Pen G 18 mU/d IV (continuous or q4h) ×4 wks PLUS gentamicin 1 mg/kg q8h IV ×2 wks	Vanco 30 mg/kg/d IV in 2 div. doses to max. 2 gm/d unless serum levels documented ×4 wks	*S. viridans, S. bovis,* nutritionally variant streptococci, tolerant strep[†] Can use cefazolin for pen G in pt with allergy that is not IgE-mediated (e.g., anaphylaxis). Alternatively, can use vanco. (*See comment above on gent and vanco*)

HEART/Infective endocarditis—Native valve—culture positive

For *S. viridans* or *S. bovis* with pen G MIC ≥1.0 and enterococci susceptible to AMP/pen G, vanco, gentamicin NOTE: Inf. Dis. consultation suggested	"Susceptible" enterococci, *S. viridans, S. bovis,* nutritionally variant streptococci [(Pen G 18–30 mu/24h IV, continuous or q4h ×4–6 wks PLUS gentamicin 1–1.5 mg/kg q8h IV ×4–6 wks]) OR (AMP 12 gm/d IV, continuous or q4h + gent as above ×4–6 wks	Vanco 30 mg/kg/d IV in 2 div. doses to max. of 2 gm/d unless serum levels measured PLUS gentamicin 1–1.5 mg/kg q8h IV ×4–6 wks	4 wks of rx if symptoms <3 mos.; 6 wks of rx if symptoms >3 mos. Vanco for pen-allergic pts; do not use cephalosporins. Do not give gent once-daily for enterococcal endocarditis. Target gent levels: peak 3 µg/mL, trough < 1 µg/mL. Vanco target serum levels: peak 20–50 µg/mL, trough 5–12 µg/mL. NOTE: Because of ↑ frequency of resistance (*see below*), all enterococci causing endocarditis should be tested in vitro for susceptibility to penicillin, β-lactamase production, gent susceptibility and vanco susceptibility.

(continued)

TABLE 25-2 (continued) Antibiotic Regimens for Treatment of Infective Endocarditis

Anatomic site, diagnosis, modifying circumstances	Etiologies (usual)	Suggested regimens		Adjunct diagnostic or therapeutic measures and comments
		Primary	Alternative	
Enterococci MIC streptomycin >2000 µg/mL; MIC genatamicin >500–2000 µg/mL; no resistance to penicillin	Enterococci, high-level aminoglycoside resistance	Pen G or AMP IV as above ×8–12 wks (approx. 50% cure)	If prolonged pen G/AMP fails, consider surgical removal of infected valve See comment	10–25% E. faecalis and 45–50% E. faecium resistant to high gent levels. May be sensitive to streptomycin, check MIC. Case report of success with combination of AMP, IMP, and vanco (Scand J Inf Dis 29:628, 1997).
Enterococci β-lactamase production test is positive and no gentamicin resistance	Enterococci, penicillin resistance	AM/SB 3.0 gm q6h IV PLUS gentamicin 1–1.5 mg/kg q8h IV ×4–6 wks	AM/SB 3.0 gm IV q6h PLUS vanco 30 mg/kg/d IV in 2 div. doses (check levels if >2 gm) ×4–6 wks	β-lactamase not detected by MIC tests with standard inocula. Detection requires testing with the chromogenic cephalosporin nitrocefin. Once-daily gentamicin rx not efficacious in animal model of E. faecalis endocardtis (JAC 39:519, 1997). Review of aminoglycoside dosage regimens. JAC 49:437, 2002.
Enterococci β-lactamase test neg.: pen G MIC >16 µg/mL; no gentamicin resistance	Enterococci, intrinsic pen G/AMP resistance	Vanco 30 mg/kg/d IV in 2 div. doses (check levels if >2 gm) PLUS gent 1–1.5 mg/kg q8h (no single dose) ×4–6 wks		Desired vanco serum levels: peak 20–50 µg/mL, trough 5–12 µg/mL

Enterococci Pen/AMP resistant + high-level gent/strep resistant + vanco resistant; usually VRE Consultation suggested	Enterococci, vanco-resistant, usually *E. faecium*	No reliable effective rx. Can try quinupristin/dalfopristin (Synercid) or linezolid‡	Teicoplanin active against a subset of vanco-resistant enterococci. Teicoplanin is not available in U.S.	Synercid activity limited to *E. faecium* and is usually bacteriostatic, therefore expect high relapse rate. Dose: 7.5 mg/kg IV (via central line) q8h. Linezolid active most enterococci, also bacteriostatic. Dose: 600 mg 2x/d. IV or PO.
Staphylococcal endocarditis Aortic and/or mitral valve infection	*Staph. aureus*, methicillin-sensitive	Nafcillin (oxacillin) 2 gm q4h IV ×4–6 wks PLUS gentamicin 1.0 mg/kg q8h IV ×3–5d	[(Cefazolin 2.0 gm q8h IV ×4–6 wks PLUS (gentamicin 1.0 mg/kg q8h IV ×3–5 d.)] OR Vanco 30 mg/kg/d IV in 2 div. doses (check levels if >2 gm/d) ×4–6 wks	Avoid cephalosporins in pts with immediate allergic reaction to penicillin; in allergic pt, vanco may not be as effective as cefazolin. No definitive data, pro or con, on once daily gentamicin for *S. aureus* endocarditis. At present, favor q8h dosing ×3–5d. ↑ recognition of IV catheter-associated *S. aureus* endocarditis. May need TEE to detect endocarditis. 23% of *S. aureus* bacteremia in association with IV catheter had endocarditis (*CID* 115:106 & 115, 1999); if TEE neg. only need 2 wks of therapy in this series.
Tricuspid valve infection (usually IVDUs): MSSA	*Staph. aureus*, methicillin-sensitive	Nafcillin (oxacillin) 2 gm q4h IV PLUS gentamicin 1 mg/kg q8h IV ×2 wks	If penicillin allergy: Not clear. High failure rate with 2 wks of vanco + gentamicin (*CID* 33: 120, 2001) Can try longer duration rx of vanco ± RIF (if sensitive).	2-week regimen not recommended if metastatic infection (e.g., osteo) or left-sided endocarditis. Cloxacillin IV without gentamicin 89% successful (*AnIM* 125:969, 1996). 2 reports of success with 4-week oral regimen: CIP 750 mg bid + RIF 300 mg bid. Less than 10% pts had MRSA (*Ln 2*: 1071, 1989; *AJM* 101:68, 1996).

(continued)

TABLE 25-2 (continued) Antibiotic Regimens for Treatment of Infective Endocarditis

Anatomic site, diagnosis, modifying circumstances	Etiologies (usual)	Suggested regimens		Adjunct diagnostic or therapeutic measures and comments
		Primary	Alternative	
Methicillin resistance (MRSA)	*Staph. aureus,* methicillin-resistant	Vanco 30 mg/kg/d IV in 2 div. doses (check levels if >2 gm/d) x4–6 wks	Fails/intolerant to vanco, can try either quinu/dalfo or linezolid#	For MRSA, no difference in duration of bateremia or fever between pts rx with vanco or vanco + RIF (*AnIM* 115:674, 1991).
Slow-growing fastidious Gm-neg. bacilli	HACEK group (*see comments*) (*Mayo Clin Proc* 72:532, 1997)	Ceftriaxone 2.0 gm qd IV x4 wks	AMP 12 gm qd (continuous or div. q4h) x4 wks + gentamicin 1.0 mg/kg q8h IV or IM x4 wks	HACEK (acronym for *Hemophilus parainfluenzae, H. aphrophilus, Actinobacillus, Cardiobacterium, Eikenella, Kingella). H. aphrophilus* resistant to vanco, clinda and methicillin. Penicillinase-positive HACEK organisms should be susceptible to AM/SB + gentamicin. For hemophilus, see *CID* 24:1087, 1997.
Bartonella species *Medicine* 80:245, 2001; *CID* 31: 131, 2000	*B. henselae, B. quintana*	Bacteremia & NO endocarditis: (Doxy 100 mg PO bid) or (erythro 500 mg PO qid) or (azithro 500 mg PO qd)—all for 4–6 wks	For endocarditis: As for no endocarditis + either gentamicin or ceftriaxone in 1st 2–3 wks. Rx 4–6 mos. May require valve replacement.	Dx: Microimmunofluorescent antibody titer ≥1:1600; blood cultures only occ. positive. Surgery: Without surgery, 1/3 cured; surgery + anti-infectives, 81% cure. *B. quintana* transmitted by body lice among homeless; asymptomatic colonization of RBCs described (*Ln* 360:226, 2002).

Infective endocarditis—culture negative

Fever, valvular disease, and ECHO vegetations ± emboli and neg. cultures

T. whippleii, Q fever, psittacosis, brucellosis, bartonella (*see above*), fungi

Emphasis is on diagnosis. See specific organism for treatment regimens.

For Q fever, see *CID* 33:1347, 2001. 4 pts with afebrile culture-neg, endocarditis had *T. whippleii* identified by PCR of resected heart valves (*AnIM* 131:112 & 144, 1999). Review Whipple's endocarditis: *CID* 33:1309, 2001.

Infective endocarditis—Prosthetic valve—empiric therapy (cultures pending)

Early (<2 months post-op)

S. epidermidis, *S. aureus* Rarely, *Enterobacteriaceae*, diphtheroids, fungi

Vanco 15 mg/kg q12h IV + gentamicin 1.0 mg/kg q8h IV + RIF 600 mg PO daily

Early surgical consultation advised. Watch for evidence of heart failure.

Late (>2 months post-op)

S. epidermidis, *S. viridans*, enterococci, *S. aureus*

Infective endocarditis—Prosthetic valve—positive blood cultures

Staph. epidermidis

Surgical consultation advised: retrospective analysis shows↓ mortality of pts with *S. aureus* endocarditis if valve replaced during antibiotic rx (*CID* 26:1302 & 1310, 1998); also, retrospective study showed ↑ risk of death 2⁰ neuro events in assoc. with Coumadin rx (*ArIM* 159:473, 1999)

(Vanco 15 mg/kg q12h IV + RIF 300 mg q8h PO) ×6 wks + gentamicin 1.0 mg q8h IV ×14 d

If *S. epidermidis* is susceptible to nafcillin/oxacillin in vitro (not common), then substitute nafcillin (or oxacillin) for vanco.

(continued)

TABLE 25-2 (continued) Antibiotic Regimens for Treatment of Infective Endocarditis

| Anatomic site, diagnosis, modifying circumstances | Etiologies (usual) | Suggested regimens | | Adjunct diagnostic or therapeutic measures and comments |
		Primary	Alternative	
	Staph. aureus	Methicillin sensitive: (Nafcillin 2.0 gm IV + RIF 300 mg q4h PO) ×6 wks + gentamicin 1.0 mg/kg q8h IV ×14 d. Methicillin resistant: (Vanco 1.0 gm q12h IV + RIF 300 mg q8h PO) ×6 wks + gentamicin 1.0 mg/kg q8h IV ×14 d.		
		See infective endocarditis, native valve, culture positive		
	Strep viridans, enterococci	Aminoglycoside (tobra if P. aeruginosa) + (AP Pen or P Ceph 3 AP or P Ceph 4)		In theory, could substitute CIP for APAG, but no clinical data.
	Enterobacteriaceae or P. aeruginosa			
	Candida, Aspergillus	Ampho B ± an azole, e.g., fluconazole		High mortality. Valve replacement plus antifungal therapy standard therapy but some success with antifungal therapy alone (CID 22:262, 1996).

*Assumes estimated creatinine clearance ≥ 80 mL/min.

†Tolerant streptococci = MBC 32-fold greater than MIC.

‡Three interesting recent reports: (1) successful rx of vanco-resistant E. faecium prosthetic valve endocarditis with Synercid without change in MIC (CID 25:163, 1997); (2) resistance to Synercid emerged during therapy of E. faecium bacteremia (CID 24:90, 1997); and (3) super-infection with E. faecalis occurred during Synercid rx of E. faecium (CID 24:91, 1997).

#Quinupristin/dalfopristin (Synercid) 7.5 mg/kg IV (via central venous line) q8h, Linezolid 600 mg IV or PO q12h.

NOTE: All dosage recommendations are for adults (unless otherwise indicated) and assume normal renal function.

Source: Adapted from Gilbert DN, Moellering RC Jr, Sande MA (eds): The Sanford Guide to Antimicrobial Therapy 2003, 33rd ed. Hyde Park, VT, Antimicrobial Therapy, 2003, p 18.

raising the possibility of 2 week once-daily therapy of IE. A recent study has concluded that a 2-week regimen of once-a-day ceftriaxone with gentamicin is as efficacious and safe for the treatment of penicillin-susceptible streptococcus endocarditis as a 4-week regimen of ceftriaxone monotherapy, and many experts offer this alternative treatment regimen.

From 15% to 20% of *S. viridans* require more than 0.1 µg/mL of penicillin for inhibition. Endocarditis caused by these organisms should be treated with penicillin for 4 weeks, combined with gentamicin for the first 2 weeks, although data are limited and clinical trials showing superior efficacy of the combined regimen over a single agent are lacking. Endocarditis due to penicillin-resistant streptococci (MIC >0.5 µg/mL) and nutritionally variant streptococci *(Streptococcus adjacens, Streptococcus defectivus)* should be treated with the antibiotic combinations recommended for enterococcal IE.

Enterococcal Endocarditis

Enterococci may cause subacute or acute IE. This occurs most commonly in women of childbearing age after obstetric procedures and in older men. This group of organisms was formerly classified as group D streptococci, but is now considered a separate genus, *Enterococcus.* Enterococci account for 5% to 20% of isolates from patients with IE. Enterococcal isolates from patients with bacterial IE include *Enterococcus faecium, Enterococcus faecalis,* and *Enterococcus durans. Streptococcus bovis* and *Streptococcus equines* are group D streptococci that may be confused with enterococci, but these streptococci usually are highly sensitive to penicillin and should be treated the same way as infections caused by *S. viridans.*

Enterococci are usually relatively resistant and highly tolerant to penicillin, exhibiting MICs of 1 to 4 µg/mL and minimum bactericidal concentrations equal to or greater than 100 µg/mL. Similar tolerance has been demonstrated for vancomycin. The cephalosporins are not clinically useful for treating these infections, although some strains of *E. faecalis* are susceptible to imipenem plus cilastatin. The MIC for penicillin, ampicillin, and vancomycin should be determined for enterococci causing IE. β-Lactamase–producing strains of enterococci have been reported over the past decade, and therapy for infections with these organisms would include vancomycin or ampicillin plus sulbactam in combination with gentamicin.

Synergistic killing has been demonstrated in vitro for most enterococci with the combination of penicillin or vancomycin and streptomycin or gentamicin. However, enterococcal isolates with high-level (MIC ≥ 500 to 2000 µg/mL) resistance to these aminoglycosides are now isolated with increasing frequency. Bactericidal synergy between a cell wall active antibiotic and aminoglycosides is lost in the presence of high-level resistance. Testing for high-level resistance to streptomycin and gentamicin is currently recommended for enterococcal IE; the other available aminoglycosides are not useful if a high-level resistance to gentamicin is demonstrated. Therefore, there is a need for newer aminoglycosides that do not incur resistance. One relatively promising aminoglycoside is arbekacin, (currently available only in Japan). This aminoglycoside is effective in vitro against 40% of the enterococci that possess the aac(6′)-Ie-aph(2″)-Ia resistance gene. This gene is by far the most prevalent gentamicin resistance gene found in clinical enterococcal isolates.

However, treatment for IE due to strains with high-level aminoglycoside resistance continues to be controversial. The standard recommendations include long-term therapy for 8 to 12 weeks with high-dose penicillin (20 to 40 million units intravenously daily in divided doses), ampicillin (2 to 3 g intravenously every 4 h or by continuous infusion), or vancomycin for patients intolerant of β-lactams. A strong consideration for valve replacement should be given for patients failing medical therapy.

Enterococci resistant to vancomycin are an increasing problem in the United States. Infection with these organisms, which are also often resistant to penicillins, has been associated with nosocomial acquisition, severe underlying disease, and previous use of antibiotics. There is no consensus about treatment of IE with multiresistant enterococci.

The recommended first therapy for vancomycin-resistant endocarditis is a high-dose ampicillin or penicillin (18 to 30 g/day) with an aminoglycoside, which may be effective if the MIC is in the range of 32 to 64. Due to the increasing prevalence of vancomycin-resistant endocarditis, there are many drugs currently under trial. Combinations of drugs have been used with some success in animal models of IE.

There are many ongoing studies to assess the antibiotic combination of quinupristin-dalfopristin (Synercid), a streptogramin combination recently approved by the U.S. Food and Drug Administration (FDA) for use in vancomycin-resistant endocarditis infections. Quinupristin plus dalfopristin seems to be a very promising drug for the treatment of vancomycin-resistant endocarditis in combination with other antimicrobials such as ampicillin, amoxicillin, doxycycline, and rifampin as indicated in various murine models. Nevertheless, quinupristin-dalfopristin is still only bacteriostatic, and in vitro resistance is a concern.

Another drug recently approved for the treatment of vancomycin-resistant endocarditis is the oxazolidinone, linezolid. A combination of linezolid with a second bactericidal antimicrobial agent seems to offer promise for the treatment of IE.

The following drugs are under investigation to be used alone or in combination for vancomycin-resistant endocarditis (MIC of ampicillin, >64) if available therapies are ineffective: teicoplanin, daptomycin, LY333328, trovafloxacin, and ramoplanin. A triple combination of high-dose penicillin, vancomycin, and gentamicin looks promising in animal models of endocarditis. Other drugs, such as evernimicin, glycylcyclines, and ketolides, are also undergoing clinical trials. Infectious disease consultation is recommended for patients with resistant enterococcal IE.

When penicillin or vancomycin can be combined with gentamicin or streptomycin, 4 weeks of therapy appears adequate for most patients. Six weeks is recommended if symptoms have been present for longer that 3 months or infection is on a prosthetic valve.

The possibility of outpatient treatment for enterococcus is also being studied. To investigate outpatient therapy for enterococcal endocarditis, a recent study compared the efficacy of teicoplanin combined with gentamicin given once a day with the standard treatment of ampicillin plus gentamicin given thrice daily. The investigators found that the combination of teicoplanin with gentamicin at 4.5 mg/kg given once a day has an efficacy equal to the "gold standard," ampicillin plus gentamicin at 1 mg/kg thrice daily. This study showed that teicoplanin plus gentamicin administered once a day may be a useful home therapy for selected cases of enterococcal endocarditis.

Endocarditis Caused by *S. aureus*

Staphylococcus aureus generally causes acute bacterial IE in patients with no prior history of valvular disease. It is the infecting agent in 25% to 45% of IE cases and may be more common at community hospitals than in university referral centers. Among intravenous drug users with IE, staphylococci account for 65% to 82% of cases. Standard therapy is a penicillinase-resistant penicillin such as nafcillin or oxacillin or a first-generation cephalosporin. The penicillins are favored because in vitro cephalosporins appear more sensitive to β-lactamase at the high organism densities (inoculum effect) expected in a valvular vegetation. It is not clear that this inoculum effect is important clinically.

Vancomycin is recommended for patients with severe allergy to β-lactams. For methicillin-sensitive *S. aureus* (MSSA) IE, there is evidence that vancomycin is not as rapidly bactericidal as nafcillin and may have higher failure rates in IE. Karchmer cautioned against using vancomycin because of dosing convenience; allergy testing and penicillin desensitization in appropriate patients should be attempted. Vancomycin is the drug of choice for IE due to MRSA, which continues to increase in the United States. The response of patients with MRSA IE appears to be slower than that of patients treated with β-lactams for MSSA disease.

For MRSA endocarditis refractory to vancomycin, rifampin or gentamicin (or both) can be added. Other possible drugs include minocycline, trimethoprim plus sulfamethoxazole, and ciprofloxacin plus rifampin, although experience in humans with these drugs is limited.

The recently licensed combination streptogramin therapy, quinupristin plus dalfopristin, has been shown to have a potential benefit when combined with a β-lactam in vitro and in rats with MRSA endocarditis. The study concluded that quinupristin plus dalfopristin in addition to cefepime could be of use for the treatment of severely ill patients who require multiple-antibiotic therapy. Another combination of quinupristin plus dalfopristin and rifampin was found to be effective in vivo.

The new antibiotic, linezolid, was recently tested in a staphylococcal endocarditis rabbit model, which showed that, like vancomycin, linezolid is effective for the treatment of experimental staphylococcal endocarditis in rabbits when plasma drug levels remain above the MIC.

Another potential therapeutic agent is lysostaphin, a potent staphylolytic agent with activity against oxacillin-resistant and -susceptible *S. aureus* (ORSA) and vancomycin–intermediate-susceptible *S. aureus* (VISA). Lysostaphin was shown to be an effective drug against experimental endocarditis due to ORSA and VISA; however, there was concern about the development of resistance. In a recent study, a β-lactam was added to lysostaphin, which easily overcame the resistance. This study suggested that lysostaphin plus nafcillin or oxacillin is a possible therapeutic option to suppress resistance and to promote antibiotic synergy.

MSSA is killed more rapidly in vitro and in animal models of IE with the combination of a penicillinase-resistant penicillin and gentamicin. In a large clinical trial, the combination of nafcillin and gentamicin for 2 weeks was associated with a more rapid clearing of bacteremia in staphylococcal IE as compared with nafcillin alone, but without improved survival and with more renal toxicity. Gentamicin is currently recommended as an optional addition to a β-lactam agent for the initial 3 to 5 days of treatment. A short course of gentamicin can be added to vancomycin for MSSA or MRSA IE, although nephrotoxicity may be more common with this combination.

Staphylococcal IE in intravenous drug users usually involves the tricuspid valve and has a significantly better prognosis than left-side disease from *S. aureus,* with a mortality rate of less than 5%. Two-week antibiotic regimens combining nafcillin plus oxacillin and an aminoglycoside have been used successfully in selected stable patients with tricuspid valve IE, with cure rates greater than 90%. There were also two studies that tested the combination of ciprofloxacin plus rifampin orally for 4 weeks for uncomplicated right-side *S. aureus* IE in patients with drug addiction. These studies also demonstrated cure rates to greater than 90%. There are few clinical data on the efficacy of cephalosporins or vancomycin in 2-week regimens, and these drugs are not recommended.

Rifampin is an extremely potent antistaphylococcal drug that achieves excellent tissue and intracellular concentrations. Resistance emerges rapidly when used as a single agent but usually not when combined with other effective drugs. In vitro, the effect of rifampin in combination with β-lactams or vancomycin is variable depending on experimental conditions. There was no advantage to vancomycin and rifampin over vancomycin alone in a clinical study of MRSA IE. Rifampin is not recommended for native valve staphylococcal endocarditis, although it does have a role in the treatment of prosthetic valve infections.

Endocarditis Caused by Less Common Pathogens

The optimal therapy for IE resulting from less common causes is still not adequately defined. HACEK organisms (haemophilus species: *Haemophilus parainfluenzae, H. aphrophilus,* and *H. paraphrophilus; Actinobacillus actinomycetemcomitans; Cardiobacterium hominis; Eikenella corrodens;* and *Kingella kingae*) account for 5% to 10% of native value IE. Third-generation cephalosporin (ceftirosone) is the principal drug used for these cases, 2 g once daily intravenously or intramuscularly for 4 weeks. Aminoglycosides and fluoroquinolones are bactericidal for *Bartonella* species. However, most patients with reported cases of IE due to *Bartonella* species are treated with a β-lactam antibiotic and an aminoglycoside but still require valve-replacement surgery for cure. Doxycycline with a second antimicrobial agent, often given for 3 to 4 years until immunoglobulin G antibody titers drop below 1:400, has been the recommended treatment for IE due to Q fever. A prospective study among 35 patients with Q fever–infective endocarditis suggested that the combination of doxycycline and hydroxychloroquine (median duration, 26 months) is associated with a lower rate of relapse than is therapy with doxycycline and a fluoroquinolone for a median of 60 months. Eradication of Q fever IE usually requires valve-replacement surgery, although relapse of infection on the replaced valve may occur. Infectious disease expert consultation is usually helpful in developing treatment regimens for these relatively unusual organisms.

In the absence of clinical clues to a specific cause, therapy for culture-negative NVE should be individualized and generally includes penicillin, ampicillin, ceftriaxone, or vancomycin, often in combination with an aminoglycoside.

Anticoagulation and Infective Endocarditis

Anticoagulant therapy has not been shown to prevent embolization in IE and may increase the risk of intracerebral hemorrhage. Anticoagulant therapy for

NVE is restricted to patients with a clear indication separate from IE; in the presence of intracranial hemorrhage or mycotic aneurysm, anticoagulant therapy should be suspended until the complications have resolved. In general, patients with IE involving a prosthetic heart valve that requires maintenance anticoagulation are cautiously given continued anticoagulant therapy during treatment of prosthetic valve endocarditis. However, in the presence of central nervous system emboli with hemorrhage, temporary discontinuation of anticoagulant therapy is appropriate.

Patients with *S. aureus* prosthetic valve endocarditis who are receiving anticoagulant therapy are particularly susceptible to central nervous system hemorrhage; indirect evidence from uncontrolled studies in a limited number of patients has suggested that anticoagulant therapy generally should be suspended in such patients during the acute phase of the illness. If cardiac surgery for IE is planned, warfarin may be discontinued and replaced with heparin to allow more rapid reversal of anticoagulation at the time of surgery. The role (if any) of aspirin and/or clopidogrel for the prevention of embolism in IE is still unclear.

The indications for anticoagulant therapy when systemic embolism occurs during the course of IE involving a native or bioprosthetic heart valve are uncertain. The therapeutic decision should consider comorbid factors, including atrial fibrillation, evidence of left atrial thrombus, evidence and size of valvular vegetations, and in particular the success of antibiotic therapy in controlling the IE.

Indication for Surgery

Valvular surgery can be life-saving for certain groups of patients with endocarditis. There is consensus that surgery is indicated in patients with active IE who have one or more of the following complications:

- Congestive heart failure that is directly related to valve dysfunction
- Persistent or uncontrolled infection while receiving appropriate antimicrobial therapy, including evidence of perivalvular extension
- Recurrent emboli, particularly in the presence of large vegetations

Several other complications are considered relative indications for surgery in selected patients with IE:

- Evidence of perivalvular infection, such as intracardiac abscess or fistula formation; this complication is usually assumed to be present in patients with mechanical prostheses
- Rupture of a sinus of Valsalva aneurysm
- Fungal endocarditis
- Endocarditis due to highly resistant microorganisms
- Relapse after a course of adequate antimicrobial therapy, particularly in prosthetic valve endocarditis (PVE)
- Culture-negative IE with fever more than 10 days after starting empiric therapy
- Large (>10 mm in diameter) hypermobile vegetations with increased risk of embolism

Most of the clinical indications for surgical treatment of endocarditis are not absolute. The risks and benefits and the timing of surgical treatment therefore must be individualized. A detailed discussion of indications for surgery in infective endocarditis is beyond the scope of this chapter.

Prophylaxis for Endocarditis

Bacteria introduced by activities of normal living, invasive medical procedures, and disease invade the bloodstream daily. Even so, endocarditis is a comparatively rare disease. When it occurs, there are often predisposing factors. Animal models have helped to identify these factors.

It has been demonstrated that the intravenous injection of a large bacterial inoculum into rabbits would cause only a transient bacteremia; normal valvular endothelium was not infected. Endocarditis would not result unless a substrate of nonbacterial thrombotic endocarditis had been induced by damaging the valvular endothelium with a catheter before inoculation. In humans, such damage can be the result of several factors. Turbulent blood flow (through a damaged prosthetic or regurgitant valve, a congenital cardiac defect, or even idiopathic hypertrophic subaortic stenosis) creates jets of flow whose impact can destroy the integrity of the endothelium, expose collagen, and result in platelet activation and adhesion. Such jets create low-pressure "sinks" distal to the origin of the jet into which bacteria are deposited.

The concept of endocarditis prophylaxis is based on identifying situations in which patients have predisposing factors for the development of endocarditis. Approximately 75% of patients with endocarditis have preexisting cardiac abnormalities. Although precise figures are lacking, the ranking of risk can be based on the frequency of each preexisting cardiac disorder in large series of patients with endocarditis who are compared with the general population. Table 25-3 lists estimates of relative risk.

Certain procedures are also associated with different amounts of risk caused by transient bacteremia. For example, dental procedures for a predisposed patient have been estimated to carry a wide-ranging risk from 9 to 1:533. For patients with prosthetic valves, the risk theoretically could be up to 1.5:100. The overall risk for endocarditis is less than 1% for each procedure, even with no antibiotic prophylaxis. However, although it has generally been thought that dental procedures carry some risk for susceptible patients, a recent population-based, case-control study concluded that dental treatment does not seem to be a risk factor for IE, even in patients with valvular abnormalities. To date, no prospective, randomized investigation has been done to answer this question, and it is not likely that one with sufficient power could be easily organized. The AHA Committee on Rheumatic Fever and Endocarditis has organized an international conference on this topic for mid-2004 to develop an international consensus on the role, if any, of antibiotic prophylaxis.

A recent article has highlighted the controversy and framed the discussion succinctly. Skepticism for continuing with prophylaxis exists because (a) there have been no published, controlled clinical trials; (b) transient bacteremias are common events; (c) individuals at risk for endocarditis are not easily identified; (d) prophylaxis provides a false sense of security for the patient and the health care provider; (e) the use of prophylactic antibiotics raises potential for increasing antimicrobial resistance; (f) inconvenience to the patient and the health care provider; (g) cost to the patient and society; and (h) poor compliance by the patient and the health care providers. The investigators also provided various reasons to promote antibiotic prophylaxis: (a) endocarditis results in high morbidity and mortality; (b) prophylaxis is a long-standing medical practice; (c) endocarditis prophylaxis follows logical prophylaxis principles (limited targeted population, limited procedures, limited pathogens, short-course regimens, reasonably safe, and inexpensive); (d) animal models support prophylaxis; and (e) medicolegal concerns abound.

TABLE 25-3 Recommendations for Prophylaxis of Endocarditis*

Cardiac conditions

   Endocarditis prophylaxis recommended
      High-risk category[†]
         Prosthetic cardiac valves, including bioprosthetic and homograft valves
         Previous bacterial endocarditis
         Complex cyanotic congenital heart disease (single-ventricle states,
            transposition of the great arteries, tetralogy of Fallot)
         Surgically constructed systemic pulmonary shunts or conduits
      Moderate-risk category
         Most congenital cardiac malformations (other than above and below)
         Acquired valvar dysfunction (rheumatic heart disease)
         Hypertrophic cardiomyopathy
         Mitral valve prolapse with valvular regurgitation and/or thickened
            leaflets
   Endocarditis prophylaxis not recommended
      Negligible-risk category (no greater risk than the general population)
         Isolated secundum atrial septal defect
         Surgical repair of atrial septal defect, ventricular septal defect, or
            patent ductus arteriosis (without residual beyond 6 mo)
         Previous coronary artery bypass graft surgery
         Mitral valve prolapse without valvular regurgitation
         Physiologic, functional, or innocent heart murmurs
         Previous Kawasaki disease without valvular dysfunction
         Previous rheumatic fever without valvular dysfunction
         Cardiac pacemakers (intravascular and epicardial) and implanted
            defibrillators
Procedures
   Endocarditis prophylaxis recommended (for moderate- and high-risk
      cardiac conditions)
      Dental[†]
         Dental extractions
         Periodontal procedures, including surgery scaling and root planing,
            probing, and recall maintenance
         Dental implant placement and reimplantation of avulsed teeth
         Endodontic (root canal) instrumentation or surgery beyond the apex
         Subgingival placement of antibiotic fibers or strips
         Initial placement of orthodontic bands but not brackets
         Intraligamentary local anesthetic injections
         Prophylactic cleaning of teeth or implants where bleeding is anticipated
         Taking of oral radiographs
         Orthodontic appliance adjustment
         Shedding of primary teeth
      Respiratory tract
         Tonsillectomy and/or adenoidectomy
         Surgical operations that involve respiratory mucosa
         Bronchoscopy with rigid bronchoscope
      Gastrointestinal tract
         Sclerotherapy for esophageal varices
         Esophageal stricture dilation
         Endoscopic retrograde cholangiography with biliary obstruction
         Biliary tract surgery
         Surgical operations that involve intestinal mucosa
      Genitourinary tract
         Prostatic surgery
         Cystoscopy
         Urethral dilation

(continued)

TABLE 25-3 *(continued)* Recommendations for Prophylaxis of Endocarditis*

Endocarditis prophylaxis not recommended
  Dental
    Restorative dentistry (operative and prosthodontic) with or without
      retraction cord
    Local anesthetic injections (non-intraligamentary)
    Intracanal endodontic treatment; post placement and buildup
    Placement of rubber dams
    Postoperative suture removal
    Placement of removable prosthodontic or orthodontic appliances
    Taking of oral impressions
    Fluoride treatments
  Respiratory tract
    Endotracheal intubation
    Bronchoscopy with a flexible bronchoscope‡ with or without biopsy
    Tympanostomy tube insertion
  Gastrointestinal tract
    Transesophageal echocardiography‡
    Endoscopy with or without gastrointestinal biopsy‡
  Genitourinary tract
    Vaginal hysterectomy‡
    Vaginal delivery‡
    Cesarean section
    In uninfected tissue
      Urethral catheterization
      Uterine dilatation and curettage
      Therapeutic abortion
      Sterilization procedures
      Insertion or removal of intrauterine devices
  Other
    Cardiac catheterization, including balloon angioplasty, implanted
      cardiac pacemaker, implanted defibrillators, and coronary stents
    Incision or biopsy of surgically scrubbed skin
    Circumcision

*This table lists selected conditions and procedures but is not meant to be all inclusive.
†Some now recommend that prophylaxis prior to dental procedures should only be
used for extractions and gingival surgery (including implant replacement) and only
for patients with high risk conditions.
‡Prophylaxis optional for high-risk patients.
Source: Adapted from Dajani AS, Taubert KA, Wilson W, et al: Prevention of
bacterial endocarditis. Recommendations by the American Heart Association.
JAMA 277:1794, 1997.

   Until new guidelines emerge, the cardiac conditions and indications for
which the AHA recommends antibiotic prophylaxis are reviewed in Table
25-3. Mitral valve prolapse deserves special comment. In a case-control study,
an eightfold increase in endocarditis risk was calculated. Other investigators
calculated a fivefold increase in the risk. However, the incidence of endocarditis remains low. According to current AHA guidelines, patients with
mitral valve prolapse with no pathologic mitral regurgitation murmur or other
evidence of mitral leak and normal leaflets are at low risk. Thus, antibiotic
prophylaxis is not necessary in this group of patients.
   The current AHA recommended prophylaxis regimens are listed in Table
25-4.

TABLE 25-4 Recommended Regimens for Chemoprophylaxis

Dental and respiratory tract and esophageal procedures*
    Amoxicillin
        Adults   2.0 g
        Children   50 mg/kg PO
    Ampicillin
        Adults   2.0 g IM or IV
        Children   50 mg/kg IM or IV
Alternates
    Clindamycin
        Adults   600 mg PO or IV
        Children   20 mg/kg PO or IV
    Clathrithromycin or azithromycin
        Adults   500 mg PO
        Children   15 mg/kg PO
    Cephalexin or cefadroxil
        Adults   2.0 g PO
        Children   50 mg/kg PO
    Cefazolin
        Adults   1.0 g IM or IV
        Children   25 mg/kg IM or IV

Gastrointestinal (excluding the esophagus) and genitourinary procedures
    Moderate-risk conditions
        Amoxicillin
            Adults   2.0 g PO
            Children   50 mg/kg PO
        Ampicillin
            Adults   2.0 g IM or IV
            Children   50 mg/kg IM or IV
    High-risk conditions
        Ampicillin
            Adults   2.0 g IM or IV + gentamicin 1.5 mg/kg (not to exceed 120 mg) within 30 min of starting the procedure; 6 h later, 1 mg IM or IV or amoxicillin 1 mg PO
           Children   50 mg/kg IM or IV (not to exceed 2.0 g) + gentamicin 1.5 mg/kg within 30 min of starting the procedure; 6 h later, ampicillin 25 mg/kg IM or IV or amoxicillin 25 mg/kg PO
    Alternate regimens for moderate
      and high-risk conditions
        Vancomycin
            Adults   1.0 g IV over 1–2 h + gentamicin[†] 1.5 mg/kg IV or IM (not to exceed 120 mg); complete injection infusion within 30 min of starting the procedure
           Children   20 mg/kg IV over 1–2 h + gentamicin[†] 1.5 mg/kgIV or IM; complete injection infusion within 30 min of starting the procedure

*These IV and PO dosages should be given 30 min and 1 h, respectively, before the procedure.
[†]Gentamicin not used in moderate-risk conditions.
Key: IM, intramuscularly; IV, intravenously; PO, orally.

Newly developed AHA guidelines for nonvalvular cardiovascular devices do not recommend secondary prophylactic coverage for the vast majority of patients with any device of this type who undergo dental, respiratory, gastrointestinal, or genitourinary procedures. Only very few exceptions are suggested, namely patients in whom less than successful device implantation has resulted in the creation or persistence of turbulent blood flow jets.

Prosthetic Valve Endocarditis

PVE is a particularly serious problem and can be difficult to treat. Classically, prosthetic valve infections have been divided into two groups: early and late. Due to the significant difference in the organisms within the first and second years of operation, the cutoff time between late and early PVE should be 1 year, although early PVE usually becomes apparent within 2 months of prosthesis insertion. In general, early PVE is caused by organisms introduced during the surgical procedure or, if the implant replaced an infected valve, residual infection. In contrast, late PVE usually is caused by the introduction of pathogens into the circulation after the time of surgery. Consequently, early PVE more commonly is caused by staphylococcal species (largely *S. epidermidis*), gram-negative organisms, and diphtheroids, whereas late disease is similar in microbial spectrum to NVE. Overall, *S. epidermidis* is the most common causative organism in PVE.

The pathology of infection is related to the class of valve used. Of 22 patients with infected mechanical valves studied at necropsy by Arnett and Roberts all had valve ring abscesses. Dehiscence, causing severe valvular regurgitation, occurred in 14 of the 22 patients, and prosthetic valve obstruction by vegetative material occurred in six. Conversely, in porcine heterografts, the infection frequently developed in the fibrin layer that covers the cusps and could spread to involve the subadjacent collagen; valve ring abscess is infrequent. Regurgitation with porcine valves occurs most often because the valve leaflets are destroyed rather than from suture line dehiscence. There are also reported cases in which fibrinous membranes developed on the atrial surface of a prosthetic mitral valve, leading to fatal obstruction of left ventricular inflow.

The diagnosis of PVE can be elusive, especially when fever and bacteremia complicate the early postoperative period. Even when an extra cardiac source can be identified, the possibility of valve seeding cannot be ignored because virtually any organism can establish a focus of infection on a newly implanted prosthetic valve. However, in a study of 32 patients who developed bacteremia postoperatively, only two (6.3%) were thought to have PVE. Bacteremia in a patient with a recently implanted prosthetic valve is an ominous sign. A recent review of six studies showed an approximately 50% overall mortality rate.

Echocardiography, in particular TEE, has become an essential test in the diagnostic workup and evaluation of PVE. Investigators have shown that TEE is more sensitive than TTE in diagnosing vegetation or abscesses. In a study of 120 patients with 148 prosthetic valves, 33 were found to have endocarditis at surgery or autopsy. TTE identified vegetations in 36% of the infected valves. TEE diagnosed 27 of 33, or 82%. These investigators also showed the superiority of TEE in diagnosing abscesses associated with endocarditis. In addition, a retrospective study of 87 patients with anatomically proven PVE found that TEE correctly identified 90% of the abscesses and 100% of the pseudoaneurysms and fistulas present.

In a large review, the mortality rate for medically treated patients was 61.4%; for those who also received surgery, the rate was 38.5%. These data were obtained from studies without controls; thus selection bias clearly played some role in determining these figures. Conversely, there was no significant difference in late mortality between the medically treated group and those who also received surgery in a retrospective study of 49 cases of definite PVE established by Duke criteria. The study, which was conducted at tertiary care centers between 1980 and 1997, also found no significant difference in the 5-year rates of recurrent endocarditis, event-related mortality, and the need for reoperation between the two groups. However, the one patient who was medically treated for staphylococcal PVE died after reoperation. Thus, the investigators proposed that patients with nonstaphylococcal PVE may be managed medically without surgery as long as the patient is hemodynamically stable and closely monitored.

For bacterial PVE, the susceptibility of the etiologic agent to antimicrobial agents is an especially important factor for outcome. PVE due to organisms resistant to conventional therapy, such as methicillin-resistant staphylococci or gram-negative bacilli, are more likely to require surgery. It also is important to note that many survivors of complicated *S. epidermidis* PVE required valve replacement within the ensuing 6 months of bacteriologic cure. In contrast, the somewhat less aggressive endocarditis caused by penicillin-susceptible streptococcal infection more often is cured medically.

A relatively unique situation in PVE is the development of infection caused by methicillin-resistant *S. epidermidis.* It has been demonstrated conclusively that these patients are more likely to survive if their antibiotic regimen includes vancomycin; moreover, the addition of rifampin and gentamicin further increased survival.

Investigators reviewed PVE in porcine bioprostheses. In this series, all patients with early PVE died. Ninety-one percent with late PVE survived with a combined medical and surgical approach. The researchers recommended a combined medical and surgical approach in PVE with *S. aureus, Candida albicans,* or gram-negative organisms.

Fungal PVE, like its counterpart on native valves, is notoriously unresponsive to medical therapy; therefore, early surgery should be performed once the diagnosis is made. Even when surgically treated, there is a high incidence of recurrent endocarditis (Table 25-5). However, a study of 16 patients with fungal PVE found that aggressive amphotericin B therapy is an important adjunct to surgery. Predisposing factors for fungal PVE other than the previous open heart surgery have been identified. Central intravascular catheter, previous bacterial endocarditis, prolonged antibiotics, total parental nutrition, and immunosuppression were the predisposing factors identified. *Candida albicans* was found to be the leading causative organism, with *Candida parapsilosis* following. Antibiotic treatment of fungal endocarditis is summarized in Table 25-2.

Antimicrobial treatment of PVE is similar to NVE treatment, with certain concepts to keep in mind. First of all, due to the larger size of the vegetations, antibiotics need to be given in doses that result in maximum, nontoxic serum concentrations so that the vegetation can be penetrated fully. Second, the duration of treatment is longer and should be determined by the MIC of the most efficient combination of antibiotics and the size of the vegetation as determined by TEE (Table 25-6). When the MIC is at least 4 µg/mL, antibiotic sterilization is unlikely.

TABLE 25-5 An Estimate of Microbiologic Cure Rates for Various Forms of Endocarditis*

	Antimicrobial therapy alone, %		Antimicrobial therapy plus surgery, %	
Native valve endocarditis				
Streptococcus spp.: viridans group, group A, S. bovis, and S. pneumoniae; Neisseria gonorrhoeae	>95		>95	
Enterococcus faecalis	90		>90	
Staphylococcus aureus (in young drug addicts)	90		>90	
Staphylococcus aureus (in older patients)	50		70	
Gram-negative aerobic bacilli†	40		65	
Fungi	<5		50	
PVE	Early PVE	Late PVE	Early PVE‡	Late PVE
Streptococcus spp.: viridans, group A, S bovis, and S pneumoniae; Neisseria gonorrhoeae	‡	80	‡	90
Enterococcus faecalis	‡	60	‡	75
Staphylococcus aureus	25	40	50	60
Staphylococcus epidermidis	20	40	60	70
Gram-negative bacilli	<10	20	40	50
Fungi	<1	<1	30	40

*Morbidity and mortality for bacteriologic cure are significantly greater than these figures indicate.
†Excluding Haemophilus spp.
‡Insufficient data to estimate rate.
Key: PVE, prosthetic valve endocarditis.
Source: Adapted from Durack DT: Infective and non-infective endocarditis, in Schlant RC, Alexander RW, O'Rourke RA, et al (eds): Hurst's the Heart, 8th ed. New York, McGraw-Hill, 1994, p 1681.

TABLE 25-6 Duration of Antimicrobial Treatment in Prosthetic Valve
Endocarditis with Respect to Vegetation Size and Minimal Inhibitory
Concentration

	Vegetation size*		
	<4 mm	5–9 mm	>10 mm
MIC ≥4 µg/L	ACU	ACU	ACU
4 µg/mL > MIC > 2 µg/mL	6 wk	ACU	ACU
2 µg/mL > MIC ≥0.5 µg/mL	6 wk	6 wk	ACU
0.5 µg/mL > MIC ≥0.1 µg/mL	6 wk	6 wk	6 wk
MIC < 0.1 µg/mL	4 wk	4 wk	6 wk

*Actual size of vegetation during treatment.
Key: ACU, antibiotic cure unlikely; MIC, minimal inhibitory concentration of the
most effective antibiotic combination.
Source: Adapted from Piper C, Korfer R, Horstkotte D: Prosthetic valve
endocarditis. Heart 85:590, 2001.

Coagulase-negative staphylococci are difficult to treat medically due to the
interaction between the organism and the synthetic material of the valve. An
example of this interaction is the irreversible adhesion and production of a
biofilm that inhibits host defense mechanisms. This protective mechanism
makes antibiotic sterilization difficult. Coagulase-negative staphylococci
may cause microabscesses, and triple therapy with rifampin (900 mg/day
divided into three doses) is recommended. Rifampin is apparently effective
inside abscesses.

Therapy for culture-negative PVE within the initial 12 months after valve
replacement often includes at least vancomycin and gentamicin. For patients
with PVE that begins 12 months or longer after valve surgery, ceftriaxone or
cefotaxime could be added to cover for so-called HACEK. If fever due to IE
persists after empirical therapy, valve replacement surgery for debridement
and to obtain material for microbiologic and pathologic evaluations may be
considered.

Valvular dysfunction caused by incompetence, stenosis of the outflow track,
or perivalvular leak is unlikely to respond to medical management and should
be treated with prompt surgery before hemodynamic compromise. The development of conduction abnormalities suggests an annular abscess. In some
studies, 69% of patients with conduction abnormalities and infection of a prosthetic aortic valve had annular abscesses. Many of these patients do not survive despite therapy. Therefore, it is prudent to follow all patients carefully and
to use the earliest sign of valvular destruction, dysfunction, myocardial invasion, or failure of bacteriologic cure as an indication for urgent surgery. The
treatment of PVE requires close consultation with a cardiac surgeon and infectious disease specialist. Several general observations can be made with regard
to the role of surgery in the management of PVE. First, the mortality of surgery is no greater (and maybe less) than the mortality of medical therapy (see
Table 25-5). The risk of recurrent PVE after surgery is usually acceptable.
Second, Baumgartner and associates reported a reinfection rate after valve
replacement for PVE of 15% over an average follow up of 3.6 years. This
reflects a linear rate of 4.1% per patient per year. Third, when prosthetic valve
replacement is clinically indicated, surgery should be performed without
delay. Indications for surgery were discussed briefly earlier in this chapter. A
detailed discussion is beyond the scope of this chapter. However, it should be

mentioned that PVE caused by selected microorganisms such as fungi, *Pseudomonas aeruginosa, S. aureus,* enterococci in the absence of bactericidal therapy and other gram-negative bacilli usually requires surgery for cure. The decision for surgery involves integration of the whole clinical picture. Multiple indications in a patient strengthens the decision to opt for surgery. Table 25-2 presents a brief summary of antibiotic treatment of PVE.

Implanted Ventricular Assist Device Infection

The introduction of implanted cardiac assist devices such as pacemakers, automatic implantable cardioverter defibrillators (AICDs), and left ventricular assist devices (LVADs) has improved survival and quality of life in seriously ill patients. However, similar to prosthetic valves, these foreign materials introduced into the human body are a nidus for infection. Infection of any of these devices is a serious complication and can be extremely difficult to manage conservatively. The reported incidences of infection are 1% to 12% for pacemakers, 1% to 6% for AICDs, and 13% to 80% for LVADs. Most investigators agree that the optimum management for pacemaker and AICD infections is explantation of the entire device and prolonged antibiotics. However, there are reported cases of pacemaker infections that were treated successfully by medical therapy alone. Explantation for LVAD infection is not a valid option unless an organ is available for transplant. LVADs are used as a bridge to transplantation. Thus, if no organ is available, the only option is medical management, which is rarely a cure. However, successful transplants have been reported in LVAD-infected individuals controlled with antibiotics.

Pacemaker endocarditis, a relatively rare but serious complication of pacemaker infection, has a mortality rate of 24%. These infections usually involve the pacemaker electrode tip, the tricuspid valve, or endocardial areas in contact with the endocardial lead. The most common organisms involved are the *Staphylococcus* species. Defining and diagnosing criteria are lacking for pacemaker endocarditis, making it difficult to diagnose. Most physicians follow criteria for IE. Two different syndromes of pacemaker endocarditis have been described, the metastatic implantation type and the more common foreign body type. The foreign body type results from the extension of a pacemaker generator pocket infection along the pacemaker wire. The implantation type results from damage to the endocardium by the transvenous pacemaker followed by bacteremic implantation. Removal of the entire pacemaker device and prolonged antibiotics for the specific pathogen comprise the optimum treatment.

RHEUMATIC FEVER

The Jones criteria for the diagnosis of rheumatic fever were updated in 1992. The guidelines include major and minor manifestations and the need for supporting evidence of antecedent group A streptococcal infection. These are summarized in Table 25-7.

There are certain circumstances in which the diagnosis of acute rheumatic fever can be made without strict adherence to the Jones criteria. Chorea, the latest of the major manifestations to appear, can present without an appearance of any other major or minor criteria of rheumatic fever, which is called *pure chorea.* Acute carditis also can develop without other manifestations

TABLE 25-7 Guidelines for the Diagnosis of Initial Attack of Rheumatic Fever (Jones Criteria, Updated 1992)*

Major manifestations	Minor manifestations	Supporting evidence of antecedent group A streptococcal infection
Carditis	Clinical findings	Positive throat culture or rapid streptococcal antigen test
Polyarthritis	Arthralgia	
Chorea	Fever	
Erythema marginatum	Laboratory findings	Elevated or rising streptococcal antibody titer
Subcutaneous nodules	Elevated acute phase reactants	
	Erythrocyte sedimentation rate	
	C-reactive protein	
	Prolonged PR interval	

*If supported by evidence of preceding group A streptococcal infection, the presence of two major manifestations or of one major and two minor manifestations indicates a high probability of acute rheumatic fever.
Source: Dajani AS, Ayoub E, Bierman FZ, et al: Guidelines for the diagnosis of rheumatic fever: Jones Criteria Update 1992. *Circulation* 87:302, 1992.

months after the initial attack. This is due to the fact that antibody titers may have decreased to normal levels, and the minor manifestations may have resolved by the time acute carditis is diagnosed.

Prevention of recurrent rheumatic fever depends on continuous prophylaxis with appropriate antibiotics. The risk of recurrence decreases with time after the previous episode. The risk increases if there are two or more previous attacks of rheumatic fever. The risk also increases in the presence of rheumatic heart disease. Parents of young children, teachers, physicians, nurses, allied medical personnel, military personnel, and other individuals living in crowded conditions have an increased risk of exposure to recurrent streptococcal infection.

The recommendations for treatment of acute streptococcal pharyngitis and prevention of rheumatic fever are summarized in Table 25-8. Penicillin remains the treatment of choice for group A streptococcal pharyngitis due to its reliability, safety, and low cost. However, recent studies have shown that a 10-day treatment with once-a-day amoxicillin is as effective as multiple daily doses of penicillin. A slightly higher rate of eradication has been reported with cephalosporins, but the cost of these drugs is higher. Other drugs, such as azithromycin, cefuroxime, cefdinir, cefixime, and cefpodoxime at 5 days, have shown results similar to those of penicillin for 10 days. Cefpodoxime and cefdinir are the only cephalosporins currently approved by the FDA for fewer than 10 days of treatment. Cefadroxil (30 mg/kg, up to 1000 mg), cefixime (8 mg/kg, up to 400 mg), cefdinir (14 mg/kg, up to 600 mg), and ceftibuten (9 mg/kg, up to 400 mg) are approved for once-daily, 10-day treatment. However, there is a consideration of cost and development of resistance with these agents. Nevertheless, because poor compliance with antibiotics increases the risk of failure in treatment and the development of acute rheumatic fever, treatment regimens that could improve compliance by decreasing daily frequency or total duration of treatment are being investigated.

In April 2000, the members of the Committee on Rheumatic Fever, Endocarditis, and Kawasaki Disease of the AHA met with a group of inter-

TABLE 25-8 Treatment of Acute Streptococcal Pharyngitis and Prevention of Rheumatic Fever

Clinical presentation of streptococcal tonsillopharyngitis		Primary prophylaxis (treatment of streptococcal tonsillopharyngitis†)			
Common finding	Findings not suggesting group A β-hemolytic streptococcal infection	Agent	Dose	Mode	Duration
Symptoms	Coryza	Betathine Penicillin G	600,000 U for patients ≤27kg (60 lb)	IM	Once
Sudden onset sore throat	Hoarseness		1,200,000 U for patients >241 g (60 lb)		
Pain on swallowing	Cough				
Fever	Diarrhea				
Headache	Conjunctivitis		or		
Abdominal pain	Anterior stomatitis				
Nausea and vomiting	Discrete ulcerative lesions				
Signs		Penicillin V (phenoxymethyl penicillin)	Children: 250 mg 2–3 times daily Adolescents and adults: 500 mg 2–3 times daily	PO	10 d
Tonsillopharyngeal erythema/exudate					
Soft palate petechiae ("doughnut" lesions)		For individuals allergic to penicillin Erythromycin Estolate	20–40 mg/kg per day 2–4 times daily (maximum,1 g/d)	PO	10 d
			or		
		Ethylsuccinate	40 mg/kg per day 2–4 times daily (maximum, 1 g/d)	PO	10 d

	Duration	Agent	Dose	Route
Rheumatic fever with carditis and residual heart disease (persistent valvular disease)*	At least 10 y since last episode and at least until age 40 y, sometimes life-long prophylaxis	Benzathine Penicillin G	1,200,000 U every 4 wk‡	IM
Rheumatic fever with carditis but no residual heart disease (no valvular disease)*	10 y since last episode or until age 25 y, whichever is longer	or Penicillin V	250 mg twice daily	PO
Rheumatic fever without carditis	5 y or until age 18 y, whichever is longer	or Sulfadiazine	0.5 g once daily for patients ≤27 kg (60 lb)	PO
			1.0 g once daily for patients > 27 kg (60 lb)	
		For individuals allergic to penicillin and sulfadiazine		
		Erythromycin	250 mg twice daily	PO

*These findings are noted primarily in children older than 3 years and adults. Symptoms and signs in younger children can be different and less specific.
†This treatment prevents rheumatic fever even if started within 7–10 days of infection. The following are not acceptable: sulfonamides, trimethoprim, tetracycline, and chloramphenicol.
‡Clinical or echocardiographic evidence. In high-risk situations, administrations every 3 weeks is justified and recommended.
Key: IM, intramuscularly; PO, orally.
Source: Adapted from Dajani A, Taubert K, Ferrieri P, et al: Treatment of acute streptococcal pharyngitis and prevention of rheumatic fever: a statement for health professionals. Pediatrics 96:158, 1995.

national experts on rheumatic fever, rheumatic heart disease, and streptococcal infections to review guidelines for the diagnosis of acute rheumatic fever according to the Jones criteria, including the 1992 statement on the "Jones Criteria Updated." In summary, the workshop participants agreed that there are insufficient data to support a revision of the Jones criteria and reaffirmed the guidelines iterated in the 1992 statement. Without a "gold standard" for the diagnosis of rheumatic fever, no single specific laboratory test exists that is pathognomic of acute rheumatic fever or its recurrences. At present, Doppler echocardiography should be used as an adjunctive technique to confirm clinical findings and to evaluate chamber sizes, ventricular function, degree of valvular regurgitation, and morphologic features of the valves. It should not be used as a major or minor criterion for establishing the diagnosis of carditis associated with acute rheumatic fever in the absence of clinical findings. Future refinements of Doppler echocardiography and prospective studies of its predictive value may prompt reassessment of its role in the diagnosis of acute rheumatic fever. The conference also concluded that data are not sufficiently compelling to designate monoarthritis as a criterion for diagnosis of acute rheumatic fever in the absence of other Jones criteria. However, it is acknowledged that this finding must be interpreted within the clinical and epidemiologic settings of rheumatic fever prevalence in various populations.

Clinical research in several areas is needed, including epidemiologic studies and determination of the prognostic implications of subclinical valvular regurgitation. In addition, research on basic pathogenetic mechanisms that result in rheumatic fever in "at-risk" individuals should continue. Future revisions of the Jones criteria statement will depend on data generated from these areas of research.

ADDITIONAL READINGS

Bisno AL. Acute pharyngitis. *N Engl J Med* 344:205, 2001.

Child JS: Diagnosis and management of infective endocarditis. *Cardiol Clin* 14:217, 1996.

Dajani AS, Ayoub E, Bierman FZ, et al: Guidelines for the diagnosis of rheumatic fever: Jones criteria update 1992. *Circulation* 87:302, 1992.

Dajani AS, Taubert KA, Wilson W, et al: Prevention of bacterial endocarditis. Recommendations by the American Heart Association. *JAMA* 277:1794, 1997.

Ferrieri P. Jones Criteria Working Group: Proceedings of the Jones Criteria Workshop. *Circ* 106:2521, 2002.

Figueroa FE, Fernandez MS, Valdez P, et al. Prospective comparison of clinical and echocardiographic diagnosis of rheumatic carditis: Long term follow up of patients with subclinical disease. *Heart* 85:407, 2001.

Green-Gastwirth V, Wiese C, Horowitz H, Frishman WH: Intravascular device infections: Epidemiology, diagnosis and management. *Heart Dis,* in press.

Gilbert DN, Moellering RC Jr, Sande MA (eds): *The Sanford Guide to Antimicrobial Therapy* 2003, 33rd ed. Hyde Park, VT, Antimicrobial Therapy, 2003.

Goldberger MH, Kalkut GE, Frishman WH: Drug treatment of infective endocarditis, in Frishman WH, Sonnenblick EH (eds): *Cardiovascular Pharmacotherapeutics.* New York, McGraw-Hill, 1997, p 1247.

Grossi EA, Goldberg JD, LaPietra A, et al: Ischemic mitral valve reconstruction and replacement: Comparison of long-term survival and complications. *J Thorac Cardiovasc Surg* 122:1107, 2001.

Hasbun R, Vikram HR, Barakat LA, et al: Complicated left-sided native valve endocarditis in adults. Risk classification for mortality. *JAMA* 289:1933, 2003.

Hyde JAJ, Darouiche RO, Costeron JW: Strategies for prophylaxis against prosthetic valve endocarditis. A review article. *J Heart Valve Dis* 7:316, 1998.

Murray BE: Vancomycin-resistant enterococcal infections. *N Engl J Med* 342:710, 2000.

Mylonakis E, Calderwood SB: Infective endocarditis in adults. *N Engl J Med* 345:1318, 2001.

O'Nunain S, Perez I, Roelke M, et al: The treatment of patients with infected implantable cardioverter-defibrillator systems. *J Thorac Cardiovasc Surg* 113:121, 1997.

Perez-Vazquez A, Farinas MC, Garcia-Palomo JD, et al: Evaluation of the Duke Criteria in 93 episodes of prosthetic valve endocarditis. *Arch Intern Med* 160:1185, 2000.

Piper C, Korfer R, Horstkotte D: Prosthetic valve endocarditis. *Heart* 85:590, 2001.

Salem DN, Daudelin DH, Levine HJ, et al: Antithrombotic therapy in valvular heart disease. *Chest* 119(suppl):207S, 2001.

Stein PD, Alpert JS, Bussey HI, et al: Antithrombotic therapy in patients with mechanical and biological prosthetic heart valves. *Chest* 19(suppl):220S, 2001.

Strom BL, Abrutyn E, Berlin JA, et al: Dental and cardiac risk factors for infective endocarditis. A population based, case-controlled study. *Ann Intern Med* 129:761, 1998.

Zarrouk V, Bozdogan B, Leclercq R, et al: Activities of the combination of quinupristin–dalfopristin with rifampin in vitro and in the experimental endocarditis due to *Staphylococcus aureus* strains with various phenotypes of resistance to macrolide-lincosamide-streptogramin antibiotics. *Antimicrob Agents Chemother* 45:1244, 2001.

Appendices

Angela Cheng-Lai *William H. Frishman*
Adam Spiegel *Pamela Charney*

APPENDIX 1 Pharmacokinetic Properties of Approved Cardiovascular Drugs

Generic name	Bio-availability, %	Protein binding, %	V_d, L/kg	$t_{1/2}$	Urinary excretion, % unchanged	Cl, mL/min per kg	Therapeutic range	References
Abciximab	NA	—	—	0.5 h	—	—	—	Faulds D, Sorkin EM: Abciximab (c7E Fab): a review of its pharmacology and therapeutic potential in ischemic heart disease. *Drugs* 48:583, 1994.
Acebutolol	37 ± 12	26 ± 3	1.2 ± 0.3	2.7 ± 0.4 h	40 ± 11	6.8 ± 0.8	—	Singh BN, Thoden WR, Wahl J: Acebutolol: a review of its pharmacology, pharmacokinetics, clinical uses, and adverse effects. *Pharmacotherapy* 6:45, 1986.
Adenosine	—	—	0.11–0.19	<10 s	—	59–152	—	Biardi P, Laghi-Pasini F, Urso R, et al: Pharmacokinetics of exogenous adenosine in man after infusion. *Eur J Clin Pharmacol* 44:505, 1993.
Alteplase	—	—	0.10–0.17	3–5 min $t_{1/2}$ is ↑ in HI	—	9.8–10.4 Cl is ↓ in HI	0.45 µg/mL	Seifried E, Tanswell P, Rijken DC, et al: Pharmacokinetics of antigen and activity of recombinant tissue-type plasminogen activator after infusion in healthy volunteers. *Arzneimittelforschung* 38:418, 1988.
Amiloride	15–25	23	17 ± 4	6–9 h $t_{1/2}$ is ↑ in RF	49 ± 10 Cl is ↓ in the elderly and RI	9.7 ± 1.9	38–48 ng/mL	Vidt DG: Mechanism of action, pharmacokinetics, adverse effects, and therapeutic uses of amiloride hydrochloride, a new potassium-sparing diuretic. *Pharmacotherapy* 1:179, 1981.

Drug								Reference
Amiodarone	46 ± 22	99.98 ± 0.01	66 ± 44	25 ± 12 d	0	1.9 ± 0.4	1.0–2.5 µg/mL	Freeman MD, Somberg JC: Pharmacology and pharmacokinetics of amiodarone. *J Clin Pharmacol* 31:1061, 1991.
Amlodipine	74 ± 17	93 ± 1	16 ± 4	39 ± 8 h $t_{1/2}$ is ↑ in the elderly and HI	10	5.9 ± 1.5 Cl is ↓ in the elderly and HI	—	Abernethy DR: The pharmacokinetic profile of amlodipine. *Am Heart J* 118:1100, 1989.
Amrinone (inamrinone)	93 ± 12	35–49	1.3 ± 0.3	4.4 ± 1.4 h (slow acetylator) 2.0 ± 0.6 h (fast acetylator) $t_{1/2}$ is ↓ in CHF and neonates	25 ± 10	4.0 ± 1.6 (slow acetylator) 8.9 ± 2.7 (fast acetylator) Cl is ↓ in CHF and neonates	3.7 µg/mL	Steinberg C, Notterman DA: Pharmacokinetics of cardiovascular drugs in children; inotropes and vasopressors. *Clin Pharmacokinet* 27:345, 1994.
Anagrelide	—	—	12	1.3 h (plasma $t_{1/2}$) 3 d (terminal elimination $t_{1/2}$)	<1	2.1	—	Spencer, CM, Brogden RN: Anagrelide: a review of its pharmacodynamic and pharmacokinetic properties, and therapeutic potential in the treatment of thrombocythaemia. *Drugs* 47:809, 1994.
Anisindione	Variable	—	—	3–5 d	—	—	—	
Anistreplase	—	—	0.084 ± 0.027	1.2 ± 0.4 h	—	0.92 ± 0.36 Cl is ↓ in HI	—	Gemmill JD, Hogg KJ, Burns JMA, et al: A comparison of the pharmacokinetic properties of streptokinase and anistreplase in acute myocardial infarction. *Br J Clin Pharmacol* 31:143, 1991.
Argatroban	NA	54	0.2	39–51 min	16	5	—	McKeage K, Plosker GL. Argatroban. *Drugs* 61:515, 2001.

(continued)

APPENDIX 1 *(continued)* Pharmacokinetic Properties of Approved Cardiovascular Drugs

Generic name	Bioavailability, %	Protein binding, %	V_d, L/kg	$t_{1/2}$	Urinary excretion, % unchanged	Cl, mL/min per kg	Therapeutic range	References
Aspirin	50–100 (depends on formulation)	76–90	0.15–0.2	2.4–19 h (depends on dose) $t_{1/2}$ is ↑ in HI	2–30 (depends on urinary pH)	0.18–0.88 Cl is ↓ in HI and neonates	150–300 µg/mL	Furst DE, Tozer TN, Melmon KL: Salicylate clearance, the resultant of protein binding and metabolism. *Clin Pharmacol Ther* 26:380, 1979.
Atenolol	50–60	5–15	0.95 ± 0.15	6.1 ± 2.0 h $t_{1/2}$ is ↑ in RI and elderly	94 ± 8	2.0 ± 0.2 Cl is ↓ in elderly and RI	0.1–1 µg/mL	Wadworth AN, Murdoch D, Brogden RN: Atenolol: a reappraisal of its pharmacological properties and therapeutic use in cardiovascular disorders. *Drugs* 42:468, 1991.
Atorvastatin	12	≥98	8	14 (11–24) h ↑ in elderly	<2	—	—	Lea AP, McTavish D: Atorvastatin: A review of its pharmacology and therapeutic potential in the management of hyperlipidaemias. *Drugs* 53:828, 1997.
Atropine	50	14–22	2.0 ± 1.1 V_d is ↑ in children	3.5 ± 1.5 h $t_{1/2}$ is ↑ in elderly and children	57 ± 8	8 ± 4 Cl is ↓ in elderly	—	Kentala E, Kaila T, Lisalo E, et al: Intramuscular atropine in healthy volunteers: a pharmacokinetic and pharmacodynamic study. *Int J Clin Pharmacol Ther Toxicol* 28:399, 1990.
Benazepril	37	95–97	0.12	0.6 h 10–11 h (active metabolic)	<1 18 (active metabolic)	0.3–0.4	—	Kaiser G, Ackermann R, Brechbukler S, et al: Pharmacokinetics of the angiotensin converting enzyme inhibitor benazepril HCl (CGS 14 824 A) in healthy volunteers after single and repeated administration. *Biopharm Drug Dispos* 10:365, 1989.

Drug								Reference
Bendroflumethiazide	100	94	1.48	3–3.9 h	30	5.3 ± 1.4	—	Beermann B, Groschinsky-Grind M, Lindstrom B: Pharmacokinetics of bendroflumethiazide. *Clin Pharmacol Ther* 22:385, 1977.
Bepridil	60	>99	8 ± 5	12–24 h	<1	5.3 ± 2.5	—	Benet LZ: Pharmacokinetics and metabolism of bepridil. *Am J Cardiol* 55:8C, 1985.
Betaxolol	76–89	50–55	4.9–9.8	14–22 $t_{1/2}$ is ↑ in elderly	15	4.7 Cl is ↓ in elderly	20–50 ng/mL	Frishman WH, Tepper D, Lazar EJ, et al: Betaxolol: A new long-acting beta1-selective adrenergic blocker. *J Clin Pharmacol* 30:686, 1990.
Bisoprolol	85–91	30–35	3.2 ± 0.5	8.2–12 h $t_{1/2}$ is ↑ in RI	50–60	3.7 ± 0.7 Cl is ↓ in RI	—	Lancaster SG, Sorkin EM: Bisoprolol: a preliminary review of its pharmacodynamic and pharmacokinetic properties, and therapeutic efficacy in hypertension and angina pectoris. *Drugs* 36:256, 1988.
Bivalirudin	40 (bioavailability of SC injection)	0	ID	25–36 min	~20	3.4	—	Fox I, Dawson A, Loynds P, et al: Anticoagulant activity of Hirulog, a direct thrombin inhibitor, in humans. *Thromb Haemost* 69:157, 1993.
Bosentan	50	>98	–0.26	5 h	<3	1.9	—	Actelion: Tracleer package insert. South San Francisco. 2002.
Bretylium	23 ± 9	0–8	5.9 ± 0.8	5–10 h $t_{1/2}$ is ↑ in RI	70–80	10.2 ± 1.9 Cl is ↓ in RI	—	Rapaport WG: Clinical pharmacokinetics of bretylium. *Clin Pharmacokinet* 10:248, 1985.

(continued)

APPENDIX 1 (continued) Pharmacokinetic Properties of Approved Cardiovascular Drugs

Generic name	Bio-availability, %	Protein binding, %	V_d, L/kg	$t_{1/2}$	Urinary excretion, % unchanged	Cl, mL/min per kg	Therapeutic range	References
Bumetanide	55–89	99 ± 0.3	0.13 ± 0.03 V_d is ↑ in RI and HI	0.3–1.5 h $t_{1/2}$ is ↑ in RI, HI, and CHF	62 ± 20	2.6 ± 0.5 Cl is ↓ in RI, HI, and CHF	—	Cook JA, Smith DE, Cornish LA, et al: Kinetics, dynamics, and bio-availability of bumetanide in healthy subjects and patients with congestive heart failure. Clin Pharmacol Ther 44:487, 1988.
Candesartan	15	>99	0.13	9–13 h	26	0.37	—	McClellan KJ, Goa KL: Candesartan cilexetil: a review of its use in essential hypertension. Drugs 56:847, 1998.
Captopril	65–75	30 ± 6	0.81 ± 0.18	2.2 ± 0.5 h $t_{1/2}$ is ↑ in RI and CHF	40–50	12.0 ± 1.4 Cl is ↓ in RI	0.05–0.5 µg/mL	Duchin KL, McKinstry DN, Cohen AI, et al: Pharmacokinetics of captopril in healthy subjects and in patients with cardiovascular diseases. Clin Pharmacokinet 14: 241, 1988.
Carteolol	85	23–30	—	5–7 h $t_{1/2}$ is ↑ in RI	50–70	—	—	Chrisp P, Sorkin EM: Ocular carteolol: A review of its pharma-cological properties, and thera-peutic use in glaucoma and ocular hypertension. Drugs Aging 2:58, 1992.
Carvedilol	25	95	1.5 ± 0.3	7–10 h (apparent mean terminal elimination $t_{1/2}$) $t_{1/2}$ is ↑ in HI	<2	8.7 ± 1.7 Cl is ↓ in HI	—	Dunn CJ, Lea AP, Wagstaff AJ: Carvedilol: A reappraisal of its pharmacological properties and therapeutic use in cardiovascular disorders. Drugs 54:161, 1997.

Drug							Reference
Chlorothiazide	10–21	20–80	0.20 ± 0.08	1.5 ± 0.2 h t½ is ↑ in RI and CHF	92 ± 5	4.5 ± 1.7 Cl is ↓ in RI	—	Osmon MA, Patel RB, Irwin DS, et al: Bioavailability of chlorothiazide from 50, 100, and 250 mg solution doses. *Biopharm Drug Dispos* 3:89, 1982.
Chlorthalidone	64 ± 10	75 ± 1	0.10 ± 0.04	47 ± 22 h t½ is ↑ in elderly	65 ± 9	0.04 ± 0.01 Cl is ↓ in elderly	—	Williams RL, Blume CD, Lin ET, et al: Relative bioavailability of chlorthalidone in humans: adverse influence of polyethylene glycol. *J Pharm Sci* 71:533, 1982.
Cilostazol	ID	95–98	ID	11–13 h	0	ID	—	Reilly MP, Mohler ER III: Cilostazol: treatment of intermittent claudication. *Ann Pharmacother* 35:48, 2001.
Clofibrate	95 ± 10	95–98	0.11 ± 0.02	12–22 h t½ is ↑ in RI	5.7 ± 2.1	0.12 ± 0.01 Cl is ↓ in RI	162–200 µg/mL	Gugler R, Kurten JW, Jensen CJ, et al: Clofibrate disposition in renal failure and acute and chronic liver disease. *Eur J Clin Pharmacol* 15:341, 1979.
Clonidine	95	20	2.1 ± 0.4	12–16 h t½ is ↑ in RI	40–60	3.1 ± 1.2 Cl is ↓ in RI	0.2–2 ng/mL	Lowenthal DT, Matzek KM, McGregor TR: Clinical pharmacokinetics of clonidine. *Clin Pharmacokinet* 14:287, 1988.
Clopidogrel	—	98	—	8 h t½ of primary metabolite (inactive carboxylic-acid derivative)	ID	—	—	Sanofi: Plavix package insert. New York, 1997.

(continued)

APPENDIX 1 (continued) Pharmacokinetic Properties of Approved Cardiovascular Drugs

Generic name	Bio-availability, %	Protein binding, %	V_d, L/kg	$t_{1/2}$	Urinary excretion, % unchanged	Cl, mL/min per kg	Therapeutic range	References
Colesevelam	NA Not hydrolyzed by digestive enzymes and not absorbed	NA	NA	NA	0.05	ID	—	Wong N: Colesevelam: a new bile acid sequestrant. Heart Dis 3:63, 2001.
Dalteparin	87	—	0.04–0.06	3–5 h $t_{1/2}$ is ↓ in RI	—	0.27–0.41	0.1–0.6 anti-Xa U/mL	Simoneau G, Bergmann JF, Kher A, et al: Pharmacokinetics of a low molecular weight heparin (Fragmin) in young and elderly subjects. Thromb Res 66:603, 1992.
Danaparoid	100 Based on plasma anti-Xa activity	—	0.11–0.13 Based on plasma anti-Xa activity	24 h Based on plasma anti-Xa activity $t_{1/2}$ is ↑ in RI	—	0.086–0.190 Total plasma Cl of plasma anti-Xa activity	0.15–0.40 U/mL Plasma anti-Xa level at 6 h post dose; further studies are needed to determine whether a therapeutic window exists for danaparoid	Skoutakis VA: Danaparoid in the prevention of thromboembolic complications. Ann Pharmacother 31:876, 1997.

(continued)

Drug								Reference
Diazoxide	NA (IV formulation)	94	0.21	48 h	ID	0.06	—	Kirsten R, Nelson K, Kirsten D, et al: Clinical pharmacokinetics of vasodilators. Part I. *Clin Pharmacokinet* 34:457, 1998.
Dicoumarol	Variable	99	—	1-2 d				
Digitoxin	>90	97 ± 0.5	0.54 ± 0.14 V_d is ↑ in children	6.7 ± 1.7 d	32 ± 15	0.055 ± 0.018 Cl is ↑ in children	14-26 ng/mL	Mooradian AD: Digitalis: an update of clinical pharmacokinetics, therapeutic monitoring techniques and treatment recommendations. *Clin Pharmacokinet* 15:165, 1988.
Digoxin	70 ± 1.3	20-25		39 ± 13 h $t_{1/2}$ ↑ RI, CHF, and elderly	60 ± 11	Cl ↑ in neonates and children	0.5-2 ng/mL	Mooradian AD: Digitalis: An update of clinical pharmacokinetics, therapeutic monitoring techniques and treatment recommendations. *Clin Pharmacokinet* 15:165, 1988.
Diltiazem	40-67	70-80	3.1 ± 1.2 V_d ↓ in RI	3.7-6 h	2-4	12 ± 4 Cl is ↓ in RI	50-200 ng/mL	Echizen H, Eichelbaum M: Clinical pharmacokinetics of verapamil, nifedipine and diltiazem. *Clin Pharmacokinet* 11:425, 1986.
Dipyridamole	37-66	91-99	—	10-12 h	<5		—	Gregov D, Jenkins A, Duncan E, et al: Dipyridamole: pharmacokinetics and effects on aspects of platelet function in man. *Br J Clin Pharmacol* 24:425, 1987.
Disopyramide	83 ± 11	68-89	0.59 ± 0.15	4-10 h $t_{1/2}$ ↑ in RI and CHF	55 ± 6	1.2 ± 0.4 Cl ↓ in MI, CHF, RI, and HI	2-4 µg/mL	Siddoway LA, Woosley RL: Clinical pharmacokinetics of disopyramide. *Clin Pharmacokinet* 11:214, 1986.

APPENDIX 1 (continued) Pharmacokinetic Properties of Approved Cardiovascular Drugs

Generic name	Bio-availability, %	Protein binding, %	V_d, L/kg	$t_{1/2}$	Urinary excretion, % unchanged	Cl, mL/min per kg	Therapeutic range	References
Dobutamine	NA	ID	0.20 ± 0.08	2.4 ± 0.7 min	0	59 ± 22 Cl ↑ in children	40–190 ng/mL	Steinberg C, Notterman DA: Pharmacokinetics of cardiovascular drugs in children: inotropes and vasopressors. Clin Pharmacokinet 27:345, 1994.
Dofetilide	>90	60–70	3–4	5–13 h	~64	5.2	—	Lenz TL, Hilleman DE: Dofetilide, a new class III antiarrhythmic agent. Pharmacotherapy 20:776, 2000.
Dopamine	NA	0	—	2 min	<5	—	—	Kulka PJ, Tryba M: Inotropic support of the critically ill patient. Drugs 45:654, 1993.
Doxazosin	63 ± 14	98.9 ± 0.5	1.5 ± 0.3	19–22 h	—	1.7 ± 0.4	—	Donelly R, Meredith PA, Elliott HL: Pharmacokinetic-pharmaco-dynamic relationships of α-adrenoceptor antagonists. Clin Pharmacokinet 17:264, 1989.
Enalapril	41 ± 15	<50	1.7 ± 0.7	1.3 h 11 h (Enalaprilat) $t_{1/2}$ is ↑ in RI and HI	54 40 (Enalaprilat)	4.9 ± 1.5 Cl is ↓ in RI, elderly, CHF, neonates, and ↑ in children	5–20 ng/mL	Louis WJ, Conway EL, Krum H, et al: Comparison of the pharmaco-kinetics and pharmacodynamics of perindopril, cilazapril and enalapril. Clin Exp Pharmacol Physiol 19(suppl 19):55, 1992.
Encainide	25–90 (depends on meta-bolic phenotype)	75–85	3.6–3.9	1–2 h (fast oxidizer) 6–11 h (slow oxidizer)	5 (fast oxidizer) 40–45 (slow oxidizer)	30 (fast oxidizer) 2.5 (slow oxidizer)	250 ng/mL	Brogden RN, Todd PA: Encainide: a review of its pharmacological properties and therapeutic efficacy. Drugs 34:519, 1987.

Enoxaparin	92	—	0.08	4.5 $t_{1/2}$ is ↑ in RI	8–20	0.3 ± 0.1 Cl is ↓ in RI	—	Bendetowicz AV, Beguin S, Caplain H, et al: Pharmacokinetics and pharmacodynamics of a low molecular weight heparin (enoxaparin) after subcutaneous injection, comparison with unfractionated heparin—a three-way crossover study in healthy volunteers. *Thromb Haemost* 71: 305, 1994.
Eplerenone	ID	≈50	0.61–1.29	4–6 h	<5	2.38	Zillich AJ, Carter BL: Eplerenone— a novel selective aldosterone blocker. *Ann Pharmacother* 36: 1567, 2002.
Eprosartan	13	98	~4.4 (this value is the population mean steady-state V_d 0.23	5–9 h	~6	11.5	Bottorff MB, Tenero DM: Pharmacokinetics of eprosartan in healthy subjects, patients with hypertension and special populations. *Pharmacotherapy* 19(4 pt 2):73S, 1999.
Eptifibatide	NA	25		2.5–2.8 h	ID	0.92–0.97	—	Goa KL, Noble S: Eptifibatide: a review of its use in patients with acute coronary syndromes and/or undergoing percutaneous coronary intervention. *Drugs* 57: 439, 1999.
Esmolol	NA	55	1.9 ± 1.3	0.13 ± 0.07 h $t_{1/2}$ is ↓ in children	<1	170 ± 70 Cl is ↓ in CAD and ↑ in children	—	Weist D: Esmolol: a review of its therapeutic efficacy and pharmacokinetic characteristics. *Clin Pharmacokinet* 28:190, 1995.

(continued)

597

APPENDIX 1 (continued) Pharmacokinetic Properties of Approved Cardiovascular Drugs

Generic name	Bio-availability, %	Protein binding, %	V_d, L/kg	$t_{1/2}$	Urinary excretion, % unchanged	Cl, mL/min per kg	Therapeutic range	References
Ethacrynic acid	100	90	—	0.5–1 h	65	—	—	Gupta EK, Ito MK: Ezetimibe: the first in a novel class of selective cholesterol-absorption inhibitors. *Heart Dis* 4:399, 2002.
Ezetimibe	ID	>90	ID	≈22 h	ID	ID		
Felodipine	20	99.6 ± 0.2	10 ± 3	10–17 h $t_{1/2}$ is ↑ in elderly and CHF	<1	12 ± 5 Cl is ↓ in elderly, HI, and CHF	—	Edgar B, Lundborg P, Regardh CG: Clinical pharmacokinetics of felodipine: a summary. *Drugs* 34 (suppl 3):16, 1987.
Fenofibrate	60–90	>99 (properties of major active metabolite fenofibric acid)	0.89 (properties of major active metabolite fenofibric acid)	19.6–26.6 h (properties of major active metabolite fenofibric acid)	ID	0.45 (plasma Cl of fenofibric acid)	—	Balfour JA, McTavish D, Heel RC: Fenofibrate. A review of its pharmacodynamic and pharmacokinetic properties and therapeutic use in dyslipidaemia. *Drugs* 40: 260, 1990.
Fenoldopam	5.7	88	0.23–0.66	0.16 h	1	24.8–38.2	3.5–14.25 µg/L	Brogden RN and Markham A: Fenoldopam: a review of its pharmacodynamic and pharmacokinetic properties and intravenous clinical potential in the management of hypertensive urgencies and emergencies. *Drugs* 54:634, 1997.

Drug							Reference
Flecainide	85–90	40–50	4.9 ± 0.4	12–30 h $t_{1/2}$ is ↑ in RI, HI, CHF, and ↓ in children	10–50	5.6 ± 1.3 Cl is ↓ in RI, HI, and CHF	0.4–0.8 µg/mL	Funck-Bretano C, Becquemont L, Kroemer HK, et al: Variable disposition kinetics and electrocardiographic effects of flecainide during repeated dosing in humans: contribution of genetic factors, dose-dependent clearance and interaction with amiodarone. *Clin Pharmacol Ther* 55:256, 1994.
Fluvastatin	9–50	98	—	1.2 h $t_{1/2}$ is ↑ in HI	<5	—	—	Tse FLS, Jaffe JM, Troendle A: Pharmacokinetics of fluvastatin after single and multiple doses in normal volunteers. *J Clin Pharmacol* 32:630, 1992.
Fonda-parinux	~100 (post SC injection)	—	0.10–0.12 (post SC injection)	13–15 h $t_{1/2}$ ↑ in elderly with reduced Cl_{Cr}	≤77	0.10–0.13 (plasma Cl) Cl is ↓ in elderly with reduced Cl_{Cr}	—	Boneu B, Necciari J, Cariou R, et al: Pharmacokinetics and tolerance of the natural pentasaccharide (SR90107/ORG31540) with high affinity to antithrombin III in man. *Thromb Haemost* 74:1468, 1995.
Fosinopril	36 ± 7	≥95	0.13 ± 0.03	11.3 ± 0.7 h (fosinoprilat) $t_{1/2}$ is ↑ in RI	<2	0.51 ± 0.10 Cl is ↓ in HI and RI	—	Hui KK, Duchin KL, Kripalani KJ, et al: Pharmacokinetics of fosinopril in patients with various degrees of renal function. *Clin Pharmacol Ther* 49:457, 1991.
Furosemide	61 ± 17	98.8 ± 0.2	0.11 ± 0.02	0.5–1.0 h $t_{1/2}$ ↑ in RI, CHF, neonates, HI, and elderly	66 ± 7	2.0 ± 0.4 Cl is ↓ in RI, CHF, neonates, and elderly	ID	Hammarlund-Udenaes M, Benet LZ: Furosemide pharmacokinetics and pharmacodynamics in health and disease—an update. *J Pharmacokinet Biopharm* 17:1, 1989.

(continued)

APPENDIX 1 (continued) Pharmacokinetic Properties of Approved Cardiovascular Drugs

Generic name	Bio-availability, %	Protein binding, %	V_d, L/kg	$t_{1/2}$	Urinary excretion, % unchanged	Cl, mL/min per kg	Therapeutic range	References
Gemfibrozil	98 ± 1	>97	0.14 ± 0.03	1.1 ± 0.2 h	<1	1.7 ± 0.4	—	Todd PA, Ward A: Gemfibrozil, a review of its pharmacodynamic and pharmacokinetic properties and therapeutic use in dyslipidaemia. Drugs 36:314, 1988.
Guanabenz	ID	95	93–147	4–14 h	<1	—	—	Holmes B, Brogden RN, Heel RC, et al: Guanabenz: a review of its pharmacodynamic properties and therapeutic efficacy in hypertension. Drugs 26:212, 1983.
Guanadrel	85	<20	—	10–12 h $t_{1/2}$ ↑ in RI	40	—	—	Finnerty FA Jr, Brogden RN: Guanadrel: a review of its pharmacodynamic and pharmacokinetic properties and therapeutic use in hypertension. Drugs 30:22, 1985.
Guanethidine	3–30	—	—	4–8 d	50	0.8	8–17 ng/mL	Woosley RL, Nies AS: Guanethidine. N Engl J Med 295:1053, 1976.
Guanfacine	80	70	6.3	10–30 h	40–75	—	5–10 ng/mL	Sorkin EM, Heel RC: Guanfacine: a review of its pharmacodynamic and pharmacokinetic properties and therapeutic efficacy in the treatment of hypertension. Drugs 31:301, 1986.
Heparin	NA	—	0.058 ± 0.01	1–2 h (increases with dose)	≤50	0.5–0.6 (plasma Cl)	—	Estes JW: Clinical pharmacokinetics of heparin. Clin Pharmacokinet 5: 204, 1980.

Drug							Reference
Hydralazine	16 ± 15 (rapid acetylator) 35 ± 4 (slow acetylator)	87	1.5 ± 1.0	2–4 h t½ is ↑ in CHF	1–15	56 ± 13 Cl is ↓ in CHF	Mulrow JP, Crawford MH: Clinical pharmacokinetics and therapeutic use of hydralazine in congestive heart failure. *Clin Pharmacokinet* 16:86, 1989.
Hydrochlorothiazide	65–75	58 ± 17	0.83 ± 0.31	2–15 h t½ is ↑ in RI, CHF, and elderly	>95	4.9 ± 1.1 Cl is ↓ in RI, CHF and elderly	Beerman B, Groschinsky Grind M: Pharmacokinetics of hydrochlorothiazide in man. *Eur J Clin Pharmacol* 12:297, 1977.
Hydroflumethiazide	50	74	—	12–27 h	40–80	—	Brors O, Jacobsen S: Pharmacokinetics of hydroflumethiazide during repeated oral administration to healthy subjects. *Eur J Pharmacol* 15:281, 1979.
Ibutilide	—	40	11	6 ± 4 h	7	29	Jungbluth GL, et al: Evaluation of the pharmacokinetics and pharmacodynamics of ibutilide fumarate and its enantiomers in healthy male volunteers (abstract). *Pharm Res* 8:S249, 1991.
Indapamide	93	71–79	0.86–1.57	14–18 h	7	—	Caruso FS, Szabadi RR, Vukovich RA: Pharmacokinetics and clinical pharmacology of indapamide. *Am Heart J* 106:212, 1983.
Irbesartan	60–80	~90	0.76–1.33	11–15 h	1	2.3–2.6	Gillis JC, Markham A: Irbesartan: a review of its pharmacodynamic and pharmacokinetic properties and therapeutic use in the management of hypertension. *Drugs* 54:885, 1997.

(continued)

APPENDIX 1 (continued) Pharmacokinetic Properties of Approved Cardiovascular Drugs

Generic name	Bio-availability, %	Protein binding, %	V_d, L/kg	$t_{1/2}$	Urinary excretion, % unchanged	Cl, mL/min per kg	Therapeutic range	References
Isosorbide dinitrate	22 ± 14 PO 45 ± 16 SL	28 ± 12	3.9 ± 1.5	1.0 ± 0.5 h	<1	45 ± 20 Cl is ↓ in HI	—	Fung HL: Pharmacokinetics and pharmacodynamics of organic nitrates. *Am J Cardiol* 60:4H, 1987.
Isosorbide mononitrate	93 ± 13	<4	0.73 ± 0.09	4.9 ± 0.8 h	<5	1.80 ± 0.24	100 ng/mL	Abshagen UWP: Pharmacokinetics of isosorbide mononitrate. *Am J Cardiol* 70:61G, 1992.
Isoxsuprine	100	ID	—	1.25 h	—	—	—	
Isradipine	17 ↑ in elderly and CHF	97	2.9	6.1–10.7 h	0	10	—	Fitton A, Benfield P: Isradipine. A review of its pharmacodynamic and pharmacokinetic properties, and therapeutic use in cardiovascular disease. *Drugs* 40:31, 1990.
Labetalol	18 ± 5 ↑ in elderly and HI	50	9.4 ± 3.4	4.9 ± 2.0 h $t_{1/2}$ ↑ in elderly	<5	25 ± 10 Cl ↓ in elderly	—	Donnelly R, Macphee GJA: Clinical pharmacokinetics and kinetic-dynamic relationships of dilevalol and labetalol. *Clin Pharmacokinet* 21:95, 1991.
Lepirudin	75–80 (after SC administration)	ID	0.13–0.46	1.3 h	~17	2.3–3.3	—	Cheng-Lai A: Hirudin. *Heart Dis* 1: 41, 1999.

Drug							Reference
Lidocaine	NA	50–70	1.1 ± 0.4	1.8 ± 0.4 h t½ is ↑ in HI and neonates	<10	9.2 ± 2.4 Cl is ↓ in CHF and HI	1.5–6 µg/mL	Thompson PD, Melmon KL, Richardson JA, et al: Lidocaine pharmacokinetics in advanced heart failure, liver disease and renal disease in humans. *Ann Intern Med* 78:499, 1973.
Lisinopril	25 ± 20 ↓ in CHF	0	2.4 ± 1.4	12 h t½ is ↑ in elderly and RI	88–100	4.2 ± 2.2 Cl is ↓ in CHF, RI, and elderly	—	Sica DA, Cutler RE, Parmer RJ, et al: Comparison of the steady-state pharmacokinetics of fosinopril, lisinopril and enalapril in patients with chronic renal insufficiency. *Clin Pharmacokinet* 20:420, 1991.
Losartan	33 ↑ in HI	98	0.49	1.5–2.5 h 6–9 h (active metabolite)	4	8.6 Cl is ↓ in HI	—	Ohtawa M, Takayama F, Saitoh K, et al: Pharmacokinetics and biochemical efficacy after single and multiple oral administration of losartan, an orally active non-peptide angiotensin II receptor antagonist, in humans. *Br J Clin Pharmacol* 35:290, 1993.
Lovastatin	<5	>95	—	3–4 h	<5	4–18 Cl is ↓ in RI	—	McKenney JM: Lovastatin: a new cholesterol-lowering agent. *Clin Pharmacol* 7:21, 1988.
Mecamyl-amine	ID	—	—	ID	50 (depends on urine pH)	—	—	
Methyldopa	42 ± 16	1–16	0.46 ± 0.15	1.8 ± 0.6 h t½ is ↑ in RI and neonates	40 ± 13	3.7 ± 1.0 Cl is ↓ in RI	—	Skerjanee A, Campbell NRC, Robertson S, et al: Pharmacokinetics and presystemic gut metabolism of methyldopa in healthy human subjects. *J Clin Pharmacol* 35:275, 1995.

(continued)

APPENDIX 1 (continued) Pharmacokinetic Properties of Approved Cardiovascular Drugs

Generic name	Bio-availability, %	Protein binding, %	V_d, L/kg	$t_{1/2}$	Urinary excretion, % unchanged	Cl, mL/min per kg	Therapeutic range	References
Metolazone	40–65	95 (50–78% bound to erythrocytes)	1.6	14 h	70–95	—	—	Tilstone WJ, Dargle H, Dargle EN, et al: Pharmacokinetics of metolazone in normal subjects and in patients with cardiac or renal failure. Clin Pharmacol Ther 16: 322, 1974.
Metoprolol	38 ± 14 ↑ in HI	11 ± 1	4.2 ± 0.7	3–4 h $t_{1/2}$ is ↑ in HI and neonates	10 ± 3	15 ± 3	50–100 ng/mL	Dayer P, Leemann T, Marmy A, et al: Interindividual variation of beta-adrenoreceptor blocking drugs, plasma concentration and effect: influence of genetic status on behavior of atenolol, bopindolol and metoprolol. Eur J Clin Pharmacol 28:149, 1985.
Mexiletine	87 ± 13	50–60	4.9 ± 0.5	9.2 ± 2.1 h $t_{1/2}$ ↑ in MI, CHF, RI, and HI	10	6.3 ± 2.7 Cl is ↓ in MI, RI (Cl$_{Cr}$ <10 mL/min) and HI	0.5–2.0 µg/mL	Monk JP, Brogden RN: Mexiletine: a review of its pharmacodynamic and pharmacokinetic properties, and therapeutic use in the treatment of arrhythmias. Drugs 40: 374, 1990.
Midodrine	90–93 (based on desglymidodrine, active metabolite of midodrine)	—	4–4.6 (based on desglymidodrine, active metabolite of midodrine)	0.5 h 3 h (based on desglymidodrine, active metabolite of midodrine)	2–4	19.7–24.3 (total-body plasma Cl of desglymidodrine)	—	McTavish D, Goa KL: Midodrine: a review of its pharmacological properties and therapeutic use in orthostatic hypotension and secondary hypotensive disorders. Drugs 38:757, 1989.

Drug								Reference
Milrinone	≥80	70	0.32 ± 0.08	0.80 ± 0.22 h $t_{1/2}$ is ↑ in CHF and RI	85 ± 10	6.1 ± 1.3 Cl is ↓ in CHF and RI	150–250 ng/mL	Young RA, Ward A: Milrinone: A preliminary review of its pharmacological properties and therapeutic use. *Drugs* 36:158, 1988.
Minoxidil	ID	0	2.7 ± 0.7	3.1 ± 0.6 h (hypertensives)	20 ± 6	24 ± 6	—	Fleishaker JC, Andreadis NA, Welshman IR, et al: The pharmacokinetics of 2.5 to 10 mg oral doses of minoxidil in healthy volunteers. *J Clin Pharmacol* 29: 162, 1989.
Moexipril	13	90	—	1.3 h 2–9 h (moexiprilat)	<10	—	—	Van Hecken A, Verbesselt R, Depre M, et al: Moexipril does not alter the pharmacokinetics or pharmacodynamics of warfarin. *Eur J Clin Pharmacol* 45:291, 1993.
Moricizine	38	95	4.4	1.5–3.5 h $t_{1/2}$ is ↑ in HI	<1	—	—	Fitton A, Buckley MM: Moricizine: A review of its pharmacological properties, and therapeutic efficacy in cardiac arrhythmias. *Drugs* 40:138, 1990.
Nadolol	34 ± 5	20 ± 4	1.9 ± 0.2	16 ± 2 h $t_{1/2}$ is ↑ in RI and children	73 ± 4	2.9 ± 0.6 Cl is ↓ in RI	—	Morrison RA, Singhvi SM, Creasey WA, et al: Dose proportionality of nadolol pharmacokinetics after intravenous administration to healthy subjects. *Eur J Clin Pharmacol* 33:625, 1988.
Nesiritide	NA	—	0.19	18 min	—	9.2	—	Cheng JWM: Nesiritide: review of clinical pharmacology and role in heart failure management. *Heart Dis* 4:199, 2002.

(continued)

APPENDIX 1 *(continued)* Pharmacokinetic Properties of Approved Cardiovascular Drugs

Generic name	Bio-availability, %	Protein binding, %	V_d, L/kg	$t_{1/2}$	Urinary excretion, % unchanged	Cl, mL/min per kg	Therapeutic range	References
Nicardipine	18 ± 11	98–99.5	1.1 ± 0.3	2–4 h $t_{1/2}$ is ↑ in HI	<1	10.4 ± 3.1 Cl is ↓ in HI	0.1 μg/mL	Singh BN, Josephson MA: Clinical pharmacology, pharmacokinetics and hemodynamic effects of nicardipine. *Am Heart J* 119:427, 1990.
Nicotinic acid	88	<20	—	0.75–1 h	—	—	—	Soons PA, Schoemaker HC, Cohen AF, et al: Intraindividual variability in nifedipine pharmacokinetics and effects in healthy subjects. *J Clin Pharmacol* 32:324, 1992.
Nifedipine	50 ± 13	96 ± 1	0.78 ± 0.22	2.5 ± 1.3 h	<1	7.0 ± 1.8	47 ± 20 ng/mL	
Nimodipine	10 ± 4 ↑ in HI	98	1.7 ± 0.6	1.1 ± 0.3 h $t_{1/2}$ is ↑ in HI and RI	<1	19 ± 6 Cl is ↓ in HI and RI	—	Langley MS, Sorkin EM: Nimodipine: A review of its pharmacodynamic and pharmacokinetic properties, and therapeutic potential in cerebrovascular disease. *Drugs* 37:669, 1989.
Nisoldipine	3.7 ↑ in HI	99	4–5	8–9 h $t_{1/2}$ is ↑ in HI	—	—	—	Baksi AK, Edwards JS, Ahr G: A comparison of the pharmacokinetics of nisoldipine in elderly and young subjects. *Br J Clin Pharmacol* 31:367, 1991.
Nitroglycerin	<1 PO 38 ± 26 SL 72 ± 20 TOP	60	2.9	1–4 min	—	—	—	Thadani U, Whitsett T: Relationship of pharmacokinetic and pharmacodynamic properties of the organic nitrates. *Clin Pharmacokinet* 15:32, 1988.

Olmesartan	28.6 (post PO administration)	99	—	10–15 h	~0.5	0.3	—	Brunner HR: The new oral angiotensin II antagonist olmesartan medoxomil: A concise overview. *J Hum Hypertens* 16(suppl 2): S13, 2002.
Penbutolol	100	80–98	<10	5 h t½ is ↑ in RI	—	—	—	Brockmeier D, Hajdu P, Henke W, et al: Penbutolol: pharmacokinetics, effect on exercise tachycardia, and in vitro inhibition of radioligand binding. *Eur J Clin Pharmacol* 35:613, 1988.
Pentoxifylline	33 ± 13 ↑ in HI	0	0	0.9 ± 0.3 h t½ is ↑ in elderly and HI	4.2 ± 0.9	60 ± 13 Cl is ↓ in elderly and HI	—	Ward A, Clissold SP: Pentoxifylline: a review of its pharmacodynamic and pharmacokinetic properties, and its therapeutic efficacy. *Drugs* 34:50, 1987.
Perindopril	~75 (properties of perindopril) ~25 (properties of perindoprilat)	60 (properties of perindopril) 10–20 (properties of perindoprilat)	3–10	0.8–1 h (properties of perindopril) 3–10 h (properties of perindoprilat) 30–120 h (prolonged terminal elimination t½ perindoprilat)	0.22 (properties of perindopril) 0.16 (properties of perindoprilat)	3.1–5.2	—	Todd PA, Fitton A: Perindopril: a review of its pharmacological properties and therapeutic use in cardiovascular disorders. Drugs 42:90, 1991.
Pindolol	75 ± 9 ↓ in RI	40–60	35–50	3.6 ± 0.6 h t½ is ↑ in RI and HI	2.3 ± 0.9	8.3 ± 1.8 Cl is ↓ in RI and HI	—	Guerret M, Cheymol G, Aubry JP, et al: Estimation of the absolute oral bioavailability of pindolol by two analytical methods. *Eur J Clin Pharmacol* 25:357, 1983.
Polythiazide	ID	84	25	25.7	—	—	—	

(continued)

APPENDIX 1 (continued) Pharmacokinetic Properties of Approved Cardiovascular Drugs

Generic name	Bio-availability, %	Protein binding, %	V_d, L/kg	$t_{1/2}$	Urinary excretion, % unchanged	Cl, mL/min per kg	Therapeutic range	References
Pravastatin	18 ± 8	43–48	0.46 ± 0.04	1.8 ± 0.8	20 h	13.5 (Cl post IV dose) Cl is ↓ in HI	—	Quion JAV, Jones PH: Clinical pharmacokinetics of pravastatin. Clin Pharmacokinet 27:94, 1994.
Prazosin	48–68	95 ± 1	0.60 ± 0.13	2.9 ± 0.8 h $t_{1/2}$ is ↑ in CHF and elderly	<1	3.0 ± 0.3 Cl is ↓ in CHF	—	Vincent J, Meredith PA, Reid JL, et al: Clinical pharmacokinetics of prazosin—1985. Clin Pharmacokinet 10:144, 1985.
Probucol	2–8	95	—	12–500 h	0	—	23.6 ± 17.2 µg/mL	
Procainamide	83 ± 16	16 ± 5	1.9 ± 0.3	3.0 ± 0.6 h $t_{1/2}$ is ↑ in RI, MI, and ↓ in children and neonates	67 ± 8	3.2 (fast acetylator) and 1.1 (slow acetylator) Cl is ↑ in children and ↓ in MI	3–10 µg/mL	Karlson E: Clinical pharmacokinetics of procainamide. Clin Pharmacokinet 3:97, 1978.
Propafenone	5–50 (dose dependent)	85–95	3.6 ± 2.1	2–10 h (fast metabolizers) 10–32 h (slow metabolizers)	<1	17 ± 8 Cl is ↓ in HI	0.2–1.5 µg/mL	Bryson HM, Palmer KJ, Langtry HD, et al: Propafenone: a reappraisal of its pharmacology, pharmacokinetics and therapeutic use in cardiac arrhythmias. Drugs 45:85, 1993.
Propranolol	26 ± 10	87 ± 6	4.3 ± 0.6	3–5 h $t_{1/2}$ is ↑ in HI	<0.5	11.4–17.1 Cl is ↓ in HI	20 ng/mL	McDevitt DG: Comparison of pharmacokinetic properties of beta-adrenoreceptor blocking drugs. Eur Heart J 8(suppl M):9, 1987.
Quinapril	60	97	0.4	2.2 ± 0.2 h (quinaprilat) $t_{1/2}$ is ↑ in elderly and RI	Trace	2.0 ± 0.6 Cl is ↓ in elderly and RI	—	Wadworth AN, Brogden RN: Quinapril: a review of its pharmacological properties and therapeutic efficacy in cardiovascular disorders. Drugs 41:378, 1991.

Drug								Reference
Quinidine	70–80 / 71 ± 17	87 ± 3	2.7 ± 1.2	6.2 ± 1.8 h t½ is ↑ in elderly	18 ± 5	4.7 ± 1.8 Cl is ↓ in RI, elderly, and severe CHF	2–6 µg/mL	Verme CN, Ludden TM, Clementi WA, et al: Pharmacokinetics of quinidine in male patients: a population analysis. *Clin Pharmacokinet* 22:468, 1992.
Ramipril	50–60	56	—	14 ± 7 h (ramiprilat) t½ is ↑ in RI	<2	1.1 ± 0.4 Cl is ↓ in RI	—	Meisel S, Shamiss A, Rosenthal T: Clinical pharmacokinetics of ramipril. *Clin Pharmacokinet* 26:7, 1994.
Reserpine	50		0.086 (apparent V_d during terminal elimination phase)	33	<1	—	—	
Reteplase	—			13–16 min (effective t½)		3.6–6.4 (plasma Cl)	2000 IU/mL (activity) 4200 µg/L (antigen)	Noble S, McTavish D: Reteplase: a review of its pharmacological properties and clinical efficacy in the management of acute myocardial infarction. *Drugs* 52:589, 1996.
Rosuvastatin	20	88	~1.9	19	~5	—	—	Cheng-Lai A: Rosuvastatin: a new HMG-CoA reductase inhibitor for the treatment of hypercholesterolemia. *Heart Dis* 5:72, 2003.
Simvastatin	<5	94	—	1.9 h	<0.5	7.6	—	Mauro VF, MacDonald JL: Simvastatin: a review of its pharmacology and clinical use. *DICP* 25:257, 1991.
Sodium nitroprusside	NA	ID	—	3–4 min 3–4 d (thiocyanate) t½ is ↑ in RI	—	—	—	Schulz V: Clinical pharmacokinetics of nitroprusside, cyanide, thiosulphate and thiocyanate. *Clin Pharmacokinet* 9:239, 1984.
Sotalol	90–100	0	2.0 ± 0.4	7–15 h t½ is ↑ in RI and elderly	80.1	2.6 ± 0.5 Cl is ↓ in RI and elderly	—	Antonaccio MJ, Gomoll A: Pharmacology, pharmacodynamics and pharmacokinetics of sotalol. *Am J Cardiol* 65:12A, 1990.

(continued)

APPENDIX 1 *(continued)* Pharmacokinetic Properties of Approved Cardiovascular Drugs

Generic name	Bio-availability, %	Protein binding, %	V_d, L/kg	$t_{1/2}$	Urinary excretion, % unchanged	Cl, mL/min per kg	Therapeutic range	References
Spironolactone	60–70	>90	—	1.3–1.4 h 13–24 h (canrenone) $t_{1/2}$ is ↑ in elderly	<1	— Cl is ↓ in elderly	—	Overdick HW, Merkus FW: The metabolism and biopharmaceutics of spironolactone in man. *Rev Drug Metab Drug Interact* 5:273, 1987.
Streptokinase	NA	—	0.08 ± 0.04	0.61 ± 0.04 h	0	1.7 ± 0.7	—	Gemmill JD, Hogg KJ, Burns JMA, et al: A comparison of the pharmacokinetic properties of streptokinase and anistreplase in acute myocardial infarction. *Br J Clin Pharmacol* 31:143, 1991.
Telmisartan	43	>99	7.1	~24 h	<1	>11	—	McClellan KJ, Markham A: Telmisartan. *Drugs* 56:1039, 1998.
Tenecteplase	NA	ID	0.09–0.21	11–20 min (α) 41–138 min (β)	ID	2.2	—	Tsikouris JP, Tsikouris AP: A review of available fibrin-specific thrombolytic agents used in acute myocardial infarction. *Pharmacotherapy* 21:207, 2001.
Terazosin	90	90–94	0.80 ± 0.18	9–12 h	12 ± 3	1.1 ± 0.2	—	Titmarsh S, Monk JP: Terazosin: a review of its pharmacodynamic and pharmacokinetic properties and therapeutic efficacy in essential hypertension. *Drugs* 33:461, 1987.
Ticlopidine	80–90	98	—	4–5 d $t_{1/2}$ is ↑ in RI	Trace	8–21 Cl is ↓ in RI	1–2 µg/mL	Saltiel E, Ward A: Ticlopidine: a review of its pharmacodynamic and pharmacokinetic properties and therapeutic efficacy in platelet-dependent disease states. *Drugs* 34:222, 1987.

Timolol	50	<10 (by equilibrium analysis; 60 (by ultrafiltration)	2.1 ± 0.8	3–5 h	15	7.3 ± 3.3	—	McGourty JC, Silas JH, Fleming JJ, et al: Pharmacokinetics and beta-blocking effects of timolol in poor and extensive metabolizers of debrisoquin. *Clin Pharmacol Ther* 38:409, 1985.
Tinzaparin	90 (based on anti-Xa activity)	ID	0.06 (based on anti-Xa activity)	3–4 h (based on anti-Xa activity)	ID	0.4 (Cl post IV administration of 4500 IU tinzaparin)	— (monitoring based on anti-Xa activity generally not advised)	Friedel HA, Balfour JA: Tinzaparin. A review of its pharmacology and clinical potential in the prevention and treatment of thromboembolic disorders. *Drugs* 48:638, 1994.
Tirofiban	NA	ID (not highly bound to plasma proteins)	0.3–0.6	~2 h	<65 (cleared from plasma largely by renal excretion with ~65 of administered dose appearing in urine, largely unchanged)	3.0–4.5	—	McClellan KJ, Goa KL: Tirofiban. A review of its use in acute coronary syndromes. *Drugs* 56:1067, 1998.
Tocainide	89 ± 5	10–15	3.0 ± 0.2	13.5 ± 2.3 h t½ is ↑ in RI	38 ± 7	2.6 ± 0.5 Cl is ↓ in CHF and RI	3–9 µg/mL	Roden DM, Woosley RL: Drug therapy: Tocainide. *N Engl J Med* 315:41, 1986.
Tolazoline	NA	—	1.61 ± 0.21	3–10 h in neonate	—	—	—	Ward RM, Daniel CH, Kendig JW, et al: Oliguria and tolazoline pharmacokinetics in the newborn. *Pediatrics* 77:307, 1986.
Torsemide	80–90	97–99	0.16	3–4 h	27	—	—	Knauf H, Spahn H, Mutschler P: The loop diuretic torsemide in chronic renal failure: Pharmacokinetic and pharmacodynamics. *Drugs* 41 (suppl 3):23, 1991.

(continued)

APPENDIX 1 *(continued)* Pharmacokinetic Properties of Approved Cardiovascular Drugs

Generic name	Bio-availability, %	Protein binding, %	V_d, L/kg	$t_{1/2}$	Urinary excretion, % unchanged	Cl, mL/min per kg	Therapeutic range	References
PTrandolapril	40–60 (trandolaprilat)	80	—	0.7–1.3 h 16–24 h (trandolaprilat) $t_{1/2}$ is ↑ in RI	—	—	—	Wiseman LR, McTavish D: Trandolapril: a review of its pharmacodynamic and pharmacokinetic properties, and therapeutic use in essential hypertension. *Drugs* 48:71, 1994.
Treprostinil	100 (SC infusion)	91	0.2	2–4 h	4	7.1	—	
Triamterene	54 ± 12	61 ± 2	13.4 ± 4.9	4.2 ± 0.7 h $t_{1/2}$ is ↑ in RI and and elderly	21	63 ± 20 Cl is ↓ in HI, RI, and elderly	—	Gilfrich HJ, Kremer G, Mohrke W, et al: Pharmacokinetics of triamterene after IV administration to man: determination of bioavailability. *Eur J Clin Pharmacol* 25:237, 1983.
Trichlor-methiazide	ID	—	—	2.3–7.3 h	ID	—	—	Sketris IS, Skoutakis VA, Acchiardo SR, et al: The pharmacokinetics of trichlormethiazide in hypertensive patients with normal and compromised renal function. *Eur J Clin Pharmacol* 20:453, 1981.
Urokinase	NA	—	—	10–20 min $t_{1/2}$ ↑ in HI	—	—	—	Maizel AS, Bookstein JJ: Streptokinase, urokinase, and tissue plasminogen activator: relative pharmacokinetics, relative advantages, and methods for maximizing rates and consistency of lysis. *Cardiovasc Intervent Radiol* 9:236, 1986.

Drug								Reference
Valsartan	25 (10–35)	95 (94–97)	0.24	6 h	<13	0.48	—	Criscione L, et al: Valsartan: pre-clinical and clinical profile of an antihypertensive angiotensin-II antagonist. *Cardiovasc Drug Rev* 13:230, 1995.
Verapamil	22 ± 8	90 ± 2	5.0 ± 2.1	4.0 ± 1.5 h t½ is ↑ in HI and elderly	<3	15 ± 6 Cl is ↓ in HI and elderly	80–300 ng/mL	McTavish D, Sorkin EM: Verapamil: an updated review of its pharma-codynamic and pharmacokinetic properties and therapeutic use in hypertension. *Drugs* 38:19, 1989.
Warfarin	93 ± 8	99 ± 1	0.14 ± 0.06	37 ± 15 h	<2	0.045 ± 0.024	— (dose should be adjusted based on desired INR range)	Chan E, McLachlan AJ, Pegg M, et al: Disposition of warfarin enantiomers and metabolites in patients during multiple dosing with *rac*-warfarin. *Br J Clin Pharmacol* 37:563, 1994.

Key: CAD, coronary artery disease; CHF, congestive heart failure; Cl, clearance; Cl_{Cr}, creatine clearance; HI, hepatic impairment; ID, insufficient data; INR, international normalized ratio; IV, intravenous; MI, myocardial infarction; NA, not applicable; PO, oral; RF, renal failure; RI, renal impairment; SC, subcutaneous; SL, sublingual; t½, half-life; TOP, topical; V_d, volume of distribution; Xa, activated factor X; ↑, increased; ↓, decreased.

APPENDIX 2 Therapeutic Use of Available Cardiovascular Drugs

α-Adrenergic blockers

Doxazosin (doxazosin, Cardura)

Indications — Hypertension, benign prostatic hyperplasia

Dosage

Adults — As an antihypertensive, initiate at 1 mg/d; dosage may be increased gradually according to blood pressure response; may increase q1–2 wk to 2, 4, 8, 16 mg/d as needed

Initiate at lowest dose and titrate to response

Elderly

Children — Safety and efficacy have not been established

Preparations — Doxazosin (generic); Cardura (Pfizer): 1-, 2-, 4-, and 8-mg tablets

Prazosin (prazosin, Minipress)

Indication — Hypertension

Dosage

Adults — As an antihypertensive, initiate therapy at 1 mg bid or tid and slowly increase to the usual maintenance dose of 6–15 mg/d in divided doses. Most patients can be maintained on a twice-daily regimen after initial titration. Doses >20 mg usually do not have increased effect; some patients may respond to up to 40 mg/d.

Initiate at lowest dose and titrate to response

Elderly

Children — Safety and efficacy have not been established; however, there has been some experience with the use of this drug in children and the following dosage regimen has been suggested: for children <7 y of age, initiate at 250 µg (0.25 mg) bid or tid and adjust to response; for children 7–12 y of age, initiate at 500 µg (0.5 mg) bid or tid and adjust to response

Preparations — Prazosin (generic); Minipress (Pfizer): 1-, 2-, 5-mg capsules

Fixed-dose combinations for the treatment of hypertension — Minizide-prazosin/polythiazide combination tablet: 1 mg/0.5 mg, 2 mg/0.5 mg, 5 mg/0.5 mg

Terazosin (terazosin, Hytrin)

Indications — Hypertension, benign prostatic hyperplasia

Dosage

Adults — As an antihypertensive, initiate therapy with 1 mg at bedtime. Dosage may be increased slowly to achieve desired response. There seems to be little benefit in exceeding a dose of 20 mg/d. Usual maintenance dose is 1–5 mg/d.

614

Elderly	Initiate at lowest dose and titrate to response
Children	Safety and efficacy have not been established
Preparations	Terazosin (generic); Hytrin (Abbott Laboratories): 1-, 2-, 5-, 10-mg capsules

Phenoxybenzamine (Dibenzyline)

Indication	Symptomatic management of pheochromocytoma

Dosage

Adults	Initiate with 10 mg bid. Dose may be increased every other day by 10 mg until the desired response is obtained. Usual dose range is 20–40 mg bid or tid. Phenoxybenzamine may be used concurrently with a beta blocker if troublesome tachycardia coexists.
Elderly	Initiate at lowest dose and titrate to response
Children	Safety and efficacy have not been established, but there has been some experience with the use of this drug in children and the following dosage regimen has been suggested: initiate at 0.2 mg/kg once daily (maximum dose, 10 mg/d); dosage may be increased gradually by 0.2-mg/kg increments until an adequate response is achieved; the usual pediatric maintenance dosage is 0.4–1.2 mg/kg daily given q6–8h; higher doses may be needed in some cases.
Preparation	Dibenzyline (Wellspring): 10-mg capsules

Phentolamine (Regitine)

Indications	Diagnosis of pheochromocytoma; prevention or control of hypertensive episodes that may occur in a patient with pheochromocytoma as a result of stress or manipulation during preoperative preparation and surgical excision; prevention or treatment of dermal necrosis and sloughing after IV administration or extravasation of norepinephrine

Dosage

Prevention or control of hypertensive episodes associated with pheochromocytoma

Adults	Preoperative: 5 mg (1 mg for children) IV or IM 1–2 h before surgery and repeat if indicated
	Intraoperative: 5 mg IV (1 mg for children) and repeat as indicated to prevent or control paroxysms of hypertension, tachycardia, respiratory depression, convulsions, or other effects related to epinephrine intoxication
Elderly	No dosage adjustment is required
Children	Use lower dose in children as described above

(continued)

APPENDIX 2 *(continued)* Therapeutic Use of Available Cardiovascular Drugs

Prevention or treatment of dermal necrosis and sloughing associated with IV norepinephrine

Adults

Prevention: 10 mg of phentolamine is added to each liter of norepinephrine solution

Treatment: Initiate within 12 h (as soon as possible) of extravasation; 5–10 mg of phentolamine in 10 mL of 0.9% sodium chloride is infiltrated into the area by using a small needle syringe

Diagnosis of pheochromocytoma (not the first test of choice; all nonessential medications should be withheld for at least 24 h before the test)

Adults

5 mg IV or IM (1 mg IV or 3 mg IM for children) is administered; 5 mg of phentolamine should be dissolved in 1 mL sterile water for injection before administration. After the IV dose, blood pressure should be monitored immediately, q30 s for the first 3 min, and every minute for the next 7 min. After the IM dose, blood pressure should be monitored q5 min for 30–45 min; blood pressure decrease ≥35 mm Hg systolic and 25 mm Hg diastolic within 2 min after IV or 20 min after IM administration of phentolamine is considered a positive test for pheochromocytoma.

Elderly   No dosage adjustment is required

Children   Use lower dose in children as described above

Preparation   Phentolamine mesylate for injection (Bedford); Regitine (Ciba): 5-mg vials

α₂-Adrenergic agonists
Clonidine (clonidine, Catapres, Catapres-TTS, Duraclon)

Indications   Hypertension (PO and transdermal formulations); severe cancer pain not adequately relieved by opioid analgesics alone (continuous epidural infusion)

Dosage

Adults

PO: Initiate therapy at 0.05–0.1 mg bid. Dose may be increased 0.1–0.2 mg/d every few days until the desired response is achieved. For rapid blood pressure reduction in patients with severe hypertension, clonidine 0.1–0.2 mg may be given, followed by 0.05–0.2 mg/h until a total dose of 0.5–0.7 mg or adequate blood pressure control is achieved. Usual dose range of clonidine is 0.2–2.4 mg/d given in 2–3 divided doses

Transdermal: Initiate with one TTS-1 (2.5 mg) patch; increase to the next largest dose q1–2 wk for additional control or use a combination of patches. Maximum dosage is 2 TTS-3 patches. *Note:* For patients already on oral clonidine, it is recommended that the oral dose be continued 1–2 d after the first transdermal system is applied.

IV: Initial dose of clonidine for continuous epidural infusion is 30 µg/h; dosage may be titrated up or down depending on pain relief and occurrence of adverse events. Experience with dosage rate >40 µg/h is limited.

Elderly — Initiate at lowest dose and titrate to response

Children — Safety and efficacy have not been established

Preparations — Clonidine (generic); Catapres (Boehringer Ingelheim): 0.1-, 0.2-, 0.3-mg tablets

Transdermal system: Catapres-TTS-1, TTS-2, TTS-3 (Boehringer Ingelheim) delivers 0.1, 0.2, 0.3 mg/d, respectively

Injection, as hydrochloride; Duraclon: 100 μg/mL (10-mL vials)

Combipres: clonidine/chlorthalidone combination tablets: 0.1 mg/15 mg, 0.2 mg/15 mg, 0.3 mg/15 mg

Fixed-dose combinations for the treatment of hypertension

Guanabenz (guanabenz, Wytensin)

Indication — Hypertension

Dosage

Adults — Initiate therapy at 4 mg bid; dose may be adjusted q1–2 wk in increments of 4-8 mg/d until adequate blood pressure control is achieved; maximum daily dose is 32 mg given in 2 divided doses

Elderly — Initiate at lowest dose and titrate to response

Children — Safety and efficacy have not been established

Preparations — Guanabenz (generic); Wytensin (Wyeth-Ayerst): 4-, 8-mg tablets

Guanfacine (guanfacine, Tenex)

Indication — Hypertension

Dosage

Adults — Initiate with 1 mg at bedtime to minimize somnolence; dose may be increased in 1-mg increments q3–4 wk until adequate blood pressure control is achieved. Maximum daily dose is 3 mg.

Elderly — Initiate at lowest dose and titrate to response

Children — Safety and efficacy have not been established

Preparations — Guanfacine (generic); Tenex (ESP Pharma): 1-, 2-mg tablets

Methyldopa (methyldopa, Aldomet)

Indication — Hypertension

Dosage

Adults — PO: Initiate therapy at 250 mg bid or tid for 2 d. Dose is then increased at intervals ≥2 d until adequate blood pressure control is achieved. Maximum PO dose is 3 g/d. *Note:* In patients receiving concomitant antihypertensive therapy other than thiazides, limit the initial dosage to 500 mg/d.

(continued)

	IV (methyldopate): Add the dose, 250–500 mg, to 100 mL 5% dextrose or give in D5W in a concentration of 10 mg/mL. Administer IV over 30–60 min q6h if necessary. Maximum dose is 1 g q6h
Elderly	Initiate at lowest dose and titrate to response
Children	Safety and efficacy have not been established, but there has been some experience with the use of this drug in children and the following dosage regimen has been suggested
	PO: Dose should be based on body weight. Initially, give 10 mg/kg daily in 2–4 divided doses. Dosage should be adjusted in daily increments of 10 mg/kg until adequate blood pressure control is achieved. Maximum daily dose is 65 mg/kg or 3 g, whichever is less.
	IV: Dose should be based on body weight: 20–40 mg/kg daily in divided doses q6h. Maximum daily dose is 65 mg/ kg or 3 g, whichever is less.
Preparations	Methyldopa (generic); Aldomet (Merck): 125-, 250-, 500-mg tablets
	Methyldopate HCl injection (generic); Aldomet injection (Merck): 50 mg/mL, 250 mg/5 mL
	Aldomet PO suspension (Merck): 250 mg/5 mL
Fixed-dose combinations for the treatment of hypertension	Aldoclor (Merck): methyldopa/chlorothiazide combination tablets: 250 mg/150 mg, 250 mg/250 mg
	Aldoril (Merck): methyldopa/hydrochlorothiazide combination tablets: 250 mg/15 mg, 250 mg/25 mg
	Aldoril D (Merck): methyldopa/hydrochlorothiazide combination tablets: 500 mg/30 mg, 500 mg/50 mg

ACE inhibitors
Benazepril (Lotensin)

Indication	Hypertension
Dosage	
Adults	Usual initial dose is 10 mg once daily. Dose can be titrated up to 40 mg/d (in 1 or 2 divided doses); maximum dose is 80 mg/d. In renovascular hypertension, renal failure, or in patients in whom diuretics have not been discontinued, the starting dose should be 5 mg.
Elderly	Dose reduction generally not required
Children	Safety and efficacy have not been established
Preparations	Lotensin (Novartis Pharmaceuticals): 5-, 10-, 20-, 40-mg tablets
Fixed-dose combinations for the treatment of hypertension	Lotensin HCT: benazepril hydrochloride/hydrochlorothiazide combination tablets: 5 mg/6.25 mg, 10 mg/12.5 mg, 20 mg/12.5 mg, 20 mg/25 mg
	Lotrel: amlodipine/benazepril hydrochloride combination capsules: 2.5 mg/10 mg, 5 mg/10 mg, 5 mg/20 mg, 10 mg/20 mg

Captopril (captopril, Capoten)

Indications

Hypertension, heart failure, left ventricular dysfunction post MI, diabetic nephropathy

Dosage

Hypertension

Adults

Initiate therapy at 12.5–25 mg bid or tid. Dosage may be increased according to response to 150 mg/d given in 3 divided doses. In renovascular hypertension, when diuretics have not been discontinued or in renal impairment, initial dose should be 6.25 mg, titrated cautiously according to response.

Elderly

Initiate at lowest dose and titrate to response

Children

Safety and efficacy have not been established, but the following regimen has been suggested: initiate with 0.3 mg/kg tid; dosage may be increased in increments of 0.3 mg/kg at intervals of 8–24 h until adequate blood pressure control is achieved

Heart failure

Adults

Initiate at 6.25–12.5 mg tid and increase dosage according to clinical response; target dose is 150 mg/d given in 3 divided doses

Diabetic nephropathy

Adults

25 mg tid in type 1 diabetes

Left ventricular dysfunction after MI

Adults

Initiate with 6.25 mg, followed by 12.5 mg tid; then increase dose to 25 mg tid during the next several days. A target dose of 50 mg tid may be achieved over the next several weeks.

Preparations

Captopril (generic): Capoten (Bristol-Myers-Squibb): 12.5-, 25-, 50-, 100-mg tablets

Fixed-dose combinations for the treatment of hypertension

Capozide (generic): captopril/hydrochlorothiazide combination tablets: 25 mg/15 mg, 25 mg/25 mg, 50 mg/15 mg, 50 mg/25 mg

Enalapril (enalapril, Vasotec) and Enalaprilat (enalaprilat, Vasotec IV)

Indications

Hypertension; heart failure; left ventricular dysfunction, asymptomatic

Dosage

Hypertension

Adults

PO: Initiate therapy at 5 mg/d. Dosage may be increased to the usual effective maintenance dose of 10–20 mg/d (maximum, 40 mg/d given in 2 divided doses). In renovascular hypertension or in patients in whom diuretics have not been discontinued 2–3 d previously, the starting dose should be 2.5 mg.

(continued)

APPENDIX 2 *(continued)* Therapeutic Use of Available Cardiovascular Drugs

	IV: Usual IV dose in hypertension is 1.25 mg q6h administered IV over 5 min. An initial dose of 0.625 mg over 5 min should be used in patients who are sodium and volume depleted or who have renal impairment (CrCl <30 mL/min). Patients should be observed 1 h after taking the dose to watch for hypotension. If response is inadequate after 1 h, the 0.625-mg dose may be repeated and therapy continued at a dose of 1.25 mg q6h.
Elderly	Initiate at lowest dose and titrate to response
Children	Safety and efficacy have not been established
Heart failure	
Adults	Initiate therapy at 2.5 mg PO once or twice per day. Dosage may be titrated according to clinical response. Usual maintenance dose is 5–40 mg/d given in 2 divided doses.
Asymptomatic left ventricular dysfunction	
Adults	Initiate therapy at 2.5 mg PO once or twice per day. Dosage may be titrated according to clinical response. The target daily dose is 20 mg/d given in 2 divided doses.
Preparations	Enalapril (generic); Vasotec (Merck): 2.5-, 5-, 10-, 20-mg tablets
	Enalaprilat (generic); Vasotec IV (Merck): 1.25 mg/mL IV solution
Fixed-dose combinations for the treatment of hypertension	Vaseretic: enalapril maleate/hydrochlorothiazide combination tablets: 5 mg/12.5 mg, 10 mg/25 mg
	Teczem (Aventis): enalapril maleate/diltiazem malate ER combination tablets: 5 mg/180 mg
	Lexxel (Astra Zeneca): enalapril maleate/felodipine ER combination tablets: 5 mg/2.5 mg, 5 mg/5 mg
Fosinopril (Monopril)	
Indications	Hypertension, heart failure
Dosage	
Hypertension	
Adults	Initiate with 10 mg/d. Dosage may be increased to the usual effective dose of 20–40 mg/d. Some patients may have a further response to 80 mg/d. Total daily dose may be divided into 2 if trough effect is inadequate. In renovascular hypertension or in patients in whom diuretics have not been discontinued, the starting dose should be 5 mg/d.
Elderly	Dose reduction generally not required
Children	Safety and efficacy have not been established
Heart failure	
Adults	Usual initial dose is 10 mg/d. The patient should be observed under medical supervision for at least 2 h for the presence of hypotension or orthostasis after the initial dose of fosinopril. An initial dose of 5 mg may be used in

patients with moderate to severe renal impairment or in those who have been vigorously diuresed. Dosage should be increased over a period of several weeks to a dose that is maximal and tolerated. Usual effective dosage range is 20–40 mg once daily.

Preparations

Fixed-dose combinations for treatment of hypertension

Monopril (Bristol-Myers-Squibb): 10-, 20-, 40-mg tablets
Monopril HCT: fosinopril/hydrochlorothiazide combination tablets: 10 mg/12.5 mg, 20 mg/12.5 mg

Lisinopril (Prinivil, Zestril)

Indications

Hypertension, heart failure, acute MI

Dosage

Hypertension

Adults

Initiate with 10 mg/d. Dosage may be adjusted to the usual effective dose of 10–40 mg/d according to response. In patients with hyponatremia, patients with renal impairment (CrCl ≤30 mL/min), or patients in whom diuretics have not been discontinued, the starting dose should be 2.5 mg/d.

Elderly

Initiate at lowest dose and titrate to response

Children

Safety and efficacy have not been established

Heart failure

Adults

Usual initial dose is 5 mg/d administered under close medical observation, especially in patients with low blood pressure. Usual effective dosage range is 5–20 mg once daily.

Acute MI

Adults

In hemodynamically stable patients, give 5 mg of lisinopril within 24 h of the onset of acute MI. Another dose of 5 mg may be given 24 h later, followed by 10 mg at 48 h, and then 10 mg once daily thereafter for 6 wk. Patients should receive, as appropriate, the standard recommended treatments, such as thrombolytics, aspirin, and beta blockers. Patients with a low systolic blood pressure (≤120 mm Hg) when treatment is initiated or during the first 3 d after the infarct should be given a lower dose of 2.5 mg. If hypotension occurs (systolic blood pressure ≤100 mm Hg), a daily maintenance dose of 5 mg may be given with temporary reductions to 2.5 mg if necessary.

Preparations

Lisinopril (generic); Prinivil (Merck): 2.5-, 5-, 10-, 20-, 40-mg tablets
Lisinopril (generic); Zestril (Astra Zeneca): 2.5-, 5-, 10-, 20-, 30-, 40-mg tablets

Fixed-dose combinations for the treatment of hypertension

Prinzide: lisinopril/hydrochlorothiazide combination tablets: 10 mg/12.5 mg, 20 mg/12.5 mg, 20 mg/25 mg
Zestoretic: lisinopril/hydrochlorothiazide combination tablets: 10 mg/12.5 mg, 20 mg/12.5 mg, 20 mg/25mg

(continued)

APPENDIX 2 (continued) Therapeutic Use of Available Cardiovascular Drugs

Moexipril (Univasc)

Indication
Hypertension

Dosage

Adults
Usual initial dose is 7.5 mg once daily in patients not receiving diuretics. Dosage may be increased gradually to a maximum of 30 mg/d (given in 1 or 2 divided doses) according to response. In renovascular hypertension or in patients in whom diuretics have not been discontinued, the recommended starting dose is 3.75 mg once daily given with close medical supervision. Similarly, for patients whose CrCl ≤40 mL/min or 1.73 m², the recommended initial dose is 3.75 mg once daily given with caution. Note: Moexipril should be taken on an empty stomach, preferably 1 h before a meal.

Elderly
Initiate at lowest dose and titrate to response

Children
Safety and efficacy have not been established

Preparations
Univasc (Schwarz Pharma): 7.5-, 15-mg tablets

Fixed-dose combinations for the treatment of hypertension
Uniretic: moexipril hydrochloride/hydrochlorothiazide combination tablets: 7.5 mg/12.5 mg, 15 mg/25 mg

Perindopril (Aceon)

Indication
Hypertension

Dosage

Adults
Usual initial dose is 4 mg once daily in patients not receiving other antihypertensives. This dose may be titrated up to a maximum of 16 mg/d based on clinical response. Usual maintenance dose is 4–8 mg once daily. For patients >70 y of age and those with CrCl of 30–60 mL/min, initiate with 2 mg once daily and titrate according to response to a maximum of 8 mg/d. Safety and efficacy of perindopril have not been established for patients with CrCl <30 mL/min.

Elderly
Initiate at lowest dose and titrate to response

Children
Safety and efficacy have not been established

Preparations
Aceon (Solvay): 2-, 4-, 8-mg tablets

Quinapril (Accupril)

Indications
Hypertension, heart failure

Dosage

Hypertension

Adults
Usual initial dose is 10 or 20 mg once daily in patients not receiving diuretics; this dose may be increased, at intervals of at least 2 wk, to a maximum of 80 mg/d (given as 1 dose or in 2 divided doses) according to

622

response. In renovascular hypertension or in patients in whom diuretics have not been discontinued, the starting dose should be 2.5–5 mg/d. For patients with CrCl of 31–60 mL/min, the initial dose should be 5 mg/d. For patients with CrCl of 10–30 mL/min, the initial dose should be 2.5 mg/d.

Elderly

Children Initiate at lowest dose and titrate to response

Heart failure

Adults Safety and efficacy have not been established

Usual initial dose is 5 mg bid titrated according to clinical response. Usual maintenance dose is 20–40 mg/d in 2 divided doses.

Preparations Accupril (Parke-Davis/Pfizer): 5-, 10-, 20-, 40-mg tablets

Fixed-dose combinations for the treatment of hypertension Accuretic: quinapril/hydrochlorothiazide combination tablets: 10 mg/12.5 mg, 20 mg/12.5 mg, 20 mg/25 mg

Ramipril (Altace)

Indications Hypertension; heart failure after MI; reduction in risk of MI, stroke, and death from cardiovascular causes

Dosage

Hypertension

Adults Usual initial dose is 2.5 mg/d; this dose may be increased gradually to a maximum of 20 mg/d (given as 1 daily dose or 2 equally divided doses) according to response. In renovascular hypertension or in patients in whom diuretics have not been discontinued, the starting dose should be 1.25 mg/d. For patients with CrCl <40 mL/min per 1.73 m², the initial dose should be 1.25 mg/d. Dosage may be titrated upward until blood pressure is controlled or to a maximum of 5 mg/d.

Elderly

Children Initiate at lowest dose and titrate to response

Heart failure after MI

Adults Safety and efficacy have not been established

Usual initial dose is 2.5 mg bid. Patients who become hypotensive at this dose may be switched to 1.25 mg bid, but all patients should then be titrated toward a target dose of 5 mg bid if tolerated. For patients with CrCl <40 mL/min per 1.73 m², the initial dose should be 1.25 mg/d. Dosage may then be increased to 1.25 mg bid up to a maximum dose of 2.5 mg bid, depending on clinical response and tolerance.

Reduction in risk of MI, stroke, and death from cardiovascular causes

Adults Initiate at 2.5 mg once daily for 1 wk, increase dose to 5 mg once daily for the next 3 wk, and then increase dose as tolerated to 10 mg once daily (may be given as divided dose).

(continued)

623

APPENDIX 2 *(continued)* Therapeutic Use of Available Cardiovascular Drugs

Preparations	Altace (Monarch): 1.25-, 2.5-, 5-, 10-mg capsules
Trandolapril (Mavik)	
Indications	Hypertension, heart failure post MI, left ventricular dysfunction post MI
Dosage	
Hypertension	
Adults	Usual initial dose is 1 mg/d in non-black patients and 2 mg/d in black patients. Dosage may be increased, according to response, at intervals of ≥1 wk to a maximum of 8 mg/d. Most patients have required dosages of 2–4 mg/d. There is little experience with doses >8 mg/d. Patients inadequately treated with once-daily dosing at 4 mg may be treated with twice-daily dosing. In renovascular hypertension or in patients in whom diuretics have not been discontinued, the starting dose should be 0.5 mg/d. Similarly, for patients with CrCl <30 mL/min or with hepatic cirrhosis, the recommended initial dose is 0.5 mg/d.
Elderly	Initiate at lowest dose and titrate to response
Children	Safety and efficacy have not been established
Heart failure or left ventricular dysfunction post MI	
Adults	Usual initial dose is 1 mg/d; this dose may be increased as tolerated to a target dose of 4 mg/d. If the 4-mg dose is not tolerated, patients can continue therapy with the greatest tolerated dose. For patients with CrCl <30 mL/min or with hepatic cirrhosis, the recommended initial dose is 0.5 mg/d.
Preparations	Mavik (Abbott): 1-, 2-, 4-mg tablets
Fixed-dose combinations for the treatment of hypertension	Tarka: trandolapril/verapamil hydrochloride ER tablets: 2 mg/180 mg, 1 mg/240 mg, 2 mg/240 mg, 4 mg/240 mg
Angiotensin II receptor blockers	
Candesartan (Atacand)	
Indication	Hypertension
Dosage	
Adults	Usual initial dose is 16 mg once daily. Dosage may be titrated within the range of 8–32 mg/d according to response. Hydrochlorothiazide has an additive effect.
Elderly	No initial dosage adjustment is required
Children	Safety and efficacy have not been established
Preparations	Atacand (AstraZeneca): 4-, 8-, 16-, 32-mg tablets

| Fixed-dose combinations for the treatment of hypertension | Atacand HCT: candesartan cilexetil/hydrochlorothiazide combination tablets: 16 mg/12.5 mg, 32 mg/12.5 mg |

Eprosartan (Teveten)

Indication

Hypertension

Dosage

Adults

Usual initial dose is 600 mg once daily. Dosage may be titrated within the range of 400–800 mg/d given in 1 or 2 divided doses.

Elderly

No initial dosage adjustment is required

Children

Safety and efficacy have not been established

Preparations

Teveten (Biovail): 400-, 600-mg tablets

Fixed-dose combinations for the treatment of hypertension

Teveten HCT: eprosartan/hydrochlorothiazide combination tablets: 600 mg/12.5 mg, 600 mg/25 mg

Irbesartan (Avapro)

Indications

Hypertension, type 2 diabetes with nephropathy to prevent end-stage renal disease

Dosage

Hypertension

Adults

Usual initial dose is 150 mg once daily. Dosage may be titrated to 300 mg once daily according to response. Hydrochlorothiazide has an additive effect.

Elderly

No initial dosage adjustment is required

Children

Safety and efficacy have not been established in children <6 y of age

Nephropathy in type 2 diabetic patients

Adults

Recommended target maintenance dose is 300 mg once daily

Children

Safety and efficacy have not been established in children <6 y of age

Preparations

Avapro (Bristol-Myers Squibb/Sanofi): 75-, 150-, 300-mg tablets

Fixed-dose combinations for the treatment of hypertension

Avalide: irbesartan/hydrochlorothiazide: 150 mg/12.5 mg, 300 mg/12.5 mg

Losartan (Cozaar)

Indications

Hypertension, type 2 diabetes with nephropathy to prevent end-stage renal disease, hypertensive patients with left ventricular hypertrophy to reduce the risk of stroke (although there is evidence that this benefit does not apply to black patients)

(continued)

625

APPENDIX 2 (continued) Therapeutic Use of Available Cardiovascular Drugs

Dosage
Adults

For hypertension, the usual initial dose is 50 mg once daily; dosage may be titrated up to 100 mg/d (in 1 or 2 divided doses). Lower initial dose of 25 mg once daily should be given to patients at high risk for hypotension, volume depletion, and those with hepatic dysfunction.

For nephropathy in type 2 diabetic patients, the usual starting dose is 50 mg once daily. Dose should be increased to 100 mg once daily based on blood pressure response.

For hypertensive patients with left ventricular hypertrophy, the usual initial dose is 50 mg once daily. Hydrochlorothiazide 12.5 mg/d should be added and/or the dose of losartan should be increased to 100 mg once daily, followed by an increase in hydrochlorothiazide to 25 mg once daily based on blood pressure response.

Elderly   No initial dosage adjustment is required
Children   Safety and efficacy have not been established
Preparations   Cozaar (Merck): 25-, 50-, 100-mg tablets
Fixed-dose combinations for the   Hyzaar: losartan/hydrochlorothiazide: 50 mg/12.5 mg, 100 mg/25 mg
treatment of hypertension

Olmesartan (Benicar)
Indication   Hypertension
Dosage
Adults   Usual recommended initial dose is 20 mg once daily when used as monotherapy in patients who are not volume contracted. If further reduction in blood pressure is required after 2 wk of therapy, the dose may be increased to 40 mg. Doses >40 mg do not appear to have greater effect. Twice-daily dosing offers no advantage over the same total dose given once daily.
Elderly   No initial dosage adjustment is required
Children   Safety and efficacy have not been established
Preparations   Benicar (Sankyo): 5-, 20-, 40-mg tablets

Telmisartan (Micardis)
Indication   Hypertension
Dosage
Adults   Usual initial dose is 40 mg once daily. Dosage may be titrated within the range of 20–80 mg/d according to response. Initiate treatment under close medical supervision for patients with hepatic impairment or biliary

626

obstructive disorders. If intravascular volume depletion is present, correct this condition before initiation of telmisartan and monitor closely.

Elderly | No initial dosage adjustment is required
Children | Safety and efficacy have not been established
Preparations | Micardis (Boehringer Ingelheim): 20-, 40-, 80-mg tablets
Fixed-dose combinations for the treatment of hypertension | Micardis HCT: telmisartan/hydrochlorothiazide: 40 mg/12.5 mg, 80 mg/12.5 mg

Valsartan (Diovan)

Indications | Hypertension, heart failure
Dosage
Hypertension
Adults | Usual initial dose is 80 mg once daily. Dosage may be increased to 160–320 mg once daily according to response.
Elderly | No initial dosage adjustment is required
Children | Safety and efficacy have not been established
Heart failure
Adults | Usual initial dose is 40 mg bid. Dosage should be titrated to 80 mg bid and then to 160 mg bid as tolerated. Maximum daily dose administered in clinical trials was 320 mg in divided doses. Reduction of concomitant diuretic dosage should be considered. Concomitant use with an ACE inhibitor and a beta blocker is not recommended.
Preparations | Diovan (Novartis): 40-, 80-, 160-, 320-mg tablets
Fixed-dose combinations for the treatment of hypertension | Diovan HCT: valsartan/hydrochlorothiazide: 80 mg/12.5 mg, 160 mg/12.5 mg

Antiarrhythmic agents
Class Ia
Disopyramide (disopyramide phosphate, Norpace)

Indications | Life-threatening ventricular arrhythmias, supraventricular arrhythmias (unlabeled use)
Dosage
Adults | Usual dosage in adults weighing >50 kg is 150 mg q6 h as conventional capsules or 300 mg q12h as ER capsules. In adults weighing <50 kg, the usual dosage is 100 mg q6h as conventional capsules or 200 mg

(continued)

627

APPENDIX 2 (continued) Therapeutic Use of Available Cardiovascular Drugs

q12h as ER capsules. When rapid control of ventricular arrhythmias is required, 300 mg of disopyramide (200 mg for patients weighing <50 kg) may be given initially, followed by the usual maintenance dose in conventional capsules. ER capsules should not be used initially when rapid control of ventricular arrhythmias is needed. In patients with cardiomyopathy or possible cardiac decompensation, the initial loading dose should not be given and an initial dosage of 100 mg q6h should not be exceeded. Dosage should be adjusted carefully while the patient is closely monitored for hypotension and/or CHF.

In patients with moderately impaired renal function (CrCl >40 mL/min) or hepatic insufficiency, the usual dosage is 100 mg q6h as conventional capsules or 200 mg q12h as ER capsules. For rapid control of a ventricular arrhythmia, an initial dose of 200 mg may be given. In patients with severely impaired renal function (CrCl ≤ 40 mL/min), the usual dosages of disopyramide (with or without an initial 150-mg dose) given as conventional capsules are as follows:

CrCl	Maintenance dose
30–40 mL/min	100 mg q8h
15–30 mL/min	100 mg q12h
<15 mL/min	100 mg q24h

Elderly   May be more sensitive to adult dose. Dose reduction is required

Children   Dosing is age specific. Total daily dose should be given in equally divided doses q6 h or at intervals according to individual requirements. Pediatric patients should be hospitalized during the initial period of therapy to allow close monitoring until maintenance dose is established.

Age	Maintenance dose
<1 y	10–30 mg/kg per day
1–4 y	10–20 mg/kg per day
4–12 y	10–15 mg/kg per day
12–18 y	6–15 mg/kg per day

Preparations   Disopyramide phosphate (generic); Norpace (Pharmacia & Upjohn): 100-, 150-mg capsules
               Disopyramide phosphate ER (generic); Norpace CR (Pharmacia & Upjohn): 100-, 150-mg ER capsules

Procainamide (procainamide HCl, Pronestyl, Pronestyl SR, Procanbid)
Indications   Ventricular arrhythmias, supraventricular arrhythmias (unlabeled use), atrial fibrillation/atrial flutter (unlabeled use)

Dosage

Adults

For initial management of arrhythmias in adults, a loading dose IV infusion of 500–600 mg may be administered at a constant rate over 25–30 min. Although it is unusual to require >600 mg to initially control an arrhythmia, the maximum recommended total dose is 1 g. Thereafter, a continuous IV infusion of 1–6 mg/min may be administered to maintain therapeutic plasma concentrations. Alternatively, a loading dose infusion of 12–17 mg/kg (at a rate of 20–30 mg/min) may be given, followed by a continuous infusion of 1–4 mg/min. Infusion rate should be lower in patients with renal impairment or hemodynamic instability. Consult procainamide package literature for information on proper dilution of procainamide before intravenous administration.

ER tablets are intended for maintenance dosing regimen. Usual maintenance dose for ventricular arrhythmias is 50 mg/kg daily in divided doses q6h for ER tablets and q12h for Procanbid. Usual maintenance dose for supraventricular arrhythmias in adults is 1 g q6h using ER tablets.

For the treatment of arrhythmias that occur during surgery and anesthesia, an IM (preferable) or IV dose of 100–500 mg can be given.

Elderly

Dosage adjustment is required for reduced renal function and other comorbid conditions (e.g., CHF).

Children

Safety and efficacy have not been established; IM injection is not recommended

Preparations

Pronestyl (Princeton Pharm): 250-, 375-, 500-mg tablets

Procainamide hydrochloride tablets (generic): 375-, 500-mg tablets

Procanbid (Monarch): 500-, 1000-mg ER tablets

Procainamide hydrochloride ER tablets (generic): 250-, 500-, 750-mg tablets

Procainamide hydrochloride capsules (generic); Pronestyl (Princeton Pharm): 250-, 375-, 500-mg capsules

Procainamide hydrochloride injection (generic): 100, 500 mg/mL

Quinidine (quinidine gluconate, Quinaglute, Dura-Tabs, quinidine sulfate, Quinidex Extentabs)

Indications

Maintenance of sinus rhythm after conversion of atrial fibrillation/flutter, atrial or ventricular premature complexes, conversion of atrial fibrillation/flutter, paroxysmal supraventricular tachycardia, paroxysmal ventricular tachycardia not associated with complete heart block, life-threatening *Plasmodium falciparum* malaria (IV quinidine gluconate)

Dosage

Adults

Quinidine is expressed in molar basis: 267 mg quinidine gluconate or 275 mg quinidine polygalacturonate is equivalent to 200 mg quinidine sulfate. The following dosages are expressed in terms of the respective salts.

(continued)

APPENDIX 2 *(continued)* Therapeutic Use of Available Cardiovascular Drugs

Quinidine sulfate: For the conversion of atrial fibrillation: 200 mg PO q2–3h for 5–8 doses. Clinicians usually used 300–400 mg PO q6h. If pharmacologic conversion back to sinus rhythm does not occur with plasma concentrations of 9 μg/mL, increase in dose would increase the risk of toxicity. For paroxysmal supraventricular tachycardia and paroxysmal ventricular tachycardia: 400–600 mg PO q2–3h until paroxysm is terminated. For the maintenance of sinus rhythm after conversion: 200–400 mg PO tid or qid or 300–600 mg ER tablets q8–12h.

Quinidine polygalacturonate: Initial dose is 275–825 mg PO followed by a second dose in 3–4h if needed. If no response after 3 or 4 equal doses, the dose may be increased by 137.5–275 mg for 3 or 4 more doses before further increasing the dosage. Usual maintenance dose is 275 mg PO bid or tid.

Quinidine gluconate: For the suppression and prevention of atrial, atrioventricular junctional, and ventricular premature complexes, administer 324–648 mg PO as ER tablets q8–12h. Maintenance dose for sinus rhythm after conversion is 324 mg q8–12h as ER tablets; increase to 648 mg q8–12h if necessary and tolerated. Quinidine gluconate injections: For atrial fibrillation/flutter (can be used for ventricular arrhythmias), administer 5–10 mg/kg at an initial rate of up to 0.25 mg/kg per min. If conversion does not occur at 10 mg/kg, attempt another means for conversion. There is a high risk for hypotension. Monitor electrocardiogram for widening of QRS and prolongation of QT intervals, disappearance of P wave, symptomatic bradycardia, or tachycardia. Consult quinidine package literature for proper dilution of intravenous injection before administration

Elderly   Initiate with lowest dose and titrate to response

Children   Safety and efficacy have not been established, but quinidine gluconate used to treat malaria in children has shown an efficacy and safety profile comparable to that in adults

Preparations   Quinidine gluconate ER tablets (generic); Quinaglute Dura-Tabs (Berlex): 324-mg ER tablets
Cardioquin (Purdue Frederick): 275-mg polygalacturonate tablets
Quinidine sulfate ER tablets (generic); Quinidex Extentabs (A. H. Robins): 300-mg ER tablets
Quinidine sulfate tablets USP (generic): 200-, 300-mg tablets
Quinidine gluconate injection: 80 mg/mL (50 mg/mL quinidine)

Class Ib
Lidocaine (lidocaine HCl, Xylocaine)
Indication   Acute treatment of ventricular tachyarrhythmias (intravenous formulation)

Dosage
Adults   *Initial IV bolus dose:* 1–1.5 mg/kg at 25–50 mg/min, may repeat 0.5–0.75 mg/kg in 5–10 min, if initial response is inadequate, up to a total dose of 3 mg/kg. No more than 200–300 mg should be administered during a 1-h period. Patients with CHF or cardiogenic shock may require a smaller dose.

	Maintenance infusion: 1–4 mg/min (20–50 μg/kg per min). A slower rate of 1–2 mg/min may be sufficient for patients with CHF, liver disease, >70 y old, or who weigh <70 kg.
Elderly	Dose reduction is required due to reduction in patient's capacity to metabolize the drug
Children	Safety and effectiveness have not been established; reduce dosage when used in children
Preparations	Lidocaine for IV admixtures (generic): 40, 100, 200 mg/mL
	Xylocaine (Astra Zeneca) for IV admixtures: 40, 200 mg/mL
	Lidocaine direct IV injection (generic); Xylocaine (Astra Zeneca): 10, 20 mg/mL
	Lidocaine hydrochloride and dextrose injection (generic): 1, 2, 4, 8 mg/mL

Mexiletine (mexiletine HCl, Mexitil)

Indication	Life-threatening ventricular arrhythmias
Dosage	
Adults	Initiate at 200 mg PO q8h; increase or decrease dosage in increments or decrements of 50–100 mg/dose q2–3 d as needed. For rapid control of ventricular arrhythmias, loading dose of 400 mg may be administered followed by a 200-mg dose 8 h later. Limit to 1200 mg/d when given q8h (i.e., 400 mg/dose) or to 900 mg/d when given q12h (i.e., 450 mg/dose).
	Patients with CHF or hepatic impairment may require dose reduction. Dosage adjustments should be made no more frequently than q2–3 d. Some patients may tolerate twice-daily dosing. For patients adequately maintained on a dose ≤300 mg q8h, total daily dose may be given divided q12h. Patients not adequately controlled by dosing q8h may respond to dosing q6h.
Elderly	Dosage adjustment is required due to reduction in patient's capacity to metabolize the drug
Children	Safety and effectiveness have not been established
Preparations	Mexiletine (generic); Mexitil (Boehringer Ingelheim): 150-, 200-, 250-mg capsules

Tocainide (Tonocard)

Indication	Life-threatening ventricular arrhythmias
Dosage	
Adults	Loading dose: 600 mg, then 400 mg after 4–6 h
	Maintenance dose: 400 mg PO q8h. Usual maintenance dose is 1.2–1.8 g/d. Maximum dose is 2.4 g/d in divided doses. Reduce initial maintenance dose by 50% in patients with hepatic dysfunction and in patients with CrCl <10 mL/min. Reduce initial maintenance dose by 25% in patients with CrCl of 10–30 mL/min.

(continued)

APPENDIX 2 *(continued)* Therapeutic Use of Available Cardiovascular Drugs

Elderly	Dosage adjustment is required due to reduction in patient's capacity to eliminate the drug
Children	Safety and effectiveness have not been established
Preparations	Tonocard (Astra Zeneca): 400-, 600-mg tablets

Class Ic

Flecainide (Tambocor)

Indications	Life-threatening ventricular arrhythmias, supraventricular tachyarrhythmias
Dosage	
Adults	For sustained ventricular tachycardia, initiate at 100 mg q12h; increase dosage in increments of 50 mg bid q4 d as needed. Usual maintenance dose is 150 mg q12h; limit to 400 mg/d. For patients with paroxysmal supraventricular tachycardia and patients with paroxysmal atrial fibrillation, initiate at 50 mg q12h. Increase dosage in increments of 50 mg bid q4 d as needed; limit to 300 mg/d in patients with paroxysmal supraventricular tachycardia.
	For patients with severe renal impairment (CrCl <35 mL/min), reduce initial dose to 50 mg q12h; increase doses at intervals of >4 d if needed and monitor plasma levels frequently to guide dosage adjustment.
Elderly	Lower doses are recommended due to age-related decline in clearance
Children	Safety and effectiveness have not been established
Preparations	Tambocor (3M Pharmaceuticals): 50-, 100-, 150-mg tablets

Propafenone (propafenone, Rythmol)

Indications	Life-threatening ventricular arrhythmias, supraventricular tachyarrhythmias (unlabeled use)
Dosage	
Adults	Initiate at 150 mg q8h. Increase dosage after 3–4 d to 225 mg q8h if needed. Dosage may be further increased to 300 mg q8h after an additional 3–4 d if needed and tolerated.
Elderly	Lower doses may be required due to reduction in patient's capacity to metabolize the drug
Children	Safety and effectiveness have not been established
Preparations	Propafenone (generic); Rythmol (Abbott): 150-, 225-, 300-mg tablets

Moricizine (Ethmozine)

Indication	Life-threatening ventricular arrhythmias
Dosage	
Adults	Usual dosage is 600–900 mg/d in 3 divided doses q8h. Dosage may be increased at 150 mg/d at 3-d intervals. Limit to 900 mg/d.

632

In patients with hepatic function impairment or significant renal impairment, an initial dose of ≤600 mg/d is recommended. In patients whose arrhythmias are well controlled, dosing q12h may aid compliance.

Elderly

Children   Lower doses may be required due to reduction in patient's capacity to metabolize the drug

Preparations   Safety and effectiveness have not been established

Class II   Ethmozine (Roberts): 200-, 250-, 300-mg tablets

β-Adrenergic blockers

Class III

Amiodarone (amiodarone, Cordarone, Pacerone)

Indications   Life-threatening ventricular arrhythmias (ventricular fibrillation or hemodynamically unstable ventricular tachycardia), supraventricular arrhythmias (not FDA approved)

Dosage

Adults   *PO: Life-threatening ventricular arrhythmias:* Loading dose is 800–1600 mg/d in divided doses for 1–3 wk (occasionally longer). Dosage should then be reduced to 600–800 mg/d in 1 to 2 divided doses for 4 wk. Maintenance dose is usually 400 mg/d. Some patients may require larger maintenance doses of 600 mg/d; others may be controlled on lower doses. Amiodarone may be administered as a single daily dose or as a twice-daily dose in patients with severe GI intolerance.

Supraventricular arrhythmias (not FDA approved): Oral loading dose of 600–800 mg/d for 7–10 d, then 200–400 mg/d as maintenance dose

IV: Life-threatening ventricular arrhythmias: Load 150 mg over 10 min (15 mg/min), then 360 mg over the next 6 h (1 mg/min). Maintenance infusion of 540 mg is then given over the next 18 h (0.5 mg/min). IV amiodarone should be used for acute treatment until the patient's ventricular arrhythmias are stabilized. Most patients require IV therapy for 48–96 h; however, the maintenance infusion of 0.5 mg/min (or less) can be administered up to 2–3 wk. A supplemental dose of 150 mg over 10 min can be given for breakthrough arrhythmias. Consult amiodarone package literature for proper dilution of drug before administration. IV amiodarone concentration should not exceed 2 mg/mL unless a central venous catheter is used.

Elderly   Dosage adjustment should be based on comorbid conditions and concurrent therapy

Children   Safety and effectiveness have not been established. Limited data suggest that amiodarone may be useful in the management of refractory supraventricular or ventricular arrhythmias in selected cases.

(continued)

APPENDIX 2 *(continued)* Therapeutic Use of Available Cardiovascular Drugs

Preparations	Amiodarone (generic); Cordarone (Wyeth-Ayerst); Pacerone (Upsher Smith): 200-mg tablets Cordarone IV (Wyeth-Ayerst): 3-mL ampule, 50 mg/mL

Bretylium (bretylium tosylate)

Indications	Life-threatening ventricular arrhythmias (ventricular fibrillation or hemodynamically unstable ventricular tachycardia unresponsive to conventional antiarrhythmic drugs)
Dosage Adults	*Immediately life-threatening ventricular arrhythmias (ventricular fibrillation or hemodynamically unstable ventricular tachycardia unresponsive to conventional antiarrhythmic drugs):* Initiate with a 5-mg/kg undiluted IV injection over approximately 1 min. CPR measures including cardioversion should be undertaken before and after bretylium administration as needed. If ventricular fibrillation persists, supplemental doses of 10 mg/kg may be given by rapid IV injection (over approximately 1 min) and repeated as needed, usually at 5- to 30-min intervals, up to a total dose of 30–35 mg/kg. *Treatment of sustained ventricular tachycardia:* A dosage of 5–10 mg/kg of bretylium diluted in 50 mL of 5% dextrose injection and given IV over 8–10 min is recommended. For continued suppression of persistently recurrent ventricular tachycardia, a continuous IV infusion of bretylium at a rate of 1–2 mg/min can be given after the initial 5- to 10-mg/kg loading dose. Alternatively, 5–10 mg/kg can be given by intermittent IV infusion over ≥8 min q6h for continued suppression of ventricular tachycardia. *Treatment of other life-threatening ventricular arrhythmias:* Administer diluted IV infusion in a dose of 5–10 mg/kg over 8–10 min and repeat this dose q1–2h if needed. Maintenance infusion can be given q6–8h, as described above. Alternatively, bretylium can be administered as a constant infusion (diluted) at a rate of 1–2 mg/min. With IM administration, give 5–10 mg/kg undiluted and repeat q1–2h as needed. Maintenance dose is 5–10 mg/kg q6–8h. Do not exceed 5-mL volume in any one site for IM injection. IM injections should not be made directly into or near a major nerve, and injection sites should be rotated.
Elderly	Dosage adjustment may be required based on renal function
Children	Safety and effectiveness have not been established
Preparations	Bretylium tosylate injection (generic): 50 mg/mL, 10-mL ampules, vials, and syringes Bretylium tosylate injection (generic): 2 mg/mL (500 mg/vial), 4 mg/mL (1000 mg/vial) in 5% dextrose injection

Dofetilide (Tikosyn)

Indications	Maintenance of normal sinus rhythm (delay in atrial fibrillation/flutter recurrence), conversion of atrial fibrillation/flutter

Dosage

Adults
Usual recommended dose of dofetilide is 500 μg bid. The dose of dofetilide must be individualized according to CrCl and QTc. Before administration of the first dose, the QTc must be determined from an average of 5–10 beats. If the QTc is >440 msec (500 msec in patients with ventricular conduction abnormalities), dofetilide is contraindicated. If heart rate is <60 beats/min, QT interval should be used. There are no data on use of dofetilide when the heart rate is <50 beats/min.

The initial dose of dofetilide is determined as follows:

CrCl	Dofetilide dose
>60 mL/min	500 μg bid
40–60 mL/min	250 μg bid
20 to <40 mL/min	125 μg bid
<20 mL/min	Dofetilide is contraindicated in these patients

At 2–3 h after administering the first dose of dofetilide, determine the QTc. If the QTc has increased >15% when compared with baseline, or if the QTc is >500 msec (550 msec in patients with ventricular conduction abnormalities), subsequent dosing should be adjusted as follows:

If the starting dose based on CrCl is:	Then the adjusted dose (for QTc prolongation) is:
500 μg bid	250 μg bid
250 μg bid	125 μg bid
125 μg bid	125 μg once a day

At 2–3 h after each subsequent dose of dofetilide, determine the QTc (for in-hospital doses 2–5). No further down titration of dofetilide based on QTc is recommended. If the QTc is >500 msec (550 msec in patients with ventricular conduction abnormalities) at any time after the second dose of dofetilide is given, dofetilide should be discontinued. Consult dofetilide package insert for complete prescribing information.

Elderly
Dosage adjustment may be required based on renal function

Children
Safety and effectiveness have not been established

Preparations
Tikosyn (Pfizer): 125-, 250-, 500-μg capsules

Ibutilide (Corvert)

Indications
Conversion of atrial fibrillation or atrial flutter of recent onset to sinus rhythm

(continued)

APPENDIX 2 *(continued)* Therapeutic Use of Available Cardiovascular Drugs

Dosage	
Adults	For patients weighing ≥60 kg, give 1 mg IV over 10 min. For patients weighing <60 kg, give 0.01 mg/kg IV over 10 min. If the arrhythmia does not terminate within 10 min after the end of the initial infusion, a second 10-min infusion of equal strength may be administered 10 min after completion of the first infusion. Ibutilide may be administered undiluted or diluted in 50 mL of 0.9% sodium chloride injection or 5% dextrose injection.
Elderly	No dosage adjustment is required
Children	Safety and effectiveness have not been established
Preparation	Corvert (Pharmacia & Upjohn): 0.1 mg/mL, 10-mL vials

Sotalol (sotalol, Betapace, Betapace AF)

Indications	Documented life-threatening ventricular arrhythmias (Betapace), maintenance of normal sinus rhythm in patients with symptomatic atrial fibrillation or atrial flutter currently in sinus rhythm (Betapace AF)
Dosage	
Adults	*Documented life-threatening ventricular arrhythmias:* Initiate with low doses and titrate up slowly. Usual starting dose is 80 mg bid. Dosage may be titrated up q3 d up to 240 or 320 mg/d given in 2–3 divided doses. Usual maintenance dose is 160–320 mg/d, but some patients may require doses as high as 480–640 mg/d. However, the higher doses should be prescribed only when the potential benefit outweighs the increased risk of adverse events. Because sotalol is excreted predominantly in urine and its elimination half-life is prolonged in patients with renal impairment, the dosing interval of sotalol should be modified according to CrCl as follows:

CrCl (mL/min)	Dosing interval
>60	12
30–59	24
10–29	36–48
<10	Dose should be individualized

In addition, dose increments in patients with renal impairment should be made after administration of at least 5–6 doses.

Maintenance of normal sinus rhythm in patients with symptomatic atrial fibrillation or atrial flutter currently in sinus rhythm: Initiate with 80 mg bid if CrCl >60 mL/min and with 80 mg once daily if CrCl is 40–60 mL/min. If CrCl <40 mL/min, sotalol (Betapace AF) is contraindicated. If the 80-mg dose level is tolerated and the QT interval remains <500 msec after at least 3 d (after 5 or 6 doses if patient is receiving once-daily dosing), the patient can be discharged. Patients should not be discharged within 12 h of electrical or pharmacologic conversion to normal sinus rhythm. Alternatively, during hospitalization, the dose can be increased to 120 mg bid or once daily depending on CrCl and the patient should be followed for 3 on this dose (followed for 5 or 6 doses if patient is receiving once daily doses). If the 120-mg dose level does not reduce the frequency of early relapse of atrial fibrillation/flutter and is tolerated without excessive QT interval prolongation (≥520 msec), an increase to 160 mg (bid or once daily depending on CrCl) can be considered.

Note: The QT interval is used to determine patient eligibility for sotalol (Betapace AF) treatment and for monitoring safety during treatment. The baseline QT interval must be ≤450 msec for a patient to be started on this medication. During initiation and titration, the QT interval should be monitored 2–4 h after each dose. If the QT interval prolongs to ≥500 msec, the dose must be reduced or the drug discontinued. During maintenance of sotalol (Betapace AF) therapy, renal function and QT should be reevaluated regularly if medically warranted. If QT ≥520 msec (JT ≥430 msec if QRS >100 msec), the dose of sotalol (Betapace AF) therapy should be reduced and patients should be carefully monitored until QT returns to <520 msec. If the QT interval is ≥520 msec while on the lowest maintenance dose level (80 mg), the drug should be discontinued.

Elderly   Dosage adjustment may be required based on renal function
Children   Safety and effectiveness have not been established
Preparations   Sotatol (generic); Betapace (Berlex): 80-, 120-, 160-, 240-mg tablets
                 Betapace AF (Berlex): 80-, 120-, 160-mg tablets

Other

Adenosine (Adenocard)

Indications   Conversion to sinus rhythm of paroxysmal supraventricular tachyarrhythmias, including that associated with Wolff-Parkinson-White syndrome

Dosage
Adults   Initiate with 6 mg as a rapid IV bolus (administered over 1–2 s). If the first dose does not result in elimination of the supraventricular tachycardia within 1–2 min, give 12 mg as a rapid IV bolus. Repeat the 12-mg dose a second time if necessary.
Adenosine injection should be given as a rapid bolus by the peripheral IV route. To ensure that the medication reaches the systemic circulation, adenosine should be administered directly into a vein or, if given into an IV line, should be given as close to the patient as possible and followed by a rapid saline flush.

(continued)

APPENDIX 2 *(continued)* Therapeutic Use of Available Cardiovascular Drugs

Elderly — Dosage adjustment is not required

Children — Safety and effectiveness have not been established

Preparations — Adenocard (Fujisawa): 3 mg/mL, 2-, 5-mL vials

Atropine (atropine sulfate)

Indications — Symptomatic sinus bradycardia (IV formulation), treatment of ventricular asystole during CPR (IV formulation)

Dosage

Adults — *Treatment of bradycardia in advanced cardiac life support during CPR:* Usual adult dose is 0.5–1 mg IV; this dose may be repeated q3–5 min until the desired heart rate is achieved. *Treatment of ventricular asystole during CPR:* 1 mg IV; this dose may be repeated in 3–5 min if needed. Total dose usually should not exceed 2.5 mg (0.04 mg/kg) in patients with severe bradycardia or ventricular asystole because a 2.5-mg dose generally results in complete vagal blockade.
Note: Atropine sulfate may be administered PO or by IM, SC, or direct IV administration. When atropine sulfate cannot be administered IV for advanced cardiac life support during CPR, the drug may be administered via an endotracheal tube or by intraosseous injection in adults and children. Some experts recommend that doses administered via endotracheal tube should be 2–2.5 times those administered IV and generally should be diluted in 10 mL of 0.9% sodium chloride or sterile water for adults, and in 1–2 mL of 0.45% or 0.9% sodium chloride for children. Such dilution may enhance tracheobronchial distribution and absorption of atropine.
When atropine sulfate is given IV, it should generally be given rapidly because slow injection of the drug may cause a paradoxical slowing of the heart rate.

Elderly — Use usual dose with caution

Children — Advanced cardiac life support during CPR: 0.02 mg/kg IV, with a minimum pediatric dose of 0.1 mg and maximum single doses of 0.5 and 1 mg in children and adolescents, respectively. The dose may be repeated at 5-min intervals to maximum total doses of 1 mg in children and 2 mg in adolescents.

Preparations — Atropine sulfate injection (generic): 0.05, 0.1, 0.3, 0.4, 0.5, 0.8, 1 mg/mL

Antithrombotics
Anticoagulants

Argatroban (Acova)

Indications — Anticoagulant for prophylaxis or treatment of thrombosis in patients with HIT, as an anticoagulant in patients with or at risk for HIT undergoing PCI

Dosage
Adults

HIT/HITTS: Usual initial dose is 2 µg/kg per min administered as a continuous infusion (the concentrated drug, 100 mg/mL, must be diluted 100-fold before infusion). Dose can be adjusted as clinically indicated and according to steady-state aPTT (1.5–3 times initial baseline value, not to exceed 100 s) up to 10 µg/kg per min. A lower initial dose of 0.5 µg/kg per min is recommended for patients with moderate hepatic impairment. The aPTT should be monitored closely and dosage adjusted as clinically indicated.

PCI in HIT/HITTS: Infusion of argatroban should be started at 25 µg/kg per min and a bolus of 350 µg/kg administered via a large bore IV line over 3–5 min. ACT should be obtained before dosing and 5–10 min after the bolus dose is completed. Procedure may proceed if the ACT >300 s.

If ACT <300 s, an additional IV bolus dose of 150 µg/kg should be administered; the infusion dose increased to 30 µg/kg per min, and the ACT checked 5–10 min later. If the ACT >450 s, the infusion rate should be decreased to 15 µg/kg per min, and the ACT checked 5–10 min later. Once a therapeutic ACT (300–450 s) has been achieved, this infusion dose should be continued for the duration of the procedure.

In case of dissection, impending abrupt closure, thrombus formation during the procedure, or inability to achieve or maintain an ACT >300 s, additional bolus doses of 150 µg/kg may be administered and the infusion dose increased to 40 µg/kg per min. The ACT should be checked after each additional bolus or change in the rate of infusion. If a patient requires anticoagulation after the procedure, argatroban may be continued, but as a lower infusion dose. Use of high doses of argatroban in PCI patients with clinically significant hepatic disease or AST/ALT levels ≥3 times the upper limit of normal should be avoided. Such patients were not studied in PCI trials.

Conversion to oral anticoagulant therapy: Because coadministration of argatroban and warfarin may cause combined effects on INR, a loading dose of warfarin should not be used. Initiate therapy with the expected daily dose of warfarin. With argatroban doses (≤2 µg/kg per min, argatroban can be discontinued when the INR is >4 on combined therapy. INR measurement should be repeated 4–6 h after discontinuation of argatroban infusion. If the repeated INR is below the desired therapeutic range, restart argatroban infusion and repeat the procedure daily until the desired therapeutic range on warfarin alone is achieved. For argatroban doses ≤2 µg/kg per min, temporarily reduce the dose of argatroban to ≤2 µg/kg per min to get a more accurate INR measurement on warfarin alone. Obtain the INR measurement on argatroban and warfarin 4–6 h after reduction of the argatroban dose and follow the process described above for administering argatroban at doses ≤2 µg/kg per min.

(continued)

639

APPENDIX 2 *(continued)* Therapeutic Use of Available Cardiovascular Drugs

Elderly	Dosage adjustment is not required
Children	Safety and effectiveness have not been established
Preparation	Argatroban injection (Glaxo SmithKline): 100 mg/mL, 2.5-mL single-use vials
Bivalirudin (Angiomax)	
Indications	Unstable angina. For use as an anticoagulant in patients with unstable angina undergoing PTCA. Bivalirudin is intended for use in patients receiving concomitant aspirin (300–325 mg/d).
Dosage	
Adults	Treatment with bivalirudin should be initiated just before PTCA. Administer an IV bolus of 1 mg/kg followed by a 4-h IV infusion at a rate of 2.5 mg/kg per h. If necessary, an additional IV bivalirudin infusion may be initiated at a rate of 0.2 mg/kg per h for ≤20 h after completion of the initial 4-h infusion. The dose may need to be reduced, and anticoagulation status monitored, in patients with renal impairment. Consult package insert for instructions on dilution of drug before administration.
Elderly	Dosage adjustment is not required
Children	Safety and effectiveness have not been established
Preparation	Angiomax (Medicines Company): 250-mg injection, lyophilized
Dalteparin sodium (Fragmin)	
Indications	Prophylaxis of deep vein thrombosis that may lead to pulmonary embolism in patients undergoing hip replacement surgery and in patients undergoing abdominal surgery who are at risk for thromboembolic complications, prevention of ischemic complications in patients with unstable angina or non-Q-wave MI (use with concurrent aspirin therapy)
Dosage	
Adults	*Abdominal surgery:* Patients with a low to moderate risk of thromboembolic complications should receive 2500 IU SC once daily for 5–10 d starting 1–2 h before surgery. Patients with a high risk of thromboembolic complications should receive 5000 IU SC once daily for 5–10 d starting the evening before surgery. Alternatively, in patients with malignancy, 2500 IU of dalteparin can be administered SC 1–2 h before surgery followed by 2500 IU SC 12 h later, and then 5000 IU once daily for 5–10 d postoperatively.
	Hip replacement surgery: Administer the first dose, 2500 IU SC, within 2 h before surgery and the second dose of 2500 IU SC in the evening of the day of surgery (≥6 h after the first dose). If surgery is performed in the

evening, omit the second dose on the day of surgery. Dalteparin 5000 IU is then administered SC once daily from first postoperative day and continued for 5–10 d. Alternatively, dalteparin 5000 IU can be administered the evening before surgery, followed by 5000 IU once daily, starting in the evening of the day of surgery and continued for 5–10 d. Up to 14 d of treatment have been well tolerated in controlled clinical trials.

Unstable angina/non-Q-wave MI: 120 IU/kg (maximum single dose of 10,000 IU) SC q12h with concurrent aspirin therapy for 5–8 d or until the patient is clinically stable.

Elderly
No data; dosage adjustment is probably not required

Children
Safety and effectiveness have not been established

Preparations
Fragmin (Pharmacia & Upjohn): 2500 anti-factor Xa IU/ 0.2 mL; 5000 anti-factor Xa IU/0.2-mL syringes; 10,000 anti-factor Xa IU/mL, 9.5-mL multiple-dose vials

Danaparoid sodium (Orgaran)

Indications
Prophylaxis of postoperative deep venous thrombosis that may lead to pulmonary embolism in patients undergoing elective hip replacement surgery

Dosage

Adults
750 anti-Xa U (0.6 mL) bid administered SC starting 1–4 h before surgery, and then not sooner than 2 h after surgery. Treatment should be continued until the patient is fully ambulatory (up to 14 d). Carefully monitor patients with serum creatinine ≥2 mg/dL. In patients with renal failure undergoing hemodialysis, reduce maintenance dosages and titrate according to predialysis plasma anti-factor Xa activity.

Elderly
Dosage adjustment is not required

Children
Safety and effectiveness have not been established

Preparations
Orgaran (Organon): 750 anti-Xa U/0.6-mL syringes, 750 anti-Xa U/0.6-mL ampules

Enoxaparin sodium (Lovenox)

Indications
Prophylaxis of deep vein thrombosis that may lead to pulmonary embolism in patients undergoing hip or knee replacement surgery, in high-risk patients undergoing abdominal surgery, and in medical patients who are at risk for thromboembolic complications due to severely restricted mobility during acute illness, treatment of acute deep vein thrombosis with or without pulmonary embolism when used in conjunction with warfarin, prevention of ischemic complications in patients with unstable angina or non-Q-wave MI with concurrent aspirin

Dosage

Adults
Hip or knee replacement surgery: 30 mg q12h SC for 7–10 d starting 12–24 h after the surgery. Up to 14 d administration has been well tolerated in clinical trials.

(continued)

Hip replacement surgery: Administer 30 mg q12h as previously stated or 40 mg once daily by SC injection. Initial dose of 40 mg once a day SC may be given approximately 12 h before surgery. After the initial phase of thrombo-prophylaxis, continued prophylaxis with enoxaparin injection 40 mg once daily for 3 wk is recommended.

Abdominal surgery: 40 mg/d by SC injection for 7–10 d starting 2 h before surgery. Up to 12 d administration has been well tolerated in clinical trials.

Treatment of deep vein thrombosis with or without pulmonary embolism: In patients with acute deep vein thrombosis without pulmonary embolism who can be treated at home, the recommended dose is 1 mg/kg q12h by SC injection. In hospitalized patients with acute deep vein thrombosis with pulmonary embolism or those with acute deep vein thrombosis without pulmonary embolism (who are not candidates for outpatient treatment), the recommended dose is 1 mg/kg q12h or 1.5 mg/kg once daily by SC injection. Therapy with warfarin should be initiated when appropriate, and enoxaparin should be continued for a minimum of 5 d and until the INR is therapeutic. Average duration of treatment is 7 d; up to 17 d of administration has been well tolerated in clinical trials.

Unstable angina and non-Q-wave MI: 1 mg/kg administered SC q12h in conjunction with PO aspirin therapy (100–325 mg once daily) for a minimum of 2 d and continued until clinical stabilization. Usual duration of treatment is 2–8 d.

Medical patients during acute illness: 40 mg once a day administered by SC injection. The usual duration of administration is 6–11 d; up to 14 d of enoxaparin injection has been well tolerated.

Dosage adjustment is not required, but dosage adjustment should be considered in patients with CrCl <30 mL/min

Elderly	
Children	Safety and effectiveness have not been established
Preparations	Lovenox (Aventis): 30 mg/0.3 mL, 40 mg/0.4 mL, 60 mg/0.6 mL, 80 mg/0.8 mL, 90 mg/0.6 mL, 100 mg/1 mL, 120 mg/0.8 mL, 150 mg/1 mL injections
Fondaparinux sodium (Arixtra)	
Indications	Prophylaxis of deep vein thrombosis that may lead to pulmonary embolism in patients undergoing hip fracture surgery, hip replacement surgery, or knee replacement surgery
Dosage	
Adults	Recommended dose of fondaparinux is 2.5 mg administered by SC injection once daily in patients undergoing hip fracture surgery, hip replacement surgery, or knee replacement surgery. After hemostasis has been established, the initial dose is given 6–8 h after surgery. Administration before 6 h after surgery has been associated with an increased risk of major bleeding.

Elderly

Usual duration of administration is 5–9 d, and up to 11 d of administration has been tolerated.
Risk of fondaparinux-associated major bleeding increases with age, with an incidence of 1.8% in patients <65 y of age, 2.2% in those 65–74 y of age, and 2.7% in those ≥75 y of age. The kidney substantially eliminates fondaparinux, and the risk of toxic reactions to fondaparinux may be greater in patients with impaired renal function. Because elderly patients are more likely to have decreased renal function, it may be useful to monitor renal function.

Children

Safety and effectiveness have not been established

Preparations

Arixtra (Organon/Sanofi-Synthelabo): 2.5-mg injection, in 0.5-mL single-dose prefilled syringes with needle

Heparin (heparin sodium)

Indications

Prophylaxis and treatment of: venous thrombosis, pulmonary embolism, atrial fibrillation with thromboembolism, and peripheral arterial embolism; prophylaxis and treatment of unstable angina, evolving stroke, acute MI (not FDA approved); prevention of clotting in cardiac/arterial surgery, blood transfusion, dialysis and other extracorporeal interventions, and disseminated intravascular coagulation

Dosage

Adults

Prophylaxis for deep venous thrombosis: 5000 U SC q8–12h until the patient is fully ambulatory.
Treatment guidelines for thromboembolic events
Continuous IV administration: 60–100 U/kg loading dose by IV injection, followed by an IV infusion of 15–25 U/kg per h and adjusted based on coagulation test results
Intermittent IV administration: Usual initial dose for a 68-kg adult is 10,000 U, followed by 5000–10,000 U q4–6h.
Deep SC injections: 10,000–20,000 U loading dose, followed by 8000–10,000 U q8h or 15,000–20,000 U q12h. Dose should be adjusted based on coagulation test results.
Open heart and vascular surgery: Minimum initial dose is 150 U/kg for patients undergoing total body perfusion for open heart surgery. For procedures <60 min, usual dose used is 300 U/kg. For procedures >60 min, usual dose used is 400 U/kg.
Heparin lock: To avoid clot formation in a heparin lock set, inject diluted heparin solution (Heparin Lock Flush Solution, USP, or 10–100 U/mL heparin solution) via the injection hub to fill the entire set to the needle tip. Replace this solution each time the heparin lock is used. Consult the set manufacturer's instructions.

Elderly

Dosage adjustment is not required

(continued)

APPENDIX 2 *(continued)* Therapeutic Use of Available Cardiovascular Drugs

Children	Dosage adjustment should be made based on weight, age, and coagulation test results
Preparations	Available in formulations of bovine or porcine origin Heparin sodium: 10, 100, 1000, 2500, 5000, 7500, 10,000, 20,000, 40,000 U/mL in various volumes as single-use or multiple-dose packages

Lepirudin (Refludan)

Indications	Prevention of further thromboembolic complications in patients with heparin-induced thrombocytopenia and associated thromboembolic disease
Dosage	
Adults	*Bolus dose:* 0.4 mg/kg (up to 44 mg) IV over 15–20 s *Maintenance dose:* 0.15 mg/kg per h (up to 16.5 mg/h) as a continuous IV infusion for 2–10 d or longer if indicated Dosage should be adjusted based on aPTT measurements. The first aPTT determination should be made 4 h after initiation of the lepirudin infusion. Follow-up aPTT determinations should be made at least once a day. Adjustments of bolus dose and maintenance dose should be made in patients receiving thrombolytic therapy concurrently and in patients with renal impairment. Consult lepirudin package insert for full prescribing information. *Concurrent warfarin therapy:* Reduce lepirudin dose to reach an aPTT ratio just above 1.5 before administering the first dose of warfarin. Lepirudin infusion should be discontinued once an INR of 2 is achieved.
Elderly	Dosage adjustment should be based on CrCl
Children	Safety and effectiveness have not been established
Preparation	Refludan (Hoechst-Marion Roussel): 50 mg/vial, powder for injection

Tinzaparin sodium (Innohep)

Indications	Treatment of acute symptomatic deep vein thrombosis with or without pulmonary embolism when administered in conjunction with warfarin
Dosage	
Adults	175 anti-factor Xa IU/kg, administered SC once daily for at least 6 d and until the patient is adequately anticoagulated with warfarin (INR ≥2 for 2 consecutive d). Use with caution in patients with renal impairment.
Elderly	Dosage adjustment is not required
Children	Safety and effectiveness have not been established
Preparation	Innohep (DuPont Pharma): 20,000 IU/mL, 2-mL vials

Warfarin (warfarin sodium, Coumadin)

Indications
Prophylaxis and treatment of venous thrombosis, pulmonary embolism, atrial fibrillation with embolization, thromboembolism associated with prosthetic heart valves

Dosage

Adults
Initiate with 5–10 mg/d for 2–4 d; adjust dose to maintain desired therapeutic INRs according to recommendations by the American College of Chest Physicians and the National Heart, Lung and Blood Institute. Warfarin injection provides an alternative administration route for patients who cannot receive oral drugs. The dose of warfarin injection is the same as the PO dose and should be administered only IV. The dose should be given as a slow bolus injection over 1–2 min into a peripheral vein.

Elderly
Initiate therapy with a lower dose; dosing is based on coagulation test results

Children
Safety and effectiveness have not been established

Preparations
Warfarin (generic); Coumadin (DuPont): 1-, 2-, 2.5-, 3-, 4-, 5-, 6-, 7.5-, 10-mg tablets
Coumadin injection (DuPont): 5 mg/vial

Antiplatelet agents
Abciximab (ReoPro)

Indications
Prevention of cardiac ischemic complications in patients undergoing PCI or in patients with unstable angina not responding to conventional medical therapy when PCI is planned within 24 h

Dosage

Adults
PCI: 0.25 mg/kg IV bolus administered 10–60 min before the start of PCI, followed by a continuous IV infusion of 0.125 µg/kg per min (to a maximum of 10 µg/min) for 12 h
Unstable angina with planned PCI within 24 h: 0.25 mg/kg IV bolus followed by an 18- to 24-h IV infusion of 10 µg/min, concluding 1 h after PCI
Note: The safety and efficacy of abciximab have been studied only with concomitant administration of heparin and aspirin. Continuous infusion of abciximab should be stopped in cases of failed PCI because there is no evidence for the efficacy of abciximab in that setting. A filter must be used during the administration of abciximab; see package insert for detailed instructions on administration.

Elderly
No dosage adjustment is required, but there may be an increased risk of major bleeding in patients >65 y of age. Caution is recommended.

Children
Safety and effectiveness have not been established

Preparation
ReoPro (Lilly): 2 mg/mL, 5-mL vials

(continued)

Anagrelide hydrochloride (Agrylin)

Indication

Treatment of essential thrombocythemia to reduce elevated platelet count and risk of thrombosis

Dosage

Adults

Initiate treatment with anagrelide under close medical supervision. Initial dose is 0.5 mg qid or 1 mg bid, which should be maintained for ≥1 wk. Dosage then should be adjusted to the lowest effective level required to reduce and maintain platelet count <600,000/μL and ideally to the normal range. Dosage should be increased by not more than 0.5 mg/d in any 1 wk. Dosage should not exceed 10 mg/d or 2.5 mg in a single dose. Most patients will experience an adequate response at a dose of 1.5–3.0 mg/d. Monitor patients with known or suspected heart disease, renal insufficiency, or hepatic dysfunction closely.

Elderly

No data; dosage adjustment is probably not required

Children

Safety and effectiveness are not established in patients <16 y of age. However, anagrelide has been used successfully in 8 pediatric patients (age range, 8–17 y), including 3 with essential thrombocythemia who were treated at a dose of 1–4 mg/d.

Preparations

Agrylin (Roberts): 0.5-, 1-mg capsules

Aspirin

Indications

Listed below are cardiovascular indications only (not all indications are FDA approved)

Prevention of arterial and venous thrombosis in: arteriovenous shunt for hemodialysis; atrial fibrillation; coronary bypass; intracoronary stent placement (in combination with clopidogrel, ticlopidine, or warfarin); MI (primary/secondary prophylaxis); prosthetic heart valves (with an oral anticoagulant and with or without dipyridamole); transient ischemic attacks; transluminal angioplasty of coronary, iliac, femoral, popliteal, or tibial artery (with or without dipyridamole); unstable angina

Dosage

Adults

Transient ischemic attacks in men: 1300 mg/d in 2–4 divided doses; doses as low as 300 mg/d may be effective if tolerance is a problem with high doses

MI/unstable angina: 80–325 mg once daily; the first dose in patients experiencing chest pain should be plain aspirin (not enteric coated), and the dose should be chewed, crushed, or dispersed in solution and administered as soon as possible for more rapid antiplatelet effect

Elderly

Dosage adjustment is not required

Children

Dosage recommendations are based on age and weight for the analgesic indication. Aspirin is not recommended in children with influenza or chickenpox due to the risk for Reye's syndrome.

Preparations
: Available in various strengths and formulations

Cilostazol (Pletal)
Indication
: Intermittent claudication

Dosage
Adults
: 100 mg bid, taken ≥30 min before or 2 h after breakfast and dinner. A lower dose of 50 mg bid should be considered during coadministration of CYP3A4 inhibitors (e.g., ketoconazole, itraconazole, erythromycin, diltiazem) and CYP2C19 inhibitors (e.g., omeprazole). Because CYP3A4 is also inhibited by grapefruit juice, patients receiving cilostazol should avoid this beverage.

Elderly
: Dosage adjustment is not required

Children
: Safety and effectiveness have not been established

Preparations
: Pletal (Otsuka, America, Pharmaceuticals/Pharmacia, Upjohn): 50-, 100-mg tablets

Clopidogrel (Plavix)
Indications
: Reduction of thrombotic events in patients with a history of recent MI, recent stroke, or established peripheral arterial disease; reduction of thrombotic events in patients with acute coronary syndrome; prevention of ischemic events, MI, stroke, and vascular death in patients with recent MI, recent stroke, or peripheral arterial disease

Dosage
Adults
: Recent MI, recent stroke or established peripheral arterial disease: 75 mg once daily
Acute coronary syndrome: For patients with acute coronary syndrome (unstable angina/non-Q-wave MI), clopidogrel should be initiated with a single 300-mg loading dose and then continued at 75 mg once daily. Aspirin (75–325 mg once daily) should be initiated and continued in combination with clopidogrel. In the CURE trial, most patients with acute coronary syndrome also received heparin acutely.

Elderly
: Dosage adjustment is not required

Children
: Safety and effectiveness have not been established

Preparation
: Plavix (Bristol Myers Squibb/Sanofi): 75-mg tablets

Dipyridamole (dipyridamole, Persantine)
Indications
: Prophylaxis of thromboembolism after cardiac valve replacement (use as an adjunct to warfarin therapy), an alternative to exercise during thallium myocardial perfusion imaging for the evaluation of coronary artery disease in patients who cannot exercise adequately

(continued)

APPENDIX 2 *(continued)* Therapeutic Use of Available Cardiovascular Drugs

Dosage

Adults
Adjunctive use in prophylaxis of thromboembolism after cardiac valve replacement: 75–100 mg four times daily (as an adjunct to warfarin therapy)

Evaluation of coronary artery disease: IV infusion: 0.14 mg/kg per min for 4 min; not to exceed 60 mg over 4 min. Radiopharmaceutical is injected within 3–5 min after completion of the dipyridamole infusion.

Elderly
Dosage adjustment is not required

Children
Safety and effectiveness have not been established in children <12 y of age

Preparations
Dipyridamole (generic); Persantine (Boehringer Ingelheim): 25-, 50-, 75-mg tablets

Persantine injection (Boehringer Ingelheim): 5 mg/mL (10 mg/2-mL ampule)

Dipyridamole and aspirin (Aggrenox)

Indication
To reduce the risk of stroke in patients who have had transient ischemia of the brain or complete ischemic stroke due to thrombosis

Dosage

Adults
Administer 1 capsule bid (1 in the morning and 1 in the evening). Capsules should be swallowed whole; do not crush or chew capsule.

Elderly
Dosage adjustment is not required

Children
Safety and effectiveness have not been established

Preparation
Aggrenox (Boehringer Ingelheim): 200 mg ER dipyridamole/25-mg aspirin capsules

Eptifibatide (Integrilin)

Indications
Treatment of patients with acute coronary syndrome (unstable angina or non-Q-wave MI), including patients who are to be managed medically and those undergoing PCI

Dosage

Adults
Acute coronary syndrome: 180 μg/kg IV bolus (over 1–2 min) administered as soon as possible after diagnosis, followed by a continuous infusion of 2 μg/kg per min until hospital discharge or initiation of coronary artery bypass graft surgery, up to 72 h. If PCI is performed during treatment with eptifibatide, consideration can be given to reducing the infusion rate to 0.5 μg/kg per min at the time of the procedure. Infusion should be continued for an additional 20–24 h after the PCI, allowing for up to 96 h of therapy. Patients weighing >121 kg have received a maximum bolus of 22.6 mg, followed by a maximum infusion rate of 15 mg/h.

PCI in patients not presenting with an acute coronary syndrome: 135 μg/kg IV bolus (over 1–2 min) administered immediately before the initiation of PCI, followed by a continuous infusion of 0.5 μg/kg per min for 20–24 h. There has been little experience in patients weighing >143 kg.

Note: The safety and efficacy of eptifibatide have been established only with concomitant administration of heparin and aspirin. Dosage adjustment is not required for patients with serum creatinine <2 mg/dL for the 180 μg/kg bolus and the 2.0 μg/kg per min infusion and <4 mg/dL for the 135 μg/kg bolus and the 0.5 μg/kg per min infusion. Plasma eptifibatide levels are expected to be higher in patients with more severe renal impairment, and data are not available for this patient population.

Elderly   Dosage adjustment is not required
Children   Safety and effectiveness have not been established
Preparations   Integrilin (COR Therapeutics, Key): 0.75 mg/mL, 100-mL vials; 2 mg/mL, 10-mL vials

Ticlopidine (ticlopidine hydrochloride, Ticlid)

Indication   To reduce the risk of thrombotic stroke in patients who have experienced stroke precursors and in patients who have had a completed thrombotic stroke

Dosage
Adults   250 mg bid with food
Elderly   Dosage adjustment is not required
Children   Safety and effectiveness have not been established
Preparation   Ticlopidine (generic); Ticlid (Roche): 250-mg tablets

Tirofiban hydrochloride (Aggrastat)

Indications   Treatment of acute coronary syndrome (in combination with heparin), including patients who are to be managed medically and those undergoing PTCA, or atherectomy

Dosage
Adults   Administer IV at an initial rate of 0.4 μg/kg per min for 30 min and then continue at 0.1 μg/kg per min. In a clinical trial, PRISM-PLUS, tirofiban was administered in combination with heparin for 48–108 h. Infusion should be continued through angiography and for 12–24 h after angioplasty or atherectomy. Patients with severe renal impairment (CrCl <30 mL/min) should receive half the usual rate of loading and maintenance infusion.
                 Note: Tirofiban was studied in a setting that included aspirin and heparin. The 250-μg/mL injection must be diluted to 50 μg/mL before administration.
Elderly   Dosage adjustment is not required
Children   Safety and effectiveness have not been established
Preparations   Aggrastat (Merck): 250 μg/mL, 50-mL vial; 50 μg/mL, 500-mL single-dose IntraVia containers

(continued)

APPENDIX 2 (continued) Therapeutic Use of Available Cardiovascular Drugs

Thrombolytic agents

Alteplase, recombinant (Activase)

Indications

Acute MI, acute ischemic stroke, pulmonary embolism, restoration of function to central venous access devices

Dosage

Adults

Acute MI: Treatment should be initiated as soon as possible after the onset of chest pain.

1. Accelerated infusion: 15 mg IV bolus, followed by 0.75 mg/kg (up to 50 mg) infused over the next 30 min, and then 0.5 mg/kg (up to 35 mg) infused over the next 60 min. Maximum total dose is 100 mg for patients who weigh >67 kg. Safety and efficacy of this accelerated infusion regimen have been investigated only with concomitant administration of heparin and aspirin.

2. 3-h infusion: 60 mg infused over 60 min (with 6–10 mg administered as a bolus over the first 1–2 min), followed by 20 mg/h infusion for the next 2 h to deliver a total dose of 100 mg. For patients weighing <65 kg, a total dose of 1.25 mg/kg given over 3 h is recommended. Although the use of anticoagulants during and after alteplase infusion has been shown to be of unclear benefit, heparin has been given concomitantly for ≥24 h in >90% of patients. Aspirin or dipyridamole has been administered either during or after heparin treatment.

Acute ischemic stroke: 0.9 mg/kg (up to 90 mg) administered IV over 60 min, with 10% of the total dose administered as a bolus over the first minute. Treatment should be initiated within 3 h after the onset of stroke symptoms. Avoid concurrent aspirin and heparin use during the first 24 h after symptom onset.

Pulmonary embolism: Administered 100 mg intravenously over 2 h. Heparin therapy should be instituted or reinstituted near the end of or immediately after the alteplase infusion when partial thromboplastin time or thrombin time returns to twice of normal or less.

Note: Alteplase must be reconstituted before administration; consult package insert for detailed instructions. In general, the adult dose can be used, but body weight should be considered. Patients >75 y of age, especially those with suspected arterial degeneration, are at an increased risk for unwanted bleeding; monitor closely.

Elderly

Children

Safety and effectiveness have not been established

Preparations

Activase (Genentech): 50 mg (29 million IU)/vial, 100 mg (58 million IU)/vial, Cathflo Activase (Genentech): 2-mg vial

Anistreplase (Eminase)

Indication

Acute MI

Dosage

Adults

Thrombolytic therapy should be initiated as soon as possible after the onset of symptoms. Dose of anistreplase is 30 U administered IV over 2–5 min.

Reconstitution: Slowly add 5 mL of sterile water for injection into the vial containing anistreplase, directing the stream of water against the side of the vial. Gently roll (do not shake) the vial to mix the powder with the liquid. The reconstituted solution should not be diluted further before administration. No other medication should be added to the vial containing anistreplase.

Elderly
Dosage adjustment is not required. Patients >75 y of age, especially those with suspected arterial degeneration, may be at risk for unwanted bleeding; monitor closely.

Children
Safety and effectiveness have not been established

Preparation
Eminase (Roberts): 30 U/single-dose vial

Reteplase, recombinant (Retavase)

Indication
Acute MI

Dosage

Adults
Treatment should be initiated as soon as possible, preferably within 12 h after the onset of chest pain. Reteplase should be administered as two 10-U bolus injections, each administered over 2 min, with the second dose given 30 min after the initiation of the first injection. Patients also should receive adjunctive therapy with heparin and aspirin. *Note:* Reteplase should be given through an IV line in which no other medications (e.g., heparin) are being injected or infused. If reteplase is to be administered through an IV line containing heparin, the line should be flushed before and after reteplase administration with 0.9% sodium chloride or 5% dextrose solution. Reteplase should be reconstituted with 10 mL sterile water for injection (without preservatives) to yield a solution of 1 U/mL. The vial should be swirled gently to dissolve the drug, taking precaution to avoid shaking. Once dissolved, 10 mL should be withdrawn from the vial into a syringe for administration to the patient. Approximately 0.7 mL will remain in the vial due to overfill.

Elderly
Dosage adjustment is not required

Children
Safety and effectiveness have not been established

Preparation
Retavase (Centocor): 10.8 U (18.8 mg)/single-use vial

Streptokinase (Streptase)

Indications
Acute MI; arterial thrombosis or embolism; cannula, arteriovenous clearance, deep vein thrombosis; pulmonary embolism

Dosage

Adults
Acute MI: Treatment should be initiated as soon as possible, preferably within 4 h after the onset of chest pain. IV infusion: Administer a total dose of 1,500,000 IU within 60 min

(continued)

651

APPENDIX 2 (continued) Therapeutic Use of Available Cardiovascular Drugs

Intracoronary infusion: Administer 20,000 IU by bolus, followed by 2000 IU/min for 60 min (total dose of 140,000 IU)

Pulmonary embolism, deep vein thrombosis, arterial thrombosis, or embolism: Administer 250,000 IU bolus infused IV over 30 min, followed by 100,000 IU/h continuous infusion for 24 h for pulmonary embolism, 72 h for deep vein thrombosis, and 24–72 h for arterial thrombosis or embolism. Treatment should be initiated as soon as possible, preferably within 7 d after onset of symptoms.

Arteriovenous cannula occlusion: Slowly instill 250,000 IU streptokinase in 2 mL solution into each occluded limb of the cannula. Clamp off cannula limb(s) for 2 h and observe closely for adverse effects. After treatment, aspirate contents of infused cannula limb(s), flush with saline, and reconnect cannula.

Note: Consult package insert for detailed instructions on reconstitution of streptokinase before administration.

Elderly
Dosage adjustment is not required. Patients >75 y of age may be more susceptible to unwanted bleeding events.

Children
Safety and effectiveness have not been established

Preparations
Streptase (Astra Zeneca): 250,000, 750,000, 1,500,000 IU/vial

Tenecteplase (TNKase)

Indication
Acute MI

Dosage

Adults
Acute MI: Treatment should be initiated as soon as possible after the onset of symptoms. Dosage of tenecteplase is based on patient's weight as follows:

Weight (kg)	Tenecteplase (mg)	Tenecteplase (mL)*
<60	30	6
≥60–<70	35	7
≥70–<80	40	8
≥80–<90	45	9
≥90	50	10

*This is the volume of tenecteplase to be administered as a single bolus dose over 5 s after one vial of tenecteplase (50 mg) is reconstituted with 10 mL of sterile water for injection. Consult tenecteplase package insert for detailed instructions on reconstitution.

Elderly
Dosage determination is based on weight. Elderly patients may be more susceptible to unwanted bleeding events.

Children
Safety and effectiveness have not been established

Preparation
TNKase (Genentech): 50 mg/vial; sterile water for injection, 10 mL

Urokinase (Abbokinase)

Indications   Coronary artery thrombosis, IV catheter clearance, pulmonary embolism

Dosage

Adults

Coronary artery thrombosis: For the treatment of coronary artery thrombi, urokinase is administered selectively into the thrombosed coronary artery via a coronary catheter. Treatment should be initiated within 6 h of the onset of symptoms. Bolus dose of heparin 2500–10,000 U should be administered by rapid IV injection, followed by intracoronary administration of urokinase at a rate of 6000 IU/min (1500 IU/mL) for up to 2 h. Duration of treatment is guided by angiography performed q15 min. Average urokinase dose used was 500,000 IU with a 60% response rate. Heparin should be continued after clot lysis.

Note: Consult urokinase package insert for detailed instructions on reconstitution of medication before administration.

Pulmonary embolism: Treatment should be initiated as soon as possible after onset of pulmonary embolism, preferably within 7 d. Administer urokinase 4400 IU/kg IV over 10 min, followed by continuous infusion of 4400 IU/kg per h for 12 h. Thrombin time should be determined 3–4 h after initiation of therapy and maintained greater than twice the normal control. Appropriate anticoagulant therapy should be initiated about 3–4 h after discontinuance of urokinase infusion (until thrombin time has decreased to less than twice the normal control value).

Note: Consult urokinase package insert for recommendations regarding rate of infusion, which is based on dilution volume of the drug.

Occluded catheter: Urokinase 5000 IU/mL is used, and only the amount that equals the internal volume of the catheter should be injected slowly into the catheter. Specific instructions provided by the manufacturer should be followed to ensure aseptic application and proper urokinase indwelling time before each aspiration attempt and to avoid the risk for air emboli.

Elderly   Dosage adjustment is not required. Elderly patients may be more susceptible to unwanted bleeding events.

Children   Safety and effectiveness have not been established

Preparations   Abbokinase Open-Cath (Abbott): 5000, 9000 IU/mL vials (urokinase for catheter clearance)

Abbokinase (Abbott): 250,000 IU/5-mL vial (urokinase for injection)

β-Adrenergic blockers

Nonselective β-Adrenergic blockers without ISA

Nadolol (nadolol, Corgard)

Indications   Angina pectoris, hypertension

(continued)

653

APPENDIX 2 *(continued)* Therapeutic Use of Available Cardiovascular Drugs

Dosage
Adults
    Hypertension: Initiate with 20–40 mg once daily; dosage may be increased gradually in increments of
    40–80 mg to a maximum of 240–320 mg/d. Usual maintenance dose is 40–80 mg once daily.
    Angina pectoris: Initiate with 40 mg once daily; dosage may be increased by 40–80 mg/d q3–7 d until
    adequate control of angina is achieved. Usual dose is 40–80 mg/d. Up to 160–240 mg/d may be needed.
    Note: Because of the long half-life of nadolol, once-daily dosing is sufficient to provide stable plasma
    concentrations. Adjustments in dosing intervals must be made for patients with renal impairment as follows:

CrCl mL/min per 1.73 m^2	Dosing interval
>50	q24 h
31–50	q24–36 h
10–30	q24–48 h
<10	q48 h or longer

Elderly
    Initiate at lowest dose and titrate to response
Children
    Safety and efficacy have not been established
Preparations
    Corgard (Monarch): 20-, 40-, 80-, 120-, 160-mg tablets
Fixed-dose combinations for
    Corzide 40/5 tablets: 40 mg nadolol and 5 mg bendroflumethiazide
the treatment of hypertension
    Corzide 80/5 tablets: 80 mg nadolol and 5 mg bendroflumethiazide

Propranolol (propranolol, Inderal, Inderal LA, InnoPran XL)

Indications
    Angina pectoris, cardiac arrhythmias, essential tremor, hypertension, hypertrophic subaortic stenosis, MI,
    migraine prophylaxis, pheochromocytoma

Dosage
Adults
    Angina pectoris
    Regular formulation: Initiate with 10–20 mg tid or qid; dosage may be increased gradually q3–7 d according
    to response to a maximum dose of 320 mg/d.
    ER formulation: Initiate with 80 mg once daily; increase dosage gradually q3–7 d as needed up to a maximum
    of 320 mg/d.
    Cardiac arrhythmias
    Regular formulation: 10–30 mg tid or qid given before meals and at bedtime.

Essential tremor

Regular formulation: Initiate with 40 mg bid; dosage may be titrated according to response to a maximum of 320 mg/d. Usual maintenance dose is 120 mg/d in divided doses.

Hypertension

Regular formulation: Initiate with 40 mg bid; dosage may be increased gradually according to response to a maximum of 640 mg/d. Usual maintenance dose is 120–240 mg/d given in 2–3 divided doses.

ER formulation: Initiate with 80 mg once daily; dosage may be increased gradually according to response to a maximum of 640 mg/d. Usual maintenance dose is 120–160 mg once daily.

InnoPran XL should be administered once daily at bedtime and should be taken consistently with or without food. Starting dose is 80 mg once daily, but dosage may be increased to 120 mg once daily.

Hypertrophic subaortic stenosis

Regular formulation: Usual dose range is 20–40 mg tid or qid given before meals and at bedtime.

ER formulation: Usual dose range is 80–160 mg once daily.

MI

Regular formulation: Usual dose range is 180–240 mg/d given in 3–4 divided doses.

Migraine prophylaxis

Regular formulation: Initiate with 80 mg/d in divided doses; dosage may be increased gradually to the usual range of 160–240 mg/d in divided doses.

ER formulation: Initiate with 80 mg once daily; dosage may be increased gradually to a maximum of 240 mg/d.

Pheochromocytoma (adjunct therapy to α-adrenergic blocker)

Regular formulation: 60 mg/d in divided doses for 3 d before surgery. To prevent severe hypertension caused by unopposed α-adrenergic stimulation, treatment with an α-adrenergic blocking agent must always be started before the use of propranolol and continued during propranolol therapy. As an adjunct to prolonged treatment of inoperable pheochromocytoma, 30 mg/d propranolol in divided doses with an α-adrenergic blocker is usually sufficient.

IV administration for life-threatening arrhythmias: Usual dose is 1–3 mg given under careful monitoring. Rate of injection should not exceed 1 mg/min. A second dose may be given after 2 min if indicated. Thereafter, do not give additional dose in <4 h.

(continued)

APPENDIX 2 (continued) Therapeutic Use of Available Cardiovascular Drugs

Elderly	Initiate at lowest dose and titrate to response
Children	Initiate with PO dosage of 0.5 mg/kg bid for treatment of hypertension. Dosage may be increased at 3- to 5-d intervals to usual range of 2–4 mg/kg daily given in divided doses. IV use is not recommended; however, a dose of 0.01–0.1 mg/kg per dose to a maximum of 1 mg/dose by slow push has been used for the management of arrhythmias.
Preparations	Propranolol (generic); Inderal (Wyeth-Ayerst): 10-, 20-, 40-, 60-, 80-mg tablets
	Propranolol ER capsules (generic); Inderal LA (Wyeth-Ayerst): 60-, 80-, 120-, 160-mg ER capsules
	Propranolol injection (generic); Inderal injection (Wyeth-Ayerst): 1 mg/mL
	InnoPran XL (Reliant): 80-, 120-mg capsules
Fixed-dose combinations	Inderide LA 80/50: propranolol 80 mg/hydrochlorothiazide 50 mg capsules
for the treatment of hypertension	Inderide LA 120/50: propranolol 120 mg/hydrochlorothiazide 50 mg capsules
	Inderide LA 160/50: propranolol 160 mg/hydrochlorothiazide 50 mg capsules
	Inderide 80/25: propranolol 80 mg/hydrochlorothiazide 25 mg tablets
	Inderide 40/25: propranolol 40 mg/hydrochlorothiazide 25 mg tablets
	Propranolol 80 mg/hydrochlorothiazide 25 mg tablets
	Propranolol 40 mg/hydrochlorothiazide 25 mg tablets

Sotalol (Betapace, Betapace AF)
Refer to *Antiarrhythmic Agents*
Timolol (timolol, Blocadren)

Indications	Hypertension, MI, migraine prophylaxis, open-angle glaucoma (ophthalmic preparation)
Dosage	
Adults	*Hypertension:* Initiate with 10 mg bid; dosage may be increased gradually (at intervals of at least 7 d) to a maximum of 60 mg/d given in 2 divided doses. Usual maintenance dose is 20–40 mg/d.
	MI: Administer 10 mg bid for long-term prophylactic use in patients who have survived a MI.
	Migraine prophylaxis: Initiate with 10 mg bid. Dose should be adjusted based on clinical response to a maximum of 30 mg/d given in divided doses. Therapy should be tapered and discontinued if a satisfactory response is not achieved after 6–8 wk of maximum daily dosage.
Elderly	Initiate at lowest dose and titrate to response
Children	Safety and effectiveness have not been established

Preparations	Timolol (generic); Blocadren (Merck): 5-, 10-, 20-mg tablets
	Timolol (generic): 0.25% and 0.50% ophthalmic solution
	Timoptic (Merck): 0.25% and 0.50% ophthalmic solution
	Timoptic XE (Merck): 0.25% and 0.50% ophthalmic gel
	Timolide 10–25: 10 mg timolol/25 mg hydrochlorothiazide tablets

Fixed-dose combinations for
the treatment of hypertension

β₁ Selective β-adrenergic blockers without ISA

Atenolol (atenolol, Tenormin)

Indications   Angina pectoris, hypertension, MI

Dosage

Adults   *Angina pectoris:* Initiate with 50 mg once daily; dosage may be increased to 100 mg/d according to response. Some patients may require 200 mg/d.

Hypertension: Initiate with 50 mg once daily, dosage may be increased (at 1- to 2-wk intervals) to 100 mg/d according to response.

MI: Treatment should be initiated with IV atenolol 5 mg administered over 5 min, followed by a second IV dose of 5 mg 10 min later. If the patient tolerates the full IV therapy, 50 mg atenolol should be administered PO 10 min after the last IV dose, followed by a second 50 mg PO dose 12 h later. Then the patient can receive PO atenolol 100 mg once daily or 50 mg bid for 6–9 d or until discharge from the hospital.

Note: Because atenolol is eliminated mainly in the kidneys as unchanged drug, dosage adjustment should be made in patients with renal impairment:

CrCl mL/min per 1.73 m²	Maximum dose
15–35	50 mg/d
<15	25 mg/d
Hemodialysis	25 or 50 mg post hemodialysis

Elderly   Initiate at lowest dose and titrate to response

Children   Safety and effectiveness have not been established

Preparations   Atenolol (generic); Tenormin (Astra Zeneca): 25-, 50-, 100-mg tablets
Tenormin injection (Astra Zeneca): 5 mg/10 mL, 10-mL ampules

Fixed-dose combinations for
the treatment of hypertension   Generic; Tenoretic 50: 50 mg atenolol/25 mg chlorthalidone tablets
Generic; Tenoretic 100: 100 mg atenolol/25 mg chlorthalidone tablets

(continued)

APPENDIX 2 *(continued)* Therapeutic Use of Available Cardiovascular Drugs

Betaxolol (betaxolol, Kerlone)

Indications

Hypertension, ocular hypertension (ophthalmic preparation), open-angle glaucoma (ophthalmic preparation)

Dosage

Adults

Hypertension: Initiate with 10 mg once daily (5 mg for elderly patients or patients with renal impairment). Dosage may be doubled q2 wk to a maximum dose of 20–40 mg/d.

Elderly

Initiate at lowest dose and titrate to response

Children

Safety and effectiveness have not been established

Preparations

Betaxolol (generic); Kerlone: 10-, 20-mg tablets

Bisoprolol (bisoprolol, Zebeta)

Indications

Hypertension

Dosage

Adults

Hypertension: Initiate with 2.5–5 mg once daily; dosage may be increased according to response to a maximum of 20 mg once daily.

Elderly

Dosage adjustment is not necessary. However, a lower initial dose of 2.5 mg should be used in patients with CrCl <40 mL/min or in patients with hepatic impairment.

Children

Safety and effectiveness have not been established

Preparations

Bisoprolol (generic); Zebeta (Lederle): 5-, 10-mg tablets

Fixed-dose combinations for the treatment of hypertension

Generic: Ziac (Lederle) bisoprolol/hydrochlorothiazide combination tablets: 2.5 mg/6.25 mg, 5 mg/6.25 mg, 10 mg/6.25 mg

Esmolol (Brevibloc)

Indications

Supraventricular tachycardia, intraoperative and postoperative tachycardia and/or hypertension

Dosage

Adults

Supraventricular tachycardia: Dosage is established by means of a series of loading and maintenance doses. Administer a loading IV infusion of 500 µg/kg per min for 1 min, followed by a maintenance IV infusion of 50 µg/kg per min for 4 min. If adequate response is not observed at the end of 5 min, repeat sequence with loading IV infusion (as above), followed by an increased maintenance infusion rate of 100 µg/kg per min. The sequence is repeated until an adequate response is obtained, with an increment of 50 µg/kg per min in the maintenance dose at each step. As desired end point (defined as desired heart rate/undesirable decrease in blood pressure) is approached, loading dose may be omitted, and increments in maintenance dose can be reduced to ≤25 µg/kg per min. Intervals between titration steps also may be increased from 5 to 10 min. Established maintenance dose usually does not exceed 200 µg/kg per min (due to the risk of hypotension) and can be given for up to 24 h (up to 48 h of therapy have been given in limited studies). Maintenance doses as low as 25 µg/kg per min and as high as 300 µg/kg per min have been used.

Intraoperative and postoperative tachycardia and/or hypertension, rapid intraoperative control: Administer 80-mg (1 mg/kg) IV bolus dose over 30 s, followed by 150 µg/kg per min infusion, and titrate the dose to maintain desired heart rate or blood pressure (up to 300 µg/kg per min).

Gradual postoperative control: Dose titration schedule is the same as the treatment in supraventricular tachycardia; however, higher dosages of up to 250–300 µg/kg per min may be needed for adequate blood pressure control.

Note: The 250 mg/mL strength of esmolol hydrochloride injection must be diluted before administration by IV infusion. The 10 mg/mL strength may be given by direct infusion. Concentrations >10 mg/mL may produce irritation. If a reaction occurs at the infusion site, the infusion should be stopped and resumed at another site. Avoid the use of butterfly needles and very small veins for infusion of esmolol.

Elderly   Initiate with a low dose and titrate according to response
Children   Safety and effectiveness have not been established
Preparations   Brevibloc (Baxter Healthcare): 10, 250 mg/mL

Metoprolol (metoprolol tartrate, Lopressor, Toprol XL)
Indications   Angina pectoris, hypertension, MI, CHF (Toprol XL)
Dosage
Adults   *Hypertension:* Initiate with 100 mg/d in single or divided doses. Dosage may be adjusted at weekly intervals (or longer) until desired blood pressure control is achieved. Effective maintenance doses range from 100 to 450 mg/d.
                 Note: ER tablets are for once-a-day administration. The same total daily dose should be used when switching from immediate-release metoprolol tablets to ER tablets.
                 Angina pectoris: Initiate with 100 mg/d in 2 divided doses. Dosage may be increased at weekly intervals until optimum clinical response is achieved. Effective maintenance doses range from 100 to 400 mg/d.
                 MI: Treatment should be initiated as soon as the patient's hemodynamic status has stabilized. Three 5-mg IV bolus injections of metoprolol should be administered at 2-min intervals. If the full 15-mg IV dose is tolerated by

(continued)

APPENDIX 2 *(continued)* Therapeutic Use of Available Cardiovascular Drugs

the patient, 50 mg of PO metoprolol (or 25 mg for those who cannot tolerate the full dose) q6 h should be initiated 15 min after the last IV dose and continued for 48 h. Thereafter, the dose may be adjusted to 100 mg bid. *CHF:* For NYHA class II patients, start with 25 mg once daily. For severe heart failure, start with 12.5 mg once daily. Titrate by doubling the dose q2 wk as tolerated; reduce dose if symptomatic bradycardia occurs. Maximal dose is 200 mg/d.

Elderly — Initiate with a low dose and titrate according to response

Children — Safety and effectiveness have not been established

Preparations — Metoprolol tartrate (generic); Lopressor (Novartis): 50-, 100-mg tablets
Toprol XL (Astra Zeneca): 25-, 50-, 100-, 200-mg ER tablets
Metoprolol tartrate injection (generic); Lopressor injection (Novartis): 1 mg/mL
Lopressor HCT tablets (Novartis): 50/25–50 mg metoprolol/25 mg hydrochlorothiazide 100/25–100 mg metoprolol/25 mg hydrochlorothiazide 100/50–100 mg metoprolol/50 mg hydrochlorothiazide

Fixed-dose combinations for the treatment of hypertension

β-Adrenergic blockers with ISA
Acebutolol (acebutolol, Sectral)

Indications — Hypertension, ventricular arrhythmia

Dosage

Adults — *Hypertension:* Initiate with 200–400 mg/d administered in 1 or 2 divided doses. Dosage may be increased gradually based on clinical response up to 600 mg bid. Most patients require 400–800 mg/d.
Ventricular arrhythmia: Initiate with 400 mg once daily or 200 mg bid. Dosage may be increased until optimal response is achieved. Usual maintenance dose is 600–1200 mg/d given in 2 divided doses.
Note: Daily dose of acebutolol should be reduced by 50% when CrCl <50 mL/min per 1.73 m². Reduce dose by 75% when CrCl <25 mL/min per 1.73 m². Use acebutolol with caution in patients with hepatic impairment.

Elderly — Initiate at lowest dose and titrate to response; avoid doses >800 mg/d

Children — Safety and effectiveness have not been established

Preparations — Acebutolol (generic); Sectral (Wyeth-Ayerst): 200-, 400-mg capsules

Carteolol (Cartrol)

Indication — Hypertension

Dosage

Adults — *Hypertension:* Initiate with 2.5 mg once daily. Dosage may be increased gradually according to response to a maximum of 10 mg once daily. Usual maintenance dose is 2.5 or 5 mg once daily.

660

Note: Guidelines for dosing intervals in patients with renal impairment are as follows:

CrCl mL/min per 1.73 m²	Dosage interval (h)
>60	24
20–60	48
<20	72

Elderly Initiate at lowest dose and titrate to response

Children Safety and effectiveness have not been established

Preparations Cartrol (Abbott): 2.5-, 5-mg tablets

Penbutolol (Levatol)

Indication Hypertension

Dosage

Adults *Hypertension:* Usual starting and maintenance doses are 20 mg once daily. Doses of 40–80 mg/d have been well tolerated but have not shown greater effect.

Elderly Initiate at lowest dose and titrate to response

Children Safety and effectiveness have not been established

Preparation Levatol (Schwarz Pharma): 20-mg tablets

Pindolol (pindolol, Visken)

Indication Hypertension

Dosage

Adults *Hypertension:* Initiate with 5 mg bid. Dosage may be increased by 10 mg/d at 3- to 4-wk intervals to a maximum of 60 mg/d if necessary.

Elderly Initiate at lowest dose and titrate to response

Children Safety and effectiveness have not been established

Preparations Pindolol, Visken (Novartis): 5-, 10-mg tablets

Dual-acting beta blockers

Carvedilol (Coreg)

Indications CHF (mild to severe), hypertension, left ventricular dysfunction after MI

Dosage

Adults *CHF:* Dosage of carvedilol must be individualized and closely monitored during the up-titration period. Dosing of digitalis, diuretics, and ACE inhibitors (if used) must be stabilized before initiation of carvedilol. Initiate

(continued)

661

APPENDIX 2 *(continued)* Therapeutic Use of Available Cardiovascular Drugs

carvedilol with 3.125 mg bid for 2 wk. If this dose is tolerated, it can then be increased to 6.25 mg bid. Dosing then should be doubled q2 wk to the highest level tolerated by the patient. Maximum recommended dose is 25 mg bid in patients weighing <85 kg and 50 mg bid in patients weighing >85 kg. If bradycardia occurs (pulse rate <55 beats/min), the dose of carvedilol should be reduced.

Hypertension: Initiate with 6.25 mg bid. Dosage may be increased to 12.5 mg bid after 7–14 d if tolerated and needed. A further increase to 25 mg bid may be made after an additional 7–14 d if necessary. Total daily dose should not exceed 50 mg.

Note: Carvedilol should be taken with food to slow the rate of absorption and reduce the incidence of orthostatic hypotension. Because carvedilol is metabolized primarily in the liver, it should not be given to patients with severe hepatic impairment. In patients with heart failure, slower titration with temporary dose reduction or withdrawal may be required based on clinical assessment; however, this should not preclude later attempts to reintroduce or increase the dose of carvedilol.

Left ventricular dysfunction after MI: Dose of carvedilol must be individualized and monitored closely during up-titration. Treatment with carvedilol may be started as an inpatient or outpatient and should be started when the patient is hemodynamically stable and fluid retention is minimized. Initiate therapy at 6.25 mg bid, which can be increased after 3–10 d to 12.5 mg bid if tolerated, and again to the target dose of 25 mg bid. A lower starting dose may be used (3.125 mg bid) and/or the rate of up-titration may be slowed if clinically indicated (e.g., due to low blood pressure or heart rate or fluid retention). Patients should be maintained on lower doses if higher doses are not tolerated. The recommended dosing regimen need not be altered in patients who received treatment with an IV or PO beta blocker during the acute phase of the MI.

Elderly
Although plasma levels of carvedilol average about 50% higher in the elderly as compared with young subjects, the manufacturer has not suggested dosage adjustment.

Children
Safety and effectiveness have not been established

Preparations
Coreg (Glaxo SmithKline): 3.125-, 6.25-, 12.5-, 25-mg tablets

Labetalol (labetalol, Normodyne, Trandate)

Indications
Hypertension, severe hypertension (IV formulation)

Dosage

Adults
Initiate with 100 mg orally twice daily; dosage may be adjusted in increments of 100 mg bid q2–3 d until desired response is reached. Usual maintenance dose is 200–400 mg bid. For severe hypertension, PO doses of 1.2–2.4 g/d in 2–3 divided doses may be needed.

Labetalol also may be administered by repeated intravenous injections. Inject 20 mg (0.25 mg/kg for an 80-kg patient) slowly over 2 min. Additional injections of 40 and 80 mg may be given at 10-min intervals until the desired blood pressure is reached or a total of 300 mg has been given. Alternatively, an IV infusion at a rate of 2 mg/min may be given (labetalol injection must be diluted properly for IV infusion); infusion rate should be adjusted according to response. Infusion should be continued until an adequate response is achieved or a total dose of 300 mg is infused. The infusion is then discontinued, and PO therapy is initiated when supine blood pressure begins to increase. Initial PO dose should be 200 mg, followed by an additional PO dose of 200 or 400 mg in 6–12 h based on blood pressure response.

Elderly Dosage adjustment based on age is not necessary

Children Safety and efficacy have not been established

Preparations Labetalol HCl (generic); Normodyne (Schering); Trandate (Prometheus): 100-, 200-, 300-mg tablets
Generic; Normodyne injection (Schering); Trandate injection (Prometheus): 5 mg/mL

Calcium antagonists
Amlodipine (Norvasc)

Indications Hypertension, chronic stable angina, vasospastic (Prinzmetal or variant) angina

Dosage

Adults *Hypertension:* Initiate with 5 mg once daily; dosage may be increased to a maximum of 10 mg once daily based on response. A lower initial dose of 2.5 mg once daily is recommended for elderly patients and patients with hepatic insufficiency.
Angina: Usual dose is 5–10 mg once daily. Use lower dose for elderly patients and patients with hepatic impairment.

Elderly Initiate at lowest dose and titrate to response

Children Safety and effectiveness have not been established

Preparations Norvasc (Pfizer): 2.5-, 5-, 10-mg tablets

Bepridil (Vascor)

Indication Chronic stable angina

Dosage

Adults Dosage should be individualized according to clinical judgment and patient's response. Usual initial dose is 200 mg once daily. Upward adjustment may be made after 10 d depending on patient's response. Usual maintenance dose is 300 mg once daily. Maximum daily dose is 400 mg.

(continued)

APPENDIX 2 (continued) Therapeutic Use of Available Cardiovascular Drugs

Elderly

Note: If nausea occurs, administer the drug with meals or at bedtime
Same initial dose as in adult patients may be used. However, elderly patients may require close monitoring due to underlying cardiac and organ system insufficiencies.

Children

Safety and effectiveness have not been established

Preparations

Vascor (Ortho-McNeil): 200-, 300-mg tablets

Diltiazem (diltiazem, Cardizem, Cardizem SR, Cardizem CD, Cardizem LA, Dilacor XR, Tiazac)

Indications

Angina pectoris, atrial fibrillation/flutter (Cardizem injectable), hypertension, paroxysmal supraventricular tachycardia (Cardizem injectable)

Dosage
Adults

Short acting (diltiazem, Cardizem): As an antianginal agent, the usual initial dose is 30 mg qid (before meals and at bedtime). Dosage should be increased gradually at 1- to 2-d intervals. Maximum daily dose is 360 mg.

SR (Cardizem SR): As monotherapy for hypertension, start with 60–120 mg bid, although some patients may respond well to lower doses. Usual dosage range is 240–360 mg/d.

SR (Cardizem CD): As monotherapy for hypertension, initiate at 180–240 mg once daily. Usual dose range in clinical trials was 240–360 mg/d. Some patients may respond to higher doses of up to 480 mg once daily. For angina, start with 120 or 180 mg once daily. Dosage may be titrated upward q7–14 d to a maximum of 480 mg once daily if necessary.

SR (Dilacor XR): For hypertension, initiate at 180–240 mg once daily. Adjust dose as needed depending on antihypertensive response. In clinical trials, the therapeutic dose range was 180–540 mg once daily. For angina, initiate at 120 mg once daily. Dosage may be titrated upward q7–14 d up to a maximum of 480 mg once daily if needed.

SR (Tiazac): Usual initial dose is 120–240 mg once daily. Maximum effect is observed after 14 d. Doses up to 540 mg daily were shown to be effective in clinical trials.

ER (Cardizem LA): When used as monotherapy for hypertension, reasonable starting doses are 180–240 mg once daily. Dosage range studied in clinical trials was 120–540 mg once daily. Cardizem LA tablets should be taken about the same time once daily in the morning or at bedtime.

Injection (diltiazem IV, Cardizem IV): For direct IV single injections (bolus), administer 0.25 mg/kg as a bolus over 2 min (20 mg is a reasonable dose for a patient with average weight). If response is inadequate, a second dose may be administered after 15 min (25 mg or 0.35 mg/kg is a reasonable dose).

IV infusion: An IV infusion may be administered for continued reduction of the heart rate (up to 24 h) in patients with atrial fibrillation or atrial flutter. Start an infusion at a rate of 10 mg/h immediately after bolus administration of 0.25 or 0.35 mg/kg. Some patients may maintain response to an initial rate of 5 mg/h. Infusion rate may be increased in 5-mg/h increments up to 15 mg/h as needed. Infusion duration >24 h and infusion rate >15 mg/h are not recommended (refer to manufacturer's package insert for proper dilution of diltiazem injection for continuous infusion).

Elderly   Initiate at lowest dose and titrate to response

Children   Safety and effectiveness have not been established

Preparations   Diltiazem (generic); Cardizem (Biovail): 30-, 60-, 90-, 120-mg tablets
Cardizem SR (Biovail): 60-, 90-, 120-mg SR capsules
Cardizem LA (Biovail): 120-, 180-, 240-, 300-, 360-, 420-mg ER tablets
Cardizem CD (Biovail): 120-, 180-, 240-, 300-, 360-mg ER capsules
Dilacor XR (Watson): 120-, 180-, 240-mg ER capsules
Tiazac (Forest): 120-, 180-, 240-, 300-, 360-, 420-mg ER capsules
Diltiazem HCl injection (generic); Cardizem injection (Biovail): 5 mg/mL (5, 10 mL)
Teczem (Hoechst Marion Roussel): 5 mg enalapril maleate/180 mg of diltiazem malate ER combination tablets

Fixed-dose combinations for the treatment of hypertension

Felodipine (Plendil)

Indication   Hypertension

Dosage

Adults   Usual initial dose is 5 mg once daily. Dosage may be increased by 5 mg at 2-wk intervals according to response. Maintenance dose ranges from 2.5 to 10 mg once daily.

Elderly   A lower initial dose of 2.5 mg once daily is recommended

Children   Safety and effectiveness have not been established

Preparations   Plendil (Astra Zeneca): 2.5-, 5-, 10-mg ER tablets

Fixed-dose combinations for the treatment of hypertension   Lexxel (Astra Pharm): 5 mg enalapril maleate/5 mg felodipine ER combination tablets

Isradipine (DynaCirc, DynaCirc CR)

Indication   Hypertension

(continued)

665

Dosage
Adults

Immediate release (DynaCirc): Initiate at 2.5 mg bid alone or in combination with a thiazide diuretic. Dosage may be adjusted in increments of 2.5–5 mg/d at 2- to 4-wk intervals if needed. Maximum daily dose is 20 mg. *Note:* Most patients show no further improvement with doses >10 mg/d; adverse reactions are increased in frequency with doses >10 mg/d.

Controlled release (DynaCirc CR): Initiate at 5 mg once daily alone or in combination with a thiazide diuretic. Dosage may be adjusted in increments of 5 mg/d at 2- to 4-wk intervals if needed. The maximum daily dose is 20 mg.

Elderly

Initiate at lowest dose and titrate to response

Children

Safety and effectiveness have not been established

Preparations

DynaCirc (Reliant): 2.5-, 5-mg capsules

DynaCirc CR (Reliant): 5-, 10-mg controlled-release tablets

Nicardipine (nicardipine, Cardene, Cardene SR)

Indications

Hypertension (Cardene, Cardene SR), short-term treatment of hypertension when PO therapy cannot be given (Cardene IV), angina (Cardene)

Dosage
Adults

Immediate release (Cardene): As an antianginal or antihypertensive agent, administer 20 mg in capsule form tid. Usual maintenance dose is 20–40 mg tid. Allow at least 3 d between dose increases. For patients with renal impairment, titrate dose beginning with 20 mg tid. For patients with hepatic impairment, titrate dose starting with 20 mg bid.

SR (Cardene SR): Initiate treatment with 30 mg bid. Effective dose ranges from 30 to 60 mg bid. For patients with renal impairment, carefully titrate dose beginning with 30 mg bid. Total daily dose of immediate-release product may not automatically be equivalent to the daily SR dose; use caution in converting.

Injection (Cardene IV): IV administered nicardipine injection must be diluted before infusion. Administer (concentration of 0.1 mg/mL) by slow, continuous infusion. Blood pressure-lowering effect is seen within minutes. For gradual blood pressure lowering, initiate at 50 mL/h (5 mg/h). Infusion rate may be increased by 25 mL/h (2.5 mg/h) q15 min to a maximum of 150 mL/h (15 mg/h). For rapid blood pressure reduction, initiate at 50 mL/h. Increase infusion rate by 25 mL/h q5 min to a maximum of 150 mL/h until desirable blood pressure lowering is reached. Infusion rate must be decreased to 30 mL/h (3 mg/h) when desirable blood pressure is achieved.

Conditions requiring infusion adjustment include hypotension and tachycardia. The IV infusion rate required to produce an average plasma concentration equivalent to a given PO dose at steady state is as follows:

PO dose (immediate release)	Equivalent IV infusion rate
20 mg q8h	0.5 mg/h
30 mg q8h	1.2 mg/h
40 mg q8h	2.2 mg/h

IV nicardipine should be transferred to PO medication for prolonged control of blood pressure as soon as the clinical condition permits. If treatment includes transfer to a PO antihypertensive agent other than nicardipine, generally initiate therapy after discontinuation of infusion. If PO nicardipine is to be used, administer the first dose of a tid regimen 1 h before discontinuation of the infusion.

Elderly Dosage adjustment is not necessary

Children Safety and effectiveness have not been established

Preparations Nicardipine HCl (generic); Cardene (Roche): 20-, 30-mg capsules
Cardene SR (Roche): 30-, 45-, 60-mg SR capsules
Cardene IV (ESP Pharma): 2.5 mg/mL injection, 10-mL ampules

Nifedipine (nifedipine, Adalat, Adalat CC, Procardia, Procardia XL)

Indications Chronic stable angina (Nifedipine, Adalat, Procardia, Procardia XL), hypertension (Adalat CC, Procardia XL), vasospastic angina (Nifedipine, Adalat, Procardia, Procardia XL)

Dosage

Adults *Short acting (Nifedipine, Adalat, Procardia):* As an antianginal, initiate nifedipine in the capsule form at 10 mg tid; dosage may be increased gradually over 7–14 d as needed. For hospitalized patients under close supervision, dosage may be increased by 10-mg increments over 4–6 h until symptoms are controlled. For elderly patients and patients with hepatic impairment, initiate treatment at 10 mg bid and monitor carefully. *Note:* Current labeling states that the short-acting product should not be used for hypertension, hypertensive crisis, acute MI, and some forms of unstable angina and chronic stable angina.
ER (Adalat CC): Initiate with 30 mg once daily and titrate over 7–14 d according to response. Usual maintenance dose is 30–60 mg once daily. Titration to doses >90 mg/d is not recommended.
ER (Procardia XL): Initiate with 30 or 60 mg once daily and titrate over 7–14 d according to response. Titration to doses >120 mg/d is not recommended. Titration may proceed more rapidly if the patient is frequently assessed. Titration to doses >120 mg/d is not

(continued)

667

APPENDIX 2 *(continued)* Therapeutic Use of Available Cardiovascular Drugs

recommended. Angina patients maintained on the short-acting formulation (nifedipine capsule) may be switched to the ER tablet at the nearest equivalent total daily dose. Experience with doses >90 mg daily in patients with angina is limited.

Elderly
: Initiate at lowest dose and titrate to response

Children
: Safety and effectiveness have not been established

Preparations
: Nifedipine (generic); Adalat (Bayer); Procardia (Pfizer): 10-, 20-mg liquid-filled capsules
Adalat CC (Bayer): 30-, 60-, 90-mg SR tablets
Procardia XL (Pfizer): 30-, 60-, 90-mg SR tablets
Generic SR tablets: 30, 60, 90 mg

Nimodipine (Nimotop)

Indication
: Subarachnoid hemorrhage

Dosage

Adults
: Usual dose is 60 mg q4h beginning within 96 h of subarachnoid hemorrhage and continuing for 21 d. Dosage should be reduced to 30 mg q4h with close monitoring of blood pressure and heart rate in patients with hepatic cirrhosis.
Note: This medication is given preferably not less than 1 h before or 2 h after meals. If the capsule cannot be swallowed (e.g., time of surgery, unconscious patient), make a hole in both ends of the capsule with an 18-gauge needle and extract the contents into a syringe. Empty the contents into the patient's in situ nasogastric tube and wash down the tube with 30 mL of normal saline.

Elderly
: Use usual dose with caution

Children
: Safety and effectiveness have not been established

Preparation
: Nimotop (Bayer): 30-mg liquid-filled capsules

Nisoldipine (Sular)

Indication
: Hypertension

Dosage

Adults
: Initiate at 20 mg PO once daily; dosage may be increased by 10 mg/wk (or at longer intervals) to attain adequate response. Usual maintenance dose is 20-40 mg once daily. Doses >60 mg/d are not recommended. For elderly patients and patients with hepatic function impairment, initiate with a dose not exceeding 10 mg/d. Monitor blood pressure closely during any dosage adjustment.

Note: Nisoldipine has been used safely with diuretics, ACE inhibitors, and beta blockers. Administration of this medication with a high-fat meal can lead to excessive peak drug concentration and should be avoided. In addition, grapefruit products should be avoided before and after dosing.

Elderly
Initiate at lower dose and titrate to response

Children
Safety and effectiveness have not been established

Preparations
Sular (First Horizon): 10-, 20-, 30-, 40-mg ER tablets

Verapamil (verapamil, verapamil SR, Calan, Calan SR, Isoptin, Isoptin SR, Verelan, Verelan PM, Covera-HS, verapamil IV, Isoptin IV)

Indications
Angina (all PO immediate-release formulations and Covera-HS), arrhythmias (all PO immediate-release formulations), hypertension (all PO formulations), supraventricular tachyarrhythmias (IV formulations)

Dosage

Adults
Immediate-release tablets (verapamil, Calan, Isoptin): As an antianginal, antiarrhythmic, and antihypertensive, initiate at 80–120 mg tid. Dosage may be increased at daily or weekly intervals as needed and tolerated. Limit to 480 mg/d in divided doses.

SR capsules (Verelan): As an antihypertensive, initiate at 120–240 mg once daily. Dosage may be adjusted in increments of 60–120 mg/d at daily or weekly intervals as needed and tolerated. Usual daily dose range is 240–480 mg.

SR tablets (verapamil SR, Calan SR, Isoptin SR): As an antihypertensive, initiate at 120–240 mg once daily with food. Dosage may be adjusted in increments of 60–120 mg/d at daily or weekly intervals as needed and as tolerated. Usual total daily dose range is 240–480 mg.

ER tablets, controlled onset (Covera-HS): Initiate with 180 mg at bedtime for hypertension and angina. If response is inadequate, the dose may be titrated upward to 540 mg/d given at bedtime.

ER capsules, controlled onset (Verelan PM): Initiate with a 200-mg dose at bedtime for hypertension; if response is inadequate, the dose may be titrated upward to 300 or 400 mg/d given at bedtime.

Injection (verapamil IV, Isoptin IV): Initiate at 5–10 mg (or 0.075–0.15 mg/kg) slowly over at least 2 min with continuous electrocardiographic and blood pressure monitoring. If response is inadequate, 10 mg (or 0.15 mg/kg) may be administered 30 min after completion of the initial dose.

Note: Fewer than 1% of patients may have life-threatening adverse responses (rapid ventricular rate in atrial flutter/fibrillation, marked hypotension, or extreme bradycardia/asystole) to verapamil injections. Monitor the initial use of IV verapamil and have resuscitation facilities available. An IV infusion (5 mg/h) has been used; precede the infusion with an IV loading dose.

(continued)

APPENDIX 2 *(continued)* Therapeutic Use of Available Cardiovascular Drugs

Elderly
Initiate the PO formulation of verapamil at lower dose and titrate to response. IV injections should be given slowly over a longer period (≥3 min) to minimize undesired effects.

Children
Safety and effectiveness have not been established, but there has been experience with the use of verapamil in the pediatric population.

Preparations
Verapamil (generic); Calan (Searle): 40-, 80-, 120-mg immediate release tablets
Verapamil (generic); Calan (Searle): 120-, 180-, 240-mg ER tablets and capsules
Calan SR (Searle); Isoptin SR (Abbott): 120-, 180-, 240-mg SR tablets
Verelan (Schwarz Pharma): 120-, 180-, 240-, 360-mg SR capsules
Covera-HS (Searle): 180-, 240-mg ER and controlled-onset tablets
Verelan PM (Schwarz Pharma): 100-, 200-, 300-mg ER and controlled-onset capsules
Verapamil HCl injection (generic): 2.5 mg/mL

Fixed-dose combination
for the treatment of hypertension
Tarka (Abbott); trandolapril/verapamil hydrochloride ER combination tablets: 2 mg/180 mg, 1 mg/240 mg, 2 mg/240 mg, 4 mg/240 mg

Diuretics
Loop diuretics
Bumetanide (bumetanide, Bumex)

Indications
Edema associated with CHF; hepatic cirrhosis or renal disease, including the nephrotic syndrome

Dosage
Adults
PO formulation: Usual dose range is 0.5–2 mg/d as a single dose. Higher dosage (>1–2 mg/d) may be required to achieve the desired therapeutic response in patients with renal insufficiency. If the initial diuresis is inadequate, repeated doses may be administered q4–6h until the desired diuretic response is achieved or until a maximum daily dosage of 10 mg is administered. An intermittent dose schedule, given on alternate days or daily for 3–4 d with rest periods of 1–2 d in between, may be used for the continued control of edema. Dosage should be kept to a minimum, with careful adjustments in dosage for patients with hepatic impairment.
IV/IM formulations: Parenteral administration of bumetanide should be reserved for patients in whom GI absorption may be impaired or in whom PO administration is not feasible. Initiate at 0.5–1 mg IV or IM. IV injection should be given over 1–2 min. If the initial diuresis is inadequate, repeated doses may be

administered q2–3h until the desired diuretic response is achieved or until a maximum daily dosage of 10 mg is administered.

Elderly   Initiate at lowest dose and titrate to response

Children   Safety and effectiveness have not been established

Preparations   Bumetanide (generic); Bumex (Roche): 0.5-, 1-, 2-mg tablets
               Bumetanide injection (generic); Bumex injection (Roche): 0.25 mg/mL

Ethacrynic acid (Edecrin, Edecrin Sodium Intravenous)

Indications   Ascites associated with malignancy, idiopathic edema, and lymphedema; edema associated with CHF, hepatic cirrhosis, or renal disease, including the nephrotic syndrome; hospitalized pediatric patients with congenital heart disease or the nephrotic syndrome (not indicated for infants)

Dosage

Adults   *PO formulation:* Initiate at 25–50 mg (lower doses should be used in patients concurrently receiving other diuretics) once daily after a meal. Dosage may be adjusted at 25- to 50-mg increments daily until the desired response is achieved or until a maximum dose of 100 mg bid is given. A dose of 200 mg bid may be required to maintain adequate diuresis in patients with severe, refractory edema. An intermittent dose schedule, given on alternate days or daily for 3–4 d with rest periods of 1–2 d in between, may be used for the continued control of edema after an effective diuresis is obtained.
               IV formulations: IV administration of ethacrynate sodium should be reserved for patients in whom a rapid onset of diuresis is desired, as in acute pulmonary edema, or when PO administration is not feasible. Usual adult IV dose is 0.5–1 mg/kg (up to 100 mg in a single IV dose) or 50 mg for an adult of average size. After reconstitution, ethacrynate sodium solution may be infused slowly (over 20–30 min) through the tubing of a running IV infusion or by direct IV injection over several minutes. If the desired diuresis is not achieved with the first dose of ethacrynate sodium, a second dose may be given after 2–3 h at a new injection site.

Elderly   Initiate at lowest dose and titrate to response

Children   Safety and effectiveness have not been established in children for IV administration and in infants for PO and IV administrations.

Preparations   Edecrin (Merck): 25-, 50-mg tablets
               Edecrin Sodium (Merck): 50 mg/vial, powder for injection

Furosemide (furosemide, Lasix)

Indications   Edema associated with CHF, hepatic cirrhosis or renal disease, including the nephrotic syndrome; hypertension (PO formulation)

(continued)

APPENDIX 2 (continued) Therapeutic Use of Available Cardiovascular Drugs

Dosage

Adults

Edema (PO formulation): Usual oral dose is 20–80 mg given as a single dose. The same dose may be repeated, or adjusted in increments of 20–40 mg q6–8h until the desired diuresis is achieved. The effective dose may then be given once or twice daily to maintain adequate fluid balance. For chronic maintenance therapy, furosemide given on alternate days or intermittently on 2–4 consecutive days each week is preferred. A maximum oral dose of 600 mg/d has been used in patients with severe fluid overload.

Edema (IV formulation): Usual dose is 20–40 mg given as a single injection. The IV route is preferred when rapid diuresis is indicated. The same dose may be repeated or adjusted in 20- to 40-mg increments q1–2h until the desired response is achieved. Each IV dose should be administered over a few minutes. Furosemide also has been administered as a continuous IV infusion in some patients to maintain adequate urine flow. A bolus of 20–40 mg should be given first, followed by an infusion with an initial rate of 0.25–0.5 mg/min. Infusion rate may be titrated up to a maximum of 4 mg/min according to clinical response.

Hypertension: Usual initial dose is 40 mg PO bid; dosage then should be adjusted according to clinical response. The maximum dose is 240 mg/d in 2–3 divided doses. Higher doses may be required for the management of edema or hypertension in patients with renal insufficiency or CHF. These patients should be monitored closely to ensure efficacy and avoid undesired toxicity.

Elderly

Initiate at lowest dose and titrate to response

Children

Safety and effectiveness have been established in children for the management of edema, but not for hypertension.

Preparations

Furosemide (generic); Lasix (Aventis): 20-, 40-, 80-mg tablets
Furosemide (generic); Lasix (Aventis): 10 mg/mL, 40 mg/5 mL PO solution
Furosemide (generic); Lasix (Aventis): 10 mg/mL injection in 2-, 4-, 10-mL single-dose vials

Torsemide (Demadex)

Indications

Edema associated with CHF, hepatic cirrhosis or renal disease, including the nephrotic syndrome; hypertension (PO formulation)

Dosage

Adults

CHF/chronic renal failure: Usual initial dose is 10–20 mg once daily via PO or IV administration. If the diuretic response is inadequate, the dose may be doubled until the desired response is achieved or until a maximum single dose of 200 mg is given.

Hepatic cirrhosis: Usual initial dose is 5–10 mg once daily administered PO or IV with an aldosterone antagonist or a potassium-sparing diuretic. If the diuretic response is inadequate, the dose may be doubled until the desired response is achieved or until a maximum single dose of 40 mg is given.

Note: Because of high bioavailability, PO and IV doses are therapeutically equivalent. Therefore, patients may be switched to and from the IV form with no change in dose. The IV injection should be administered slowly over 2 min.

Hypertension: Usual initial dose is 5 mg/d PO. If adequate reduction in blood pressure is not achieved in 4–6 wk, the dose may be increased up to 10 mg once daily. If the blood pressure response is still inadequate, an additional antihypertensive agent should be added.

Elderly	Initiate at lowest dose and titrate to response
Children	Safety and effectiveness have not been established
Preparations	Demadex (Roche): 5-, 10-, 20-, 100-mg tablets Demadex injection (Roche): 10 mg/mL

Thiazide diuretics
Bendroflumethiazide (bendroflumethiazide, Naturetin)
Indications   Edema, hypertension

Dosage

Adults   *Edema:* Initiate at 5–20 mg/d given once daily in the morning or in 2 divided doses. Usual maintenance dose is 2.5–5 mg once daily in the morning. Electrolyte imbalance may occur less frequently by administering bendroflumethiazide every other day or on a 3–5 d/wk schedule during maintenance therapy.

Hypertension: Initiate at 5–20 mg/d once daily in the morning or in 2 divided doses. Usual maintenance dose is 2.5–15 mg once daily given in the morning.

Elderly	Initiate at lowest dose and titrate to response
Children	Safety and effectiveness have not been established
Preparations	Naturetin (Apothecon): 2.5-, 5-, 10-mg tablets Bendroflumethiazide 4 mg/*Rauwolfia serpentina* 50 mg
Fixed-dose combinations for the treatment of hypertension	Corzide 80/5: Bendroflumethiazide 5 mg/Nadolol 80 mg Corzide 40/5: Bendroflumethiazide 5 mg/Nadolol 40 mg

Benzthiazide (Exna)
Indications   Edema, hypertension

(continued)

APPENDIX 2 (continued) Therapeutic Use of Available Cardiovascular Drugs

Dosage	
Adults	*Edema:* Initiate at 50–200 mg/d given in 1–2 doses for a few days until the desired diuresis is achieved (dosages >100 mg/d should be divided and administered in 2 daily doses). Usual maintenance dose is 50–150 mg/d. Electrolyte imbalance may occur less frequently by administering benzthiazide every other day or on a 3–5 d/wk schedule during maintenance therapy.
	Hypertension: Initiate at 25–50 mg bid after breakfast and lunch; dosage may be titrated up to a maximum of 100 mg bid if necessary.
Elderly	Initiate at lowest dose and titrate to response
Children	Safety and effectiveness have not been established
Preparation	Exna (Robins): 50-mg tablets
Chlorothiazide (chlorothiazide, Diuril, Sodium Diuril)	
Indications	Edema, hypertension (PO formulation)
Dosage	
Adults	*Edema:* Administer 500–1000 mg once daily in the morning or twice daily PO or IV (the IV route should be reserved for patients who are unable to take PO medication or for emergency situations). Electrolyte imbalance may occur less frequently by administering chlorothiazide every other day or on a 3- to 5-d/wk schedule during maintenance therapy.
	Hypertension: Initiate at 250–500 mg once daily in the morning or twice daily; dosage may be titrated up to a maximum of 2000 mg (2 g)/d given in divided doses.
Elderly	Initiate at lowest dose and titrate to response
Children	Safety and effectiveness have been established for the PO formulation, but not for the IV formulation
Preparations	Chlorothiazide (generic); Diuril (Merck): 250-, 500-mg tablets
	Diuril (Merck): 250 mg/5 mL PO suspension
	Sodium Diuril (Merck): 500 mg, powder for injection
Fixed-dose combinations for the treatment of hypertension	Diupres 500: chlorothiazide 500 mg/reserpine 0.125 mg
	Diupres 250: chlorothiazide 250 mg/reserpine 0.125 mg
	Aldoclor 250: chlorothiazide 250 mg/methyldopa 250 mg
	Aldoclor 150: chlorothiazide 150 mg/methyldopa 250 mg

Chlorthalidone (chlorthalidone, Hygroton, Thalitone)

Indications
Edema, hypertension

Dosage

Adults
Edema: Administer 50–100 mg (Thalitone, 30–60 mg) daily or 100 mg (Thalitone, 60 mg) on alternate days. Some patients may require doses up to 200 mg (Thalitone, 120 mg) daily.

Hypertension: Initiate at 25 mg (Thalitone, 15 mg) once daily. Dosage may be increased gradually to a maximum of 100 mg once daily (Thalitone, 50 mg) if needed.

Note: Dosages >25 mg/d (Thalitone, 15 mg/d) are likely to potentiate potassium waste, but provide no further benefit in sodium excretion or blood pressure reduction.

Initiate at lowest dose and titrate to response

Elderly
Children
Safety and effectiveness have not been established

Preparations
Chlorthalidone (generic): 25-, 50-, 100-mg tablets
Thalitone (Monarch): 15-, 25-mg tablets
Hygroton (RPR): 50-, 100-mg tablets

Fixed-dose combinations for the treatment of hypertension
Clorpres: chlorthalidone/clonidine combination tablets, 15 mg/0.1 mg, 15 mg/0.2 mg, 15 mg/0.3 mg
Combipres 0.1: chlorthalidone 15 mg/clonidine 0.1 mg combination tablets
Combipres 0.2: chlorthalidone 15 mg/clonidine 0.2 mg combination tablets
Combipres 0.3: chlorthalidone 15 mg/clonidine 0.3 mg combination tablets
Tenoretic 50: chlorthalidone 25 mg/atenolol 50 mg combination tablets
Tenoretic 100: chlorthalidone 25 mg/atenolol 100 mg combination tablets

Hydrochlorothiazide (hydrochlorothiazide, HydroDIURIL, Microzide)

Indications
Edema, hypertension

Dosage

Adults
Edema: Administer 25–200 mg/d in 1–3 divided doses for a few days until the desired diuresis is achieved. Usual maintenance dose is 25–100 mg/d. Electrolyte imbalance may occur less frequently by administering hydrochlorothiazide every other day or on a 3- to 5-d/wk schedule during maintenance therapy.

Hypertension: Initiate at 12.5–25 mg once daily in the morning. Dosage may be titrated up to 50 mg once daily according to response. Doses >50 mg often are associated with significant reductions in serum potassium.

Elderly
Initiate at lowest dose and titrate to response

(continued)

APPENDIX 2 *(continued)* Therapeutic Use of Available Cardiovascular Drugs

Children	Hydrochlorothiazide should be dosed based on body weight and clinical response
Preparations	Hydrochlorothiazide (generic); HydroDIURIL (Merck): 25-, 50-mg tablets
	Microzide (Watson): 12.5-mg capsules
	Hydrochlorothiazide (generic): 50 mg/5 mL PO solution
	Various sources
Fixed-dose combinations for the treatment of hypertension	Hydrochlorothiazide 50 mg/reserpine 0.125 mg combination tablets
	Hydrochlorothiazide 25 mg/reserpine 0.125 mg combination tablets
	Hydrap-ES; Marpres; Ser-Ap-Es tablets: hydrochlorothiazide 15 mg/reserpine 0.1 mg/hydralazine 25 mg
	Hydrazide capsules
	Hydrochlorothiazide 50 mg/hydralazine 100 mg
	Hydrochlorothiazide 50 mg/hydralazine 50 mg
	Hydrochlorothiazide 25 mg/hydralazine 25 mg
	Ziac tablets
	Hydrochlorothiazide 6.25 mg/bisoprolol 2.5 mg
	Hydrochlorothiazide 6.25 mg/bisoprolol 5 mg
	Hydrochlorothiazide 6.25 mg/bisoprolol 10 mg
	Timolide 10-25 tablets: hydrochlorothiazide 25 mg/timolol 10 mg
	Inderide LA capsules
	Hydrochlorothiazide 50 mg/propranolol 160 mg
	Hydrochlorothiazide 50 mg/propranolol 120 mg
	Hydrochlorothiazide 50 mg/propranolol 80 mg
	Inderide tablets and various sources
	Hydrochlorothiazide 25 mg/propranolol 80 mg
	Hydrochlorothiazide 25 mg/propranolol 40 mg
	Aldoril tablets and various sources
	Hydrochlorothiazide 50 mg/methyldopa 500 mg
	Hydrochlorothiazide 30 mg/methyldopa 500 mg
	Hydrochlorothiazide 25 mg/methyldopa 250 mg
	Hydrochlorothiazide 15 mg/methyldopa 250 mg

Lopressor HCT tablets
Hydrochlorothiazide 50 mg/metoprolol 100 mg
Hydrochlorothiazide 25 mg/metoprolol 100 mg
Hydrochlorothiazide 25 mg/metoprolol 50 mg
Capozide tablets
Hydrochlorothiazide 25 mg/captopril 50 mg
Hydrochlorothiazide 25 mg/captopril 25 mg
Hydrochlorothiazide 15 mg/captopril 50 mg
Hydrochlorothiazide 15 mg/captopril 25 mg
Lotensin HCT tablets
Hydrochlorothiazide 25 mg/benazepril 20 mg
Hydrochlorothiazide 12.5 mg/benazepril 20 mg
Hydrochlorothiazide 12.5 mg/benazepril 10 mg
Hydrochlorothiazide 6.25 mg/benazepril 5 mg
Monopril HCT tablets
Hydrochlorothiazide 12.5 mg/fosinopril 10 mg
Hydrochlorothiazide 12.5 mg/fosinopril 20 mg
Uniretic tablets
Hydrochlorothiazide 12.5 mg/moexipril 7.5 mg
Hydrochlorothiazide 12.5 mg/moexipril 15 mg
Hydrochlorothiazide 25 mg/moexipril 15 mg
Vaseretic 10-25 tablets: hydrochlorothiazide 25 mg/enalapril 10 mg
Prinzide and Zestoretic tablets
Hydrochlorothiazide 25 mg/lisinopril 20 mg
Hydrochlorothiazide 12.5 mg/lisinopril 20 mg
Atacand HCT tablets
Hydrochlorothiazide 12.5 mg/candesartan 16 mg
Hydrochlorothiazide 12.5 mg/candesartan 32 mg
Avalide tablets
Hydrochlorothiazide 12.5 mg/irbesartan 150 mg

(continued)

APPENDIX 2 (continued) Therapeutic Use of Available Cardiovascular Drugs

Hydrochlorothiazide 12.5 mg/irbesartan 300 mg
Diovan HCT tablets
    Hydrochlorothiazide 12.5 mg/valsartan 80 mg
    Hydrochlorothiazide 25 mg/valsartan 160 mg
Hyzaar tablets
    Hydrochlorothiazide 12.5 mg/losartan 50 mg
    Hydrochlorothiazide 25 mg/losartan 100 mg
Micardis HCT tablets
    Hydrochlorothiazide 12.5 mg/telmisartan 40 mg
    Hydrochlorothiazide 12.5 mg/telmisartan 80 mg
Esimil tablets: hydrochlorothiazide 25 mg/guanethidine 10 mg

Hydroflumethiazide (hydroflumethiazide, Diucardin, Saluron)

Indications
    Edema, hypertension

Dosage

Adults
    Edema: Initiate at 50 mg once or twice a day. Usual maintenance dose ranges from 25 to 200 mg/d (administer in 2 divided doses when dosage exceeds 100 mg/d). Electrolyte imbalance may occur less frequently by administering hydroflumethiazide every other day or on a 3- to 5-d/wk schedule during maintenance therapy.
    Hypertension: Usual maintenance dose is 50–100 mg/d. Do not exceed 200 mg/d

Elderly
    Initiate at lowest dose and titrate to response

Children
    Safety and effectiveness have not been established

Preparations
    Hydroflumethiazide (generic); Diucardin (Wyeth-Ayerst); Saluron (Apothecon): 50-mg tablets

Fixed-dose combinations for the treatment of hypertension
    Salutensin tablets: hydroflumethiazide 50 mg/reserpine 0.125 mg

Indapamide (indapamide, Lozol)

Indications
    Edema, hypertension

Dosage

Adults
    Edema: Initiate at 2.5 mg once daily in the morning. Dosage may be increased to 5 mg once daily according to response. Electrolyte imbalance may occur less frequently by administering indapamide every other day or on a 3–5 d/wk schedule during maintenance therapy.

	Hypertension: Initiate at 1.25 mg once daily in the morning. Dosage may be increased gradually to 5 mg once daily according to response.
Elderly	Initiate at lowest dose and titrate to response
Children	Safety and effectiveness have not been established
Preparations	Indapamide (generic): 2.5-mg tablets Lozol (Aventis): 1.25-, 2.5-mg tablets

Methyclothiazide (methyclothiazide, Enduron)

Indications	Edema, hypertension
Dosage	
Adults	*Edema*: Initiate at 2.5–10 mg once daily in the morning. Usual maintenance dose is 2.5–5 mg once daily. Electrolyte imbalance may occur less frequently by administering methyclothiazide every other day or on a 3–5 d/wk schedule during maintenance therapy. *Hypertension*: Administer 2.5–5 mg once daily in the morning
Elderly	Initiate at lowest dose and titrate to response
Children	Safety and effectiveness have not been established
Preparations	Methyclothiazide (generic): 2.5-, 5-mg tablets Aquatensen (Wallace); Enduron (Abbott): 5-mg tablets
Fixed-dose combinations for the treatment of hypertension	Diutensen-R Tablets (Wallace): methyclothiazide 2.5 mg/reserpine 0.1 mg

Metolazone (Mykrox, Zaroxolyn)

Indications	Edema (Zaroxolyn only), hypertension (Mykrox and Zaroxolyn)
Dosage	
Adults	*Edema*: Administer Zaroxolyn at 5–10 mg/d given once daily in the morning. Dosage up to 20 mg once daily may be used in patients with renal insufficiency. Usual maintenance dose for Zaroxolyn is 2.5–10 mg given once daily in the morning. Electrolyte imbalance may occur less frequently by administering metolazone every other day or on a 3–5 d/wk schedule during maintenance therapy. *Hypertension*: Administer 2.5–5 mg of Zaroxolyn or 0.5–1 mg of Mykrox once daily in the morning. *Note*: The metolazone formulations are not bioequivalent or therapeutically equivalent at the same doses. When switching from Zaroxolyn to Mykrox, determine the dose by titration starting at 0.5 mg once daily and increasing to 1 mg once daily according to response.

(continued)

679

APPENDIX 2 *(continued)* Therapeutic Use of Available Cardiovascular Drugs

Elderly — Initiate at lowest dose and titrate to response
Children — Safety and effectiveness have not been established
Preparations — Mykrox (Celltech): 0.5-mg tablets
Zaroxolyn (Celltech): 2.5, 5, 10 mg

Polythiazide (Renese)
Indications — Edema, hypertension
Dosage
Adults — *Edema:* Administer 1–4 mg once daily in the morning. Electrolyte imbalance may occur less frequently by administering polythiazide every other day or on a 3–5 d/wk schedule during maintenance therapy.
Hypertension: Administer 2–4 mg once daily in the morning.
Elderly — Initiate at lowest dose and titrate to response
Children — Safety and effectiveness have not been established
Preparations — Renese (Pfizer): 1-, 2-, 4-mg tablets
Minizide capsules
Polythiazide 0.5 mg/prazosin 1 mg
Polythiazide 0.5 mg/prazosin 2 mg
Polythiazide 0.5 mg/prazosin 5 mg
Fixed-dose combinations for the treatment of hypertension — Renese-R tablets: polythiazide 2 mg/reserpine 0.25 mg

Quinethazone (Hydromox)
Indications — Edema, hypertension
Dosage
Adults — *Edema:* Administer 25–200 mg/d as a single dose in the morning or in 2 divided doses. Electrolyte imbalance may occur less frequently by administering quinethazone every other day or on a 3–5 d/wk schedule during maintenance therapy.
Hypertension: Administer 25–100 mg/d as a single dose in the morning or in 2 divided doses.
Elderly — Initiate at lowest dose and titrate to response
Children — Safety and effectiveness have not been established
Preparation — Hydromox (Lederle): 50-mg tablets

Trichlormethiazide (trichlormethiazide, Diurese, Metahydrin, Naqua)

Indications
Edema, hypertension

Dosage

Adults
Edema: Administer 2–4 mg once daily in the morning. Electrolyte imbalance may occur less frequently by administering trichlormethiazide every other day or on a 3–5 d/wk schedule during maintenance therapy.
Hypertension: Administer 2–4 mg/d as a single dose in the morning or in 2 divided doses.

Elderly
Initiate at lowest dose and titrate to response

Children
Safety and effectiveness have not been established

Preparations
Trichlormethiazide (generic); Diurese (American Urologicals): 4-mg tablets
Metahydrin (Aventis); Naqua (Schering): 2-, 4-mg tablets

Fixed-dose combinations for the treatment of hypertension
Metatensin #4 Tablets (Aventis): trichlormethiazide 4 mg/reserpine 0.1 mg
Metatensin #2 Tablets (Aventis): trichlormethiazide 2 mg/reserpine 0.1 mg

Potassium-sparing diuretics

Amiloride (amiloride, Midamor)

Indications
As adjunctive therapy with thiazide or other kaliuretic diuretics in CHF or hypertension to prevent excessive potassium loss

Dosage

Adults
Administer 5–10 mg once daily. Although dosages >10 mg/d usually are not necessary, higher doses (up to 20 mg/d) have been used occasionally in some patients with persistent hypokalemia.

Elderly
Initiate at lowest dose and titrate to response

Children
Safety and effectiveness have not been established

Preparations
Amiloride (generic); Midamor (Merck): 5-mg tablets

Fixed-dose combinations for the treatment of hypertension
Moduretic tablets and various generic products: amiloride 5 mg/hydrochlorothiazide 50 mg

Eplerenone

Indication
Hypertension

Dosage

Adults
Starting dose is 50 mg once daily; if inadequate blood pressure response, does can be increased to 50 mg twice daily.

Elderly
Initiate at lowest dose and titrate to response

(continued)

681

APPENDIX 2 *(continued)* Therapeutic Use of Available Cardiovascular Drugs

Children	Safety and effectiveness have not been established
Preparation	Inspra (Pharmacia): 25 mg tablets

Spironolactone (spironolactone, Aldactone)

Indications	Edema associated with CHF, liver cirrhosis, or nephrotic syndrome; hypokalemia; hypertension (usually used in conjunction with other agents such as a thiazide diuretic); primary hyperaldosteronism
Dosage	
Adults	*Edema:* Initiate at 100 mg/d (range, 25–200 mg/d) administered as a singe dose or in divided doses. If spironolactone is used as a sole agent, treatment should be continued for at least 5 d. Thereafter, the dose may be adjusted based on response or a more potent diuretic may be added.
	Diuretic-induced hypokalemia: Usual dose ranges from 25 to 100 mg/d.
	Hypertension: Initiate at 50–100 mg/d in single or divided doses. Usual dose ranges from 25 to 100 mg/d.
	Primary hyperaldosteronism (diagnostic test)
	Long test: Spironolactone 400 mg is administered daily for 3–4 wk. Correction of hypokalemia and hypertension provides presumptive evidence for the diagnosis.
	Short test: Spironolactone 400 mg is administered daily for 4 d. If serum potassium level increases during the therapy but declines after discontinuation of the drug, a presumptive diagnosis should be considered.
	Hyperaldosteronism (maintenance therapy): Administer 100–400 mg/d in preparation for surgery. For patients not suitable for surgery, long-term therapy with spironolactone may be used. Dosage should be titrated individually (maintain at the lowest possible dose).
Elderly	Initiate at lowest dose and titrate to response
Children	Safety and effectiveness have been established for the management of edema only
Preparations	Spironolactone (generic): 25-mg tablets
	Aldactone (Pharmacia & Upjohn): 25-, 50-, 100-mg tablets
Fixed-dose combinations for the treatment of hypertension	Aldactazide tablets and various generic products
	Spironolactone 25 mg/hydrochlorothiazide 25 mg
	Spironolactone 50 mg/hydrochlorothiazide 50 mg

Triamterene (Dyrenium)

Indications	Edema associated with CHF, hepatic cirrhosis, nephrotic syndrome, steroid use, or secondary hyperaldosteronism

Dosage	
Adults	When used as a single agent, the usual initial dose is 100 mg bid after meals. Dosage should not exceed 300 mg/d. Once edema is controlled, most patients can be maintained on 100 mg/d or every other day. When used in combination with a kaliuretic diuretic, the initial dose is 50 mg once daily. The dose should be titrated based on response to a maximum of 100 mg/d.
Elderly	Initiate at lowest dose and titrate to response
Children	Safety and effectiveness have not been established
Preparations	Dyrenium (Wellspring): 50-, 100-mg capsules
Fixed-dose combinations for the treatment of hypertension	Dyazide capsules: triamterene 37.5 mg/hydrochlorothiazide 25 mg
	Maxzide capsules: triamterene 37.5 mg/hydrochlorothiazide 25 mg
	Maxzide capsules: triamterene 75 mg/hydrochlorothiazide 50 mg
	Various generic triamterene/hydrochlorothiazide tablets and capsules

Endothelin receptor antagonist
Bosentan (Tracleer)

Indication	Treatment of pulmonary arterial hypertension in patients with World Health Organization class III or IV symptoms, to improve exercise ability and decrease the rate of clinical worsening
Dosage	
Adults	Initiate at 62.5 mg bid for 4 wk and then increase to the maintenance dose of 125 mg bid. Doses >125 mg bid did not appear to confer additional benefit sufficient to offset the increased risk of liver injury. Refer to Tracleer package insert for recommendations on dosage adjustment and monitoring in patients developing aminotransferase abnormalities during therapy.
	Note: Because of potential liver injury and in an effort to make the chance of fetal exposure to bosentan as small as possible, bosentan may be prescribed only through the TRACLEER Access Program.
Elderly	Clinical experience has not identified differences in responses between elderly and younger patients
Children	Safety and efficacy in pediatric patients have not been established. In patients weighing <40 kg but >12 y of age, the recommended initial and maintenance dose is 62.5 mg bid.
Preparations	Tracleer (Actelion): 62.5-, 125-mg tablets

(continued)

APPENDIX 2 *(continued)* Therapeutic Use of Available Cardiovascular Drugs

Inotropic and vasopressor agents

Phosphodiesterase inhibitors

Inamrinone lactate (inamrinone lactate, Inocor)

Indications — CHF, short-term management

Dosage

Adults — Initiate with an IV bolus dose of 0.75 mg/kg administered slowly over 2–3 min, followed by a continuous infusion of 5–10 µg/kg per min. A second bolus of 0.75 mg/kg may be given 30 min after the initial bolus dose. Total dose should not exceed 10 mg/kg per d. Rate of administration and duration of therapy should be determined by the responsiveness of the patient.

Elderly — Initiate at lowest dose and titrate to response

Children — Safety and effectiveness have not been established

Preparation — Inamrinone Lactate (Abbott Hospital): 5 mg/mL, 20-mL ampules
Inocor (Sanofi Winthrop): 5 mg/mL, 20-mL ampules

Milrinone lactate (milrinone lactate, Primacor)

Indications — CHF, short-term management

Dosage

Adults — Initiate with an IV loading dose of 50 µg/kg administered slowly over 10 min, followed by a continuous infusion of 0.375 µg/kg per min. Rate of administration and duration of therapy should be determined by the responsiveness of the patient. Total dose should not exceed 1.13 mg/kg/d, or 0.75 µg/kg per min. The following infusion rates are recommended for patients with renal impairment:

CrCl mL/min per 1.73 m^2	Infusion rate µg/kg per min
50	0.43
40	0.38
30	0.33
20	0.28
10	0.23
5	0.20

Elderly — Dosage should be adjusted based on renal function

Children — Safety and effectiveness have not been established

Preparations — Milrinone lactate injections (generic); Primacor Injections (Sanofi/Synthelabo): 1 mg/mL, 10-, 20-mL single-dose vials; 200 µg/mL in 100 mL of 5% dextrose injection; 200 µg/mL in 200 mL of 5% dextrose injection

Adrenergic receptor agonists
Dobutamine (dobutamine, Dobutrex)

Indication   Short-term inotropic support in patients with cardiac decompensation due to depressed contractility
Dosage
Adults   Rate of infusion required to increase cardiac output usually ranges from 2.5 to 15 µg/kg per min. Infusion rate and duration of therapy should be determined based on clinical response.
             Note: Consult manufacturer's package insert for instructions on proper dilution of dobutamine injection before infusion.
Elderly   Initiate at lowest dose and titrate to response
Children   Safety and effectiveness have not been established
Preparations Dobutamine(generic); Dobutrex (Lilly): 12.5-mg/mL injection, 20-mL vials

Dopamine (dopamine, Intropin)
Indication   Hemodynamic imbalances after adequate fluid resuscitation
Dosage
Adults   Initially give dopamine IV at an infusion rate of 1-5 µg/kg per min. Adjust by increments of 1–4 µg/kg per min at intervals of 10–30 min according to clinical response. Lower initial doses are recommended for patients with chronic heart failure (0.5–2 µg/kg per min) and for patients with occlusive vascular disease (≤1 µg/kg per min). Most patients respond to a dose <20 µg/kg per min. Severely ill patients should be given a higher initial dose of 5 µg/kg per min. Dosage may be increased gradually according to response by using 5–10 µg/kg per min increments, up to a maximum rate of 20–50 µg/kg per min.
             Note: Consult manufacturer's package insert for instructions on proper dilution of dopamine injection before infusion.
Elderly   Initiate at lowest dose and titrate to response
Children   Safety and effectiveness have not been established
Preparations Dopamine (generic); Intropin (Faulding): 40, 80, 160-mg/mL injections
             Dopamine in 5% dextrose (Abbott): 80, 160, 320 mg/100 mL

(continued)

685

APPENDIX 2 *(continued)* Therapeutic Use of Available Cardiovascular Drugs

Isoproterenol (isoproterenol, Isuprel)

Indications
Emergency treatment of cardiac arrhythmias, shock, bronchospasm

Dosage
Adults
Emergency treatment of cardiac arrhythmias: Usual initial adult IV bolus dose is 0.02–0.06 mg (1–3 mL of a 1:50,000 dilution); subsequent doses range from 0.01 to 0.2 mg (0.5–10 mL of a 1:50,000 dilution). For IV infusion, the initial rate of administration is 5 µg/min (1.25 mL of a 1:250,000 dilution/min or 2.5 mL of a 1:500,000 dilution/min); subsequent dosage is adjusted based on the patient's response and generally ranges from 2 to 20 µg/min.
Shock: As an adjunct therapy for the management of shock, isoproterenol is administered by IV infusion. IV infusion rates of 0.5–5 µg (0.25–2.5 mL of a 1:500,000 dilution) per minute have been recommended; rate of infusion should be adjusted based on the patient's response. Rates >30 µg/min have been used in advanced stages of shock. Some clinicians have recommended that isoproterenol be administered only for a short time (≤1 h) to patients with septic shock.
Bronchospasm: For the control of bronchospasm occurring during anesthesia, administer 0.01–0.02 mg (0.5–1 mL of a 1:50,000 dilution) IV isoproterenol. This dose may be repeated if necessary.

Elderly
Initiate at lowest dose and titrate to response

Children
Safety and effectiveness have not been established, but IV isoproterenol has been used in children with asthma or in postoperative cardiac patients with bradycardia.

Preparations
Isoproterenol injection (generic); Isuprel injection (Sanofi): 1:5000 solution (0.2 mg/mL)
Isuprel injection (Sanofi): 1:50,000 (0.02 mg/mL)

Epinephrine (epinephrine, Adrenalin, various sources)

Indications
Cardiac arrest; symptomatic bradycardia; anaphylaxis; severe allergic reactions

Dosage
Adults
Cardiac arrest, ventricular fibrillation and pulseless ventricular tachycardia, pulseless electrical activity, or asystole in advanced cardiac life support: Usual IV dose is 0.5–1 mg (usually as 5–10 mL of a 1:10,000 injection) repeated q3–5 min if needed. Each dose of epinephrine given by peripheral injection should be followed by a 20-mL flush of IV fluid to ensure delivery of the drug into the central compartment. The extremity where the drug is injected should be elevated for 10–20 s.
Higher doses of 3–5 mg (~0.1 mg/kg) repeated q3–5 min as necessary may be considered if the 1-mg dose has failed. Doses as high as 0.2 mg/kg have been given, but caution with potentially severe adverse effects

686

should be used when high doses are used. Alternatively, the initial IV administration may be followed by a continuous infusion, at an initial rate of 1 µg/min and titrated up to 3–4 µg/min as needed. IV infusions of epinephrine should be administered via central venous access whenever possible to reduce the risk of extravasation and to ensure good bioavailability. If intravenous access is not available, epinephrine may be administered via the endotracheal tube. A dose of 2–2.5 mg diluted in 10 mL of 0.9% sodium chloride has been recommended.

Symptomatic bradycardia: Usual initial dose is 1 µg/min [infusion solution of 2 µg/mL may be prepared by adding 1 mg (1 mL of a 1:1000 injection) of epinephrine to 500 mL of a compatible IV solution] by continuous infusion. Rate of infusion is titrated based on clinical response and usually ranges from 2 to 10 µg/min.

Elderly	Initiate at lowest dose and titrate to response
Children	Administer with caution to infants and children. Dosage should be adjusted based on weight.
Preparations	Syringes: 1 mg/mL (1:1,000) in 0.3, 1, 2 mL; 0.5 mg/mL (1:2,000) in 0.3 mL; 0.1 mg/mL (1:10,000) in 10 mL
	Ampules: 5 mg/mL (1:200) in 0.3 mL; 1 mg/mL (1:1000) in 1 mL
	Vials: 5 mg/mL (1:200) in 5 mL; 1 mg/mL (1:1000) in 30 mL

Metaraminol (Aramine)

Indications Hypotension associated with spinal anesthesia; hypotension due to hemorrhage, reactions to medications, surgical complications; shock associated with brain damage due to trauma or tumor

Dosage

Adults *Prevention of hypotension:* Usual IM dose ranges from 2 to 10 mg. The lowest effective dose for the shortest possible time should be used. At least 10 min should elapse before additional doses are administered. *Note:* SC administration of metaraminol has been used. However, this mode of administration is not recommended because of increased risk of local tissue injury. When given IV, metaraminol is given preferably in the large veins of the antecubital fossa or the thigh.

Severe hypotension or shock: Usual dose for a single direct IV injection ranges from 0.5 to 5 mg. If necessary, the direct IV injection may be followed by a continuous infusion (15–100 mg in 500 mL of compatible diluent), with the rate adjusted according to blood pressure response.

Elderly	Initiate at lowest dose and titrate to response
Children	Safety and effectiveness have not been established
Preparation	Aramine (Merck): 10 mg/mL (1% as bitartrate), 10-mL vials

(continued)

APPENDIX 2 (continued) Therapeutic Use of Available Cardiovascular Drugs

Methoxamine (Vasoxyl)

Indications
: Hypotension associated with anesthesia, paroxysmal supraventricular tachycardia associated with hypotension or shock

Dosage

Adults
: *Hypotension:* IM dose ranges from 5 to 20 mg. A dose of 5–10 mg may be adequate when only moderate hypotension is present. In an emergency, 3–5 mg of methoxamine may be administered slowly by direct IV injection. IV administration may be supplemented with an IM dose of 10–15 mg to provide more prolonged effects.
  Prevention of hypotension during anesthesia: Usual dose is 10–15 mg (up to 20 mg may be required at high levels of anesthesia) given IM shortly before or at the time of administration of the spinal anesthetic. This dose may be repeated at intervals of at least 15 min if needed.
  Paroxysmal supraventricular tachycardia: Administer 10 mg (range, 5–15 mg) IV over 3–5 min. Alternatively, 10–20 mg IM may be injected. Systolic blood pressure should not be raised above 160 mmHg.

Elderly
: Initiate at lowest dose and titrate to response

Children
: Safety and effectiveness have not been established

Preparation
: Vasoxyl (Glaxo SmithKline): 20-mg/mL injection

Midodrine (ProAmatine)

Indication
: Orthostatic hypotension

Dosage

Adults
: Recommended dose is 10 mg tid (doses may be given at 3- to 4-h intervals). Dosing should take place during the daytime hours, when the patient is upright and pursuing daily activities. Do not give midodrine after the evening meal or <4 h before bedtime due to the risk of supine hypertension.

Elderly
: Dosage adjustment based on age is not necessary. However, lower initial doses of 2.5 mg should be administered to patients with renal impairment.

Children
: Safety and effectiveness have not been established

Preparations
: ProAmatine (Shire): 2.5-, 5-mg tablets

Norepinephrine (norepinephrine, Levophed)

Indications
: Hypotensive state, cardiac arrest (as an adjunct for severe hypotension)

Dosage	
Adults	Norepinephrine is administered by continuous IV infusion. The infusion solution is usually prepared by adding 4 mg norepinephrine bitartrate (4 mL of the commercially available injection) to 1 L of 5% dextrose injection to yield a solution that contains 4 μg of base/mL. Usual initial dosage of norepinephrine is 8–12 μg of base/min and the usual maintenance dosage is 2–4 μg of base/min. Dosage should be titrated according to the patient's response. Alternatively, norepinephrine may be initiated at a rate of 0.5–1 μg of base/min and titrated to maintain a desired blood pressure response. A few hypotensive patients have required as much as 68 mg/d of norepinephrine bitartrate. In patients requiring very large dosages of norepinephrine, occult blood volume depletion should be suspected and corrected if present; central venous pressure monitoring may be helpful in detecting and managing this situation.
Elderly	Dosage should be adjusted based on clinical response
Children	Safety and effectiveness have not been established, although there has been experience with the use of norepinephrine in the pediatric population.
Preparation	Norepinephrine injection (generic); Levophed (Sanofi): 1 mg (as bitartrate)/mL, 4-mL ampules

Phenylephrine (phenylephrine, Neo-Synephrine)

Indications	Management of vascular failure in shock, shock-like states, drug-induced hypotension, or hypersensitivity; termination of paroxysmal supraventricular tachycardia attacks; maintenance of adequate blood pressure during spinal and inhalation anesthesia

Dosage	
Adults	*Mild or moderate hypotension:* Usual dose is 2–5 mg (range, 1–10 mg) administered SC or IM. Initial dose should not exceed 5 mg. Additional IM or SC doses may be given in 1–2 h if needed. Alternatively, phenylephrine may be administered by slow IV injection in a dose ranging from 0.1 to 0.5 mg (0.2 mg is the usual dose). The IV dose may be repeated after 10–15 min if necessary. For convenience in administration by IV injection, 1 mL phenylephrine injection containing 10 mg/mL may be diluted with 9 mL sterile water for injection to yield a solution containing 1 mg/mL.
	Severe hypotension: A continuous IV infusion at a rate of 100–180 μg/min should be initiated and titrated based on clinical response. Once the blood pressure is stabilized, a maintenance infusion rate of 40–60 μg/min is usually sufficient. Infusion solutions may be prepared by adding 10 mg phenylephrine to 500 mL diluent.
	Hypotension associated with spinal anesthesia: For prevention of hypotension during spinal anesthesia, a dose of 2 or 3 mg should be administered IM or SC 3–4 min before administration of the anesthetic agent.

(continued)

APPENDIX 2 (continued) Therapeutic Use of Available Cardiovascular Drugs

For management of hypotensive emergencies during spinal anesthesia, an initial dose of 0.2 mg IV may be given. Any subsequent dose should not exceed the previous dose by 0.1–0.2 mg, and a single dose should not exceed 0.5 mg.

Paroxysmal supraventricular tachycardia: Up to 0.5 mg phenylephrine may be given by rapid IV injection (over 20–30 s). Subsequent doses may be given in increments of 0.1–0.2 mg if indicated and should not exceed 1 mg in a single dose.

Elderly   Dosage should be adjusted based on clinical response
Children   Dosage should be adjusted based on weight and clinical response
Preparations   Phenylephrine HCl (generic): Neo-Synephrine (Sanofi): 1% (10 mg/mL) injection

Other inotropic agents
Digoxin (digoxin, Lanoxicaps, Lanoxin)

Indications   CHF, atrial fibrillation

Dosage   *Rapid digitalization:* A full digitalizing dosage of digoxin may be given if other cardiac glycosides have not been administered within the previous 2 wk. Total dosages for rapid digitalization are listed below. Peak body digoxin stores of 8–12 µg/kg are generally required for therapeutic effect with minimum risk of toxicity in most patients with heart failure and normal sinus rhythm. Higher body digoxin stores of 10–15 µg/kg often are required for control of ventricular rate in patients with atrial flutter/fibrillation. Lower loading doses (i.e., 6–10 µg/kg) should be considered in patients with severe renal impairment.

Usual digitalizing dosages based on lean body weight in patients with normal renal function

Age	Capsules*	Elixir†	Injection*	Tablets†
Premature neonates	—	20–30 µg/kg	15–25 µg/kg	20–30 µg/kg
Full-term neonates	—	25–35 µg/kg	20–30 µg/kg	25–35 µg/kg
1–24 mo	—	35–60 µg/kg	30–50 µg/kg	35–60 µg/kg
2–5 y	25–35 µg/kg	30–40 µg/kg	25–35 µg/kg	30–40 µg/kg
5–10 y	15–30 µg/kg	20–35 µg/kg	15–30 µg/kg	20–35 µg/kg
>10 y	8–12 µg/kg	10–15 µg/kg	8–12 µg/kg	10–15 µg/kg

*This loading dose is usually given in 3 divided doses, with 50% of the total dose given as the first dose and two additional doses (25% each) given at 4- to 8-h intervals after assessing clinical response. For IV administration, digoxin injection is given undiluted over ≥5 min or diluted with a fourfold or greater volume of sterile water for injection, 5% dextrose injection, or 0.9% sodium chloride injection and given ≥5 min.

†This loading dose is usually given in 3 divided doses, with 50% of the total dose given as the first dose and two additional doses (25% each) given at 6- to 8-h intervals after assessing clinical response.

Slow digitalization or maintenance therapy: Usual maintenance dosage in adults is 100–375 µg/d. For slow digitalization in children <10 y of age, 25–35% of the total dose of digoxin for rapid digitalization is administered daily. Slow digitalization is the preferred regimen in patients with heart failure, and the dose should be administered orally whenever possible. Dosage requirement for each individual should be adjusted based on clinical response and renal function. It may take 1–3 wk for a patient to reach steady-state serum digoxin concentrations, depending on renal function. In patients with severe renal impairment, a maintenance dose given q2–3 d may be adequate to maintain desired serum digoxin concentrations.

Elderly	Dosage should be adjusted based on renal function, clinical response, and serum concentration.
Children	Dosage should be adjusted based on age, weight, renal function, clinical response, and serum concentration.
Preparations	Digoxin (generic): 0.125-, 0.25-mg tablets
	Lanoxin (Glaxo SmithKline): 0.125-, 0.25-mg tablets
	Digitek (Bertek): 0.125-, 0.25-mg tablets
	Lanoxicaps (Glaxo SmithKline): 0.05-, 0.1-, 0.2-mg capsules
	Digoxin elixir (generic); Lanoxin (Glaxo SmithKline): 50 µg/mL
	Digoxin injection (generic): 250 µg/mL
	Lanoxin injection (Glaxo SmithKline): 100, 250 µg/mL

Lipid-lowering agents
Bile acid sequestrants
Cholestyramine (cholestyramine, Questran, Questran Light, Prevalite)

Indications	As adjunctive therapy to diet in patients with elevated LDL cholesterol (type 2 hyperlipidemia), relief of pruritus associated with partial biliary obstruction
Dosage	
Adults	Initiate at 4 g (anhydrous cholestyramine resin) 1–2 times daily at mealtime. The contents of 1 powder packet or 1 level scoop must be mixed with 60–180 mL water or noncarbonated beverage before administration. Maintenance dose is up to 4 g (anhydrous cholestyramine resin) 6 times daily at mealtime and at bedtime. Maximum recommended daily dose is 24 g (anhydrous cholestyramine resin). *Note:* Administration time for cholestyramine should be modified to avoid interference with the absorption of other medications. Because cholestyramine may worsen constipation, patients who are constipated should be

(continued)

APPENDIX 2 (continued) Therapeutic Use of Available Cardiovascular Drugs

	started on dosages of 1 packet or scoop once daily for 5–7 d that are increased by 1 dose/d every month up to a maximum of 6 doses/d.
Elderly	Dosage adjustment is not necessary
Children	Optimal dosing has not been established; long-term effects are not known in this population.
Preparations	Cholestyramine (generic); Questran (Apothecon): 4 g anhydrous cholestyramine resin/9 g powder
	Cholestyramine Light (generic): 4 g anhydrous cholestyramine resin/dose
	Questran Light (Apothecon): 4 g (as anhydrous cholestyramine resin)/5 g powder
	Prevalite (Upsher Smith): 4 g (as anhydrous cholestyramine resin)/5.5 g powder

Colestipol (Colestid)

Indication	As adjunctive therapy to diet in patients with elevated LDL cholesterol (type 2 hyperlipidemia)
Dosage	
Adults	Granules: Initiate at 5 g once or twice daily; dosage may be increased by 5 g daily at 1- to 2-mo intervals. Usual daily dose is 5–30 g given once or in divided doses. The prescribed amount of granules must be mixed with a glassful of liquid before administration; do not take dry.
	Tablets: Initiate at 2 g once or twice daily; dosage may be increased by 2 g once or twice daily at 1- to 2-mo intervals. Usual daily dose is 2–16 g given once or in divided doses. Tablets should be swallowed whole, one at a time, with plenty of water or other appropriate fluids.
	Note: Administration time for colestipol should be modified to avoid interference with the absorption of other medications. Because colestipol may worsen constipation, patients who are constipated should be started on a once-daily dose for 5–7 d that increases by 1 dose/d every month up to a maximum of 6 doses/d.
Elderly	Dosage adjustment is not necessary
Children	Safety and effectiveness have not been established
Preparations	Colestid granules (Pharmacia & Upjohn): 5 g colestipol HCl/dose, 5 g colestipol HCl/7.5 g powder
	Colestid tablets (Pharmacia & Upjohn): 1 g

Colesevelam (Welchol)

Indications	As adjunctive therapy to diet and exercise used alone or in combination with an HMG-CoA reductase inhibitor to reduce elevated LDL cholesterol in patients with primary hypercholesterolemia (type 2a hyperlipidemia)
Dosage	
Adults	*Monotherapy:* Recommended initial dose is 3 tablets taken bid with meals (and water or other appropriate fluids) or 6 tablets once daily with a meal. Dose may be increased to 7 tablets daily as needed.

692

Combination therapy: When colesevelam is administered concurrently with an HMG-CoA reductase inhibitor, the recommended dose is 3 tablets taken bid with meals (and water or other appropriate fluids) or 6 tablets taken once daily with a meal. Doses of 4–6 tablets/d are safe and effective when coadministered with an HMG-CoA reductase inhibitor or when the 2 drugs are dosed apart.

Elderly — Dosage adjustment is not necessary

Children — Safety and effectiveness have not been established

Preparation — Welchol (Sankyo Parke Davis): 625-mg tablets

Fibric acid derivatives
Clofibrate (Atromid-S)

Indications — As adjunctive therapy to diet in patients with type 3 hyperlipidemia, as adjunctive therapy to diet in patients with elevated triglyceride concentrations (type 4 and 5 hyperlipidemias) who are at risk for pancreatitis

Dosage

Adults — Usual dosage is 1 g bid. Some patients may respond to lower dosages.

Elderly — Dosage adjustment is not necessary

Children — Safety and effectiveness have not been established

Preparation — Atromid-S (Wyeth-Ayerst): 500-mg capsules

Fenofibrate (Lofibra, Tricor)

Indications — As adjunctive therapy to diet for the reduction of LDL cholesterol, total cholesterol, triglycerides, and apolipoprotein B and to increase HDL cholesterol in patients with primary hypercholesterolemia or mixed dyslipidemia (type 2a and 2b hyperlipidemias); as adjunctive therapy to diet for the reduction of elevated triglyceride concentrations (type 4 and 5 hyperlipidemias)

Dosage

Adults — *Primary hypercholesterolemia/mixed hyperlipidemia:* Initial dose is 160 mg/d.
Hypertriglyceridemia: Initial dose ranges from 54 to 160 mg/d. Dosage should be individualized according to patient response and adjust if necessary after repeat lipid determinations at 4- to 8-wk intervals. Maximum dose is 160 mg/d.
Note: A dose of 54 mg/d should be initiated in patients with impaired renal function.

Elderly — Initiate with a dose of 54 mg/d

Children — Safety and effectiveness have not been established

(continued)

693

APPENDIX 2 *(continued)* Therapeutic Use of Available Cardiovascular Drugs

Gemfibrozil (gemfibrozil, Lopid)

Preparations	Tricor (Abbott): 54-, 160-mg tablets; Lofibra (Gates): 67, 134, 200 mg tablets
Indications	As adjunctive therapy to diet in patients with elevated triglyceride concentrations (type 4 and 5 hyperlipidemias) who are at risk for pancreatitis, reducing the risk of developing coronary heart disease in patients with type 2b hypercholesterolemia with low HDL cholesterol and no history or symptoms of coronary heart disease after other treatments have failed
Dosage	
Adults	Usual dosage is 600 mg bid 30 min before the morning and evening meals.
	Note: Gemfibrozil may worsen renal impairment in patients with serum creatinine concentrations >2.0 mg/dL and therefore should be used cautiously in this group.
Elderly	Dosage adjustment is not required
Children	Safety and effectiveness have not been established
Preparations	Gemfibrozil (generic); Lopid (Parke-Davis): 600-mg tablets

Nicotinic acid

Nicotinic acid (Niacor, Niaspan, Slo-Niacin)

Indications	As adjunctive therapy to diet for reduction of elevated total cholesterol, LDL cholesterol, apolipoprotein B, and triglyceride concentrations and to increase HDL cholesterol in patients with primary hypercholesterolemia (heterozygous familial and nonfamilial) and mixed dyslipidemia (types 2a and 2b); as adjunctive therapy in the management of elevated triglyceride concentrations (type 4 and 5 hyperlipidemias) in patients at risk for pancreatitis; as adjunctive therapy to diet to reduce the risk of recurrent nonfatal MI in patients with a history of MI and hypercholesterolemia (ER niacin, Niaspan); as combination therapy with a bile acid sequestrant to slow the progression or promote regression of atherosclerosis in patients with clinical evidence of coronary heart disease who have elevated cholesterol concentrations (ER niacin, Niaspan)
Dosage	
Adults	*Immediate-release preparations:* Usual dose of immediate-release niacin (Niacor) is 1–2 g bid or tid with meals. Initiate with 250 mg/d as a single dose after the evening meal and increase the frequency of dosing and total daily dose at 4- to 7-d intervals until the desired LDL or triglyceride level is reached or the first-level therapeutic dose of 1.5–2 g/d is reached. If hyperlipidemia is not adequately controlled after 2 mo at this level, dosage may be further increased at 2- to 4-wk intervals to 3 g/d (1 g tid). Maximum dose is 6 g/d.

ER preparations: Usual initial dosage of ER niacin preparation (Niaspan) is 500 mg/d at bedtime. Dosage may be increased by no more than 500 mg daily at 4-wk intervals as needed until the desired response is achieved. Maximum daily dose is 2 g.

Note: Immediate-release and ER preparations are not interchangeable. For patients switching from an immediate-release to an ER preparation, therapy should be instituted with the recommended initial dose and gradually titrated upward.

Elderly   Dosage adjustment is not necessary

Children   Safety and effectiveness have not been established

Preparations   Niacor (Upsher-Smith): 500-mg tablets (scored)

Niaspan (Kos Pharmaceuticals): 500-, 750-, 1000-mg ER tablets

Niacin SR (generic): 125-, 250-mg ER tablets

Slo-Niacin (Upsher-Smith): 250-, 500-, 750-mg ER tablets

Fixed-dose combinations for   Advicor (Kos Pharmaceuticals): niacin ER/lovastatin combination tablets: 500 mg/20 mg, 750 mg/20 mg,
treatment of primary hypercholes-   1000 mg/20 mg
terolemia and mixed dyslipidemia

HMG-CoA reductase inhibitors

Atorvastatin (Lipitor)

Indications   As adjunctive therapy to diet for reduction of elevated total cholesterol, LDL cholesterol, apolipoprotein B, and triglyceride concentrations and to increase HDL cholesterol in patients with primary hypercholesterolemia (heterozygous familial and nonfamilial) and mixed dyslipidemia (types 2a and 2b); as adjunctive therapy to diet for the management of elevated triglyceride concentrations (type 4 hyperlipidemia); for treatment of patients with primary dysbetalipoproteinemia (type 3 hyperlipidemia) who do not respond adequately to diet; to reduce total and LDL cholesterol levels in patients with homozygous familial hypercholesterolemia as an adjunct to other lipid-lowering treatments (e.g., LDL apheresis) or if such treatments are unavailable; as adjunctive therapy to diet for reduction of elevated total cholesterol, LDL cholesterol, and apolipoprotein B levels in boys and post-menarchal girls 10–17 y of age with heterozygous familial hypercholesterolemia if, after an adequate trial of diet therapy, the following findings are present: LDL cholesterol remains ≥190 mg/dL or LDL remains ≥160 mg/dL and there is a positive family history of premature CVD or ≥2 other CVD risk factors are present in the pediatric patient

(continued)

APPENDIX 2 *(continued)* Therapeutic Use of Available Cardiovascular Drugs

Dosage

Adults Usual initial dosage is 10–20 mg once daily. Dosage may be titrated q2–4 wk up to 80 mg once daily.

Elderly Dosage adjustment is not necessary

Children *Heterozygous familial hypercholesterolemia in pediatric patients 10–17 y of age:* Usual initial dosage is 10 mg once daily; dosage may be increased to 20 mg once daily if response is inadequate after 4 wk of treatment at the lower dose

Preparations Lipitor (Pfizer): 10-, 20-, 40-, 80-mg tablets

Fluvastatin (Lescol, Lescol XL)

Indications As adjunctive therapy to diet for reduction of elevated total cholesterol, LDL cholesterol, apolipoprotein B, and triglyceride concentrations and to increase HDL cholesterol levels in patients with primary hypercholesterolemia and mixed dyslipidemia (types 2a and 2b) whose response to dietary restriction of saturated fat and cholesterol and other nonpharmacologic measures alone has not been adequate; to slow the progression of coronary atherosclerosis in patients with coronary heart disease as part of a treatment strategy to lower total and LDL cholesterol to target levels; for reducing the risk of undergoing coronary revascularization procedures in patients with coronary heart disease.

Dosage

Adults Initiate therapy at 20–40 mg once daily at bedtime. Dosage may be titrated q4 wk based on response up to a maximum dose of 80 mg/d. If 80 mg/d is required, the dose may be given as a single daily dose by using the ER preparation or in divided doses as a 40-mg capsule bid.

Elderly Dosage adjustment is not necessary

Children Safety and effectiveness have not been established

Preparations Lescol (Novartis/Reliant): 20-, 40-mg capsules
Lescol XL (Novartis/Reliant): 80-mg ER tablets

Lovastatin (lovastatin, Mevacor)

Indications As adjunctive therapy to diet for reduction of elevated total and LDL cholesterol levels in patients with primary hypercholesterolemia (types 2a and 2b) whose response to dietary restriction of saturated fat and cholesterol and to other nonpharmacologic measures alone has not been adequate (immediate release only); to slow the progression of coronary atherosclerosis in patients with coronary heart disease as part of a treatment strategy to lower total and LDL cholesterol levels to target levels; to reduce the risk of MI, unstable angina, and coronary revascularization procedures in individuals without symptomatic CVD who have average to moderately elevated total cholesterol and LDL cholesterol levels and below average HDL cholesterol concentrations; as adjunctive therapy to diet for reduction of elevated total cholesterol, LDL cholesterol, and apolipoprotein B levels in adolescent boys and girls who are at least 1 y postmenarche, 10–17 y of age, with heterozygous familial hypercholesterolemia if, after an adequate trial of diet therapy, the following findings are present: LDL cholesterol remains ≥190 mg/dL or LDL remains ≥160 mg/dL and there is a positive family history of premature CVD or ≥2 other CVD risk factors are present in the adolescent patient; as adjunctive therapy to diet for the reduction of elevated total and LDL cholesterol, apolipoprotein B, and triglyceride concentrations and to increase HDL cholesterol in patients with primary hypercholesterolemia (heterozygous familial and nonfamilial) and mixed dyslipidemia (types 2a and 2b) when the response to a diet restricted in saturated fat and cholesterol and to other nonpharmacologic measures alone has been inadequate (ER only)

Dosage	
Adults	*Immediate release:* Usual initial dosage is 20 mg once daily for patients requiring ≥20% reductions in LDL cholesterol and 10 mg once daily for patients requiring LDL reductions of <20%, administered with the evening meal. Dosage may be titrated q4 wk or more up to a maximum of 80 mg given once daily or in 2 divided doses. If used in combination with cyclosporine, therapy should begin with 10 mg lovastatin and should not exceed 20 mg/d. If used in combination with fibrates or niacin, the dose of lovastatin should not exceed 20 mg. In patients taking amiodarone or verapamil concomitantly with lovastatin, the dose should not exceed 40 mg/d. *ER:* Usual starting dose is 20, 40, or 60 mg once daily given in the evening at bedtime. Recommended dosing range is 10–60 mg/d in single doses. Individualize dose according to the recommended goal of therapy and concomitant medications.
Elderly	Dosage adjustment is not necessary
Children	Adolescents 10–17 y of age with heterozygous familial hypercholesterolemia (immediate release only): Recommended dosing range is 10–40 mg/d; the maximum recommended dose is 40 mg/d.
Preparations	Lovastatin (generic); Mevacor (Merck): 10-, 20-, 40-mg tablets Altocor (Andrx Pharmaceuticals): 10-, 20-, 40-, 60-mg ER tablets
Fixed-dose combinations for the treatment of primary hyper-cholesterolemia and mixed dyslipidemia	Advicor (Kos Pharmaceuticals): niacin ER/lovastatin combination tablets: 500 mg/20 mg, 750 mg/20 mg, 1000 mg/20 mg

(continued)

APPENDIX 2 *(continued)* Therapeutic Use of Available Cardiovascular Drugs

Pravastatin (Pravachol)

Indications

As adjunctive therapy to diet for reduction of elevated total and LDL cholesterol, apolipoprotein B, and triglyceride concentrations and to increase HDL cholesterol in patients with primary hypercholesterolemia and mixed dyslipidemia (types 2a and 2b); as adjunctive therapy to diet in the management of elevated triglyceride concentrations (type 4 hyperlipidemia); for the treatment of patients with primary dysbetalipoproteinemia (type 3 hyperlipidemia) who do not respond adequately to diet; to reduce the risks of MI, undergoing myocardial revascularization procedures, and cardiovascular mortality with no increase in death from noncardiovascular causes in hypercholesterolemic patients without clinically evident coronary heart disease (primary prevention of coronary events); to reduce the risk of total mortality by reducing coronary death, MI, undergoing myocardial revascularization procedures, stroke, and stroke/transient ischemic attack and slow the progression of coronary atherosclerosis in patients with clinically evident coronary heart disease (secondary prevention of cardiovascular events); as an adjunct to diet and lifestyle modifications for treatment of heterozygous familial hypercholesterolemia in children and adolescents ≥8 y of age if, after an adequate trial of diet, the following findings are present: LDL cholesterol remains ≥190 mg/dL or LDL cholesterol remains ≥160 mg/dL and there is a positive family history of premature CVD or ≥2 other CVD risk factors are present in the patient

Dosage

Adults

Recommended starting dose is 40 mg once daily. If a daily dose of 40 mg does not achieve desired cholesterol concentrations, 80 mg once daily may be given. Dosage should be titrated based on response at 4-wk intervals. A lower starting dose of 10 mg is recommended for patients with significant renal or hepatic impairment. If used in combination with cyclosporine, therapy should begin with 10 mg pravastatin once daily at bedtime and generally should not exceed 20 mg/d (dosage must be titrated with caution).

Elderly

Dosage adjustment is not necessary

Children 8–13 y

Recommended dose is 20 mg once daily. Doses >20 mg have not been studied.

Adolescents 14–18 y

Recommended starting dose is 40 mg once daily. Doses >40 mg have not been studied.

Preparations

Pravachol (Bristol-Myers Squibb): 10-, 20-, 40-, 80-mg tablets

Fixed-dose combination: Pravigard (Bristol Myers Squibb): aspirin/pravastatin combination tablets: 81 mg/20 mg, 81 mg/40 mg, 325 mg/20 mg, 325 mg/40 mg, 325 mg/80 mg

Rosuvastatin (Crestor)

Indications

As adjunctive therapy to diet for reduction of elevated total and LDL cholesterol, apolipoprotein B, non-HDL cholesterol and triglyceride levels and to increase HDL cholesterol in patients with primary hypercholesterolemia (heterozygous familian and non-familial) and mixed dyslipidemias (types 2a and 2b); as an adjunct to diet for patients with elevated serum triglyceride levels (type 4); to reduce LDL cholesterol, total cholesterol, and apolipoprotein B in patients with homozygous familial hypercholesterolemia; as an adjunct to other lipid-lowering treatment (LDL apheresis) or if such treatments are unavailable.

The usual initial dose is 10 mg once daily. Initiation of therapy with 5 mg once daily may be considered for patients requiring less aggressive LDL-cholesterol reduction or those who have predisposing factors to myopathy. For patients with marked hypercholesterolemia (LDL cholesterol > 190 mg/dL) and aggressive lipid targets, a 20 mg starting dose may be considered. The 40 mg dose should be reserved for those patients not achieving goal LDL cholesterol at 20 mg.

Dosage adjustment is not necessary

Safety and effectiveness have not been established.

Crestor (Astra Zeneca): 5-, 10-, 20-, 40-mg tablets

Simvastatin (Zocor)

As adjunctive therapy to diet for reduction of elevated total and LDL cholesterol, apolipoprotein B, and triglyceride concentrations and to increase HDL cholesterol in patients with primary hypercholesterolemia (heterozygous familial and nonfamilial) and mixed dyslipidemia (types 2a and 2b); as adjunctive therapy to diet in the management of elevated triglyceride concentrations (type 4 hyperlipidemia); for the treatment of patients with primary dysbetalipoproteinemia (type 3 hyperlipidemia); to reduce total and LDL cholesterol levels in patients with homozygous familial hypercholesterolemia as an adjunct to other lipid-lowering treatments (e.g., LDL apheresis) or if such treatments are unavailable; to reduce the risks of death, nonfatal MI, stroke, or transient ischemic attack and to reduce the risk for undergoing myocardial revascularization procedures in patients with coronary heart disease and hypercholesterolemia

Usual initial dosage is 20 mg once daily in the evening or 40 mg once daily for patients requiring a large reduction in LDL cholesterol (>45%). Dosage may be titrated q4 wk or more often up to a maximum dosage of 80 mg every evening. Patients taking cyclosporine or who have severe renal insufficiency should be started on 5 mg/d. Recommended dosage for patients with homozygous familial hypercholesterolemia is 40 mg every evening or 80 mg/d in 3 divided doses (20 and 20 mg and an evening dose of 40 mg). If used in combination

(continued)

APPENDIX 2 (continued) Therapeutic Use of Available Cardiovascular Drugs

with cyclosporine, fibrates, or niacin, the daily dosage of simvastatin should not exceed 10 mg. In patients taking amiodarone or verapamil concomitantly with simvastatin, the dose should not exceed 20 mg/d.

Elderly   Dosages ≤20 mg/d are generally sufficient for maximum LDL reduction
Children   Safety and effectiveness have not been established
Preparations   Zocor (Merck): 5-, 10-, 20-, 40-, 80-mg tablets

Selective Cholesterol Absorption Inhibitor

Ezetimibe (Zetia)

Indications   As monotherapy or in combination with an HMG-CoA reductase inhibitor as adjunctive therapy to diet for the reduction of elevated total cholesterol, LDL cholesterol, and apolipoprotein B in patients with familial and non-familial hypercholesterolemia; as adjunctive therapy to diet for the reduction of elevated sitosterol and campesterol levels in patients with familial sitosterolemia.

Dosage
Adults   Usual dose is 10 mg once daily with or without food. The drug can be administered with an HMG-CoA reductase inhibitor for increment effect. Drugs should be given either ≥2 h before or ≥4 h after administration of a BAS.

Elderly   Dosage adjustment is not necessary.
Children   Safety and effectiveness have not been established.
Preparation   Zetia (Schering, Merck/Schering Plough): 10-mg capsule

Natriuretic Peptide

Nesiritide (Natrecor)

Indication   Treatment of patients with acutely decompensated CHF who have dyspnea at rest or with minimal activity

Dosage
Adults   The recommended dose of nesiritide is an IV bolus of 2 µg/kg followed by a continuous infusion of 0.01 µg/kg per min. Nesiritide should not be initiated at a dose that is above the recommended dose. The dose-limiting side effect of nesiritide is hypotension. Blood pressure should be monitored closely during administration. If hypotension occurs during the administration of nesiritide, the dose should be reduced or discontinued and other measures to support blood pressure should be started (IV fluids, changes in body position). In the VMAC trial, when symptomatic hypotension occurred, nesiritide was discontinued and subsequently could be restarted at a dose that was reduced by 30% (with no bolus administration) once the patient was stabilized.

In the VMAC trial, there was limited experience with increasing the dose of nesiritide above the recommended dose. In those patients, the infusion dose of nesiritide was increased by 0.005 μg/kg per min (preceded by a bolus of 1 μg/kg) no more frequently than q3 h up to a maximum dose of 0.03 μg/kg per min. Experience with administering nesiritide for longer than 48 h is limited. Refer to the Natrecor package insert for complete prescribing information.

Elderly   Use usual dose with caution
Children   Safety and effectiveness have not been established
Preparations   Natrecor (Scios): powder for injection, lyophilized: 1.5-mg single-use vials

Neuronal and ganglionic blockers

Guanadrel (Hylorel)

Indication   Hypertension
Dosage
Adults   Initiate at 5 mg bid. Dosage may be adjusted at weekly or monthly intervals until blood pressure is controlled. Usual maintenance dose is 20–75 mg/d in 2–4 divided doses. For patients with CrCl of 30–60 mL/min, initiate therapy with 5 mg q24 h. For patients with CrCL <30 mL/min, increase dosage interval to 48 h. Dosage increments should be made cautiously at intervals ≥7 d for patients with moderate renal insufficiency and ≥14 d for patients with severe renal insufficiency.
Elderly   Initiate at lowest dose and titrate to response
Children   Safety and effectiveness have not been established
Preparations   Hylorel (Fisons): 10-, 25-mg tablets

Guanethidine (Ismelin)

Indications   Moderate to severe hypertension, renal hypertension
Dosage
Adults   Initiate at 10 or 12.5 mg/d. Dosage may be increased gradually according to response (10- to 12.5-mg increments at weekly intervals). Usual maintenance dose is 25–50 mg/d. Dosage may be increased more rapidly and with larger increments under careful hospital supervision.
Elderly   Initiate at lowest dose and titrate to response
Children   Initiate with a 0.2 mg/kg per 24 h as a single oral dose. Daily dose may be increased by 0.2 mg/kg at 7–10 d intervals if needed.
Preparations   Guanethidine (generic), Ismelin (Ciba): 10-, 25-mg tablets (both are scored)

(continued)

APPENDIX 2 *(continued)* Therapeutic Use of Available Cardiovascular Drugs

Mecamylamine (Inversine)

Indication

Severe hypertension

Dosage

Adults

Initiate at 2.5 mg bid. Dosage may be adjusted in increments of 2.5 mg at intervals of at least q2 d according to response. The smallest dose should be taken in the morning to limit the orthostatic adverse effects of the drug. Usual maintenance dose is 25 mg/d in 3 divided doses.

Note: It is recommended that mecamylamine be administered at consistent times in relation to meals because hypotension may occur after a meal. Ingestion of mecamylamine with meals may slow the drug's absorption and thereby produce desired gradual correction of severe hypertension. Therapy with mecamylamine should not be discontinued abruptly.

Elderly

Initiate at lowest dose and titrate to response

Children

Safety and effectiveness have not been established

Preparation

Inversine (Layton): 2.5-mg tablets

Reserpine (reserpine)

Indications

Hypertension, psychotic disorders

Dosage

Adults

Usual maintenance dose for hypertension is 0.1–0.25 mg/d, taken with meals to avoid gastric irritation

Elderly

Initiate at lowest dose and titrate to response

Children

Safety and effectiveness have not been established

Preparations

Reserpine (generic): 0.1-, 0.25-mg tablets

Fixed-dose combinations for the treatment of hypertension

Diupres: reserpine/chlorothiazide combination tablets: 0.125 mg/250 mg; 0.125 mg/500 mg

Regroton: reserpine/chlorthalidone combination tablets: 0.25 mg/50 mg

Demi-Regroton: reserpine/chlorthalidone combination tablets: 0.125 mg/25 mg

Hydropres: reserpine/hydrochlorothiazide combination tablets: 0.125 mg/25 mg, 0.125 mg/50 mg

Salutensin: reserpine/hydroflumethiazide combination tablets: 0.125 mg/50 mg

Diutensen-R (Wallace): reserpine/methyclothiazide combination tablets: 0.1 mg/2.5 mg

Metatensin: reserpine/trichlormethiazide combination tablets: 0.1 mg/2 mg, 0.1 mg/4 mg

Renese-R: reserpine/trichlormethiazide combination tablets: 0.25 mg/2 mg

Hydrap-ES; Marpres; Ser-Ap-Es; Tri-Hydroserpine: reserpine/hydrochlorothiazide/hydralazine HCl combination tablets: 0.1 mg/15 mg/25 mg

Trimethaphan (Arfonad)

Indications

Production of controlled hypotension during surgery; short-term acute control of blood pressure in hypertensive emergencies; emergency treatment of pulmonary edema in patients with pulmonary hypertension associated with systemic hypertension

Dosage

Adults

For controlled hypotension during surgery, initiate therapy as an IV infusion at 3–4 mg/min. Infusion rate should be adjusted according to response to a maintenance dose of 0.2–6 mg/min. Trimethaphan should be administered after the patient is anesthetized, and this drug should be discontinued before wound closure to allow blood pressure to return toward normal. For hypertensive emergency, initiate trimethaphan at 0.5–1 mg/min and adjust the infusion rate according to response. Usual maintenance infusion rate is 1–5 mg/min.

Note: Trimethaphan should be diluted in the proper amount of compatible fluid before IV infusion (500 mg in 10 mL trimethaphan may be diluted in 500 mL of 5% dextrose injection to yield to final solution containing 1 mg/mL of trimethaphan).

Elderly

Initiate at lowest dose and titrate to response

Children

Dosage is based on body weight; use with caution

Preparation

Arfonad (Roche): 50-mg/mL injection

Vasodilators

Cilostazol (Pletal)

Refer to *Antiplatelet Agents* for the summary of this agent

Diazoxide (Hyperstat IV)

Indications

Hypertensive emergencies (IV formulation), hypoglycemia (PO formulation)

Dosage

Adults

Hypertensive emergencies: Administer 1–3 mg/kg (up to 150 mg in a single injection) by rapid IV injection q5–15 min as needed to obtain the desired blood pressure response. Further doses may be given q4–24 h as needed to maintain desired blood pressure until PO antihypertensive medication can be instituted. Continued treatment for >4–5 d usually is not necessary; do not use for >10 d.

Note: IV injection should be administered only into a peripheral vein. Treatment is most effective when IV administration is completed in ≤30 s. The solution's alkalinity is irritating to tissue; avoid extravasation. Patient should remain recumbent during and for 15–30 min after medication administration.

(continued)

Elderly

Children

Hypoglycemia: Initiate therapy with the PO formulation at 1 mg/kg q8h; adjust dosage according to clinical response. Usual maintenance dose is 3–8 mg/kg per d given in 2–3 divided doses.

Initiate at lowest dose and titrate to response

Dosing is based on weight; drug-induced edema may occur in infants given the PO formulation of diazoxide

Preparations

Hyperstat IV (Schering): 15-mg/mL injection, 20-mL ampules

Proglycem (Baker Norton): 50-mg capsules; 50 mg/mL PO suspension

Epoprostenol (Flolan)

Indication

Primary pulmonary hypertension (epoprostenol is indicated for the long-term IV treatment of primary pulmonary hypertension in NYHA class III and IV patients)

Dosage

Adults

Acute dose ranging: Infusion rate is initiated at 2 ng/kg per min and adjusted in increments of 2 ng/kg per min q15 min or longer until dose-limiting pharmacologic effects occur. The most common dose-limiting pharmacologic effects are nausea, vomiting, headache, hypotension, and flushing. During acute dose ranging in clinical trials, the mean maximum dose that did not result in dose-limiting pharmacologic effects was 8.6 ± 0.3 ng/kg per min.

Note: Epoprostenol must be reconstituted only with sterile diluent for epoprostenol. Reconstituted solutions of epoprostenol must not be diluted or administered with other parenteral solutions or medications.

Continuous chronic infusion: Chronic infusions of epoprostenol should be initiated at 4 ng/kg per min less than the maximum tolerated infusion rate determined during acute dose ranging. If the maximum tolerated infusion rate is <5 ng/kg per min, the chronic infusion should be initiated at one-half the maximum tolerated infusion rate. During clinical trials, the mean initial chronic infusion rate was 5 ng/kg per min.

Note: Chronic continuous infusion of epoprostenol should be administered through a central venous catheter. Temporary peripheral intravenous infusions may be used until a central access is established

Dosage adjustments: Adjustments in the chronic infusion rate should be based on persistence, recurrence, or worsening of the patient's symptoms of primary pulmonary hypertension and the occurrence of adverse events due to excessive doses of epoprostenol. In general, increases in dose from the initial chronic dose should be expected. Increments in dose should be considered if symptoms of primary pulmonary hypertension persist or recur after improving. Infusion should be adjusted by 1–2 ng/kg per min in increments at intervals sufficient to allow assessment of clinical response; these intervals should be at least 15 min. In contrast, reduced dosage of epoprostenol should be considered when dose-related pharmacologic events occur. Dosage reductions should be made gradually in decrements of 2 ng/kg per min q15 min or longer until the dose-limiting adverse effects resolve

Note: Abrupt withdrawal of epoprostenol or sudden large reductions in infusion rates should be avoided with the exception of life-threatening situations such as unconsciousness or collapse. Consult manufacturer's package insert for detailed information on administration and reconstitution of epoprostenol.

Elderly
Use usual dose with caution

Children
Safety and effectiveness have not been established

Preparations
Flolan (Glaxo SmithKline): 0.5, 1.5 mg powder for reconstitution and 50-mL vials of sterile diluent for Flolan

Fenoldopam (Corlopam)

Indications
In-hospital, short-term (up to 48 h) management of severe hypertension when rapid, but quickly reversible, emergency reduction of blood pressure is indicated, including malignant hypertension with deteriorating end-organ function

Dosage

Adults
Initial dose of fenoldopam is chosen according to the desired magnitude and rate of blood pressure reduction in a given clinical situation. In general, there is a greater and more rapid blood pressure reduction as the initial dose is increased. Lower initial doses (0.03–0.1 µg/kg per min) titrated slowly have been associated with less reflex tachycardia than have higher initial doses (≥0.3 µg/kg per min). Recommended increments for titration are 0.05–0.1 µg/kg per min at intervals of ≥15 min. Doses <0.1 µg/kg per min have very modest effects and appear only marginally useful in patients with severe hypertension. Doses of 0.01–1.6 µg/kg per min have been studied in clinical trials. Most of the effect of a given infusion rate is attained within 15 min. Fenoldopam infusion can be abruptly discontinued or gradually tapered before discontinuation. Oral antihypertensive agents can be added during fenoldopam infusion (after blood pressure is stable) or after its discontinuation.
Note: Fenoldopam should be administered by continuous IV infusion only. A bolus dose should not be used. The fenoldopam injection ampule concentrate must be diluted with the appropriate amount of compatible fluid before infusion. Consult manufacturer's package insert for instructions on proper dilution of fenoldopam.

Elderly
Dosage adjustment is not necessary

Children
Safety and effectiveness have not been established

Preparation
Corlopam (Abbott): 10-mg/mL injection, concentrate

Hydralazine (hydralazine, Apresoline)

Indications
Essential hypertension (PO formulation), severe essential hypertension when the drug cannot be given orally or when the need to lower blood pressure is urgent (parenteral formulation)

(continued)

APPENDIX 2 *(continued)* Therapeutic Use of Available Cardiovascular Drugs

Dosage	
Adults	*PO formulation:* Initiate therapy at 10 mg qid for the first 2–4 d; increase to 25 mg qid for the rest of the first week. Thereafter, the dosage may be increased to 50 mg qid during the second and subsequent weeks. Dosage should be maintained at the lowest effective level. Maximum dose is 300 mg/d. Higher doses have been used in the treatment of CHF.
	Parenteral administration: Usual dose is 10–20 mg administered IV or 10–50 mg administered IM; low doses in these ranges should be used initially. Parenteral doses may be repeated as necessary and may be increased within the above ranges based on blood pressure response.
	Note: Because hydralazine interacts with stainless steel, resulting in a pink discoloration, injections should be used as quickly as possible after being drawn through a needle or syringe; stainless steel filters should also be avoided. In addition, hydralazine should not be diluted with solutions containing dextrose or other sugars.
Elderly	Initiate at lowest dose and titrate to response
Children	Safety and effectiveness have not been established, although there is experience with the use of hydralazine in children
Preparations	Hydralazine (generic), Apresoline (Novartis): 10-, 25-, 50-, 100-mg tablets
	Hydralazine (generic): 20-mg/mL injection, 1-mL vials
Fixed-dose combinations for the treatment of hypertension	Hydra-Zide: hydralazine hydrochloride/hydrochlorothiazide combination capsules: 25 mg/25 mg, 50 mg/50 mg, 100 mg/50 mg
	Hydrap-ES; Marpres; Ser-Ap-Es; Tri-Hydroserpine: reserpine/hydrochlorothiazide/hydralazine HCl combination tablets: 0.1 mg/15 mg/25 mg

Isosorbide dinitrate (isosorbide dinitrate, Isordil, Isordil Titradose, Isordil Tembids, Sorbitrate, Dilatrate SR)

Indication	Angina pectoris (treatment and prevention)
Dosage	
Adults	*Short-acting oral tablets (isosorbide dinitrate, Isordil Titradose):* Administer 5–20 mg tid; dosage may be adjusted as needed and tolerated. Usual dose is 10–40 mg tid. Use with caution in patients with hepatic or renal impairment.
	Note: A daily nitrate-free interval ≥14 h has been recommended to minimize tolerance. The optimal nitrate-free interval may vary among different patients, doses, and regimens.

706

SR PO tablets and capsules (isosorbide dinitrate, Isordil Tembids, Dilatrate-SR): Administer SR preparations once daily or twice daily in doses given 6 h apart (i.e., 8 A.M. and 2 P.M.). Do not exceed 160 mg/d.

SL and chewable tablets (isosorbide dinitrate, Isordil, Sorbitrate): Usual initial dose is 2.5–5 mg for SL tablets and 5 mg for chewable tablets. Dosage may be titrated upward until angina is relieved or until dose-related adverse effects occur. For acute prophylaxis, 5–10 mg of SL or chewable tablets may be administered q2–3 h. Use of SL or chewable isosorbide dinitrate for the termination of acute anginal attacks should be reserved for patients intolerant of or unresponsive to SL nitroglycerin.

Elderly   Initiate at lowest dose and titrate to response
Children   Safety and effectiveness have not been established
Preparations   Tablets, short acting (isosorbide dinitrate): 5, 10, 20, 30 mg
Tablets, short acting (Isordil Titradose, Sorbitrate): 5, 10, 20, 30, 40 mg
Tablets, SL (isosorbide dinitrate, Isordil): 2.5, 5, 10 mg
Tablets, SL (Sorbitrate): 2.5, 5 mg
Tablets, chewable (Sorbitrate): 5, 10 mg
Tablets, SR (isosorbide dinitrate, Isordil Tembids): 40 mg
Capsules, SR (Dilatrate SR, Isordil Tembids): 40 mg

Isosorbide mononitrate (isosorbide mononitrate, ISMO, Monoket, Imdur)
Indication   Angina pectoris (prevention)
Dosage
Adults   *Tablets (isosorbide mononitrate, Monoket, ISMO):* Administer 20 mg bid with doses given 7 h apart. An initial dose of 5 mg bid may be appropriate for persons of small stature; dosage should be increased to at least 10 mg by the second or third day of therapy.
ER tablets (isosorbide mononitrate, Imdur): Initiate at 30 or 60 mg once daily. Dosage may be increased to 120 mg once daily after several days if necessary. Rarely, 240 mg may be required in some patients.
Elderly   Dosage adjustment is not necessary
Children   Safety and effectiveness have not been established
Preparations   Tablets (isosorbide mononitrate, ISMO): 20 mg
Tablets (Monoket): 10, 20 mg
Tablets, ER (isosorbide mononitrate): 60 mg
Tablets, ER (Imdur): 30, 60, 120 mg

(continued)

707

APPENDIX 2 *(continued)* Therapeutic Use of Available Cardiovascular Drugs

Minoxidil (minoxidil, Loniten)

Indications

Severe hypertension (PO formulation), male pattern baldness of the vertex of the scalp (topical formulation)

Dosage

Adults

PO formulation: Initiate therapy at 5 mg once daily; dosage may be increased by 10 mg at intervals of ≥3 d as needed. Usual maintenance dose is 10–40 mg/d in 1–2 divided doses. Maximum dose is 100 mg/d.
Topical formulation: Apply 1 mL to affected areas of the scalp twice daily (morning and night). Wash hands after applying.

Elderly

Initiate at lowest dose and titrate to response

Children

Safety and effectiveness have not been established, although there is experience with the use of minoxidil in children

Preparations

Minoxidil (generic); Loniten (Pharmacia & Upjohn): 2.5-, 10-mg tablets
Rogaine topical solution (Pharmacia & Upjohn): 2%/60 mL, 5%/60 mL

Nitroglycerin (various sources)

Indications

Prevention of angina pectoris (PO SR tablets and capsules, transdermal system), prevention and treatment of angina pectoris (SL tablets, translingual spray, transmucosal tablets, topical ointment), control of blood pressure in perioperative hypertension (IV formulation), CHF associated with acute MI (IV formulation), angina pectoris unresponsive to recommended doses of organic nitrates or beta blockers (IV formulation), controlled hypotension during surgical procedures (IV formulation)

Dosage

Adults

SL tablets (Nitrostat): Dissolve 1 tablet under the tongue or in the buccal pouch at first sign of an acute anginal attack. Repeat approximately q5 min until relief is obtained. No more than 3 tablets should be taken in 15 min. If pain persists, notify physician or get to the emergency room immediately. SL tablets also may be used prophylactically 5–10 min before activities that might trigger an acute attack.
Translingual spray (Nitrolingual pump spray): At the onset of an attack, spray 1–2 metered doses onto or under the tongue. No more than 3 metered doses should be administered within 15 min. If chest pain continues, seek immediate medical attention. Translingual spray also may be used prophylactically 5–10 min before activities that might trigger an acute attack. Do not inhale spray.
Transmucosal, buccal tablets (Nitrogard): Administer 1 mg q3–5 h during waking hours. Place tablet between lip and gum above incisors or between cheek and gum. Do not chew or swallow tablet.

SR capsules (nitroglycerin, Nitro-Bid Plateau Caps): Initiate therapy at 2.5 mg tid. Dosage may be titrated upward to an effective dose or until dose-related adverse effects occur. Tolerance may develop when nitroglycerin is administered without a nitrate-free interval. Consider administering on a reduced schedule (once or twice daily).

SR tablets (Nitrong): Initiate therapy at 2.6 mg tid. Dosage may be titrated upward to an effective dose or until dose-related adverse effects occur. Tolerance may develop when nitroglycerin is administered without a nitrate-free interval. Consider administering on a reduced schedule (once or twice daily).

Topical ointment (nitroglycerin, Nitro-Bid): Initiate therapy at 15–30 mg (1–2 in.), q8 h; dosage may be increased by 0.5 inch per application q6 h to a maximum of 75 mg (5 in.) per application q4 h.

Note: Any regimen of nitroglycerin ointment administration should include a daily nitrate-free interval of about 10–12 h to avoid tolerance. To apply the ointment using the dose-measuring paper applicator, place the applicator on a flat surface, printed side down. Squeeze the necessary amount of ointment from the tube onto the applicator, place the applicator (ointment side down) on the desired area of skin (usually on non-hairy skin of chest or back), and tape the applicator into place. Do not rub in.

Transdermal systems (Nitroglycerin Transdermal, Minitran, Nitro-Dur): Initiate therapy with a 0.1- or 0.2-mg/h patch. Apply patch for 12–14 h; remove for 10–12 h before applying a new patch. Patch should be applied onto clean, dry, hairless skin of chest, inner upper arm, or shoulder. Avoid placing below knee or elbow. Change site of placement to decrease skin irritation. Apply a new patch if the first patch loosens or falls off.

IV formulations (nitroglycerin IV, Tridil IV, Nitro-Bid IV, nitroglycerin in 5% dextrose): Initiate IV infusion at 5 μg/min; increase by increments of 5 μg/min at 3- to 5-min intervals until desired effect is obtained or to 20 μg/min. Dosage may be increased beyond 20 μg/min by 10-μg/min increments at 3- to 5-min intervals and then by 20-μg/min increments until desired effect is achieved. Reduce dosage increments and frequency of dosage increments as partial effects are noted. There is no fixed optimum dose. Continuously monitor physiologic parameters, such as blood pressure and heart rate, and other measurements, such as pulmonary capillary wedge pressure, to achieve accurate dose. Maintain adequate blood and coronary perfusion pressures.

Note: IV infusion must be given through a special non-polyvinylchloride IV infusion set or infusion pump. Consult manufacturer's package insert for instructions on dilution and administration of IV nitroglycerin.

Elderly — Initiate at lowest dose and titrate to response

Children — Safety and effectiveness have not been established

(continued)

APPENDIX 2 (continued) Therapeutic Use of Available Cardiovascular Drugs

Preparations

SL tablets (Nitrostat): 0.3, 0.4, 0.6 mg
Translingual spray (Nitrolingual pump spray): 0.4 mg/metered dose
Transmucosal tablets, controlled release: 1, 2, 3 mg
Capsules, SR (nitroglycerin, Nitro-Bid Plateau Caps): 2.5, 6.5, 9 mg
Capsules, SR (Nitroglyn): 13 mg
Tablets, SR (Nitrong): 2.6, 6.5, 9 mg
Topical ointment (nitroglycerin, Nitro-Bid): 2% in a lanolin petrolatum base
Transdermal systems (nitroglycerin): 0.1, 0.2, 0.4, 0.6 mg/h
Transdermal systems (Deponit): 0.2, 0.4 mg/h
Transdermal systems (Nitrodisc, Nitro-Dur): 0.3 mg/h
Transdermal systems (Minitran, Nitro-Dur): 0.1, 0.2, 0.3, 0.4, 0.6 mg/h
Transdermal systems (Nitro-Dur, Transderm-Nitro, Nitro-Derm): 0.8 mg/h
IV (nitroglycerin IV, Nitro-Bid IV, Tridil IV): 5 mg/mL (1-, 5-, 10-mL vials)
IV (Tridil IV): 0.5 mg/mL, 10-mL ampules
IV (nitroglycerin in 5% dextrose): 25 mg in 250 mL, 50 mg in 250 and 500 mL, 100 mg in 250 mL, 200 mg in 500 mL

Papaverine (papaverine, SR)

Indications

Relief of cerebral and peripheral ischemia associated with arterial spasm and myocardial ischemia complicated by arrhythmias

Dosage
Adults

PO formulation: Administer 150 mg in an ER formulation q8–12 h or 300 mg q12 h.
Note: It is uncertain if effective plasma concentrations are maintained for 12 h with ER preparations. In the past, the FDA has recommended that papaverine products be withdrawn from the market.
Parenteral administration: Papaverine may be administered IM or by slow IV injection over 1–2 min. The IV route is preferred when an immediate effect is desired. Usual parenteral dose is 30 mg; however, a dosage of 30–120 mg may be repeated q3 h as needed. In the treatment of cardiac extrasystoles, 2 doses may be given 10 min apart.

Elderly

Initiate at lowest dose and titrate to response

Children

Safety and effectiveness have not been established

Preparations

Papaverine HCl (generic): 150-mg ER capsules
Papaverine HCl (generic): 30-mg/mL injection

Pentoxifylline (pentoxifylline, Trental)

Indication
Intermittent claudication

Dosage

Adults
Initiate therapy at 400 mg tid with meals; dosage may be reduced to 400 mg bid if GI or central nervous system adverse effects occur. Although therapeutic effects may be observed within 2–4 wk, continue treatment for ≥8 wk.

Elderly
Use usual dose with caution

Children
Safety and effectiveness have not been established

Preparations
Pentoxifylline (generic): 400-mg tablets
Pentoxifylline (generic): 400-mg ER tablets
Trental (Aventis): 400-mg ER tablets

Nitroprusside (sodium nitroprusside, Nitropress)

Indications
Hypertensive crises, production of controlled hypotension to reduce bleeding during surgery, acute CHF

Dosage

Adults
Usual initial dose is 0.3 µg/kg per min (range, 0.1–0.5 µg/kg per min) as an IV infusion. Dosage may be adjusted slowly in increments of 0.5 µg/kg per min according to response. Usual infusion rate is 3 µg/kg per min. Maximum recommended infusion rate is 10 µg/kg per min; infusion at the maximum dose rate should never last >10 min. To keep the steady-state thiocyanate concentration <1 mmol/L, the rate of a prolonged infusion should not exceed 3 µg/kg per min (1 µg/kg per min in anuric patients). When >500 µg/kg nitroprusside is administered faster than 2 µg/kg per min, cyanide is generated faster than the unaided patient can eliminate it. *Note:* After reconstitution with the appropriate diluent, sodium nitroprusside injection is not suitable for direct injection. The reconstituted solution must be further diluted in the appropriate amount of sterile 5% dextrose injection before infusion. The diluted solution should be protected from light by promptly wrapping the medication container with the supplied opaque sleeve. Sodium nitroprusside should be administered through an infusion pump, preferably a volumetric pump. Consult the manufacturer's package insert for complete prescribing information.

Elderly
Use usual dose with caution

Children
Appropriate studies have not been performed; however, pediatrics-specific problems that would limit the usefulness of this agent in children are not expected.

(continued)

711

APPENDIX 2 Therapeutic Use of Available Cardiovascular Drugs *(continued)*

Preparations	Sodium nitroprusside (generic); Nitropress (Abbott): 50 mg/vial, powder for injection
Treprostinil (Remodulin)	
Indications	For the treatment of pulmonary arterial hypertension in patients with NYHA class II to IV symptoms, to diminish symptoms associated with exercise
Dosage	
Adults	Infusion rate is initiated at 1.25 ng/kg per min SC continuous infusion. Infusion rate is reduced to 0.625 ng/kg per min if not tolerated. The dose can then be titrated by no more than 1.25 ng/kg per min per week for the first 4 wk and then by no more than 2.5 ng/kg per min per week thereafter, depending on the clinical response. The dose should be decreased with excessive pharmacologic effects or with unacceptable infusion site reactions (pain).
Elderly	Use usual dose with caution
Children	Safety and effectiveness have not been established
Preparations	Remodulin (United Therapeutics): injection 1, 2.5, 5, 10 mg/mL (20 mL)

Key: ACE, angiotensin-converting enzyme; ACT, activated clotting time; aPTT, activated partial thromboplastin time; bid, twice daily; CHF, congestive heart failure; CPR, cardiopulmonary resuscitation; CrCl, creatinine clearance; CURE, Clopidogrel in Unstable Angina to Prevent Recurrent Events; CVD, cardiovascular disease; CYP, cytochrome P450; D5W, 5% dextrose in water; ER, extended release; FDA, U.S. Food and Drug Administration; GI, gastrointestinal; HDL, high-density lipoprotein; HIT, heparin-induced thrombocytopenia; HITTS, heparin-induced thrombocytopenia and thrombosis syndrome; HMG-CoA, hydroxymethylglutaryl coenzyme A; IM, intramuscular; INR, international normalized ratio; ISA, intrinsic sympathomimetic activity; IV, intravenous; LDL, low-density lipoprotein; MI, myocardial infarction; NYHA, New York Heart Association; PCI, percutaneous coronary intervention; PRISM-PLUS, the Platelet Receptor Inhibition in Ischemic Syndrome Management in Patients Limited by Unstable signs and symptoms study; PTCA, percutaneous transluminal coronary angioplasty; qid, four times daily; SC, subcutaneous; SL, sublingual; SR, sustained release; tid, three times daily; U, units; VMAC, Vasodilation in the Management of Acute CHF.

APPENDIX 3 Guide to Cardiovascular Drugs Used in Pregnancy and with Nursing

Drug	Use in pregnancy	Use during lactation	Classification*
α-Adrenergic antagonists			
Doxazosin	Weigh benefits vs. risk	Breast feeding not recommended; excretion in milk unknown	C
Phenoxybenzamine	Weigh benefits vs. risk	Breast feeding not recommended; excretion in milk unknown	C
Phentolamine	Weigh benefits vs. risk	Breast feeding not recommended; excretion in milk unknown	C
Prazosin	Weigh benefits vs. risk	Breast feed with caution; drug excreted in breast milk	C
Terazosin	Weigh benefits vs. risk	Breast feeding not recommended; excretion in milk unknown	C
α₂-Adrenergic agonists			
Clonidine	Weigh benefits vs. risk	Breast feed with caution; drug excreted in breast milk	C
Guanabenz	Weigh benefits vs. risk	Breast feeding not recommended; excretion in milk unknown	C
Guanfacine	Use only if clearly indicated	Breast feeding not recommended; excretion in milk unknown	C
Methyldopa	Weigh benefits vs. risk	Breast feed with caution; drug excreted in breast milk	B (PO), C (IV)
ACE inhibitors	Use of ACE inhibitors during the second and third trimesters of pregnancy has been associated with fetal and neonatal injury, including hypotension, neonatal skull hypoplasia, anuria, reversible or irreversible renal failure, and death		
Benazepril		Breast feeding not recommended; excretion in milk unknown	
Captopril		Breast feeding not recommended; drug excreted in breast milk	
Enalapril		Breast feeding not recommended; drug excreted in breast milk	
Fosinopril		Breast feeding not recommended; drug excreted in breast milk	
Lisinopril		Breast feeding not recommended; excretion in milk unknown	
Moexipril		Breast feeding not recommended; excretion in milk unknown	
Perindopril		Breast feeding not recommended; excretion in milk unknown	
Quinapril		Breast feeding not recommended; drug excreted in breast milk	
Ramipril		Breast feeding not recommended; excretion in milk unknown	
Trandolapril		Breast feeding not recommended; excretion in milk unknown	
Angiotensin II receptor blockers	Use of medications that act directly on the RAS during the second and third trimesters of		
Candesartan		Breast feeding not recommended; excretion in milk unknown	C (first trimester)
Eprosartan		Breast feeding not recommended; excretion in milk unknown	D (second and third trimesters)

ACE inhibitors classification: C (first trimester), D (second and third trimesters)

(continued)

713

APPENDIX 3 *(continued)* Guide to Cardiovascular Drugs Used in Pregnancy and with Nursing

Drug	Use in pregnancy	Use during lactation	Classification*
Irbesartan	pregnancy has been associated with fetal and neonatal injury, including hypotension, neonatal skull hypoplasia, anuria, reversible or irreversible renal failure, and death	Breast feeding not recommended; excretion in milk unknown	C
Losartan		Breast feeding not recommended; excretion in milk unknown	C
Olmesartan		Breast feeding not recommended; excretion in milk unknown	C
Telmisartan		Breast feeding not recommended; excretion in milk unknown	C
Valsartan		Breast feeding not recommended; excretion in milk unknown	C
Antiarrhythmic agents			
Class Ia			
Disopyramide	Weigh benefits vs. risk	Breast feeding not recommended; drug excreted in breast milk	C
Procainamide	Weigh benefits vs. risk	Breast feeding not recommended; drug excreted in breast milk	C
Quinidine	Weigh benefits vs. risk	Breast feeding not recommended; drug excreted in breast milk	C
Class Ib			
Lidocaine	Use only if clearly indicated	Breast feed with caution; drug excreted in breast milk	B
Mexiletine	Weigh benefits vs. risk	Breast feeding not recommended; drug excreted in breast milk	C
Tocainide	Weigh benefits vs. risk	Breast feeding not recommended; drug excreted in breast milk	C
Class Ic			
Flecainide	Weigh benefits vs. risk	Breast feeding not recommended; drug excreted in breast milk	C
Moricizine	Use only if clearly indicated	Breast feeding not recommended; drug excreted in breast milk	B
Propafenone	Weigh benefits vs. risk	Breast feeding not recommended; excretion in breast milk unknown	C
Class II (beta blockers)			
Acebutolol	Use only if clearly indicated	Breast feeding not recommended; drug excreted in breast milk	B
Atenolol	Weigh benefits vs. risk	Breast feeding not recommended; drug excreted in breast milk	C
Betaxolol	Weigh benefits vs. risk	Breast feed with caution; drug excreted in breast milk	C
Bisoprolol	Weigh benefits vs. risk	Breast feeding not recommended; excretion in milk unknown	C
Carteolol	Weigh benefits vs. risk	Breast feeding not recommended; excretion in milk unknown	C
Carvedilol	Weigh benefits vs. risk	Breast feeding not recommended; excretion in milk unknown	C
Esmolol	Weigh benefits vs. risk	Breast feeding not recommended; excretion in milk unknown	C

Labetalol	Weigh benefits vs. risk	Breast feed with caution; drug excreted in breast milk	C
Metoprolol	Weigh benefits vs. risk	Breast feeding not recommended; drug excreted in breast milk	C
Nadolol	Weigh benefits vs. risk	Breast feed with caution; drug excreted in breast milk	C
Penbutolol	Weigh benefits vs. risk	Breast feeding not recommended; excretion in milk unknown	C
Pindolol	Use only if clearly indicated	Breast feed with caution; drug excreted in breast milk	B
Propranolol	Weigh benefits vs. risk	Breast feed with caution; drug excreted in breast milk	C
Timolol	Weigh benefits vs. risk	Breast feed with caution; drug excreted in breast milk	C
Class III			
Amiodarone	Not recommended	Breast feeding not recommended; drug excreted in breast milk	D
Bretylium	Weigh benefits vs. risk	Breast feeding not recommended; excretion in milk unknown	C
Dofetilide	Weigh benefits vs. risk	Breast feeding not recommended; excretion in milk unknown	C
Ibutilide	Weigh benefits vs. risk	Breast feeding not recommended; excretion in milk unknown	C
Sotalol	Use only if clearly indicated	Breast feeding not recommended; drug excreted in breast milk	B
Class IV (calcium antagonists)†			
Amlodipine	Weigh benefits vs. risk	Breast feeding not recommended; excretion in milk unknown	C
Bepridil	Weigh benefits vs. risk	Breast feeding not recommended; drug excreted in breast milk	C
Diltiazem	Weigh benefits vs. risk	Breast feeding not recommended; drug excreted in breast milk	C
Felodipine	Weigh benefits vs. risk	Breast feeding not recommended; excretion in milk unknown	C
Isradipine	Weigh benefits vs. risk	Breast feeding not recommended; excretion in milk unknown	C
Nicardipine	Weigh benefits vs. risk	Breast feeding not recommended; excretion in milk unknown	C
Nifedipine	Weigh benefits vs. risk	Breast feeding not recommended; drug excreted in breast milk	C
Nimodipine	Weigh benefits vs. risk	Breast feeding not recommended; excretion in milk unknown	C
Nisoldipine	Weigh benefits vs. risk	Breast feeding not recommended; excretion in milk unknown	C
Verapamil	Weigh benefits vs. risk	Breast feeding not recommended; drug excreted in breast milk	C
Antithrombotic agents			
Anticoagulants			
Argatroban	Use only if clearly needed	Breast feeding not recommended; excretion in milk unknown	B

(continued)

APPENDIX 3 (continued) Guide to Cardiovascular Drugs Used in Pregnancy and with Nursing

Drug	Use in pregnancy	Use during lactation	Classification*
Bivalirudin	Use only if clearly needed	Breast feeding not recommended; excretion in milk unknown	B
Dalteparin	Use only if clearly needed	Breast feeding not recommended; excretion in milk unknown	B
Danaparoid	Use only if clearly needed	Breast feeding not recommended; excretion in milk unknown	B
Enoxaparin	Use only if clearly needed	Breast feeding not recommended; excretion in milk unknown	B
Fondaparinux	Use only if clearly needed	Breast feeding not recommended; excretion in milk unknown	B
Heparin	Weigh benefits vs. risk	Not excreted in breast milk	C
Lepirudin	Use only if clearly needed	Breast feeding not recommended; excretion in milk unknown	B
Tinzaparin	Use only if clearly needed	Breast feeding not recommended; excretion in milk unknown	B
Warfarin	Contraindicated	Breast feeding not recommended; drug excreted in breast milk	X
Antiplatelets			
Anagrelide	Weigh benefits vs. risk	Breast feeding not recommended; excretion in milk unknown	C
Aspirin	Contraindicated in third trimester	Breast feed with caution; drug excreted in breast milk	D
Abciximab	Weigh benefits vs. risk	Breast feeding not recommended; excretion in milk unknown	C
Clopidogrel	Use only if clearly needed	Breast feeding not recommended; excretion in milk unknown	B
Dipyridamole	Use only if clearly needed	Breast feed with caution; drug excreted in breast milk	B
Eptifibatide	Use only if clearly needed	Breast feeding not recommended; excretion in milk unknown	B
Ticlopidine	Use only if clearly needed	Breast feeding not recommended; excretion in milk unknown	B
Tirofiban	Use only if clearly needed	Breast feeding not recommended; excretion in milk unknown	B
Thrombolytics			
Alteplase (t-PA)	Weigh benefits vs. risk	Breast feeding not recommended; excretion in milk unknown	C
Anistreplase	Weigh benefits vs. risk	Breast feeding not recommended; excretion in milk unknown	C
Reteplase	Weigh benefits vs. risk	Breast feeding not recommended; excretion in milk unknown	C
Streptokinase	Weigh benefits vs. risk	Breast feeding not recommended; excretion in milk unknown	C
Tenecteplase	Weigh benefits vs. risk	Breast feeding not recommended; excretion in milk unknown	C
Urokinase	Use only if clearly needed	Breast feeding not recommended; excretion in milk unknown	B

Diuretics

Loop

Bumetanide	Weigh benefits vs. risk	Breast feeding not recommended; excretion in milk unknown	C
Ethacrynic acid	Use only if clearly needed	Breast feeding not recommended; excretion in milk unknown	B
Furosemide	Weigh benefits vs. risk	Breast feeding not recommended; drug excreted in breast milk	C
Torsemide	Use only if clearly needed	Breast feeding not recommended; excretion in milk unknown	B

Thiazides

Bendroflumethiazide	Weigh benefits vs. risk	Breast feed with caution; drug excreted in breast milk	C
Benzthiazide	Weigh benefits vs. risk	Breast feed with caution; drug excreted in breast milk	C
Chlorothiazide	Use only if clearly needed	Breast feed with caution; drug excreted in breast milk	B
Chlorthalidone	Use only if clearly needed	Breast feeding not recommended; drug excreted in breast milk	B
Hydrochlorothiazide	Use only if clearly needed	Breast feed with caution; drug excreted in breast milk	B
Hydroflumethiazide	Weigh benefits vs. risk	Breast feeding not recommended; drug excreted in breast milk	C
Indapamide	Use only if clearly needed	Breast feeding not recommended; drug excreted in breast milk	B
Methyclothiazide‡	Use only if clearly needed	Breast feeding not recommended; drug excreted in breast milk	B
Metolazone	Use only if clearly needed	Breast feeding not recommended; drug excreted in breast milk	B
Polythiazide	Weigh benefits vs. risk	Breast feed with caution; drug excreted in breast milk	D
Quinethazone	Weigh benefits vs. risk	Breast feed with caution; drug excreted in breast milk	D
Trichlormethiazide	Weigh benefits vs. risk	Breast feed with caution; drug excreted in breast milk	C

Potassium sparing

Amiloride	Use only if clearly needed	Breast feeding not recommended; excretion in milk unknown	B
Eplerenone	Use only if clearly needed	Breast feeding not recommended; excretion in milk unknown	B
Spironolactone	Weigh benefits vs. risk	Breast feeding not recommended; drug excreted in breast milk	D
Triamterene	Use only if clearly needed	Breast feeding not recommended; excretion in milk unknown	B

Endothelin receptor antagonist

Bosentan	Contraindicated	Breast feeding not recommended; excretion in milk unknown	X

(continued)

APPENDIX 3 (continued) Guide to Cardiovascular Drugs Used in Pregnancy and with Nursing

Drug	Use in pregnancy	Use during lactation	Classification*
Inotropic and vasopressor agents			
Digoxin	Weigh benefits vs. risk	Breast feed with caution: drug excreted in breast milk	C
Amrinone (Inaminone)	Weigh benefits vs. risks	Breast feeding not recommended; excretion in milk unknown	C
Milrinone	Weigh benefits vs. risk	Breast feeding not recommended; excretion in milk unknown	C
Dobutamine	Use only if clearly needed	Breast feeding not recommended; excretion in milk unknown	B
Dopamine	Weigh benefits vs. risk	Breast feeding not recommended; excretion in milk unknown	C
Isoproterenol	Weigh benefits vs. risk	Breast feeding not recommended; excretion in milk unknown	C
Epinephrine	Weigh benefits vs. risk	Breast feed with caution; drug excreted in breast milk	C
Metaraminol	Weigh benefits vs. risk	Breast feeding not recommended; excretion in milk unknown	C
Methoxamine	Weigh benefits vs. risk	Breast feeding not recommended; excretion in milk unknown	C
Midodrine	Weigh benefits vs. risk	Breast feeding not recommended; excretion in milk unknown	C
Norepinephrine	Weigh benefits vs. risk	Breast feeding not recommended; excretion in milk unknown	C
Phenylephrine	Weigh benefits vs. risk	Limited absorption in GI tract; excretion in milk unknown	C
Lipid-lowering agents			
BAS			
Cholestyramine	Weigh benefits vs. risk	Breast feed with caution; excretion in breast milk unknown	C
Colestipol	Weigh benefits vs. risk	Breast feed with caution; excretion in breast milk unknown	Not evaluated
Colesevelam	Use only if clearly needed	Breast feed with caution; excretion in breast milk unknown	B
FAD			
Clofibrate	Weigh benefits vs. risk	Breast feeding not recommended; excretion in milk unknown	C
Fenofibrate	Weigh benefits vs. risk	Breast feeding not recommended; excretion in milk unknown	C
Gemfibrozil	Weigh benefits vs. risk	Breast feeding not recommended; excretion in milk unknown	C
Nicotinic acid	Weigh benefits vs. risk	Breast feed with caution; excretion in milk unknown	C
HMG-CoA reductase inhibitors			
Atorvastatin	Contraindicated	Breast feeding not recommended; excretion in milk unknown	X
Fluvastatin	Contraindicated	Breast feeding not recommended; drug excreted in breast milk	X

Lovastatin	Contraindicated	Breast feeding not recommended; excretion in milk unknown	X
Pravastatin	Contraindicated	Breast feeding not recommended; drug excreted in breast milk	X
Rosuvastatin	Contraindicated	Breast feeding not recommended; excretion in milk unknown	X
Simvastatin	Contraindicated	Breast feeding not recommended; excretion in milk unknown	X

Selective cholesterol absorption inhibitor

Ezetimibe	Weigh benefits vs. risk	Breast feeding not recommended; excretion in milk unknown	C

Natriuretic peptide

Nesiritide	Weigh benefits vs. risk	Breast feeding not recommended; excretion in milk unknown	C

Neuronal and ganglionic blockers

Guanadrel	Use only if clearly needed	Breast feeding not recommended; excretion in milk unknown	B
Guanethidine	Weigh benefits vs. risk	Breast feeding not recommended; drug excreted in breast milk	C
Mecamylamine	Weigh benefits vs. risk	Breast feeding not recommended; excretion in milk unknown	C
Reserpine	Weigh benefits vs. risk	Breast feeding not recommended; drug excreted in breast milk	C
Trimethaphan	Not recommended	Breast feeding not recommended; excretion in milk unknown	D

Vasodilators

Cilostazol	Weigh benefits vs. risk	Breast feeding not recommended; excretion in milk unknown	C
Diazoxide	Weigh benefits vs. risk	Breast feeding not recommended; excretion in milk unknown	C
Epoprostenol	Use only if clearly needed	Breast feeding not recommended; excretion in milk unknown	B
Fenoldopam	Use only if clearly needed	Breast feeding not recommended; excretion in milk unknown	B
Hydralazine	Weigh benefits vs. risk	Breast feeding not recommended; drug excreted in breast milk	C
Isosorbide Dinitrate	Weigh benefits vs. risk	Breast feeding not recommended; excretion in milk unknown	C
Isosorbide Mononitrate	Weigh benefits vs. risk	Breast feeding not recommended; excretion in milk unknown	C
Isoxsuprine	Weigh benefits vs. risk	Breast feeding not recommended; excretion in milk unknown	C
Minoxidil	Weigh benefits vs. risk	Breast feeding not recommended; drug excreted in breast milk	C
Nitroglycerin	Weigh benefits vs. risk	Breast feeding not recommended; excretion in milk unknown	C
Nitroprusside	Weigh benefits vs. risk	Breast feeding not recommended; excretion in milk unknown	C
Papaverine	Weigh benefits vs. risk	Breast feeding not recommended; excretion in milk unknown	C

(continued)

APPENDIX 3 (continued) Guide to Cardiovascular Drugs Used in Pregnancy and with Nursing

Drug	Use in pregnancy	Use during lactation	Classification*
Pentoxifylline	Weigh benefits vs. risk	Breast feeding not recommended; drug excreted in breast milk	C
Tolazoline	Weigh benefits vs. risk	Breast feeding not recommended; excretion in milk unknown	C
Treprostinil	Use only if clearly needed	Breast feeding not recommended; excretion in milk unknown	B

*Pregnancy Categories/U.S. Food and Drug Administration Pregnancy Risk Classification: B, Animal reproduction studies have not demonstrated fetal risk or have not shown an adverse effect (other than a decrease in fertility). However, there are no controlled studies of pregnant women in the first trimester to confirm these findings and no evidence of risk in the later trimesters. C, Animal studies have shown adverse effects (teratogenic or embryocidal), but there are no confirmatory studies in women, or studies in animals and women are not available. Because of the potential risk to the fetus, drugs should be given only if justified by potentially greater benefits. D, Evidence of human fetal risk is available. Despite the risk, benefits from use in pregnant women may be justifiable in select circumstances (e.g., if the drug is needed in a life-threatening situation and/or no other safer acceptable drugs are effective). An appropriate "warning" statement will appear on the labeling. X, Studies in animals and humans have demonstrated fetal abnormalities and/or evidence of fetal risk based on human experience. Thus, the risk of drug use and consequent fetal harm outweighs any potential benefit, and the drug is contraindicated in pregnant women. An appropriate "contraindicated" statement will appear on the labeling.

†Only diltiazem and verapamil are indicated for arrhythmias.

‡The pregnancy category of methyclothiazide has ranged from B to D.

Key: ACE, angiotensin-converting enzyme; BAS, bile acid sequestrants; FAD, fibric acid derivatives; GI, gastrointestinal; HMG-CoA, hydroxymethylglutaryl coenzyme A; IV, intravenously; PO, orally; RAS, renin-angiotensin system; t-PA, tissue-type plasminogen activator.

Source: Adapted from Ngo A, Frishman WH, Elkayam E: Cardiovascular pharmacotherapeutic considerations during pregnancy and lactation, in Frishman WH, Sonnenblick EH (eds): Cardiovascular Pharmacotherapeutics. New York, McGraw-Hill, 1997, p 1309.

APPENDIX 4 Dosing Recommendations of Cardiovascular Drugs in Patients with Hepatic Disease and/or Congestive Heart Failure

Drug	Cirrhosis	CHF
α-Adrenergic antagonists		
Doxazosin	Usual dose with frequent monitoring	Usual dose with frequent monitoring
Phenoxybenzamine	Usual dose with frequent monitoring	Usual dose with frequent monitoring
Phentolamine	Usual dose with frequent monitoring	Usual dose with frequent monitoring
Prazosin	Usual dose with frequent monitoring	Usual dose with frequent monitoring
Terazosin	Usual dose with frequent monitoring	Usual dose with frequent monitoring
α₂-Adrenergic agonists		
Clonidine	Usual dose with frequent monitoring	Usual dose with frequent monitoring
Guanabenz	Initiate with lower dose	Usual dose with frequent monitoring
Guanfacine	Initiate with lower dose	Usual dose with frequent monitoring
Methyldopa	Initiate with lower dose	Usual dose with frequent monitoring
ACE inhibitors		
Benazepril	Usual dose with frequent monitoring	Usual dose with frequent monitoring
Captopril	Usual dose with frequent monitoring	Usual dose with frequent monitoring
Enalapril	Usual dose with frequent monitoring	Usual dose with frequent monitoring
Fosinopril	Usual dose with frequent monitoring	Usual dose with frequent monitoring
Lisinopril	Usual dose with frequent monitoring	Usual dose with frequent monitoring
Moexipril	Dose reduction may be necessary	Usual dose with frequent monitoring
Perindopril	Usual dose with frequent monitoring	Usual dose with frequent monitoring
Quinapril	Usual dose with frequent monitoring	Usual dose with frequent monitoring
Ramipril	Usual dose with frequent monitoring	Usual dose with frequent monitoring
Trandolapril	Initiate with lower dose	Usual dose with frequent monitoring
Angiotensin II receptor antagonists		
Candesartan	Usual dose with frequent monitoring	Usual dose with frequent monitoring
Eprosartan	Usual dose with frequent monitoring	Usual dose with frequent monitoring
Irbesartan	Usual dose with frequent monitoring	Usual dose with frequent monitoring
Losartan	Initiate with lower dose	Usual dose with frequent monitoring
Olmesartan	Usual dose with frequent monitoring	Usual dose with frequent monitoring

(continued)

APPENDIX 4 *(continued)* Dosing Recommendations of Cardiovascular Drugs in Patients with Hepatic Disease and/or Congestive Heart Failure

Drug	Cirrhosis	CHF
Telmisartan	Dose reduction may be necessary; consider alternative treatment	Dose reduction may be necessary
Valsartan	Usual dose with frequent monitoring	Usual dose with frequent monitoring
Antiarrhythmics		
Adenosine	Usual dose with frequent monitoring	Usual dose with frequent monitoring
Amiodarone	Usual dose with frequent monitoring	Usual dose with frequent monitoring
Atropine	Usual dose with frequent monitoring	Usual dose with frequent monitoring
Bretylium	Usual dose with frequent monitoring	Usual dose with frequent monitoring
Disopyramide	Initiate with lower dose	Dose reduction may be necessary
Dofetilide	Usual dose with frequent monitoring	Usual dose with frequent monitoring
Flecainide	Use lower dose or alternative treatment	Dose reduction may be necessary
Ibutilide	Usual dose with frequent monitoring	Usual dose with frequent monitoring
Lidocaine	Initiate with lower dose	Initiate with lower dose
Mexiletine	Initiate with lower dose	Initiate with lower dose
Moricizine	Use lower dose or alternative treatment	Dose reduction may be necessary
Procainamide	Dose reduction may be necessary	Dose reduction may be necessary
Propafenone	Initiate with lower dose	Contraindicated in uncontrolled CHF
Quinidine	Reduce maintenance dose and monitor serum concentration*	Contraindicated in uncontrolled CHF
Sotalol	Usual dose with frequent monitoring	Contraindicated in uncontrolled CHF
Tocainide	Avoid loading dose; limit dose to 1200 mg/d	Dose reduction may be necessary
Antithrombotics		
Anticoagulants		
Argatroban	Initiate with lower dose	Usual dose with frequent monitoring
Bivalirudin	Usual dose with frequent monitoring	Usual dose with frequent monitoring
Dalteparin	Usual dose with frequent monitoring	Usual dose with frequent monitoring
Danaparoid	Usual dose with frequent monitoring	Usual dose with frequent monitoring
Enoxaparin	Usual dose with frequent monitoring	Usual dose with frequent monitoring
Fondaparinux	Usual dose with frequent monitoring	Usual dose with frequent monitoring

(continued)

Drug		
Heparin	Dose reduction may be necessary; titrate dose based on coagulation test result	Usual dose with frequent monitoring
Lepirudin	Usual dose with frequent monitoring	Usual dose with frequent monitoring
Tinzaparin	Usual dose with frequent monitoring	Usual dose with frequent monitoring
Warfarin	Initiate at lower dose	Dose reduction may be necessary
Antiplatelets		
Anagrelide	Dose reduction may be necessary; weigh benefits vs. risk when LFT >1.5 times the upper limit of normal	Weigh benefits vs. risk; use of anagrelide may cause CHF
Aspirin	Usual dose with frequent monitoring	Usual dose with frequent monitoring
Dipyridamole	Reduce dose with biliary obstruction	Usual dose with frequent monitoring
Ticlopidine	Contraindicated	Usual dose with frequent monitoring
Clopidogrel	Usual dose with frequent monitoring	Usual dose with frequent monitoring
Abciximab	Usual dose with frequent monitoring	Usual dose with frequent monitoring
Eptifibatide	Usual dose with frequent monitoring	Usual dose with frequent monitoring
Tirofiban	Initiate at lower dose	Usual dose with frequent monitoring
Thrombolytics		
Alteplase	Usual dose with frequent monitoring	Usual dose with frequent monitoring
Anistreplase	Dose reduction may be necessary	Usual dose with frequent monitoring
Streptokinase	Dose reduction may be necessary	Usual dose with frequent monitoring
Urokinase	Dose reduction may be necessary	Usual dose with frequent monitoring
Reteplase	Usual dose with frequent monitoring	Usual dose with frequent monitoring
Tenecteplase	Use usual dose with caution; risk of bleeding may increase	Usual dose with frequent monitoring
β-Adrenergic blockers		
Nonselective		
Nadolol	Usual dose with frequent monitoring	Usual dose with frequent monitoring
Propranolol	Initiate with lower dose	Usual dose with frequent monitoring
Sotalol	Usual dose with frequent monitoring	Usual dose with frequent monitoring

APPENDIX 4 *(continued)* Dosing Recommendations of Cardiovascular Drugs in Patients with Hepatic Disease and/or Congestive Heart Failure

Drug	Cirrhosis	CHF
Timolol	Initiate with lower dose	Usual dose with frequent monitoring
β₁ Selective		
Atenolol	Usual dose with frequent monitoring	Usual dose with frequent monitoring
Betaxolol	Usual dose with frequent monitoring	Usual dose with frequent monitoring
Bisoprolol	Initiate with lower dose	Usual dose with frequent monitoring
Esmolol	Usual dose with frequent monitoring	Usual dose with frequent monitoring
Metoprolol	Dose reduction may be necessary	Usual dose with frequent monitoring
With ISA: nonselective		
Carteolol	Usual dose with frequent monitoring	Usual dose with frequent monitoring
Penbutolol	Dose reduction may be necessary	Usual dose with frequent monitoring
Pindolol	Dose reduction may be necessary	Usual dose with frequent monitoring
With ISA: β₁ selective		
Acebutolol	Usual dose with frequent monitoring	Usual dose with frequent monitoring
Dual acting		
Carvedilol	Initiate with lower dose	Initiate at lower dose; contraindicated in severely decompensated CHF
Labetalol	Dose reduction may be necessary	Usual dose with frequent monitoring
Calcium channel blockers		
Amlodipine	Initiate with lower dose	Usual dose with frequent monitoring
Bepridil	Dose reduction may be necessary	Contraindicated in uncompensated cardiac insufficiency
Diltiazem	Dose reduction may be necessary	Usual dose with frequent monitoring
Felodipine	Dose reduction may be necessary	Usual dose with frequent monitoring
Isradipine	Dose reduction may be necessary	Usual dose with frequent monitoring
Nicardipine	Initiate with lower dose	Usual dose with frequent monitoring
Nifedipine	Dose reduction may be necessary	Usual dose with frequent monitoring
Nimodipine	Initiate with lower dose	Usual dose with frequent monitoring

Nisoldipine	Initiate with lower dose
Verapamil	Initiate with lower dose
	Usual dose with frequent monitoring
	Avoid in patients with severe left ventricular dysfunction
Diuretics	
Loop	
Bumetanide, ethacrynic acid, furosemide, torsemide	May precipitate hepatic coma; dose reduction is probably not necessary; titrate dosage based on clinical response
	Usual dose with frequent monitoring
Thiazide	
Bendroflumethiazide, benzthiazide, chlorothiazide, hydrochlorothiazide, hydroflumethiazide, methyclothiazide, polythiazide, quinethazone	May precipitate hepatic coma; diuretic effect is decreased in patients with renal insufficiency (CrCl <30 mL/min); dosage adjustment is probably not required in HI; titrate dosage based on clinical response
	Usual dose with frequent monitoring
Trichlormethiazide	
Indapamide	Dose reduction may be necessary
	Usual dose with frequent monitoring
Metolazone	May precipitate hepatic coma; diuretic effect is preserved in patients with renal insufficiency; dosage adjustment is probably not required in HI
	Usual dose with frequent monitoring
Potassium sparing	
Amiloride	Dose reduction may be necessary
Eplerenone	Usual dose with frequent monitoring
Spironolactone	Usual dose with frequent monitoring
	Usual dose with frequent monitoring
Triamterene	Usual dose with frequent monitoring
	Usual dose with frequent monitoring
Endothelin receptor antagonist	
Bosentan	Caution should be exercised during the use of bosentan in patients with mildly impaired liver function; bosentan generally should be avoided in patients with moderate or severe HI
	Usual dose with frequent monitoring

(continued)

APPENDIX 4 *(continued)* Dosing Recommendations of Cardiovascular Drugs in Patients with Hepatic Disease and/or Congestive Heart Failure

Drug	Cirrhosis	CHF
Inotropic agents and vasopressors		
Amrinone (inamrinone)	Dose reduction may be necessary	Usual dose with frequent monitoring
Digoxin, dobutamine	Usual dose with frequent monitoring	Usual dose with frequent monitoring
Dopamine, milrinone	Usual dose with frequent monitoring	Usual dose with frequent monitoring; initiate dopamine at lower dose in patients with chronic heart failure
Midodrine	Usual dose with frequent monitoring	Usual dose with frequent monitoring
Norepinephrine, epinephrine	Usual dose with frequent monitoring	Usual dose with frequent monitoring
Isoproterenol, metaraminol	Usual dose with frequent monitoring	Usual dose with frequent monitoring
Methoxamine, phenylephrine	Usual dose with frequent monitoring	Usual dose with frequent monitoring
Lipid lowering		
BAS		
Cholestyramine	Contraindicated in total biliary obstruction	Usual dose with frequent monitoring
Colestipol	Contraindicated in total biliary obstruction	Usual dose with frequent monitoring
Colesevelam	Contraindicated in total biliary obstruction	Usual dose with frequent monitoring
FAD		
Clofibrate	Contraindicated in clinically significant hepatic dysfunction	Usual dose with frequent monitoring
Fenofibrate	Contraindicated in clinically significant hepatic dysfunction, including primary biliary cirrhosis and in patients with unexplained persistent transaminase elevation	Unknown
Gemfibrozil	Contraindicated in clinically significant hepatic dysfunction, including primary biliary cirrhosis	Unknown
HMG-CoA reductase inhibitors Atorvastatin, fluvastatin, lovastatin, pravastatin, rosuvastatin, simvastatin	Start at lowest dose and titrate cautiously; contra-indicated in patients with active liver disease or unexplained persistent transaminase elevation	Usual dose with frequent monitoring
Nicotinic acid	Use with caution; contraindicated in patients with active liver disease or unexplained persistent transaminase elevation	Usual dose with frequent monitoring

Selective cholesterol absorption inhibitors

Ezetimibe — Usual dose with frequent monitoring

Natriuretic peptide

Nesiritide — Not recommended in patients with moderate or severe HI

Cirrhotic patients with ascites and avid sodium retention were shown to have blunted natriuretic response to low-dose brain natriuretic peptide — Usual dose with frequent monitoring

Neuronal and ganglionic blockers

Guanadrel — Usual dose with frequent monitoring — Contraindicated in frank CHF

Guanethidine — Dose reduction may be necessary — Contraindicated in frank CHF

Mecamylamine — Usual dose with frequent monitoring — Usual dose with frequent monitoring

Reserpine — Dose reduction may be necessary — Usual dose with frequent monitoring

Trimethaphan — Dose reduction may be necessary — Contraindicated in severe cardiac disease

Vasodilators

Alprostadil — Usual dose with frequent monitoring — Usual dose with frequent monitoring

Cilostazol — Usual dose with frequent monitoring — Contraindicated

Diazoxide — Dose reduction may be necessary — Contraindicated in uncompensated CHF

Epoprostenol — Usual dose with frequent monitoring — Contraindicated in severe left ventricular systolic dysfunction

Fenoldopam — Usual dose with frequent monitoring — Usual dose with frequent monitoring

Hydralazine — Dose reduction may be necessary — Higher doses have been used

Isosorbide dinitrate — Use lower dose; avoid in severe HI — Used in combination with hydralazine

Isosorbide mononitrate — Caution in severe HI — Avoid in acute CHF

Isoxsuprine — Dose reduction may be necessary — Usual dose with frequent monitoring

Minoxidil — Usual dose with frequent monitoring — Usual dose with frequent monitoring

Nitroglycerin — Dose reduction may be necessary; avoid in severe HI — Usual dose with frequent monitoring

Sodium nitroprusside — Initiate with lower dose — Usual dose with frequent monitoring

Papaverine — Dose reduction may be necessary — Usual dose with frequent monitoring

(continued)

727

APPENDIX 4 *(continued)* Dosing Recommendations of Cardiovascular Drugs in Patients with Hepatic Disease and/or Congestive Heart Failure

Drug	Cirrhosis	CHF
Pentoxifylline	Usual dose with frequent monitoring	Unknown
Sildenafil	Initiate with lower dose	Usual dose with frequent monitoring
Tolazoline	Unknown	Unknown
Treprostinil	Reduce initial dose in patients with mild-moderate HI; use of treprostinil has not been studied in patients with severe HI.	Usual dose with frequent monitoring

*Due to an increased volume of distribution, a larger loading dose of quinidine may be indicated.

Key: ACE, angiotensin-converting enzyme; BAS, bile acid sequestrants; CHF, congestive heart failure; CrCl, creatine clearance; FAD, fibric acid derivatives; HMG-CoA, hydroxymethylglutaryl coenzyme A; HI, hepatic impairment; ISA, intrinsic sympathomimetic activity; LFT, liver function test.

Source: Adapted from Frishman WH, Sokol SI: Cardiovascular drug therapy in patients with intrinsic hepatic disease and impaired hepatic function secondary to congestive heart failure, in Frishman WH, Sonnenblick EH (eds): *Cardiovascular Pharmacotherapeutics.* New York, McGraw-Hill, 1997, p 1561.

APPENDIX 5 Dose Adjustment in Patients with Renal Insufficiency

Drug	CrCl 30–60 mL/min	CrCl <30 mL/min	Dialyzability (hemodialysis)
α-Adrenergic antagonists			
Doxazosin	Use usual dose	Use usual dose	No
Phenoxybenzamine	Use usual dose	Use usual dose	No
Phentolamine	Use usual dose	Use usual dose	No
Prazosin	Use usual dose	Start with low dose and titrate based on response	No
Terazosin	Use usual dose	Use usual dose	No
α₂-Adrenergic agonists			
Clonidine	Use usual dose	Start with low dose and titrate based on response	No
Guanabenz	Use usual dose	Use usual dose	Unknown
Guanfacine	Use usual dose	Start with low dose and titrate based on response	No
Methyldopa	Use usual dose	Start with low dose and titrate based on response	Yes
ACE inhibitors			
Benazepril	Use usual dose	Start with low dose and titrate based on response	No*
Captopril	Start with low dose and titrate based on response	Start with low dose and titrate based on response	Yes
Enalapril	Use usual dose	Start with low dose and titrate based on response	Yes
Fosinopril	Use usual dose	Start with low dose and titrate based on response	No
Lisinopril	Use usual dose	Start with low dose and titrate based on response	Yes

(continued)

APPENDIX 5 *(continued)* Dose Adjustment in Patients with Renal Insufficiency

Drug	CrCl 30–60 mL/min	CrCl <30 mL/min	Dialyzability (hemodialysis)
Moexipril	For patients with CrCl ≥40 mL/min, start with low dose and titrate based on response	Start with low dose and titrate based on response	Unknown
Perindopril	Start with low dose and titrate based on response	The use of this drug is not recommended because of significant perindoprilat accumulation	Yes
Quinapril	Start with low dose and titrate based on response	Start with low dose and titrate based on response	No
Ramipril	For patients with CrCl <40 mL/min, start with low dose and titrate based on response	Start with low dose and titrate based on response; up to a maximum of 5 mg/d	Unknown
Trandolapril	Use usual dose	Start with low dose and titrate based on response	Yes (trandolaprilat)
Angiotensin II receptor blockers			
Candesartan	Use usual dose	Start with low dose and titrate based on response	No
Eprosartan	Use usual dose	Start with low dose and titrate based on response	No
Irbesartan	Use usual dose	Use usual dose	No
Losartan	Use usual dose	Use usual dose	No
Olmesartan	Use usual dose	Start with low dose and titrate based on response; maximum dose should not exceed 20 mg	Unknown
Telmisartan	Use usual dose	Use usual dose with caution	No
Valsartan	Use usual dose	Use usual dose with caution	Unknown (probably no)
Antiarrhythmic agents			
Adenosine	Use usual dose	Use usual dose	No
Atropine	Use usual dose with caution	Use usual dose with caution	No

Class Ia		
Disopyramide	Decrease loading dose by 25% to 50% Decrease maintenance dose by 25% or give 100 mg (nonsustained release) q6–8 h	No*
Procainamide	Increase dosing interval to q4–6 h	Decrease loading dose by 50% to 75% Decrease maintenance dose by 50% to 75% or give 100 mg (nonsustained release) q12–24h Increase dosing interval to q8–24h	Yes (give maintenance dose after dialysis or supplement with 250 mg post hemodialysis)
Quinidine	Use usual dose	Use usual dose with caution; decrease maintenance dose by 25% if CrCl <10 mL/min	Yes (give maintenance dose after dialysis or supplement with 200 mg post hemodialysis)
Class Ib		
Lidocaine	Use usual dose	Use usual dose with caution	No
Mexiletine	Use usual dose	Reduce dose if CrCl <10 mL/min	No
Tocainide	Use usual dose	Decrease 25–50% or increase dosing interval to q24h	Yes (give maintenance dose after dialysis or supplement with 25% of maintenance dose post hemodialysis)
Class Ic		
Flecainide	Use usual dose	Initiate with 100 mg q24h or 50 mg q12h; titrate based on response	No
Moricizine	Use usual dose	Start with low dose and titrate based on response	Unknown
Propafenone	Use usual dose	Use usual dose with caution	No

(continued)

APPENDIX 5 *(continued)* Dose Adjustment in Patients with Renal Insufficiency

Drug	CrCl 30–60 mL/min	CrCl <30 mL/min	Dialyzability (hemodialysis)
Class II (β-adrenergic antagonists)			
Acebutolol	Decrease 50%	Decrease 75%	Yes—acebutolol and diacetolol
Atenolol	Use usual dose with caution	Up to a maximum of 50 mg q24–48h	No
Betaxolol	Use usual dose with caution	Up to a maximum of 20 mg q24h	No
Bisoprolol	Use usual dose with caution	Start with low dose and titrate based on response	No
Carteolol	Increase dosing interval to q48h	Increase dosing interval to q48–72h	Unknown
Carvedilol	Use usual dose with caution	Start with low dose and titrate based on response	No
Esmolol	Use usual dose	Use usual dose	No
Labetalol	Use usual dose	Use usual dose	No
Metoprolol	Use usual dose	Use usual dose	No
Nadolol	Use usual dose with caution	Increase dosing interval to q48–72h	Yes
Penbutolol	Use usual dose	Use usual dose	No
Pindolol	Use usual dose	Use usual dose	Unknown
Propranolol	Use usual dose	Use usual dose	No
Timolol	Use usual dose	Use usual dose	No
Class III			
Amiodarone	Use usual dose	Use usual dose	No
Bretylium	Decrease 50%	Decrease 50–75%	No
Dofetilide	Start with lower dose and titrate based on response	Start with lower dose and titrate based on response; dofetilide is contraindicated in patients with CrCl of <20 mL/min	Unknown
Ibutilide	Use usual dose	Use usual dose with caution	Unknown (probably no)
Sotalol	Increase dosing interval to q24h	Increase dosing interval to q36–48h; individualize dosage for patients with	Yes (give maintenance dose after dialysis or supplement

		CrCl <10 mL/min	with 80 mg post hemodialysis
Class IV (calcium antagonists†)			
Amlodipine	Use usual dose	Use usual dose with caution	No
Bepridil	Use usual dose	Use usual dose with caution	No
Diltiazem	Use usual dose	Use usual dose with caution	No
Felodipine	Use usual dose	Use usual dose	No
Isradipine	Use usual dose	Use usual dose with caution	No
Nicardipine	Use usual dose	Use usual dose; titrate dose carefully	No
Nifedipine	Use usual dose	Use usual dose	No
Nimodipine	Use usual dose	Use usual dose	No
Nisoldipine	Use usual dose	Use usual dose	No
Verapamil	Use usual dose	Use usual dose with caution	No
Antithrombotic agents			
Antiplatelet agents			
Abciximab	Use usual dose	Use usual dose with caution	No
Anagrelide	Weigh benefit vs. risk when SCr ≥2 mg/dL	Weigh benefit vs. risk when SCr ≥2 mg/dL	Unknown
Aspirin	Use usual dose	Use usual dose with caution	Yes
Clopidogrel	Use usual dose	Use usual dose	No
Dipyridamole	Use usual dose	Use usual dose	No
Eptifibatide	Use lower dose if SCr >2 mg/dL	Contraindicated if SCr >4 mg/dL	Yes
Ticlopidine	Use usual dose	Use with caution; dose reduction may be required	No
Tirofiban	Use usual dose with caution	Decrease 50%	Yes
Anticoagulants			
Argatroban	Use usual dose	Use usual dose	Unknown
Bivalirudin	Reduce infusion dose by ≈20%	Reduce infusion dose by 60–90%	Yes (≈25% removed)

(continued)

APPENDIX 5 (continued) Dose Adjustment in Patients with Renal Insufficiency

Drug	CrCl 30–60 mL/min	CrCl <30 mL/min	Dialyzability (hemodialysis)
Dalteparin	Use usual dose	Use usual dose with caution; specific recommendations on dosage adjustments are not available	No
Danaparoid	Use usual dose	Use usual dose with caution if SCr ≥2 mg/dL	No
Enoxaparin	Use usual dose	Use with caution; dose reduction may be required (decrease 20–30%)	No
Fondaparinux	Use usual dose with caution	Contraindicated	Yes
Heparin	Use usual dose	Use usual dose with caution	No
Lepirudin	Bolus dose: 0.2 mg/kg; infusion rate: 30–50% of usual dose	Bolus dose: 0.2 mg/kg; infusion rate: 15% of usual dose; contraindicated if SCr >6 mg/dL	Yes
Tinzaparin	Use usual dose	Use usual dose with caution; specific recommendations on dosage adjustments are not available	No
Warfarin	Use usual dose	Use usual dose with caution	No
Thrombolytic agents			
Alteplase	Use usual dose with caution	Use usual dose with caution	No
Anistreplase	Use usual dose with caution	Use usual dose with caution	No
Reteplase	Use usual dose with caution	Use usual dose with caution	No
Streptokinase	Use usual dose with caution	Use usual dose with caution	No
Tenecteplase	Use usual dose with caution	Use usual dose with caution	No
Urokinase	Use usual dose with caution	Use usual dose with caution	No
Diuretics (contraindicated in anuric patients)			
Loop diuretics			
Bumetanide	Use usual dose	Use usual dose with caution	No
Ethacrynic Acid	Use usual dose	Use usual dose with caution	No
Furosemide	Use usual dose	Use usual dose with caution	No

Torsemide	Use usual dose	Use usual dose with caution	No
Thiazide diuretics			
Chlorthalidone	Use usual dose with caution	Ineffective	No
Hydrochlorothiazide and similar agents	Use usual dose with caution	Ineffective	No
Indapamide	Use usual dose with caution	Ineffective if CrCl <15 mL/min	No
Metolazone	Use usual dose with caution	Use usual dose with caution	No
Potassium-sparing diuretics			
Amiloride	Use usual dose with caution	Contraindicated	Unknown
Eplerenone	Use usual dose	Use usual dose	No
Spironolactone	Use usual dose with caution	Contraindicated	No
Triamterene	Use usual dose with caution	Contraindicated	Unknown
Endothelin receptor antagonist			
Bosentan	Use usual dose	Use usual dose	Unknown (probably no)
Inotropic agents and vasopressors			
Amrinone (inamrinone)	Start with low dose and titrate based on response	Start with low dose and titrate based on response	No
Digoxin	Use usual dose and titrate based on response	Start with low dose, many patients only need a dose q48–72 h; if loading dose is indicated, decrease 25%	No
Dobutamine	Use usual dose and titrate based on response	Use usual dose and titrate based on response	Unknown
Dopamine	Use usual dose and titrate based on response	Use usual dose and titrate based on response	No
Epinephrine	Use usual dose with caution	Use usual dose with caution	Unknown
Isoproterenol	Use usual dose with caution	Use usual dose with caution	Unknown
Metaraminol	Start with low dose and titrate to response	Start with low dose and titrate to response	Unknown

(continued)

APPENDIX 5 (continued) Dose Adjustment in Patients with Renal Insufficiency

Drug	CrCl 30–60 mL/min	CrCl <30 mL/min	Dialyzability (hemodialysis)
Methoxamine	Use usual dose with caution	Use usual dose with caution	Unknown
Midodrine	Start with low dose and titrate based on response	Start with low dose and titrate based on response	Yes—midodrine and desglymidodrine
Milrinone	Decrease 25–50%; start with low dose and titrate based on response	Decrease 50–75%; start with low dose and titrate based on response	Unknown
Norepinephrine	Use usual dose with caution	Use usual dose with caution	Yes
Phenylephrine	Use usual dose with caution	Use usual dose with caution	Unknown
Lipid-lowering agents			
BAS			
Cholestyramine, colestipol, colesevelam	Possibility of hyperchloremic acidosis is increased in patients with renal insufficiency; use usual dose with caution		
FAD			
Clofibrate	Increase dosing interval to q6–12 h	Increase dosing interval to q12–24 h; avoid use if CrCl <10 mL/min	No
Fenofibrate	Start with low dose and titrate based on response	Start with low dose and titrate based on response	No
Gemfibrozil	Use usual dose with caution	Use usual dose with caution	No
HMG-CoA reductase inhibitors			
Atorvastatin	Use usual dose	Use usual dose	No
Fluvastatin	Use usual dose	Use usual dose with caution	No
Lovastatin	Use usual dose	Use usual dose with caution	No
Pravastatin	Use usual dose	Use usual dose with caution	No
Rosuvastatin	Use usual dose	Start with low dose (5 mg QD) and titrate; not to exceed 10 mg	Unknown
Simvastatin	Use usual dose	Start with low dose and titrate based on response	No

736

Drug			
Nicotinic acid	Start with low dose and titrate based on response; use with caution	Start with low dose and titrate based on response; use with caution	Unknown
Selective cholesterol absorption inhibitor			
Ezetimibe	Use usual dose	Use usual dose	Unknown (probably no)
Natriuretic peptide			
Nesiritide	Use usual dose	Use usual dose with caution	Unknown (probably no)
Neuronal and ganglionic blockers			
Guanadrel	Increase dosing interval to q24 h; dosage increments should be made cautiously at intervals ≥7 d	Increase dosing interval to q48 h; dosage increments should be made cautiously at intervals	Unknown (probably no)
Guanethidine	Start with low dose and titrate based on response	Start with low dose and titrate based on response; use with caution	Unknown
Mecamylamine	Start with low dose and titrate based on response	Start with low dose and titrate based on response; use with caution	Unknown
Reserpine	Use usual dose	Use usual dose with caution; avoid use if CrCl <10 mL/min	No
Trimethaphan	Start with low dose and titrate based on response	Start with low dose and titrate based on response; use with caution	Unknown
Vasodilators			
Alprostadil	Individualize dose	Individualize dose	Unknown
Cilostazol	Use usual dose	Use usual dose with caution; patients on hemodialysis have not been studied	No
Diazoxide	Start with low dose and titrate based on response	Start with low dose and titrate based on response; use with caution	No
Epoprostenol	Individualize dose	Individualize dose	Unknown
Fenoldopam	Individualize dose	Individualize dose	Unknown
Hydralazine	Increase dosing interval to q6–8 h	Increase dosing interval to q8–24 h	No

(continued)

APPENDIX 5 *(continued)* Dose Adjustment in Patients with Renal Insufficiency

Drug	CrCl 30–60 mL/min	CrCl <30 mL/min	Dialyzability (hemodialysis)
Isosorbide dinitrate	Use usual dose	Start with low dose and titrate based on response; use with caution	Unknown
Isosorbide mononitrate	Use usual dose	Use usual dose with caution	No
Isoxsuprine	Start with low dose and titrate based on response	Start with low dose and titrate based on response; use with caution	Unknown
Minoxidil	Use usual dose	Start with low dose and titrate based on response	No
Nitroglycerin	Use usual dose	Use usual dose with caution	No
Nitroprusside	Start with low dose and titrate based on response; use with caution	Start with low dose and titrate based on response; use with caution	Yes
Papaverine	Use usual dose	Use usual dose with caution	Unknown
Pentoxifylline	Use usual dose	Use usual dose with caution	Unknown
Sildenafil	Use usual dose	Start with low dose and titrate based on response	No
Tolazoline	Start with low dose and titrate based on response; use with caution; specific dosing guidelines are lacking	Start with low dose and titrate based on response; use with caution; specific dosing guidelines are lacking	Unknown
Treprostinil	Use with caution; no studies have been performed in patients with renal insufficiency	Use with caution; no studies have been performed in patients with renal insufficiency	Unknown

*Hemodialysis does not remove appreciable amounts of this drug. However, dialysis may be considered in overdosed patients with severe renal impairment.
†Only diltiazem and verapamil are indicated for arrhythmias.
Key: ACE, angiotensin-converting enzyme; BAS, bile acid sequestrants; CrCl, creatinine clearance; FAD, fibric acid derivatives; HMG-CoA, hydroxymethylglutaryl coenzyme A; SCr, serum creatinine.
Source: Adapted from Feinfeld DA: Renal considerations in cardiovascular drug therapy, in Frishman WH, Sonnenblick EH (eds): *Cardiovascular Pharmacotherapeutics.* New York, McGraw-Hill, 1997, p 1283.

APPENDIX 6 Selected Cardiovascular Medications and Gender Issues

Drug	Evidence for efficacy in women	Considerations when treating women
Antiplatelet drugs		
Aspirin	Primary prevention: U.S. Nurses' Cohort shows decreased MI*	Women have higher rates of hemorrhagic stroke than do men
	Secondary CAD prevention: decreases reinfarction†	Physician's Health Study showed an increased risk of bleeding when on aspirin; increased risk of bleeding at term in pregnancy; present in breast milk
Glycoprotein IIb/IIIa antagonists	Effective in women undergoing PTCA	Women have higher risk than men with PTCA, but benefit as much from treatment
Agents that affect blood pressure		
ACE inhibitors	Post-MI: decreased mortality†	Cough is 2-3 times greater in women; increased fetal abnormalities possible; present in breast milk
	CHF: decreased mortality†	
Angiotensin II receptor blockers		Increased fetal abnormalities possible
Beta blockers	Antihypertension: effective in preventing MI, CVA, and death in women†	Present in breast milk; blood levels of propranolol may be higher in men
	Post-MI: decreases mortality†	
	Increased risk of MI in women†	
Calcium blockers	Increased effect of amlodipine in women in reducing blood pressure†	Edema may be more common in women; verapamil clearance may be greater in women than in men; present in breast milk
Clonidine	No data about efficacy in women	Inability to achieve orgasm; possible decreased craving for tobacco more common in women†

(continued)

739

APPENDIX 6 (continued) Selected Cardiovascular Medications and Gender Issues

Drug	Evidence for efficacy in women	Considerations when treating women
Thiazide diuretics	Decreased CVA, MI, death†	Decreased urinary calcium excretion; women have greater increase in risk of gout; acute pulmonary edema and allergic interstitial
		Pneumonitis is more common in women; excreted in breast milk
Guanethidine		Orthostatic hypotension more common in women
Hydralazine	Effective in hypertension in pregnancy and peripartum	SLE more common in women than in men; present in breast milk
Methyldopa	Often preferred in pregnancy for treating hypertension	Painful breast enlargement; decreased libido
Nitrates	Decreased mortality after MI†	Potential for difference in metabolism in women
Antiarrhythmic agents		
Disopyramide	No data looking at efficacy in women	Complication of torsade de pointes more frequent in women†
Procainamide	No gender-specific data available	Drug-induced SLE more common in women
Quinidine	No sex-specific data available	Torsade de pointes more common in women; clearance may be faster in women; present in breast milk
Conjugated estrogens	Increased HDL cholesterol decreases total cholesterol and LDL cholesterol	Need for progestin in women with intact uterus to prevent endometrial abnormalities
	Post-MI: not effective*	
	Primary CAD prevention: ineffective	

Hypolipidemic agents		
Colestipol	No effect on primary prevention†	
Clofibrate	Effective in secondary prevention in women†	
HMG-CoA Reductase Inhibitors	Primary and secondary prevention Possible efficacy in women† Decreases cholesterol and slows plaque progression without respect to sex	Gastrointestinal side effects more common in women
Nicotine preparations	Gum equally effective in women† Patch effective in women†	Gum may suppress weight gain; not recommended in pregnancy

*Studies of efficacy in women.

†Studies of efficacy in men and women, with analysis by sex.

Key: ACE, angiotensin-converting enzyme; CAD, coronary artery disease; CHF, congestive heart failure; CVA, cerebrovascular accident; HDL, high-density lipoprotein; HMG-CoA, hydroxymethylglutaryl coenzyme A; LDL, low-density lipoprotein; MI, myocardial infarction; PTCA, percutaneous transluminal coronary angioplasty; SLE, systemic lupus erythematosus.

Source: Adapted from Charney P, Meyer BR, Frishman WH, et al: Gender, race and genetic issues in cardiovascular pharmacotherapy, in Frishman WH, Sonnenblick EH (eds): *Cardiovascular Pharmacotherapeutics.* New York, McGraw-Hill, 1997, p 1350.

APPENDIX 7 Pharmacokinetic Changes, Routes of Elimination, and Dosage Adjustments of Selected Cardiovascular Drugs in the Elderly

Drug	$t_{1/2}$	V_D	Cl	Primary routes of elimination	Dosage adjustment
α-Adrenergic antagonists					
Doxazosin	↑	↑	↑*	Hepatic	Initiate at lowest dose; titrate to response
Prazosin	↑	—	—	Hepatic	Initiate at lowest dose; titrate to response
Terazosin	↑	—	—	Hepatic	Initiate at lowest dose; titrate to response
α₂-Adrenergic agonists					
Clonidine	—	—	—	Hepatic/renal	Initiate at lowest dose; titrate to response
Guanabenz	↑	—	—	Hepatic	Initiate at lowest dose; titrate to response
Guanfacine	—	—	↓	Hepatic/renal	Initiate at lowest dose; titrate to response
Methyldopa	—	—	—	Hepatic	Initiate at lowest dose; titrate to response
ACE inhibitors					
Benazepril	↑	—	↓	Renal	No initial dosage adjustment is needed
Captopril	NS	—	↓	Renal	Initiate at lowest dose; titrate to response
Enalapril	—	—	—	Renal	Initiate at lowest dose; titrate to response
Fosinopril	—	NS	—	Hepatic/renal	No initial dosage adjustment is needed
Lisinopril	↑	—	↓	Renal	Initiate at lowest dose; titrate to response
Moexipril	—	—	—	Hepatic/renal	Initiate at lowest dose; titrate to response
Perindopril	—	—	—	Renal	Initiate at lowest dose; titrate to response
Quinapril	—	—	—	Renal	Initiate at lowest dose; titrate to response
Ramipril	—	—	—	Renal	Initiate at lowest dose; titrate to response
Trandolapril	—	—	—	Hepatic/renal	Initiate at lowest dose; titrate to response
Angiotensin II receptor blockers					
Candesartan	—	—	—	Hepatic/renal	No initial dosage adjustment is needed
Eprosartan	NS	—	—	Hepatic/biliary/renal	No initial dosage adjustment is needed
Irbesartan	—	—	—	Hepatic	No initial dosage adjustment is needed
Losartan	—	—	—	Hepatic	No initial dosage adjustment is needed
Olmesartan	—	—	—	Renal/biliary	No initial dosage adjustment is needed

Telmisartan	—	←	Hepatic/biliary	No initial dosage adjustment is needed
Valsartan	—	—	Hepatic	No initial dosage adjustment is needed
Antiarrhythmic agents				
Class I				
Disopyramide	←	→	Renal	Initiate at lowest dose; titrate to response
Flecainide	←	←	Hepatic/renal	Initiate at lowest dose; titrate to response
Lidocaine	←	NS	Hepatic	Initiate at lowest dose; titrate to response
Mexiletine	—	—	Hepatic	Initiate at lowest dose; titrate to response
Moricizine	—	→	Hepatic	Initiate at lowest dose; titrate to response
Procainamide	—	—	Renal	Initiate at lowest dose; titrate to response
Propafenone	—	NS	Hepatic	Initiate at lowest dose; titrate to response
Quinidine	←	→	Hepatic	Initiate at lowest dose; titrate to response
Tocainide	←	→	Hepatic/renal	Initiate at lowest dose; titrate to response
Class II (see Beta blockers)				
Class III				
Amiodarone	—	—	Hepatic/biliary	Initiate at lowest dose; titrate to response
Bretylium	—	—	Renal	Initiate at lowest dose; titrate to response
Dofetilide	—	—	Renal	Adjust dose based on renal function
Ibutilide	—	—	Hepatic	No adjustment needed
Sotalol	—	—	Renal	Adjust dose based on renal function
Class IV (see Calcium channel blockers)				
Other antiarrhythmics				
Adenosine	—	—	Erythrocytes/vascular endothelial cells	No adjustment needed
Atropine	—	—	Hepatic/renal	Use usual dose with caution

(continued)

APPENDIX 7 *(continued)* Pharmacokinetic Changes, Routes of Elimination, and Dosage Adjustments of Selected Cardiovascular Drugs in the Elderly

Drug	$t_{1/2}$	V_D	Cl	Primary routes of elimination	Dosage adjustment
Antithrombotics					
Anticoagulants					
Argatroban	—	—	—	Hepatic/biliary	Use usual dose with caution
Bivalirudin	—	—	—	Renal/proteolytic cleavage	Adjust dose based on renal function
Dalteparin	—	—	—	Renal	Use usual dose with caution
Danaparoid	NS	NS	NS	Renal	Use usual dose with caution
Enoxaparin	←	—	→	Renal	Use usual dose with caution
Fondaparinux	—	—	—	Renal	Use usual dose with caution
Heparin	←	—	→	Hepatic/reticuloendothelial system	Use usual dose with caution
Lepirudin	←	—	→	Renal	Adjust dose based on renal function
Tinzaparin	—	—	—	Renal	Use usual dose with caution
Warfarin	NS	NS	NS	Hepatic	Initiate at lowest dose; titrate to response
Antiplatelets					
Abciximab	—	—	—	Unknown	Use usual dose with caution
Anagrelide	—	—	→	Hepatic/renal	Use usual dose with caution
Aspirin	NS	—	—	Hepatic/renal	Use usual dose with caution
Clopidogrel	—	—	—	Hepatic	Use usual dose with caution
Dipyridamole	—	—	—	Hepatic/biliary	Use usual dose with caution
Eptifibatide	—	—	→	Renal/plasma	Use usual dose with caution
Ticlopidine	←	—	→	Hepatic	Use usual dose with caution
Tirofiban	—	—	—	Hepatic	Use usual dose with caution
Thrombolytics					
Alteplase	—	—	—	Hepatic	Use usual dose with caution
Anistreplase	—	—	—	Unknown	Use usual dose with caution
Reteplase	—	—	—	Hepatic	Use usual dose with caution
Streptokinase	—	—	—	Circulating antibodies/reticuloendothelial system	Use usual dose with caution
Tenecteplase	—	—	—	Hepatic	Use usual dose with caution
Urokinase	—	—	—	Hepatic	Use usual dose with caution

β-Adrenergic blockers					
Nonselective without ISA					
Nadolol	NS	—	—	Renal	Initiate at lowest dose; titrate to response
Propranolol	↑	NS	↓	Hepatic	Initiate at lowest dose; titrate to response
Timolol	—	—	—	Hepatic	Initiate at lowest dose; titrate to response
β₁ selective without ISA					
Atenolol	↓	NS	↓	Renal	Initiate at lowest dose; titrate to response
Betaxolol	—	—	—	Hepatic	Initiate at lowest dose; titrate to response
Bisoprolol	—	—	—	Hepatic/renal	Initiate at lowest dose; titrate to response
Esmolol	—	—	—	Erythrocytes	Use usual dose with caution
Metoprolol	NS	NS	NS	Hepatic	Initiate at lowest dose; titrate to response
Nonselective with ISA					
Carteolol	—	—	—	Renal	Initiate at lowest dose; titrate to response
Penbutolol	—	—	—	Hepatic	Use usual dose with caution
Pindolol	—	—	—	Hepatic/renal	Initiate at lowest dose; titrate to response
β₁ selective with ISA					
Acebutolol	↓	↑	—	Hepatic/biliary	Initiate at lowest dose; titrate to response
Dual acting					
Carvedilol	—	—	—	Hepatic/biliary	Initiate at lowest dose; titrate to response
Labetalol	—	—	NS	Hepatic	No initial dosage adjustment is needed
Calcium channel blockers					
Amlodipine	↓	—	↑	Hepatic	Initiate at lowest dose; titrate to response
Bepridil	—	—	—	Hepatic	Use usual dose with caution
Diltiazem	↓	NS	↑	Hepatic	Initiate at lowest dose; titrate to response
Felodipine	—	NS	↑	Hepatic	Initiate at lowest dose; titrate to response
Isradipine	—	—	↑	Hepatic	Initiate at lowest dose; titrate to response
Nicardipine	NS	NS	—	Hepatic	No initial dosage adjustment is needed
Nifedipine	↑	—	↓	Hepatic	Initiate at lowest dose; titrate to response
Nimodipine	—	—	—	Hepatic	Use usual dose with caution
Nisoldipine	—	—	—	Hepatic	Initiate at lowest dose; titrate to response
Verapamil	↓	NS	↑	Hepatic	Initiate at lowest dose; titrate to response

(continued)

APPENDIX 7 *(continued)* Pharmacokinetic Changes, Routes of Elimination, and Dosage Adjustments of Selected Cardiovascular Drugs in the Elderly

Drug	t½	V_D	Cl	Primary routes of elimination	Dosage adjustment
Diuretics					
Loop					
Bumetanide	—	NS	—	Renal/hepatic	Initiate at lowest dose; titrate to response
Ethacrynic acid	—	—	↓	Hepatic	Initiate at lowest dose; titrate to response
Furosemide	↑	NS	—	Renal	Initiate at lowest dose; titrate to response
Torsemide	—	—	—	Hepatic	Initiate at lowest dose; titrate to response
Thiazides					
Bendroflumethiazide	—	—	—	Renal	Initiate at lowest dose; titrate to response
Benzthiazide	—	—	—	Unknown	Initiate at lowest dose; titrate to response
Chlorothiazide	—	—	—	Renal	Initiate at lowest dose; titrate to response
Chlorthalidone	—	—	↓	Renal	Initiate at lowest dose; titrate to response
Hydrochlorothiazide	—	—	—	Renal	Initiate at lowest dose; titrate to response
Hydroflumethiazide	—	—	—	Unknown	Initiate at lowest dose; titrate to response
Indapamide	—	—	—	Hepatic	Initiate at lowest dose; titrate to response
Methyclothiazide	—	—	—	Renal	Initiate at lowest dose; titrate to response
Metolazone	—	—	—	Renal	Initiate at lowest dose; titrate to response
Polythiazide	—	—	—	Unknown	Initiate at lowest dose; titrate to response
Quinethazone	—	—	—	Unknown	Initiate at lowest dose; titrate to response
Trichlormethiazide	—	—	—	Unknown	Initiate at lowest dose; titrate to response
Potassium sparing					
Amiloride	—	—	↓	Renal	Initiate at lowest dose; titrate to response
Eplerenone	—	—	—	Hepatic	No initial dosage adjustment is necessary
Spironolactone	—	—	—	Hepatic/biliary/renal	Initiate at lowest dose; titrate to response
Triamterene	↓	—	—	Hepatic/renal	Initiate at lowest dose; titrate to response
Endothelin receptor antagonist					
Bosentan	—	—	—	Hepatic/biliary	Use usual dose with caution

Drug		Metabolism/excretion	Dosage recommendation
Inotropic and vasopressor agents			
Amrinone (inamrinone)	—	Hepatic/renal	Initiate at lowest dose; titrate to response
Digoxin	↓	Renal	Initiate at lowest dose; titrate to response
Dobutamine	—	Hepatic/tissue	Initiate at lowest dose; titrate to response
Dopamine	—	Renal/hepatic/plasma	Initiate at lowest dose; titrate to response
Epinephrine	—	Sympathetic nerve endings/hepatic/plasma	Initiate at lowest dose; titrate to response
Isoproterenol	—	Renal	Initiate at lowest dose; titrate to response
Metaraminol	—	Hepatic/biliary/renal	Initiate at lowest dose; titrate to response
Methoxamine	—	Unknown	Initiate at lowest dose; titrate to response
Midodrine	—	Tissue/hepatic/renal	No initial dosage adjustment is needed
Milrinone	—	Renal	Adjust based on renal function
Norepinephrine	—	Sympathetic nerve endings/hepatic/plasma	Initiate at lowest dose; titrate to response
Phenylephrine	—	Hepatic/intestinal	Initiate at lowest dose; titrate to response
Lipid-lowering drugs			
BAS			
Cholestyramine	—	Not absorbed from GI tract	No adjustment needed
Colestipol	—	Not absorbed from GI tract	No adjustment needed
Colesevelam	—	Not absorbed from GI tract	No adjustment needed
FAD			
Clofibrate	—	Hepatic/renal	Adjust based on renal function
Fenofibrate	—	Renal	No adjustment necessary
Gemfibrozil	—	Hepatic/renal	No adjustment necessary
Nicotinic acid	—	Hepatic/renal	No initial dosage adjustment is needed
HMG-CoA reductase inhibitors			
Atorvastatin	↓	Hepatic/biliary	No initial dosage adjustment is needed
Fluvastatin	—	Hepatic	No initial dosage adjustment is needed
Lovastatin	—	Hepatic/fecal	No initial dosage adjustment is needed
Pravastatin	—	Hepatic	No initial dosage adjustment is needed
Rosuvastatin	—	Hepatic/fecal	Initiate at lowest dose; titrate to response
Simvastatin	—	Hepatic/fecal	No initial dosage adjustment is needed

(continued)

APPENDIX 7 (continued) Pharmacokinetic Changes, Routes of Elimination, and Dosage Adjustments of Selected Cardiovascular Drugs in the Elderly

Drug	$t_{1/2}$	V_D	Cl	Primary routes of elimination	Dosage adjustment
Selective cholesterol absorption inhibitor					
Ezetimibe	—	—	—	Small intestine/hepatic/biliary	No adjustment needed
Natriuretic peptide					
Nesiritide	—	—	—	Cellular internalization fill and lysosomal proteolysis/proteolytic cleavage/renal filtration	Use usual dose with caution
Neuronal and ganglionic blockers					
Guanadrel	—	—	—	Hepatic/renal	Initiate at lowest dose; titrate to response
Guanethidine	—	—	—	Hepatic/renal	Initiate at lowest dose; titrate to response
Mecamylamine	—	—	—	Renal	Initiate at lowest dose; titrate to response
Reserpine	—	—	—	Hepatic/fecal	Initiate at lowest dose; titrate to response
Trimethaphan	—	—	—	Hepatic/renal	Initiate at lowest dose; titrate to response
Vasodilators					
Alprostadil	—	—	—	Pulmonary/renal	Initiate at lowest dose; titrate to response
Cilostazol	—	—	—	Hepatic	No adjustment necessary
Diazoxide	—	—	—	Hepatic/renal	Initiate at lowest dose; titrate to response
Epoprostenol	—	—	—	Hepatic/renal	Initiate at usual dose with caution
Fenoldopam	—	—	—	Hepatic	No adjustment necessary
Hydralazine	—	—	—	Hepatic	Initiate at lowest dose; titrate to response
ISDN	—	—	—	Hepatic	Initiate at lowest dose; titrate to response
ISMN	NS	—	NS	Hepatic	No adjustment necessary
Isoxsuprine	—	—	—	Renal	Initiate at lowest dose; titrate to response
Minoxidil	—	—	—	Hepatic	Initiate at lowest dose; titrate to response
Nitroglycerin	—	—	—	Hepatic	Initiate at lowest dose; titrate to response

Drug				Elimination	Recommendation
Nitroprusside	—	—	—	Hepatic/renal/erythrocytes	Use usual dose with caution
Papaverine	—	—	—	Hepatic	Initiate at lowest dose; titrate to response
Pentoxifylline	—	—	→	Hepatic/renal	Use usual dose with caution
Sildenafil	—	—	—	Hepatic/fecal	Initiate at lowest dose; titrate to response
Treprostinil	—	—	—	Hepatic/renal	Use usual dose with caution; dose reduction may be necessary

*The increase in Cl is small when compared with the increase in V_D.

Key: ↓, decrease; ↑, increase; —, no information or not relevant; ACE, angiotensin-converting enzyme; BAS, bile acid sequestrants; Cl, clearance; FAD, fibric acid derivatives; GI, gastrointestinal; HMG-CoA, hydroxymethylglutaryl coenzyme A; ISA, intrinsic sympathomimetic activity; ISDN, isosorbide dinitrate; ISMN, isosorbide mononitrate; NS, no significant change; $t_{1/2}$, half-life; V_D, volume of distribution.

APPENDIX 8 Selected Cardiovascular Medications and Ethnic Issues

Drug or drug class	Evidence of efficacy in different ethnic groups	Consideration in treatment
α-Adrenergic antagonists	Prazosin is less effective in blacks	Blacks may need higher doses, generally a second-line agent
Beta blockers Propranolol	No difference in plasma concentrations of propranolol between Malays, Indians, and Chinese	Blacks may need larger doses of propranolol to achieve same effects as in whites
	Compared with white patients, black patients have lower plasma concentration of propranolol when this drug is taken orally	
	S-isomer clears more slowly than the R-isomer; all metabolic pathways have higher metabolic rates in blacks as than in whites	
	Chinese have lower plasma concentrations and higher clearance of propranolol, mainly secondary to increased ring oxidation and conjugation	
Metoprolol	No differences in metabolism of metoprolol between whites and blacks in the United States; Chinese have a higher incidence of slow metabolizers (with 1 or 2 copies of CYP2D6*10) and have significantly higher plasma concentrations of R- and S-isomers of metoprolol	Lower doses of metoprolol are required in Chinese
	The S-isomer (which confers beta-blocking activity) reaches higher concentrations than the R-isomer; in poor metabolizers, there is a lasting effect after 24 h, which correlates with reduced clearance of the S-isomer	

Others	Response of blacks to other beta blockers is similar to that of whites
	Labetalol seems to be effective in blacks
	Carvedilol was effective in CHF treatment in all subgroups
	In blacks, bucindolol was worse than placebo in advanced heart failure
	Unusually high plasma concentrations of alprenolol and timolol have been found in subjects with the CYP2D6-poor metabolizer phenotype
	Plasma concentrations and degree of beta-blockade were greater in subjects with the CYP2D6-PM phenotype taking timolol
	Carvedilol can be used in blacks for heart failure; bucindolol should be avoided in blacks with advanced heart failure
Calcium channel blockers	Nifedipine clearance is faster in whites than in blacks; South Asians, Mexicans, and Nigerians have higher drug exposure and longer half-life, when compared with whites
	Diltiazem is less effective in younger white men when compared to blacks
	Nifedipine might be a good initial treatment for hypertension in Asians, Hispanics, and blacks
	Diltiazem may not be a good choice in young white patients
Diuretics	Blacks respond better than whites to thiazide diuretics
	Good initial choice for antihypertensive therapy in blacks

(continued)

APPENDIX 8 (continued) Selected Cardiovascular Medications and Ethnic Issues

Drug or drug class	Evidence of efficacy in different ethnic groups	Consideration in treatment
Antiarrhythmics	Propafenone concentrations were elevated in poor metabolizers of dextromorphan in a Chinese population and CNS side effects were more frequent	Close observation of side effects may be warranted in CYP2D6-intermediate metabolizers, such as many Asians, and in CYP2D6-poor metabolizers
	Poor metabolizers of propafenone have a higher incidence of side effects	
	Extensive metabolizers of encainide accumulate active metabolites that lead to greater QRS widening	
	Poor metabolizers of flecainide have higher drug exposure and longer half-lives	
Warfarin	Mean maintenance dose of warfarin in Chinese subjects is ~3.1 mg vs. 6.1 mg in whites	Use lower warfarin doses in Chinese
Aspirin	In Nigerians, overall excretion (particularly the glucuronide conjugate) is higher in males than in females	Some populations may have increased side effects or decreased effectiveness
ACE inhibitors and ARBs	Fosinoprilat has lower clearance and distribution volume in Chinese than in whites	Chinese may need lower doses
	Less antihypertensive effect in blacks at lower doses; however, the antihypertensive effect of ACE inhibitors is increased when a diuretic is given concurrently	Blacks may need an additional drug (e.g., a diuretic) to achieve blood pressure control
	ACE inhibitors may not be as effective in blacks as in whites for heart failure, which may partly explain the worse outcome of left ventricular dysfunction in blacks	Alternative or additional therapy in blacks with left ventricular dysfunction may be needed
Statins	Chinese and Japanese have higher plasma levels of rosuvastatin	Lower doses of rosuvastatin are required in Chinese and Japanese patients

Key: ACE, angiotensin-converting enzyme; ARB, angiotensin receptor blocker; CHF, congestive heart failure; CNS, central nervous system.

Index

Page numbers followed by *t* denote tables. Page numbers followed by *f* denote figures.